General Ophthalmology

10th edition

General Ophthalmology

DANIEL VAUGHAN, MD

Clinical Professor of Ophthalmology
University of California, San Francisco
Member, Francis I. Proctor Foundation
for Research in Ophthalmology

TAYLOR ASBURY, MD

Clinical Professor of Ophthalmology
College of Medicine
University of Cincinnati

Illustrated by
LAUREL V. SCHAUBERT

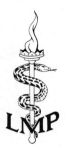

LANGE Medical Publications   Los Altos, California 94022

International Standard Book Number: 0-87041-105-5
Library of Congress Catalogue Card Number: 82-84778

General Ophthalmology, 10th ed. $17.00
Copyright © 1958, 1960, 1962, 1965, 1968, 1971, 1974, 1977, 1980, 1983

A Concise Medical Library for Practitioner and Student

Current Medical Diagnosis & Treatment 1983 (annual revision). Edited by M.A. Krupp   1983
  and M.J. Chatton. 1130 pp.

Current Pediatric Diagnosis & Treatment, 7th ed. Edited by C.H. Kempe, H.K. Silver,   1982
  and D. O'Brien. 1106 pp, *illus.*

Current Surgical Diagnosis & Treatment, 5th ed. Edited by J.E. Dunphy and L.W. Way.   1981
  1138 pp, *illus.*

Current Obstetric & Gynecologic Diagnosis & Treatment, 4th ed. Edited by   1982
  R.C. Benson. 1038 pp, *illus.*

Harper's Review of Biochemistry (formerly **Review of Physiological Chemistry**),   1981
  18th ed. D.W. Martin, Jr., P.A. Mayes, and V.W. Rodwell. 614 pp, *illus.*

Review of Medical Physiology, 10th ed. W.F. Ganong. 628 pp, *illus.*   1981

Review of Medical Microbiology, 15th ed. E. Jawetz, J.L. Melnick, and E.A. Adelberg.   1982
  553 pp, *illus.*

Basic & Clinical Pharmacology. Edited by B.G. Katzung. 815 pp, *illus.*   1982

Basic & Clinical Immunology, 4th ed. Edited by D.P. Stites, J.D. Stobo,   1982
  H.H. Fudenberg, and J.V. Wells. 775 pp, *illus.*

Basic Histology, 3rd ed. L.C. Junqueira and J. Carneiro. 504 pp, *illus.*   1980

Clinical Cardiology, 3rd ed. M. Sokolow and M.B. McIlroy. 763 pp, *illus.*   1981

General Urology, 10th ed. D.R. Smith. 598 pp, *illus.*   1981

Correlative Neuroanatomy & Functional Neurology, 18th ed. J.G. Chusid. 476 pp, *illus.*   1982

Principles of Clinical Electrocardiography, 11th ed. M.J. Goldman. 438 pp, *illus.*   1982

Handbook of Obstetrics & Gynecology, 7th ed. R.C. Benson. 808 pp, *illus.*   1980

Physician's Handbook, 20th ed. M.A. Krupp, L.M. Tierney, Jr., E. Jawetz, R.L. Roe,   1982
  and C.A. Camargo. 774 pp, *illus.*

Handbook of Pediatrics, 13th ed. H.K. Silver, C.H. Kempe, and H.B. Bruyn. 735 pp, *illus.*   1980

Handbook of Poisoning: Prevention, Diagnosis, & Treatment, 11th ed. R.H. Dreisbach.   1983
  632 pp.

This edition of
General Ophthalmology
is dedicated to
Phillips Thygeson and Ruth Lee Thygeson

Table of Contents

7. Conjunctiva (cont'd)

Foreword

This tenth edition of *General Ophthalmology* chronicles important changes in its subject that have occurred since 1980. The entire book has in fact been carefully reviewed with the assistance of many authorities in special fields, and certain parts have been extensively revised, especially the chapters on optics, preventive ophthalmology, and the ocular manifestations of systemic disease. The eye is the "window of the body," showing us in so many ways the state of the body systems—vascular, neurologic, metabolic, etc. Today's medical students and all physicians—nonophthalmologists as well as ophthalmologists—must know how to use such simple ophthalmologic instruments as the ophthalmoscope, the magnifying loupe, and the tonometer. Only by means of them can the student or practitioner hope to acquire easily many of the important items of diagnostic information that may be vital to his patient's general health. In addition to early experience with these instruments and some knowledge of what can be learned from their intelligent use, the student and physician need a simple but comprehensive text on the desk or office bookshelf for reference and refreshment. For this purpose, among its many others, *General Ophthalmology* would seem ideally suited.

Publishing costs have escalated fantastically since the first edition of this excellent work was published more than 20 years ago, but Lange Medical Publications has managed to keep its cost well within the purchasing power of almost any young student or physician. That it fills a widespread need in the world of medicine in general and of ophthalmology in particular is attested by the worldwide acceptance of what has become the most popular textbook of ophthalmology and the numerous foreign translations in which it appears. A German translation is now completed and will be published in 1983.

Phillips Thygeson

Preface

This tenth edition is a substantial revision of the preceding one, but the intended function of *General Ophthalmology* is as before: to serve as a concise and current review of the subject for medical students, ophthalmology residents, practicing ophthalmologists, and our colleagues in other fields of medicine and surgery.

As in preceding editions, the authors have continued and even expanded their policy of seeking help from established authorities in special fields. Their names are listed on the page following, but we especially want to acknowledge the contributions of some experts who have contributed major portions of the new edition. We hope the users and reviewers of this book will recognize that Dr Orson White has presented for the first time in the literature of our specialty a mathematically precise exposition of the optical principles that have been understood and used for years by optical engineers. Dr White makes another original contribution in his exposition of the pressure dynamics of glaucoma in that chapter, which is also reviewed and brought up to 1983 standard by Dr Robert Shaffer.

Dr Philip Ellis, himself an author of a leading text on therapeutics in ophthalmology, has reviewed and revised our appendix on drug therapy. Dr Barry Skarf, under the direction of Dr William Hoyt, has revised the chapter on neuro-ophthalmology, and Dr Phillips Thygeson has updated his superb chapters on diseases of the conjunctiva and cornea.

Once again we have pleasure in expressing our gratitude to Dr Khalid Tabbara for serving as consultant editor for the entire text. Dr Tabbara also contributes the chapter on tears.

We are happy to be able to announce that a monumental effort by Dr Heinrich König has now culminated in a German translation of our book, which is now translated into five languages. It is a pleasure also to note that Dr Taj Kirmani of Karachi, Pakistan, will soon produce an introductory English language book on ophthalmology for health workers in developing areas of the world which will contain a number of chapters borrowed from *General Ophthalmology*.

Daniel Vaughan
Taylor Asbury

March, 1983

Acknowledgments

Arthur K. Asbury
Crowell Beard
Diane Beeston
Lindsay Bibler
Roderick Biswell
Laurie Vaughan Campbell
J. Brooks Crawford
Patricia Cunnane
Chandler Dawson
Paul Riordan Eva
Hans Beat Gassmann
Elizabeth Graham
Margaret Henry
Harry Hind
Creig S. Hoyt
Geraldine Hruby
Marianne Thalmann Huslid

Vicente Jocson
Raga Malaty
G. Richard O'Connor
James O'Donnell
Conor C. O'Malley
Patrick O'Malley
Bruce Ostler
Patricia Pascoe
Kenneth D. Rogers
Joel G. Sacks
Michael Sanders
John P. Shock
Lionel W. Sorenson
John H. Sullivan
Ralph T. Sutton
Renate Unsöld
H.Ward Wick

General Ophthalmology

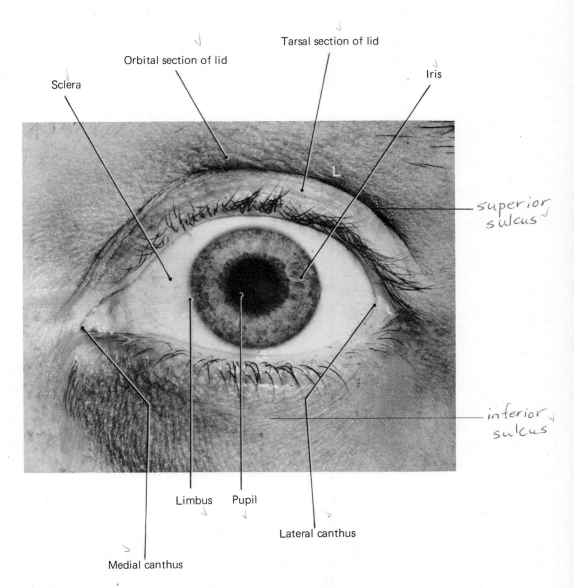

Sclera

Orbital section of lid

Tarsal section of lid

Iris

L

superior
sulcus

inferior
sulcus

Limbus   Pupil

Lateral canthus

Medial canthus

Figure 1–1. External landmarks of the eye. The sclera is covered by transparent conjunctiva. (Photo by HL Gibson, from: *Medical Radiography and Photography*. Labeling modified slightly.)

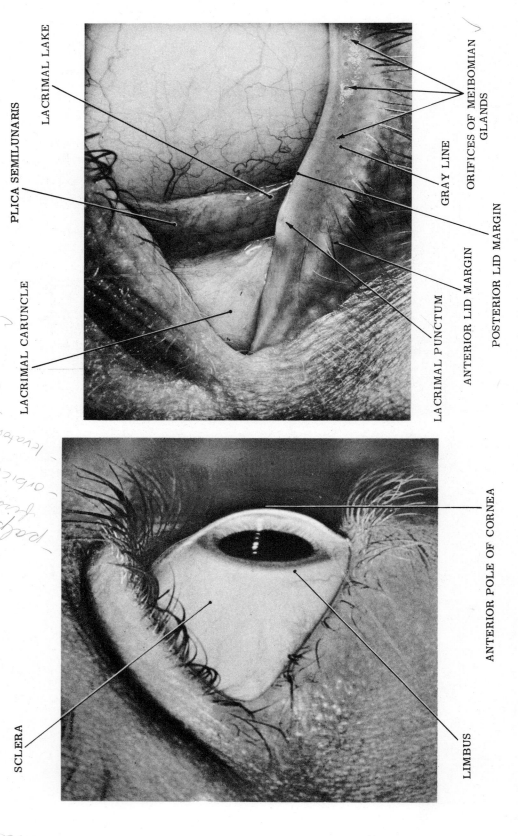

Figure 1–2. External landmarks of the eye. The sclera is covered by transparent conjunctiva. (Photos by HL Gibson, from: *Medical Radiography and Photography*. Labeling modified slightly.)

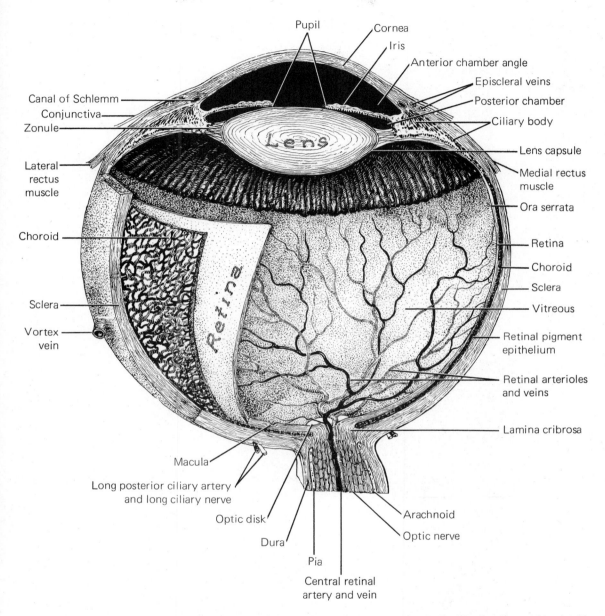

Figure 1–3. Internal structures of the human eye. (Redrawn from an original drawing by Paul Peck and reproduced, with permission, from: *The Anatomy of the Eye*. Courtesy of Lederle Laboratories.)

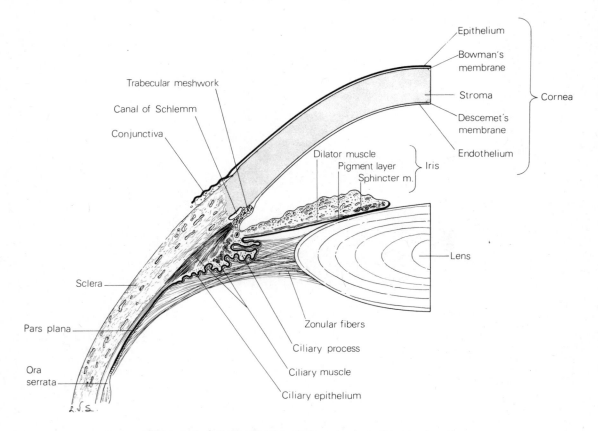

Figure 1–4. Anterior chamber angle and surrounding structures.

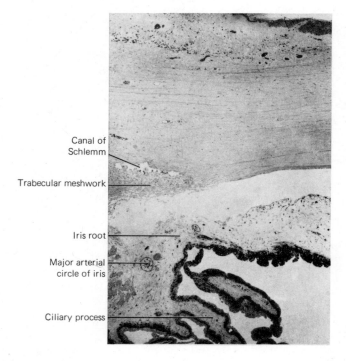

Figure 1–5. Photomicrograph of anterior chamber angle and related structures. (Courtesy of I Wood and L Garron).

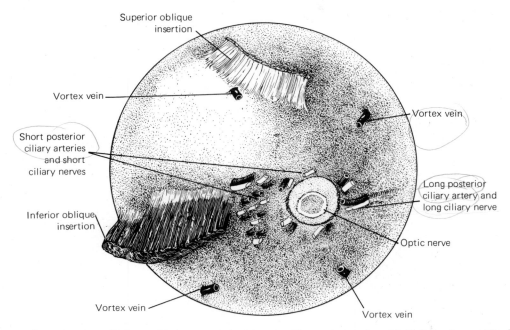

Figure 1–6. Posterior view of left eye. (Redrawn and reproduced, with permission, from Wolff E: *Anatomy of the Eye and Orbit,* 4th ed. Blakiston-McGraw, 1954.)

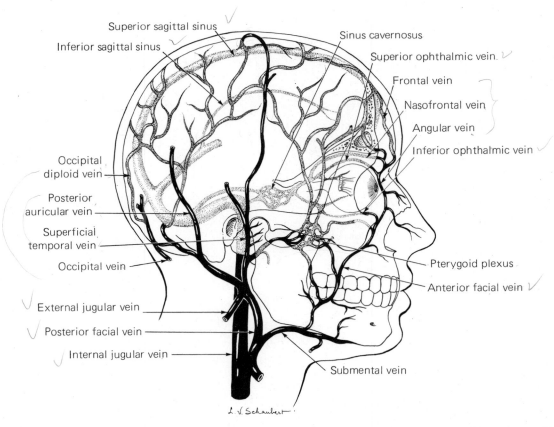

Figure 1–7. Venous drainage system of the eye. (Redrawn and reproduced, with permission, from Wolff E: *Anatomy of the Eye and Orbit,* 4th ed. Blakiston-McGraw, 1954.)

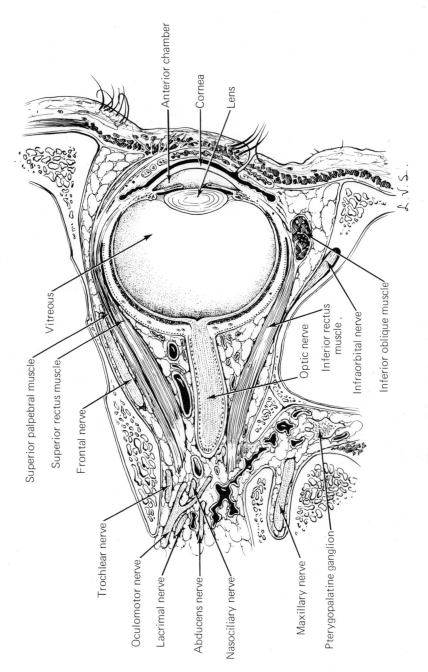

Figure 1-8. Lateral view of eye and surrounding structures.

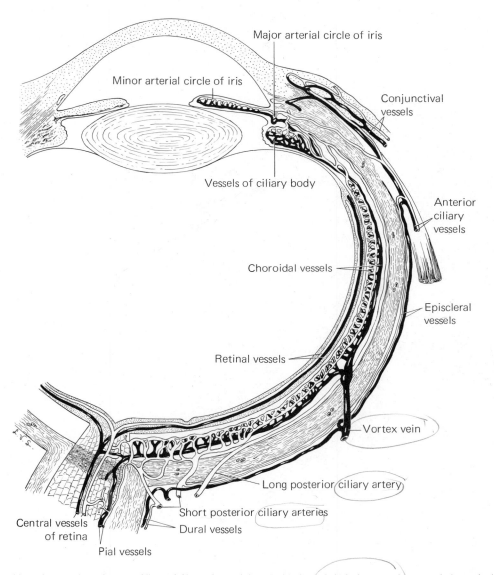

Figure 1–9. Vascular supply to the eye. All arterial branches originate with the ophthalmic artery. Venous drainage is through the cavernous sinus and the pterygoid plexus.

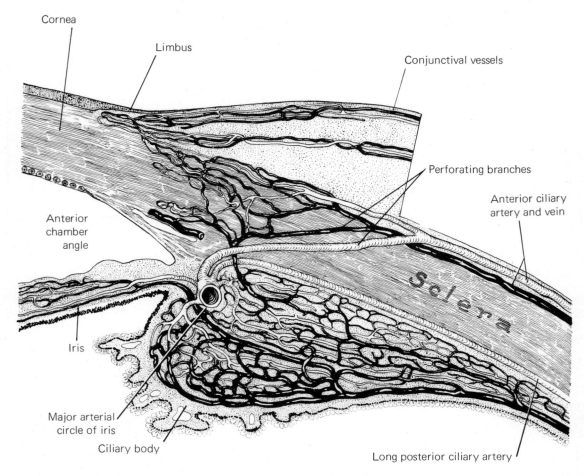

Figure 1–10. Vascular supply of the anterior segment. (Modified, redrawn, and reproduced, with permission, from Wolff E: *Anatomy of the Eye and Orbit,* 4th ed. Blakiston-McGraw, 1954.)

EMBRYOLOGY OF THE EYE
(Fig 2–1)

OPTIC VESICLE STAGE

The earliest embryonic stage at which ocular structures can be differentiated from the rest of the fetus is the embryonic plate stage. The site of the eye is indicated by flattened areas on both sides of the anterior end of the neural groove. The edges of the neural groove (2.5-mm stage or 2-week stage) thicken to form the neural folds. The folds fuse to form the neural tube, which sinks into the underlying mesoderm and detaches from the surface ectoderm. Before the anterior end of the neural tube is completely closed, buds of neural ectoderm grow toward the surface ectoderm on either side to form the spherical optic vesicles (4-mm or 3-week stage). These vesicles are connected to the forebrain by the optic stalks. At the 4-mm stage, a thickening of the surface ectoderm, the lens plate, begins to form just opposite the ends of the optic vesicles.

OPTIC CUP STAGE

The optic vesicle invaginates to produce the optic cup, so that the original outer wall of the optic vesicle becomes approximated to its inner wall. Invagination of the lower surface of the optic stalk and the optic vesicle occurs simultaneously, creating a groove known as the choroidal (fetal) fissure. At the same time, the lens plate also invaginates to form first a cup and then a hollow sphere known as the lens vesicle. By the 9-mm (4-week) stage, the lens vesicle separates completely from the surface ectoderm to lie free in the rim of the optic cup.

The choroidal fissure permits entrance into the optic stalk of the vascular mesoderm that eventually forms the hyaloid system. As invagination becomes complete, the choroidal fissure narrows until it becomes completely closed (13-mm or 6-week stage), leaving one small permanent opening at the anterior end of the optic stalk through which pass the hyaloid artery until the 100-mm (4-month) stage and the central retinal artery and vein thereafter.

At this point, the ultimate general structure of the eye has been determined. Further development consists of differentiation into individual structures. In general, differentiation occurs relatively more rapidly in the posterior than in the anterior segment early in gestation and more rapidly in the anterior segment later in gestation.

EMBRYONIC ORIGINS OF INDIVIDUAL EYE STRUCTURES*

Surface Ectoderm
Lens; epithelium of cornea, conjunctiva, lacrimal gland and drainage system; vitreous (mesoderm also contributes to vitreous).

Neural Ectoderm
Vitreous, retina; epithelium of iris, ciliary body, and retina; pupillary muscle sphincter and dilator, optic nerve.

Mesoderm
Sclera; stroma of cornea, conjunctiva, iris, ciliary body, choroid; extraocular muscles, lids (except epithelium and conjunctiva), hyaloid system (gone by birth), sheaths of the optic nerve; connective tissue and blood supply of eye, bony orbit, and vitreous.

EMBRYOLOGY OF SPECIFIC STRUCTURES

Lens
Soon after the lens vesicle lies free in the rim of the optic cup (13-mm or 6-week stage), the cells of its posterior wall elongate, encroach on the empty cavity, and finally fill it in (26-mm or 7-week stage). At about this stage (13-mm or 6-week), a hyaline capsule is secreted by the lens cells. Secondary lens fibers elongate from the equatorial region and grow forward under the subcapsular epithelium, which remains as a single layer of cuboid epithelial cells, and backward under the lens capsule. These fibers meet to form the lens sutures (upright "Y" anteriorly and inverted "Y" posteriorly), which are complete by the seventh

---

*Endoderm does not contribute to the formation of the eye.

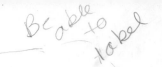

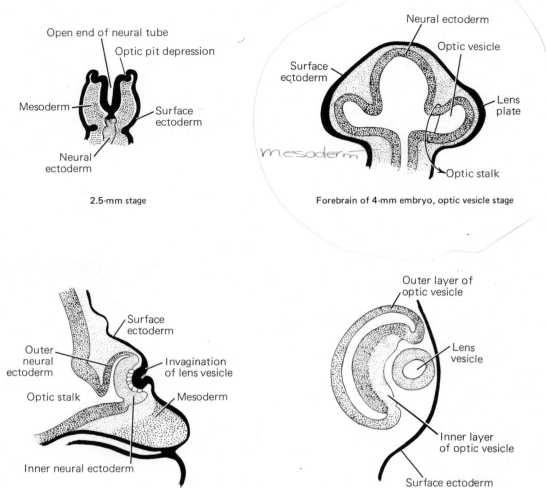

Optic pit depression

Open end of neural tube

Mesoderm

Surface ectoderm

Neural ectoderm

2.5-mm stage

Neural ectoderm

Optic vesicle

Surface ectoderm

Lens plate

mesoderm

Optic stalk

Forebrain of 4-mm embryo, optic vesicle stage

Surface ectoderm

Outer neural ectoderm

Invagination of lens vesicle

Optic stalk

Mesoderm

Inner neural ectoderm

5-mm stage. Beginning formation of optic cup by invagination.

Outer layer of optic vesicle

Lens vesicle

Inner layer of optic vesicle

Surface ectoderm

9-mm stage. Lens vesicle has separated from surface ectoderm and lies free in rim of optic cup.

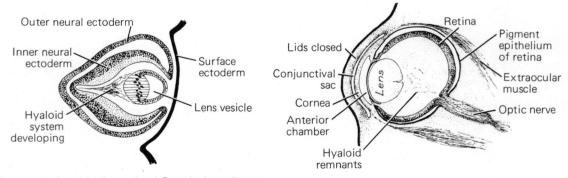

Outer neural ectoderm

Inner neural ectoderm

Surface ectoderm

Hyaloid system developing

Lens vesicle

13-mm stage. Choroidal fissure closed. Posterior lens cells growing forward.

Retina

Lids closed

Pigment epithelium of retina

Conjunctival sac

Cornea

Anterior chamber

Extraocular muscle

Optic nerve

Lens

Hyaloid remnants

65-mm stage (3 months)

Figure 2–1. Embryologic development of ocular structures. (Redrawn and reproduced, with permission, from Mann IC: *The Development of the Human Eye,* 2nd ed. British Medical Association, 1950.)

month. (This growth and proliferation of secondary lens fibers continues at a decreasing rate throughout life; the lens therefore continues to enlarge slowly, causing compression of the lens fibers.)

Retina

The outer layer of the optic cup remains as a single layer and becomes the pigment epithelium of the retina. Pigmentation begins at the 10-mm (5-week) stage. The inner layer undergoes a complicated differentiation into the other 9 layers of the retina. This occurs slowly throughout gestation. By the seventh month, the outermost cell layer (consisting of the nuclei of the rods and cones) is present as well as the bipolar, amacrine, and ganglion cells and nerve fibers. The macular region is thicker than the rest of the retina until the eighth month, when macular depression begins to develop. Macular development is not complete until 6 months after birth.

Optic Nerve

The axons of the ganglion cell layer of the retina form the inner nerve fiber layer. The fibers slowly form the optic stalk and then the optic nerve (26-mm or 7-week stage). Mesodermal elements enter the surrounding tissue to form the vascular septa of the nerve. Medullation extends from the brain peripherally down the optic nerve, and at birth has reached the lamina cribrosa. Medullation is completed by age 3 months.

Iris & Ciliary Body

During the third month (50-mm stage), the rim of the optic cup grows forward in front of the lens as a double row of epithelium and lies posterior to mesoderm, which becomes the stroma of the iris. These 2 epithelial layers become pigmented in the iris, whereas only the outer layer is pigmented in the ciliary body. Folds appear in the epithelial layers of the ciliary body; mesoderm grows into this fold to form the ciliary processes. By the fifth month (150-mm stage), the sphincter muscle of the pupil is developing from a bud of nonpigmented epithelium derived from the anterior epithelial layer of the iris near the pupillary margin. Soon after the sixth month, the dilator muscle appears in the anterior epithelial layer near the ciliary body.

Choroid

At the 6-mm (3½-week) stage, a network of capillaries encircles the optic cup and develops into the choroid. By the 13-mm (6-week) stage, the outer neural epithelial layer has secreted Bruch's membrane. By the third month, the intermediate and large venous channels of the choroid are developed and drain into the vortex veins to exit from the eye.

Vitreous (Fig 2–2)

A. First Stage: (Primary vitreous, 4.5- to 13-mm or 3- to 6-week stage.) At about the 4.5-mm stage, fibrils grow in from the inner layer of the optic vesicle to join elements from the lens vesicle that—along with some mesoderm fibrils associated with the hyaloid

artery—form the primary vitreous. This stage ends as the lens capsule appears, precluding any further lens participation in vitreous formation. The primary vitreous does not atrophy and ultimately lies just behind the posterior pole of the lens as the hyaloid canal.

B. Second Stage: (Secondary vitreous, 13- to 65-mm or 3- to 10-week stage.) Müller's fibers of the retina become continuous with vitreous fibrils, so that the secondary vitreous is mainly derived from retinal ectoderm. The hyaloid system develops a set of vitreous vessels as well as vessels on the lens capsule surface (tunica vasculosa lentis). The hyaloid system is at its height at 40 mm and then atrophies from posterior to anterior.

C. Third Stage: (Tertiary vitreous, 65 mm or 10 weeks on.) During the third month, the marginal bundle of Drualt is forming. This consists of vitreous fibrillar condensations extending from the future ciliary epithelium of the optic cup to the equator of the lens. Condensations then form the suspensory ligament of the lens, which is well developed by the 100-mm or 4-month stage. The hyaloid system atrophies completely during this stage.

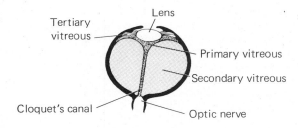

Figure 2–2. The vitreous. (Redrawn and reproduced, with permission, from Duke-Elder WS: *Textbook of Ophthalmology.* Vol 1. Mosby, 1942.)

Blood Vessels

Long ciliary arteries bud off from the hyaloid at the 16-mm (6-week) stage and anastomose around the optic cup margin with the major circle of the iris by the 30-mm (7-week) stage.

The hyaloid system (see Vitreous) atrophies completely by the eighth month. The hyaloid artery gives rise to the central retinal artery and its branches (100-mm or 4-month stage). Buds begin to grow into the retina and develop the retinal circulation, which reaches the ora serrata at 8 months. The branches of the central retinal vein develop simultaneously.

Cornea

The epithelium is derived from surface ectoderm, whereas the rest of the cornea comes from mesodermal structures. The earliest differentiation is seen at about the 12-mm (5-week) stage, when endothelial cells appear. Descemet's membrane is secreted by the flattened endothelial cells by the 75-mm (12-week) stage. The stroma slowly thickens, largely by an increase in the number of elastic fibers, and forms an anterior condensation just under the epithelium that is recognizable at 100 mm (4 months) as Bowman's membrane. A definite corneoscleral junction is present at 4 months.

Anterior Chamber

The anterior chamber of the eye first appears at 20 mm (7 weeks) and remains very shallow until birth. At 65 mm (9–10 weeks), Schlemm's canal appears as a vascular channel at the level of the recess of the angle and gradually assumes a relatively more anterior location as the angle recess develops. The iris, which in the early stages of development is quite anterior, gradually lies relatively more posteriorly as the chamber angle recess develops, most likely because of the difference in rate of growth of the anterior segment structures. The trabecular meshwork develops from the loose vascular mesodermal tissue lying originally at the margin of the optic cup. The aqueous drainage system is ready to function before birth.

Sclera & Extraocular Muscles

The sclera and extraocular muscles are formed from condensations of mesoderm encircling the optic cup and are first identifiable at the 20-mm (7-week) stage. Development of these structures is well advanced by the fourth month. Tenon's capsule appears about the insertions of the rectus muscles at the 80-mm (12-week) stage and is complete at 5 months.

Lids & Lacrimal Apparatus

The lids develop from mesoderm except for the skin and conjunctiva. The lid buds are first seen at 16 mm (6 weeks) growing in front of the eye, where they meet and fuse at the 37-mm (8-week) stage. They separate during the fifth month, and lashes and meibomian and other lid glands develop. The lacrimal gland (including the accessory glands and the conjunctiva) and drainage system develop from ectoderm. The canaliculi, lacrimal sac, and nasolacrimal duct are developed by burying a solid epithelial cord between the maxillary and nasal processes. This cord canalizes just before birth.

PATHOLOGY OF CONGENITAL OCULAR ABNORMALITIES

Congenital defects of the ocular structures have been described under 2 main headings: (1) developmental anomalies or dysplasias of embryonal origin and (2) tissue reactions to intrauterine inflammation in the latter months of gestation. Examples of the first type are the colobomas, dermoid tumors, anophthalmos, and microphthalmos. In the second category belong certain lesions of chorioretinitis similar to those seen in postnatal life and some forms of cataract. Heredity plays a major role in many congenital deformities.

In reviewing the embryologic development of the eye, with its complex folds to form the optic vesicles, cornea, lens, and anterior chamber, it is obvious that any failure of regression of primitive vascular tissue at the proper stage, or failure of fusion of embryonic tissue, would lead to a defect of development, eg, of the iris or choroid (coloboma). These developmental defects commonly occur at any point from a segment of the optic nerve itself at the disk, along the choroidal structure and the ciliary body, or in an iris segment. These defects are often seen grossly as a missing wedge of iris tissue or may be seen with the ophthalmoscope as a large white strip extending radially along the inner surface of the eye toward the periphery.

An eye may be missing (anophthalmos) or smaller than normal (microphthalmos). A small eye is quite often deficient in function.

Congenital lens opacities may occur at any time during the formation of the lens, and the stage at which the opacity began to develop is often measurable by the depth of the opacity. The innermost fetal nucleus of the lens forms early in embryonal life and is surrounded by the embryonal nucleus. Adult addition to the lens is a peripheral subcapsular growth in postnatal life. Certain types of congenital cataracts are familial, whereas others may occur as reactions to intrauterine influences.

Congenital rests, such as dermoids, occur frequently in the ocular structures.

GROWTH & DEVELOPMENT

Eyeball

At birth, the eye is larger in relation to the rest of the body than is the case in children and adults. In relation to its ultimate size (reached at 7–8 years), it is comparatively short, averaging 17.3 mm in anteroposterior length (the only optically significant dimension). This would make the eye quite hyperopic if it were not for the refractive power of the nearly spherical lens.

Cornea

The newborn infant has a relatively large cornea that reaches adult size by the age of 2 years. It is flatter than the adult cornea, and its curvature is greater at the periphery than in the center. (The reverse is true in adults.)

Almost all astigmatic refractive errors are produced by differences in curvature in the various meridians of the cornea. In the infant, the vertical meridian usually has the greatest curvature. In adult life the cornea tends to flatten, and the flattening is more marked in the vertical than the horizontal, changing the axis of astigmatism. However, the degree of astigmatism changes very little throughout life.

Lens

At birth, the lens is more nearly spherical in shape than later in life, producing a greater refractive power that helps to compensate for the short anteroposterior diameter of the eye. The lens grows throughout life as new fibers are added to the periphery, making it flatter.

The consistency of the lens material changes throughout life. At birth, it may be compared with soft plastic; in old age, the lens is of a glasslike consistency. This accounts for the greater resistance to change of shape in accommodation as one grows older.

Refractive State

About 80% of children are born hyperopic, 5% myopic, and 15% emmetropic. Hyperopia increases until about 7–8 years of age and then gradually decreases until 19 or 20 years of age. After age 7 or 8, myopia gradually increases until about 25 years. (Hyperopia decreases much less than myopia increases.) There is usually little change in refractive error during the third and fourth decades. Presbyopia occurs in almost all people at age 42–46.

Iris

At birth, there is little or no pigment on the anterior surface of the iris; the posterior pigment layer showing through the translucent tissue gives the eyes of most infants a bluish color. As the pigment begins to appear on the anterior surface, the iris assumes its definitive color. If considerable pigment is deposited, the eyes become brown. Less iris stroma pigmentation results in blue, hazel, or green.

Position

During the first 3 months of age, eye movements may be so poorly coordinated (because of the normally slow development of reflexes) that doubt may exist about the straightness of the eyes. Most of the binocular reflexes should be well developed by 6 months of age. Deviation that persists beyond age 6 months should be investigated (see Chapter 15).

Nasolacrimal Apparatus

The cord of cells that hollows out to form the nasolacrimal duct between the tear sac and the nose usually becomes patent at about the time of birth. Failure to function may not be noticed for some time because of lack of tear secretion in the first few weeks of life. Failure of tear production by 3 months of age demands attention.

Optic Nerve

The completion of the medullation process around the optic nerve fibers usually occurs within a few weeks after birth.

AGING CHANGES IN THE EYE

Eyelids

Aging of the skin tissues produces gradual loss of elasticity, with wrinkling and drooping folds (dermatochalasis). There may be fatty alteration of the tissues (xanthelasma).

Conjunctiva

Senile plaques and degenerative infiltrates occasionally are found.

Cornea

The cornea may show circular infiltration of degenerative material within the limbus ("arcus senilis"). A flattening of curvature of the vertical meridian tends to produce distorted vision.

Lens

The lens continues to grow throughout life, although in senescence the rate of growth decreases. The consistency changes from the soft plastic juvenile lens to an almost "glasslike" character, with increasing difficulty in change of shape with attempted accommodation (presbyopia).

Disturbances of lens metabolism may produce tissue changes with resultant loss of transparency (cataract). Most older people have some degree of cataract.

Vitreous

Increase in "floaters" (muscae volitantes) due to fibrillar condensations, exudates, degenerative deposits, or asteroid hyalosis; detachment and liquefaction of vitreous.

Choroid & Retina

Arteriosclerosis of the vessels of the choroid and retina may be followed by degenerative changes in these tissues.

3 | Examination*

ROUTINE EYE EXAMINATION

The routine ophthalmologic examination consists of careful elicitation of the patient's history, physical examination of the eyes, and assessment of visual function. The history should include not only the patient's ocular manifestations but general information about age, occupation, and physical health. Special examinations may be required to determine ocular pathophysiology or to establish the pressure of associated systemic disease. The patient's pertinent past medical records should be obtained whenever possible.

GENERAL INFORMATION

Age

The age of the patient is important not only as an etiologic factor in senile changes but also for the purpose of comparing individual abilities with established norms for the age group and in helping to determine what one might expect in the way of performance without discomfort. For example, in cases of amblyopia, occlusive treatment should improve the visual acuity of a child under age 6, whereas the same treatment in a child over 6 would be less effective. In a young child it is not too important to correct the visual acuity to 6/6 (20/20), since demands for clear distance visual acuity are much less at an early age than is the case with older school children or adults. Age also plays a role in the rate of progression of myopia, which tends to increase during the teens and levels off in the third decade.

Age is also an important factor in visual disability in the prepresbyopic or early presbyopic period, as the symptoms of presbyopia are often quite disconcerting to a person who has had good eyesight throughout life. Proper explanation of these symptoms to the patient may postpone the need for the first pair of reading glasses or facilitate the adjustment to the first pair.

Occupation

Occupational demands for visual acuity are im-

*Ophthalmoscopic examination: See pp 343–362.

portant in determining the treatment of visual symptoms. Special requirements, such as those involved in working with small objects or at unusual working distances, must be considered in the work-fatigue balance of the visual effort. Even in the same age group, marked differences in symptoms may be noted between 2 individuals with the same refractive error whose work makes widely different demands on their eyes. Small refractive errors that produce discomfort in an accountant, for example, may be unnoticed by a laborer.

In presbyopic patients requiring occupational bifocals, special work requirements play an important role in the prescription of bifocal segments.

In industrial injuries a careful record should be made of time and circumstances of injury, previous emergency treatment, and visual acuity.

SYMPTOMS & SIGNS

Most of the presenting manifestations of eye involvement fall into one of 5 categories: (1) subnormal visual acuity; (2) pain or discomfort; (3) change of appearance of lids, orbit, or eye; (4) diplopia or dizziness; and (5) discharge or increased conjunctival secretion. Some of the important features of each complaint are discussed below.

Subnormal Visual Acuity

A. Duration: Is visual acuity the same as it has been for most of the patient's life? Was the change noted recently? Was it found by accidentally covering one eye? Has there been a gradual diminution of acuity over months or years?

B. Difference in Visual Acuity in the 2 Eyes: Is the patient certain that visual acuity was formerly the same in both eyes? Has the patient passed an eye examination as part of a driver's test or military physical examination? At that time was the visual acuity the same in both eyes?

C. Disturbances of Vision:

1. Distortion of the normal shapes of objects (metamorphopsia) is most often due to astigmatism or macular lesions.

2. Photophobia is commonly due to corneal inflammation, aphakia, iritis, and ocular albinism. Some

drugs may produce increased light sensitivity (eg, chloroquine, acetazolamide).

3. Color change (chromatopsia), such as yellow, white, or red vision, may be due to chorioretinal lesions or lenticular changes, or may be associated with systemic disturbances (eg, yellow vision of jaundice) or certain medications (eg, yellow or white vision in digitalis toxicity).

4. Halos, or rings seen when viewing lights or bright objects, are typically thought of as accompanying glaucoma but are also found with other processes causing corneal edema or infiltration as well as with lens changes. Incipient cataract is the most common cause of halos.

5. "Spots" before the eyes, seen as dots or filaments that move with the eye, are almost always due to benign vitreous opacities.

6. Visual field defects may be due to disorders of the cornea, media, retina, optic nerve, or brain. Quivering or scintillating blind spots (scotomas) may occur transiently as a result of localized constriction of cerebral or retinal arteries.

7. Night blindness, or difficulty seeing in the dark (nyctalopia), may be congenital (retinitis pigmentosa, hereditary optic atrophy) or acquired (vitamin A deficiency, glaucoma, optic atrophy, cataract, retinal degeneration).

8. Momentary loss of vision (amaurosis fugax) may imply impending cerebrovascular accident, spasm of the central retinal artery, or partial occlusion of the internal carotid artery.

Pain or Discomfort

The usual painful symptoms mentioned are headache, "eye-ache," and burning or itching of the eyes or eyelids. Photophobia (sensitivity to light) may cause great discomfort; fatigue symptoms such as "pull," "tired eyes," and "a feeling of pressure" may be described. Acute localized pain intensified by movement of the eye or lid suggests a foreign body or corneal abrasion.

Aside from poor visual acuity, **headache** is the most common complaint that causes a patient to go to an ophthalmologist for an eye examination. If the eye examination discloses no pathologic abnormalities that may account for the symptom, a careful description of the type of headache and a history of its onset, relationship to use of the eyes, duration, and associated symptoms may not only rule out eye disease as a probable cause but may indicate the proper diagnosis.

For example, the headache that occurs upon arising in the morning and disappears soon afterward is seldom caused by eye disorders; a general medical examination is indicated. On the other hand, mild to moderate headaches that occur toward the end of a day of exacting eye work and that are relieved by a few hours of rest or sleep are more probably due to ocular disorders. Any case of severe headache that is becoming worse should suggest an intracranial lesion; visual field tests, ophthalmoscopy, and neurologic consultation are indicated.

"Eye-ache" often accompanies extreme fatigue with or without excessive use of the eyes. It is more common in patients with muscle imbalances, but it may be present with inflammatory lesions involving the episclera, iris, or choroid. The eyes may also ache with the increased pressure of glaucoma. In severe acute congestive glaucoma, the pain may be so intense as to radiate throughout the cranium and be accompanied by nausea and vomiting. Ocular pain may also be caused by fever, neuralgia, retrobulbar neuritis, and temporal arteritis. Aching eyes constitute one of the first symptoms of severe influenza and dengue.

Burning and itching may be a symptom of eyestrain, but the most frequent cause is inflammation of the lids or conjunctiva, eg, chronic blepharitis, conjunctivitis, and allergic reactions of the hay fever type. Itching, in particular, is a symptom of ocular allergy.

A sensation of "pull" is often described in adjusting to a new lens prescription, particularly if the prescription incorporates a change in astigmatic correction. There may also be sensations of pull or actual ache in adjusting to the first pair of bifocals.

Change in Appearance

A. Discoloration: Redness or congestion of the lids, conjunctiva, or scleras may be due to an acute inflammatory reaction to infection, trauma, or allergy or to acute glaucoma. Subconjunctival hemorrhage is sudden in onset and bright red in appearance. (Gross intraocular hemorrhage gives no external ocular sign.) Change of color of the cornea may occur with corneal ulcer or intraocular infection, producing cloudiness of the anterior chamber or an actual level of purulent material in the anterior chamber (hypopyon). Change of color of the "white" of the eye may be noted. Yellow scleras are usually seen with jaundice or antimalarial drug toxicity (eg, quinacrine). Blue scleras are associated with osteogenesis imperfecta. Dark discoloration may follow prolonged local or systemic use of silver compounds (rare) or may be due to scleral thinning and degeneration.

B. Swelling: One or both lids may be swollen. Swelling of one lid suggests a local abscess; bilateral swelling indicates a more generalized reaction such as blepharitis, allergy, myxedema, or malignant exophthalmos.

C. Mass: An orbital mass may occur, causing displacement of the globe.

D. Displacement: The eyes may be displaced forward or in other directions. There may be a change of position of the lids, either drooping (ptosis) or retracted (elevated).

Diplopia & Vertigo

It is difficult to differentiate diplopia and vertigo without a careful history. Both may be described by the patient as "dizziness." If double vision is described, it is important to know the time of onset, whether it is constant or intermittent, whether it occurs in certain positions of gaze or at certain distances, and whether the 2 objects seen are horizontal or vertical. Monocular diplopia occurs in lenticular changes, macular lesions, malingering, or hysteria.

Vertigo or light-headedness is often (but seldom justifiably) ascribed to eye disorders, since the patient frequently notes that during this time it is difficult to focus on any object or that "things seem to go around." The attacks are frequently associated with sudden changes in posture, such as arising suddenly from a lying or seated position, or sudden changes in the position of the head or neck muscles.

Discharge (Exudate or Epiphora)

It is important to know the type and amount of discharge, when it occurs, and whether chronic crusting or "granulation" of the lid margins occurs. If the discharge is watery (epiphora) and not associated with redness or pain, it is usually due to excessive formation of tears or obstruction of the lacrimal drainage system. The patency of the drainage system may be examined by irrigating the canaliculi and nasolacrimal ducts. If the discharge is watery but accompanied by photophobia or burning, viral conjunctivitis or keratoconjunctivitis may be present. A purulent discharge usually indicates a bacterial infection. A discharge seen with allergic conditions often contains a large number of eosinophils. Samples of the exudate may be stained with methylene blue, Giemsa's, Gram's, or other stains for microscopic identification of cell types and bacteria. If necessary, further identification of bacteria may be done by culture.

Decreased or Increased Lacrimation

Many systemic disorders are marked by decreased tearing. Dryness of the eyes is a frequent complaint in elderly patients and also occurs in several of the collagen disorders (eg, Sjögren's syndrome) and in patients taking tranquilizers. Excessive tearing (epiphora) may be due to chemical irritation (eg, smog), allergy, acute inflammatory disease of the eye, or tear duct obstruction.

PHYSICAL EXAMINATION OF THE EYE BY THE GENERAL PHYSICIAN

VISUAL ACUITY

Visual acuity determination should be part of the routine examination of all patients—not only those who present with eye complaints.

Technique

The usual method of testing visual acuity is with one of various types of special charts of test letters. (The Snellen chart is most commonly used.)

The patient faces the test chart at a distance of 6 meters (or 20 feet). A clean card or occluder is placed

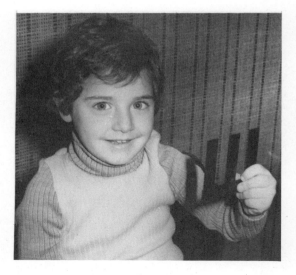

Figure 3–1. E game: Measuring visual acuity in preschool children.

in front of the left eye without pressure on the globe, and the patient is asked to read as far down the chart as possible with the right eye. If the patient is able to read the line marked 6/6 (20/20), this is recorded and the same procedure repeated for the left eye. If the patient can read the large letters at the top of the chart but cannot read down to the 6/6 (20/20) line, the value that corresponds to the smallest line that can be read is recorded. A patient who is unable to read the large letters at the top of the chart should be moved progressively closer to the chart until they can be read; this distance is then recorded as the distance from the chart over 12 meters (40 feet) or 60 meters (200 feet), ie, x/12 (if meters are used), x/40 (if feet are used). If glasses for distance are worn, the test should be repeated with glasses on and the results recorded as "uncorrected" and "corrected." Corrected visual acuity is far more important than uncorrected visual acuity.

Preschool children or illiterates should be instructed in the "E" game, then tested with the illiterate E chart (Fig 3–1). In this test the patient is taught to point a finger in the same direction as the bars of the E. The average 4-year-old child can cooperate satisfactorily in this test. Charts with test pictures have been devised but are not as accurate.

A corrected visual acuity of less than 6/9 (20/30) is abnormal.

INSPECTION

Inspection of external ocular structures (lids, conjunctiva, corneas, scleras, and lacrimal apparatus) should include everting the upper eyelids for inspection of the conjunctival surface with the patient looking down. This can be done easily by grasping the lashes of the upper eyelid with one hand, pulling out and down

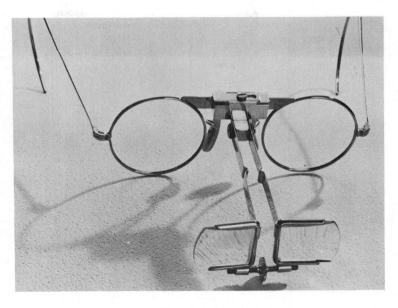

Figure 3–2. Bausch and Lomb Duoloupe.

slightly to put the tissue on stretch, and then pressing on the lid with a thin applicator stick at the superior border of the tarsal plate.

The exposed surfaces are inspected for defects, foreign bodies, inflammation, discharge, epiphora, dryness, clarity, color, or any other abnormality.

With a history of injury in which the coats of the eye may have been lacerated, great care should be taken in opening the lids to avoid pressure upon the eyeball. In the presence of pain and lid spasm, it may be necessary to instill a few drops of sterile anesthetic solution in order to examine the eye. In small children it may even be necessary to give a short-acting, light general anesthetic.

Pupils

The pupils should be inspected for size, color, shape, reaction to the stimulation of light, the effect of accommodation, and the presence or absence of the consensual light response. (Light directed into the pupil of one eye normally constricts the pupils of both eyes.) Examination for reaction to light is best performed in a darkened room with the examiner to the side of the patient. The pupils may be markedly constricted (miotic) due to the effects of bright illumination, central nervous system syphilis, or narcotic or parasympathomimetic drugs. They may be dilated as a result of dim illumination, myopia, or sympathomimetic drugs. Unequal pupils (anisocoria) may be normal but suggest neurologic disease if one or both pupils do not react well to light. Argyll Robertson pupil is one in which there is failure of direct and consensual light response with retention of the normal response of pupillary constriction on accommodation (focusing on a near object). The tonic pupil of Adie's syndrome (see

p 215) must be differentiated from Argyll Robertson pupil.

Position of the Eyes

Note the size (microphthalmos or enophthalmos), prominence (exophthalmos), and position (orbital tumor, strabismus) of the eyes. Palpation may be helpful in locating orbital tumors and determining their size, consistency, and pulsation.

The eyes should be observed for alignment as well as for movement of the eyes together in all fields of gaze. Any limitation can be further investigated as described in the section on strabismus evaluation in Chapter 15.

CONFRONTATION VISUAL FIELD TESTS

Many conditions are associated with loss of side vision. If special instruments for a careful perimetric field study are not available, the simple confrontation test should be performed as a rough test for gross defects.

Equipment & Materials

The only equipment needed is a simple wand, such as a pencil with a white eraser, a small white bead, or the examiner's finger.

Technique

The observer and patient face each other at arm's length. The patient is then told to hold one hand lightly over the left eye and look with the right eye at the examiner's left eye. The examiner then holds the target as far to the side as possible at middle distance from the

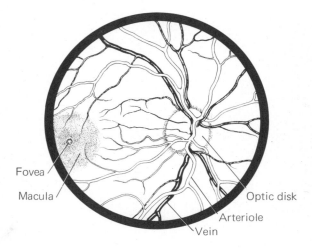
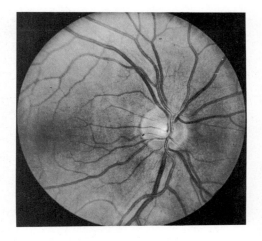

Fovea
Macula
Optic disk
Arteriole
Vein

Figure 3–3. The normal fundus. Diagram at left shows landmarks of photograph at right. (Photo by Diane Beeston.)

patient. The target is then slowly brought into the line of sight, and the patient is instructed to respond as soon as the target can be identified. This is repeated at intervals of 30–45 degrees around the 360-degree periphery. The fullness of the reported field is compared to that of the observer's. The test is then repeated for the other eye.

Interpretation of Findings

Gross hemianopia, bitemporal defects, or large unilateral defects can be detected by confrontation. The test should not be considered a substitute for a careful tangent screen or perimetric visual field examination but merely as a gross screening test.

SPECIAL OPHTHALMOLOGIC EXAMINATIONS

SLIT LAMP EXAMINATION
(Biomicroscopy)

The slit lamp consists of a microscope and special light source. Slit lamp examination is indicated in any condition of the eyelids or eyeball that can be better diagnosed and treated by having a well illuminated and highly magnified view of the area involved (eg, dendritic keratitis, corneal foreign body, iris tumor).

Equipment & Materials

A slit lamp is shown in Fig 3–4.

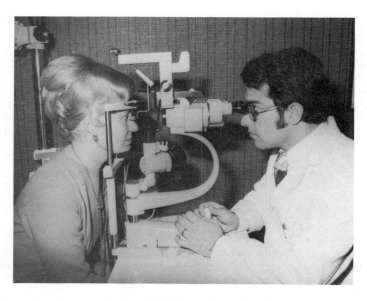

Figure 3–4. Eye examination with Zeiss slit lamp. (Photo by Diane Beeston.)

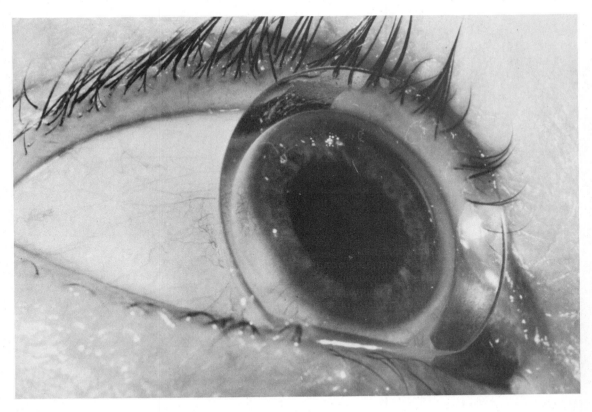

Figure 3–5. O'Malley self-adhering corneal contact lens.

Technique

Both the patient and the examiner are seated. The patient places chin on chin rest and forehead against frame while the examiner views the eyes through the microscope.

The lids, cornea, anterior chamber, and iris can be easily and quickly studied by moving the focus of both the microscope and the light back and forth. Since the strong light of the slit lamp causes the iris to contract, a mydriatic may be necessary to study lens detail.

For detailed binocular viewing of the vitreous, optic nerve, posterior and peripheral retina, and choroid, the 15-mm O'Malley self-adhering corneal contact lens is recommended (Fig 3–5).

To facilitate the examination, a local anesthetic (not always necessary) is instilled and the pupil is widely dilated with a combination of mydriatic and cycloplegic.

VISUAL FIELD EXAMINATION

The functions of the retina, optic nerve, and optic pathways are tested by performing peripheral and central visual field tests. Peripheral field examination is most useful in detecting disorders that cause constriction of peripheral vision in one or both eyes (as in retinal detachment, retinitis pigmentosa, or syphilis). Central field examination is useful in detecting disorders causing loss of a portion of the central visual field, particularly in glaucoma, optic neuritis, macular disease, malingering, or hysteria. If intracranial disease is suspected, examination of both the central and peripheral fields is indicated.

Equipment & Materials

Perimeter, tangent screen, light source, and test objects.

Technique

The test must be explained carefully to the patient, since it is important to obtain accurate responses.

A. Peripheral Fields: The patient is seated at a perimeter and the left eye covered with a bandage that does not exert pressure on the eyeball. The patient focuses with the right eye on a spot in the central portion of the perimeter 0.33 m from the eye. A white test object is brought in from the side at 15-degree intervals through the 360 degrees, and the patient is asked to signal when the test object is visible. The test object is then passed back along the same meridian from a seeing to a nonseeing area and the patient is asked to signal when it disappears. Both eyes are tested and the visual field plotted on a special chart (see p 380). With the Goldmann perimeter, both the central and peripheral visual fields can be charted in one examination.

There are now available some new, highly sophisticated and expensive automated perimeters that have yet to prove their value, particularly if a good technician is available to do the conventional examination.

B. Central Fields: The central field examination is of greater diagnostic and clinical importance than peripheral field tests. The patient is seated 1–2 m from a 1.8- by 2.4-m black felt tangent screen, and each eye is covered alternately. The blind spots are outlined, using a 2- to 3-mm white test object. The entire central visual field is then tested in each eye for visual defects (scotomas). The technique is similar to that employed in the peripheral field examination.

Normal & Abnormal Findings

The peripheral and central visual fields are measured in degrees. Normal values are shown on p 380. The normal blind spot is located at eye level about 13–18 degrees temporal to central fixation and just slightly (one-third disk diameter) inferior to the fixation point. An abnormally large blind spot can be due to papilledema or glaucoma.

Visual field defects must be carefully studied and correlated with other clinical findings to determine the exact site and nature of the lesions causing the defect. These are discussed in Chapter 17.

SCHIOTZ TONOMETRY

Tonometry is the determination of intraocular pressure by means of an instrument that measures the amount of corneal indentation produced by a given weight. It should be part of the general physical examination by internists and general physicians as well as ophthalmologists.

Indications

Tonometer readings should be taken on all patients over the age of 20 having a routine eye examination or general physical examination and on any patient suspected of having increased intraocular pressure for any reason.

Contraindications & Precautions

Tonometry should be done with great caution on patients with corneal ulcers. It is extremely important to clean the tonometer before each use by carefully wiping the footplate with a moist sterile cotton swab and to sterilize the instrument once a day (dry heat).

Corneal abrasions are rarely caused by Schiotz tonometry. Epidemic keratoconjunctivitis can be spread by tonometry, and this can be prevented if the tonometer is cleaned before each use and the physician washes hands between patients.

Equipment & Materials

Local anesthetic solution and a Schiotz tonometer (Fig 3–6).

Technique

Anesthetic solution is instilled into each eye. The patient lies supine and is asked to stare at a spot on the ceiling with both eyes or at a finger placed directly in the line of gaze overhead. The tonometer is then placed on the corneal surface of each eye and the scale reading taken from the tonometer. The intraocular pressure is determined by referring to a chart that converts the

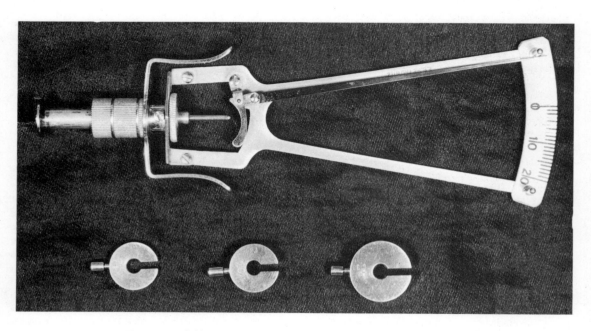

Figure 3–6. Schiotz tonometer and weights. (Photo by Diane Beeston.)

scale reading to millimeters of mercury. If the scale reading is 4 or less, the 7.5 and 10 g weights are added separately to gain further information concerning the intraocular pressure.

Normal Findings
12–20 mm Hg.

Interpretation of Abnormalities
If the intraocular pressure is 20–30 mm Hg or more, further investigation is indicated to determine whether or not glaucoma is present—ie, tonometry is a screening device to select patients for glaucoma testing. Visual field and ophthalmoscopic examinations should be done and the tonometer readings repeated several times at different hours of the day or on different days before the diagnosis of glaucoma can be regarded as established. If the pressure remains high on successive readings and there is a visual field defect or cupping of the optic disks, the diagnosis of glaucoma can be definitely established. In borderline cases, tonography may be helpful in establishing the presence or absence of glaucoma (see Chapter 14).

Accuracy of Method & Sources of Error
Schiotz tonometry (Fig 3–7) is accurate for clinical purposes. Sources of error include scleral rigidity, a poorly calibrated tonometer, improper application of the tonometer to the cornea, or an uncooperative patient who squeezes the eyelids shut. (The abnormal pressure of the orbicularis muscles on the eye artificially elevates the intraocular pressure.)

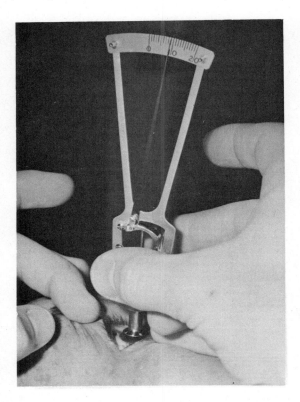

Figure 3–7. Measuring the intraocular pressure with a Schiotz tonometer. (Photo by Diane Beeston.)

APPLANATION TONOMETRY

Applanation tonometry (Fig 3–8) measures the force required to flatten rather than indent a small area of the central cornea and is more accurate than Schiotz tonometry. Applanation tonometry is widely used by ophthalmologists, but the equipment is impractical for the nonophthalmologist because it is fairly sophisticated and very expensive.

GONIOSCOPY

Gonioscopy consists of direct visualization of the anterior chamber angle (Fig 3–9). It should be performed in all cases of suspected glaucoma. It is also useful to estimate the extent of involvement of tumors of the iris, to look for suspected foreign bodies in the anterior chamber angle, and to search for aberrant blood vessels, which must be avoided if glaucoma surgery becomes necessary.

Equipment & Materials
Local anesthetic solution, a goniolens, and a source of illumination depending on the type of goniolens.

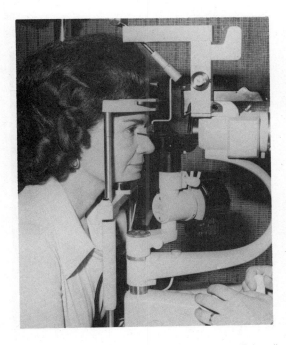

Figure 3–8. Applanation tonometer mounted on a Zeiss slit lamp. (Photo by Diane Beeston.)

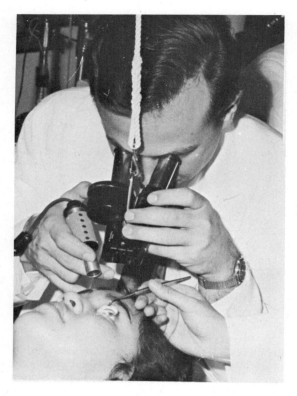

Figure 3–9. Gonioscopy. Examination of the anterior chamber angle with focal illuminator, goniolens, and hand microscope. (Photo by Diane Beeston.)

Technique

With the goniolens in place and the patient's gaze fixed on a light or spot on the ceiling, the examiner holds the microscope and the illuminating source and views the contents of the anterior chamber, particularly the anterior chamber angle, through a circumference of 360 degrees.

In recent years, gonioscopy has been performed more frequently using a contact lens containing a prism. The patient is seated, and the slit lamp is used as a source of illumination and magnification.

Normal & Abnormal Findings

Normally (and in most cases of chronic glaucoma), the structures of the anterior chamber angle can be clearly visualized. If the angle is extremely narrow and the intraocular pressure is normal, the patient is at risk of developing angle-closure glaucoma, an ocular emergency.

AQUEOUS OUTFLOW STUDY
(Tonography)

Tonography permits a rough calculation of the rate of outflow of aqueous from the eye. The test is based upon the change in the intraocular pressure that

occurs when an electronic tonometer is applied to the eye for 4 minutes.

Serious questions have been raised in recent years concerning the clinical usefulness of tonography, and it is being used less often in the evaluation of glaucoma patients.

SCHIRMER TEST

The Schirmer test is a gross measurement of the quantity of tear fluid in the conjunctival sac. It is indicated in any patient who complains of dry or chronically irritated eyes. The test is performed with standardized 5- by 35-mm Schirmer strips. One end of the filter paper is bent and inserted into the conjunctival sac near the inner angle and left for 5 minutes with the eyes closed.

The tears from the conjunctival sac should wet at least 15 mm of the filter paper strip in 5 minutes. If less than 15 mm of wetting occurs on repeated examinations, this is evidence of decreased tear production (see Chapter 6).

CORNEAL STAINING

Corneal staining consists of the instillation of fluorescein or other dyes (eg, rose bengal) into the conjunctival sac to outline irregularities of the corneal surface. Staining is indicated in corneal trauma or other corneal disorders (eg, herpes simplex keratitis) when examination with a loupe or slit lamp in the absence of a stain has not been satisfactory.

Precautions

Because the corneal epithelium, the chief barrier to corneal infection, is usually interrupted when corneal staining is indicated, be certain that whatever dye is used (particularly fluorescein) is sterile.

Equipment & Materials

Note: Fluorescein must be sterile. Fluorescein on papers or sterile individual dropper units are safest. Fluorescein solution may be used, but the physician runs the risk of introducing a new organism into the eye.

Technique

The individually wrapped fluorescein paper is wetted with sterile saline or touched to the wet conjunctiva so that a thin film of fluorescein spreads over the corneal surface. Any irregularity in the cornea is stained by the fluorescein and is thus more easily visualized.

Normal & Abnormal Findings

If there is no superficial corneal irregularity, a uniform film of dye covers the cornea. If the corneal surface has been altered, the affected area absorbs more of the dye and will stain a deeper green. It is customary to sketch the staining area on the patient's record for later comparison to show the progress of healing.

MEASUREMENT OF THE REFRACTIVE POWER OF THE CORNEA

Although originally designed for measuring corneal astigmatism as part of refraction, the keratometer is now used primarily to measure the radii of anterior corneal curvature (in millimeters) for contact lens fitting. It is also a helpful diagnostic aid in some corneal conditions, particularly keratoconus.

THE KLEIN KERATOSCOPE

The Klein keratoscope is used to study the regularity of the corneal light reflection in the examination of suspected keratoconus. It is a round disk with alternating black and white concentric rings and a hole in the center. The cornea is examined through the Klein keratoscope much as one would use an ophthalmoscope.

The reflections of the rings are not distorted in a normally curved cornea. Typical distortions in keratoconus are shown in Fig 3–10.

IRRIGATION OF THE LACRIMAL DRAINAGE SYSTEM

Irrigation of the lacrimal drainage system is a diagnostic or therapeutic procedure that consists of injecting fluid through the upper or lower punctum into the upper or lower canaliculus, whence it will normally flow into the lacrimal sac and down through the nasolacrimal duct into the nasopharynx. Irrigation is done in patients of all ages who complain of tearing. In infants who are not cured of dacryocystitis by massage and irrigation of the lacrimal sac and by antibacterial drops, probing of the nasolacrimal duct is indicated.

Equipment & Materials

Local anesthetic solution, a punctum dilator, a 2-mL syringe with a lacrimal irrigation cannula, and sterile water or physiologic saline solution (Fig 3–11). One must be certain that the cannula has a dull tip so that the wall of the canaliculus will not be punctured.

Technique

Adults require one instillation of anesthetic solution in the conjunctival sac.

The upper and lower puncta in the affected eye are first dilated and the lacrimal needle then passed into the canaliculus. Sterile water or saline solution injected into the canaliculus and tear sac normally passes down the nasolacrimal duct into the nose.

Normal & Abnormal Findings

If the lacrimal drainage system is patent and an individual sits with head back, the fluid will be im-

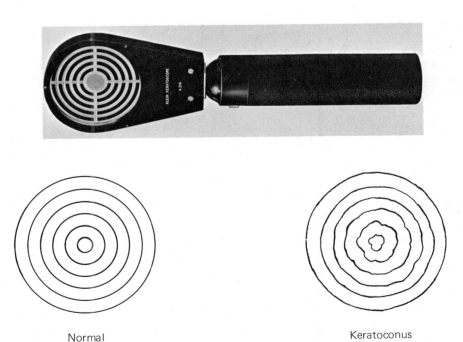

Normal   Keratoconus

Figure 3–10. *Top:* Klein keratoscope. *Bottom:* Pattern of rings in normal eye and eye with keratoconus.

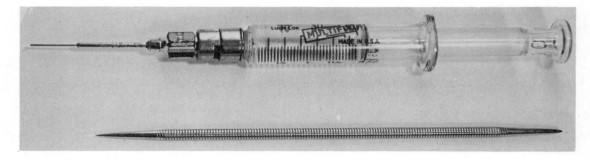

Figure 3–11. Syringe with gold cannula and punctum dilator.

mediately felt in the throat; if one sits with head forward, the fluid will run out of the nose. If the fluid is injected into the lower punctum and comes out of the upper punctum and does not go into the nose or throat, the site of obstruction is in the nasolacrimal duct or the common canaliculus at the entrance to the tear sac. If the fluid will not enter the canaliculus under pressure and does not come out of the opposite punctum or in the throat, the site of obstruction is in the canaliculus.

PROBING OF THE LACRIMAL DRAINAGE SYSTEM

Probing the lacrimal drainage system consists of passing a metal (preferably silver) probe of uniform caliber through the upper or lower punctum and the upper or lower canaliculus into the tear sac and down the nasolacrimal duct into the nose. It is indicated in obstruction of the upper or lower canaliculus or the nasolacrimal duct (particularly in infants) that is not relieved by irrigation.

Probing of the lacrimal drainage system should not be done in patients with acute dacryocystitis. It should always be done gently in order to avoid making a false passage through the canaliculus or lacrimal sac.

Equipment & Materials

Local anesthetic solution, a punctum dilator, and a flexible silver probe about 15 cm long should be used. The probes vary in diameter (Fig 3–12) and are numbered accordingly from No. 1 (smallest) upward to No. 8.

Technique

In adults, anesthetic drops are instilled into the conjunctival sac and the area of the tear sac is infiltrated with anesthetic.

The upper and lower puncta are dilated and the probe is passed into the tear sac. Lateral pressure on the lid is maintained until the probe is obstructed by the bony nasal wall; the probe is then withdrawn slightly, turned approximately 90 degrees, and passed through the nasolacrimal duct.

Normal & Abnormal Findings

The probe should pass freely and easily through all of the lacrimal passages and should be easily visualized with a nasal speculum in the inferior meatus of the nose. The point of obstruction may be noted when the probe cannot be passed farther with undue force. The most common site of obstruction in patients of all ages is the nasolacrimal duct.

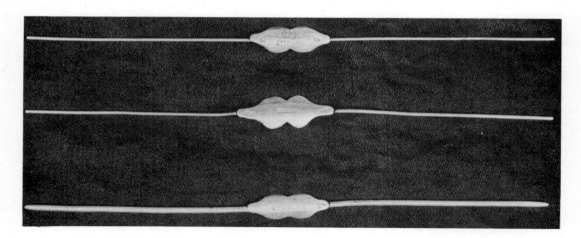

Figure 3–12. Lacrimal probes of various diameters. (Photo by Diane Beeston.)

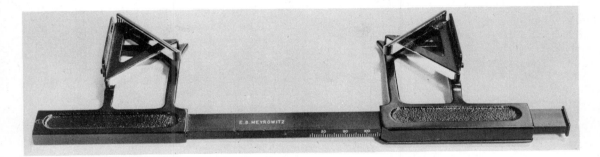

Figure 3–13. Hertel exophthalmometer. (Courtesy of Jenkel-Davidson Optical Co.)

Probing is almost always successful in relieving the obstruction in infants but is seldom successful in adults, for whom dacryocystorhinostomy is usually required.

LIGHT & COLOR PERCEPTION

Gross tests of retinal function may be performed by stimulating the macula with light or by merely testing light and color perception. Retinal function testing is indicated principally in patients with corneal or lens opacities that preclude a view of the retina and for whom surgery is contemplated.

Technique
A. Test of Macular Function: The patient sits with eyes closed as the examiner massages the eyeball gently with the lighted end of a small flashlight. The patient is then asked to describe what is seen. If the macula is functioning properly, the patient will see a red central area surrounded by the retinal blood vessels. If macular function is impaired, the central area will be dark rather than red and no blood vessels will be seen. Two disadvantages of the test are that it is highly subjective and is difficult for some elderly patients to comprehend.

B. Color Perception and Light Projection: A bandage is placed over one eye and the patient's hand is placed over the bandage to exclude all light. The patient is then asked to look straight ahead with the other eye. A light is held in 4 different quadrants and the patient is asked to identify the direction from which the light is approaching the eye. A red lens is then held in front of the light, and the patient is asked to differentiate the red from the white light. If all questions are answered correctly, it is reasonably certain that the retina is functioning normally.

Accuracy of Method & Sources of Error
The methods are reasonably accurate as gross tests of retinal function. However, if the opacities of the media are unusually dense, the tests must be cautiously interpreted, since it may be that not enough light is reaching the retina to give it proper stimulation.

EXOPHTHALMOMETRY

The exophthalmometer is an instrument for determining the degree of anterior projection of the eyes. This is an accurate method of diagnosing and, more particularly, following the course of a patient with exophthalmos.

Equipment & Materials
An exophthalmometer is shown in Fig 3–13.

Technique
The patient stands with his or her back against the wall and looks into the examiner's eyes. The 2 small concave parts of the exophthalmometer are placed against the lateral orbital margins and the bar reading is noted. This reading represents the distance between the lateral orbital walls. It must be constant for successive examinations if the course is to be judged accurately.

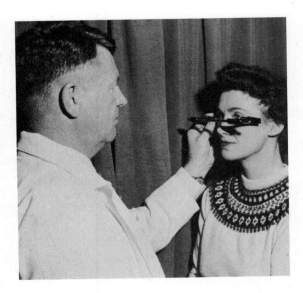

Figure 3–14. Measuring ocular protrusion with the Hertel exophthalmometer.

The examiner then views the cornea of the patient's right eye in the mirror with the patient fixing the right eye on the examiner's left eye. The cornea is simultaneously lined up in the mirror with a scale that reads directly in millimeters. The left eye is then observed in the same way, with the patient fixing the left eye on the examiner's right eye. Both the bar reading and the degree of exophthalmos are recorded in millimeters. (A typical reading: with a bar reading of 96 mm, RE = 17 mm, LE = 17 mm.)

Normal & Abnormal Findings

The normal range of bar readings is 12–20 mm. The reading is usually the same in each eye and indicates the anterior distances from the corneas to the lateral orbital margins. When exophthalmos is diagnosed (bar readings over 20 mm), one must look for some underlying cause, eg, thyroid disease or orbital tumor. Periodic exophthalmometer readings aid greatly thereafter in observing the course of the disease.

COLOR VISION TESTS

Determination of a person's ability to perceive the primary colors and shades thereof is performed as part of the physical examination of military recruits, transportation workers, and others whose occupations require the best possible color perception.

The term color blindness is something of a misnomer. Because color blindness is such a relative thing, color deficient might be a more descriptive term. No one is ever disabled by being color deficient. People are merely tested by our somewhat crude methods and are excluded from certain job categories if they fail the tests.

Equipment & Materials

The most commonly used polychromatic plates are those of Ishihara, Stilling, and Hardy-Rand-Rittler (Fig 3–15). The plates are made up of dots of the primary colors printed on a background of similar dots in a confusion of colors. The dots are set in patterns (eg, numbers) that are indiscernible by persons with color perception defects.

Technique

Under adequate illumination, the various polychromatic plates are presented to the patient, who is asked to identify the patterns.

Normal & Abnormal Findings

All of the patterns are recognizable to the person with normal color vision. A color-blind person is unable to identify the various figures and forms on the polychromatic plates. The type of color blindness is diagnosed according to the plates used. Red-green blindness is diagnosed in about 8% of the male population and 0.4% of the female population. Blue-yellow or violet blindness is extremely rare.

Accuracy of Method & Sources of Error

An experienced color-defective person may have memorized the plates. If this is suspected, some other test, such as examination with the Eldridge-Green lamp, should be used. Abnormalities of the ocular media, the retina, or the optic nerve can affect the test and should be ruled out if color blindness is discovered.

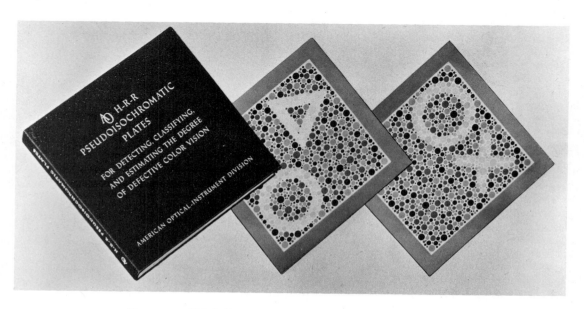

Figure 3–15. H-R-R (Hardy-Rand-Rittler) pseudoisochromatic plates.

TESTS FOR MALINGERING

Utilizing the refractor, place a strong convex lens in front of the good eye and a weak convex lens in front of the ''blind'' eye. If the patient reads small letters on the test chart, the eye under consideration is not blind. This test can be more subtly done with the refractor than with the trial frame, since the strong convex lens is not visible to the patient when the refractor is used.

Place a 10-diopter base-out prism in front of the ''blind'' eye. If there is sight in the eye, diplopia will result and the eye will be seen to move inward to correct the diplopia.

Place a pair of red-green glasses on the patient, with the red lens in front of the right eye and the green lens in front of the left eye. If the left eye is the suspected eye and the patient can read green letters with this eye, the eye is not blind; the green letters will not be transmitted through the red lens in front of the right eye.

BINOCULAR INDIRECT
OPHTHALMOSCOPY

Binocular indirect ophthalmoscopy (Fig 3–16) is a means of observing the posterior segment of the eye with a strong source of illumination and a convex lens held before the patient's eye. The observer views an inverted image of the retina that is formed between the lens and the observer's eye.

Binocular indirect ophthalmoscopy can be used to advantage whenever ophthalmoscopic examination is indicated. The advantages of this technique over direct ophthalmoscopy are that the field is larger, the view is stereoscopic, there is more illumination, and the peripheral retina can be more easily visualized. The

disadvantages are the inverted image, decreased magnification, and the fact that the pupil must be dilated with a mydriatic strong enough to overcome the pupillary constrictive effect of the bright light. Retinal surgeons rely heavily on indirect ophthalmoscopy both for preoperative diagnostic evaluation and during retinal detachment surgery.

OPHTHALMODYNAMOMETRY

Ophthalmodynamometry gives an approximate measurement of the relative pressures in the central retinal arteries and is an indirect means of assessing the carotid artery flow on either side. The test consists of exerting pressure on the sclera with a spring plunger while observing with an ophthalmoscope the vessels emerging from the optic disk. The pressure is gradually increased until the central retinal artery begins to pulsate at the point where it or one of its branches leaves the disk. This reading represents the diastolic pressure in the ophthalmic artery on that side, and this pressure is approximately half the brachial blood pressure. The procedure is then repeated in the other eye. The 2 readings are recorded directly from the scale in millimeters of mercury.

Examination with Bailliart's ophthalmodynamometer is shown in Fig 3–17. The test is performed with the patient in a sitting position with the head supported.

Ophthalmodynamometry is indicated in the neurologic evaluation of patients who complain of ''blacking out'' (amaurosis fugax) in one eye, spells of weakness on one side of the body, or other symptoms of impending cerebrovascular accident. No significant complications have been reported with its use.

A difference of more than 20% in the diastolic

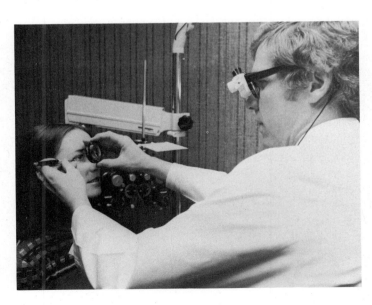

Figure 3–16. Schultz-Crock binocular indirect ophthalmoscope. (Photo by Diane Beeston.)

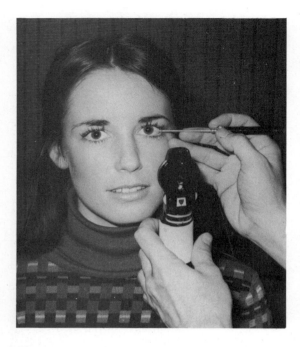

Figure 3–17. Measuring central retinal artery pressure with Bailliart's ophthalmodynamometer. (Photo by Diane Beeston.)

pressures between the 2 eyes suggests insufficiency of the carotid arterial system on the side with the lower reading.

TRANSCORNEAL TRANSILLUMINATION

Transcorneal transillumination is an excellent method for visualizing tumors, injury, or hemorrhage of the ciliary body or anterior choroid, not only when the media are clear enough to permit indirect ophthalmoscopy but even in the presence of gross opacities of the cornea, lens, and vitreous.

In all but the most heavily pigmented individuals, the form and relationships of the vitreous base (which straddles the ora serrata, not externally visible), the pars plana of the ciliary body, and the thickened portion (corona) of the ciliary body are visible through the sclera in fine detail (Fig 3–18).

Equipment & Materials
Use a topical anesthetic solution, a mydriatic, and a transcorneal transilluminator (Figs 3–19 and 3–20).

Technique
Cover the anesthetized cornea completely with the rubber cap in a darkened room so that all of the light is directed through the widely dilated pupil. This produces total illumination (the normal eye lights up like an incandescent bulb) of the entire eyeball, except for the corona ciliaris and vitreous base, which are clearly

visible through the sclera as dark circumferential bands; the light area between the bands is the pars plana. The ora serrata is located in the mid portion of the vitreous base but is not visible as a separate line or shadow.

Normal & Abnormal Findings
A tumor, hemorrhage, or foreign body in the ciliary body or choroid will not transilluminate and will appear dark.

FLUORESCEIN ANGIOGRAPHY

Ophthalmoscopy following the intravenous injection of fluorescein has gained great diagnostic importance in ophthalmology. This specialized technique provides sequential evaluation of the anatomic and physiologic status of the choroidal and retinal vasculature.

Equipment & Materials
The following items are needed: sterile aqueous sodium fluorescein solution, 10%; 5-mL syringe with 21-gauge needle; indirect ophthalmoscope with cobalt filter; and, if permanent photographic records are to be made, a fundus camera with appropriately paired filters, eg, Nos. 47 and 15 Kodak Wratten filters.

Technique
Following maximum mydriasis, 5 mL of 10% aqueous sodium fluorescein is rapidly injected into the antecubital vein with the patient in a sitting position. Black and white photographs are taken with a camera equipped with a motorized film advance and a high-intensity flash generator capable of recycling at approximately 1-second intervals. Photographs are taken

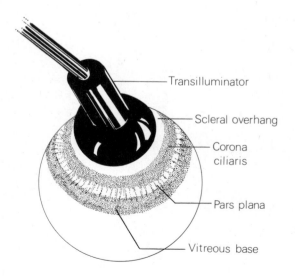

Transilluminator

Scleral overhang

Corona ciliaris

Pars plana

Vitreous base

Figure 3–18. Details of transcorneal transillumination with O'Malley transilluminator.

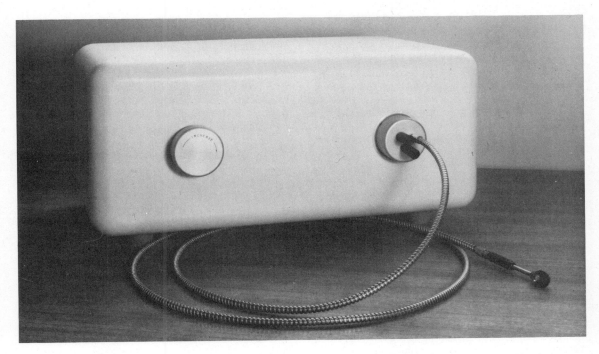

Figure 3—19. Skia light source, fiberoptic cable, and O'Malley transilluminator. (Photo by Terry King.)

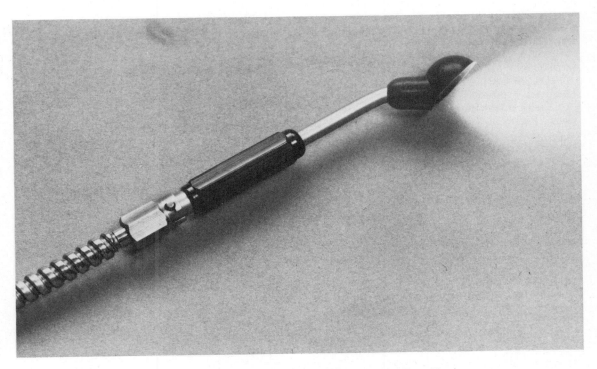

Figure 3—20. O'Malley-Skia transilluminator. (Photo by Terry King.)

prior to injection and then at half-second intervals for 20 seconds. Additional exposures are made at 3 minutes, 30 minutes, and 60 minutes. Valuable information can be obtained by simply observing the fundus after the injection of fluorescein (fluorescein angioscopy). A cobalt or Wratten 47A filter should be placed before the light source of the indirect ophthalmoscope.

Normal Findings

The normal pattern of fluorescein angiography can be divided into 3 phases:

A. Filling Phase: (8–20 seconds.) The choroidal circulation (choroidal flush) precedes retinal arterial filling. It is first seen in the macular area and spreads toward the periphery. A cilioretinal artery is observed at this stage. The fluorescein leaks from the choroidal vessels to the extravascular space.

The retinal arterial filling phase starts 0.5 second after the choroidal flush (Fig 3–21). This is followed by capillary transition and a venous drainage phase.

The retinal pigment epithelium acts as a physical and optical barrier to fluorescein. It prevents leakage of the dye into the inner retina and, except in albino patients, masks most of the fluorescence of the underlying choroidal circulation.

B. Recirculation Phase: (3–5 minutes.) The fluorescein concentration in the choroidal intravascular and extravascular spaces is equal. In the normal retina, fluorescein is confined to the intravascular space and there is no leakage to surrounding tissue.

C. Late Phase: (30–60 minutes.) There is little or no fluorescein in the retinal vessels. There may be very faint staining in the choroid and lamina cribrosa. This stage marks the elimination of fluorescein from the body.

Abnormal Findings

Vascular abnormalities such as arteriovenous shunts, microaneurysms, and neovascularization are detected early in the filling phase. Vascular leakage can be observed later. Window defects in the retinal pigment epithelium eliminate the optical barrier between the retina and choroid and transmit underlying fluorescence. Hyperpigmented areas and retinal hemorrhages, on the other hand, obscure the underlying fluorescence. Serous choroidal fluid accumulated under the retinal pigment epithelium shows early fluorescence. Serous fluid between the sensory and pigment epithelium fluoresces more slowly and at a later stage. Retinal edema or inflammation and fibrous tissue may show variable degrees of fluorescence. Suspected papilledema can be confirmed by vascular leakage in the area of the disk.

AMSLER GRID

The Amsler grid is useful for detecting and following central scotomas.

Equipment & Materials

The Amsler grid is shown in Fig 3–23.

Technique

With one eye occluded, the patient holds the Amsler grid chart at the customary reading distance with glasses on. While fixating the central dot, the individual is asked to describe and outline any area of distortion or absence of the grid.

This test may be used by patients at home to detect progression of macular disease.

Normal & Abnormal Findings

Abnormal findings include all positive and negative scotomas. The patient may describe a gray area, an area where the lines are missing, or an area where the grid is distorted (metamorphopsia).

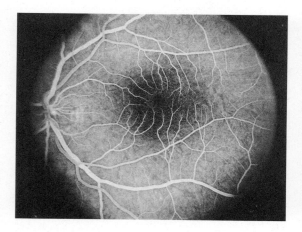

Figure 3–21. Normal angiogram, mid venous phase. (Photo courtesy of Roger Griffith and Terry King.)

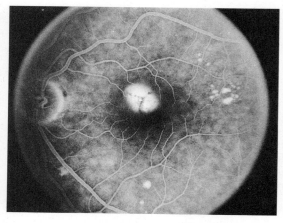

Figure 3–22. Abnormal angiogram showing prominent perifoveal detachment of the retinal pigment epithelium. (Photo courtesy of Roger Griffith and Terry King.)

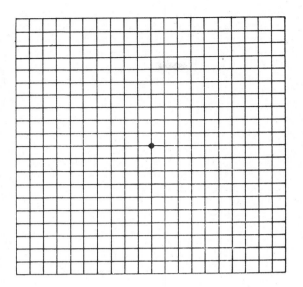

Figure 3–23. Amsler recording chart. A replica of Chart No. 1, printed in black on white for convenience of recording. (Courtesy of H.O.V. Optical Co.)

X-RAY EXAMINATION*

X-ray examination of the eye and orbit should be done in unilateral exophthalmos, optic nerve disease of unknown cause, intraocular or orbital foreign body, or suspected orbital fractures or tumors.

By utilizing radiopaque markers on the cornea and taking x-rays at different angles, one can accurately localize intraocular foreign bodies. It is often important to determine if a foreign body is intraocular or intraorbital; if it is not visible ophthalmoscopically, x-ray is the best means of localizing the object. Interpretation of x-rays taken about the eye and orbit in other conditions is beyond the scope of this book.

ELECTRORETINOGRAPHY

The normal retina exhibits certain electrical changes when exposed to light. Measurement of the changes in potential under the influence of light is known as electroretinography. The recorded electroretinogram (ERG) represents the difference in potential between an electrode placed in a corneal contact lens and an electrode placed on the forehead. The ERG is a composite curve resulting from several superimposed events and consists of 4 waves:

a **wave:** The initial negative response after a latency period following the light stimulus (photoreceptor cell layer).

b **wave:** The positive deflection (bipolar cell layer).

c **wave:** A slight positive deflection.

d **wave (off effect):** A positive potential occurring when the light is turned off.

The ganglion cell layer and the nerve fiber layer do not contribute to the ERG.

Electroretinography is usually performed under both photopic (light-adapted) and scotopic (dark-adapted) conditions.

In recent years there has been a resurgence of interest in the clinical application of the ERG. It may be a helpful diagnostic aid in patients with *diffuse* retinal damage with or without ophthalmoscopic changes. It is also of great help in the evaluation of the retina if the optical media are opaque. Local macular diseases are not detected by electroretinography. The ERG is being widely used in ophthalmic research laboratories.

THE BERMAN METAL LOCATOR

The Berman metal locator is an electromagnetic detecting device for localization of metallic foreign bodies. It is used to determine the position of a magnetic metallic foreign body in the eye or orbit that cannot be well localized by x-ray or by ophthalmoscopy. It has a sterilizable tip and is particularly useful during surgical removal of a metallic intraocular foreign body.

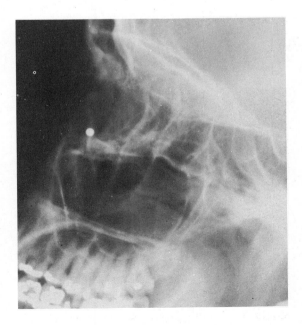

Figure 3–24. Intraocular metallic foreign body as seen by x-ray. (Left lateral view.)

*CT scans are illustrated and discussed on pp 363–370.

VISUAL EVOKED RESPONSE (VER)
(Visual Evoked Potential [VEP])

When a flash of light strikes the retina, it evokes a volley of nerve impulses that are transmitted along the visual pathways to the occipital cortex. The response to the light stimulus can be recognized only after an averaging computer eliminates asynchronous spontaneous activity and thus enhances the response to repeated (50–100) light stimulations.

Fig 3–25 shows the normal response to 100 flash stimuli recorded from over the occipital lobes. The first upward deflection at a latency of 40–50 ms gives data on the velocity and quality of conduction along the visual pathways. Later components show the response as the visual information is processed in the brain.

By stimulating each eye separately, optic nerve lesions can be recognized in the absence of hemisphere response from the affected nerve (Fig 3–26). Partial optic nerve lesions result in delayed conduction and reduced amplitude. Retrochiasmatic lesions are recognized by the different hemispheric responses (Fig 3–27).

Visual evoked response is becoming an important tool in the objective investigation of the visual system in babies or nonresponsive patients. It is of recognized value in the detection of subclinical lesions in the visual pathways, eg, as may occur in multiple sclerosis. By the use of a patterned light of various gratings, the VER has become a major tool in research on amblyopia.

ULTRASONOGRAPHY
(Diagnostic Ultrasound, Echography, Echo-ophthalmography)

Recent advances in ultrasonic diagnostic methods have made echography an important diagnostic aid in ophthalmology. Echography helps in differentiating orbital tumors and supplements or sometimes replaces ophthalmoscopy whenever opacities of the ocular media prevent visualization of the ocular fundus.

The ultrasound machine utilizes extremely high-frequency sound waves (8–10 MHz) to detect echoes reflected from soft tissues of varying density. A probe is placed on the eyelid, and the ultrasound waves are reflected back to the sound probe to form an echogram. There are 2 main methods of ultrasonography, using different types of instruments: A scan and B scan. The A scan is a pinlike beam of sound that traverses the tissues, and the echo appears as a deviation of a line against time to provide accurate quantitative graphic evidence of amplitude changes. The B scan makes sections through the entire tissue (literally the sum of multiple A scans) and depicts the shape and location of existing lesions in 2-dimensional form.

Ultrasonography may be used to examine the posterior portion of the eye when the media are opaque (eg, due to cataract). The method can detect retinal

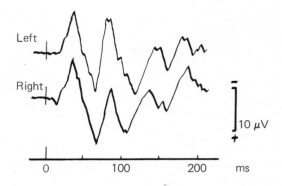

Figure 3–25. Normal VER recorded from over the left and right occipital poles. (Courtesy of M Feinsod.)

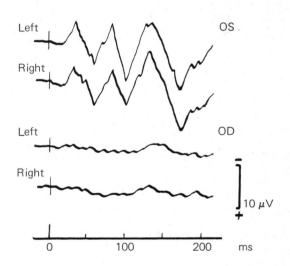

Figure 3–26. Complete right optic nerve lesion. No response is evoked by stimulating the right eye (OD). (Courtesy of M Feinsod.)

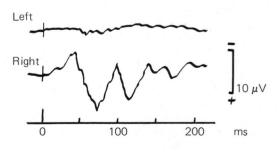

Figure 3–27. Right homonymous hemianopia. No response is recorded from over the left hemisphere. (Courtesy of M Feinsod.)

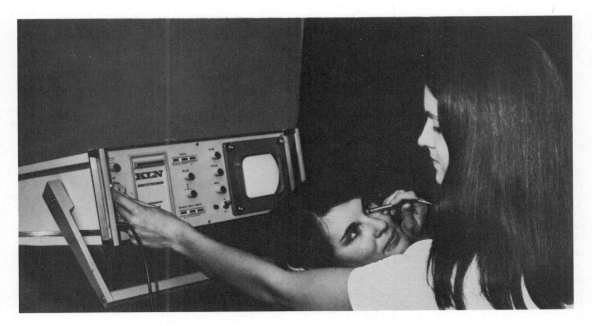

Figure 3–28. 7200 MA ultrasonoscope for echo-ophthalmography. (Courtesy of Rohé Scientific Corp.)

detachment, lesions behind a retinal detachment, density and amount of extraneous material in the vitreous, ocular tumors and foreign bodies, and orbital lesions.

Echography is gradually assuming a more important place in ophthalmology as an aid to the diagnosis of intraocular and orbital diseases.

● ● ●

References

Braley AE et al: *Stereoscopic Atlas of Slit-lamp Biomicroscopy.* 2 vols. Mosby, 1970.

Bodis-Wollner I, Yahar MD: Measurements of visual evoked potentials in Parkinson's disease. *Brain* 1978;**101**:661.

Boyd BF (editor): *Highlights of Ophthalmology.* 2 vols. Highlights of Ophthalmology Press, 1981.

Bronson NR: Contribution of ultrasonography. Page 555 in: *Highlights of Ophthalmology 1978–1979.* Boyd BF (editor). Clinica Boyd, 1979.

Bronson NR et al: *Ophthalmic Contact B-Scan Ultrasonography for the Clinician.* Intercontinental Publications, Inc, 1976.

Dallow RL: Reliability of orbital tests: Ultrasonography, computerized tomography, and radiography. *Ophthalmology* 1978;**85**:1218.

Davidorf FH: A simplified B-scan ultrasonoscope for ocular diagnosis. *Ann Ophthalmol* 1975;**7**:927.

Feinsod M et al: Visually evoked response. *Arch Ophthalmol* 1976;**94**:237.

Fuller DG et al: Ultrasonographic features of choroidal malignant melanomas. *Arch Ophthalmol* 1979;**97**:1465.

Harrington DO: *The Visual Fields: A Textbook and Atlas of Clinical Perimetry,* 5th ed. Mosby, 1981.

Heijl A et al: A clinical comparison of three computerized automatic perimeters in the detection of glaucoma defects. *Arch Ophthalmol* 1981;**99**:832.

Keeney AH: *Ocular Examination: Basis and Technique,* 2nd ed. Mosby, 1976.

Krimsky E: Simple eye tests. *Postgrad Med* (Dec) 1966;**40**:697.

McQuown DS: Ocular and orbital echography. *Radiol Clin North Am* 1975;**13**:523.

Miller BW: A review of practical tests for ocular malingering and hysteria. *Surv Ophthalmol* 1973;**17**:241.

Moses R: *Adler's Physiology of the Eye,* 7th ed. Mosby, 1981.

Norton EWD (editor): Symposium: The value of fluorescein angiography in the study of choroidal and pigment epithelial disease. *Trans Am Acad Ophthalmol Otolaryngol* 1973;**77**:724.

Perkins ES: Tonometry. *Proc R Soc Med* 1976;**60**:63.

Pinschmidt NW: Evaluation of the Schirmer tear test. *South Med J* 1970;**63**:1256.

Quickert MH: A fluorescein-anesthetic solution for applanation tonometry. *Arch Ophthalmol* 1967;**77**:734.

Smith SE: Mydriatic drugs for routine fundal inspection. *Ophthalmol Digest* 1972;**34**:10.

4 | Principles of Management of Common Ocular Disorders

It is not necessary to refer every patient with an eye disease to an ophthalmologist for treatment. In general, sties, bacterial conjunctivitis, superficial trauma to the lids, cornea, and conjunctiva, and superficial corneal foreign bodies can be treated just as effectively by the internist or general physician as by the ophthalmologist. On the other hand, more serious eye diseases or symptoms such as the following should be referred as soon as possible for specialized care: iritis, glaucoma, retinal detachment, strabismus, eye pain or blurred vision of undetermined origin, double vision, and corneal trauma or infection.

In the management of acute ocular disorders, it is most important to establish a definitive diagnosis before prescribing treatment. "All red eyes are not pinkeye," is a useful maxim, and the physician must be alert for the more serious iritis, keratitis, or glaucoma (see chart on inside front cover). The common practice of prescribing "shotgun" topical antibiotic combinations containing corticosteroids is to be discouraged, principally because of the inherent danger of incautious steroid treatment.

This chapter is an attempt to summarize for the nonspecialist the basic principles and techniques of diagnosis and management of common ocular problems. All of the disorders discussed here are dealt with in greater detail elsewhere in this book.

OFFICE EQUIPMENT & SUPPLIES

Basic Equipment

A great many specialized instruments have been devised for the investigation of eye disorders. However, most diseases of the eye can be diagnosed with the aid of a few relatively simple instruments:

(1) Hand flashlight.
(2) Binocular loupe.
(3) Ophthalmoscope.
(4) Visual acuity chart (Snellen).
(5) Tonometer. (Tonometry should be done on all patients over 20 years of age having a physical examination.)

Basic Medications
A. Local Anesthetics:
1. Proparacaine, 0.5%.
2. Tetracaine, 0.5%.

B. Dyes: Sterile fluorescein papers, rose bengal solution.

C. Mydriatics: Phenylephrine, 2.5%, is a satisfactory mydriatic when the examiner wishes to obtain a clearer view of the lens, vitreous, or ocular fundus.

D. Miotics: Pilocarpine, 1%, should be instilled at the end of the examination in all eyes that have been dilated with phenylephrine. This is to prevent an attack of acute angle-closure glaucoma if the anterior chamber angle is narrow.

E. Antibacterial Agents: Sulfisoxazole, 4% ophthalmic solution or ointment; and gentamicin, 0.3% solution or ointment.

HISTORY & PHYSICAL EXAMINATION

History

When taking a history from a patient who presents with an eye problem, a useful initial question is, "How do your eyes bother you?" After the patient has described the present difficulty, inquire specifically about glasses, blurred vision, pain, red eyes, double vision, trauma to the eyes or head, headaches, and "eyestrain." Information concerning the patient's general health is also relevant, particularly with regard to diabetes mellitus and hypertension. Since many eye diseases have a genetic pattern, the family history should be obtained. The patient's age and occupation are important factors in many ocular difficulties. Patients with glasses should be asked how long it has been since their prescription was changed.

Physical Examination

An adequate gross physical examination of the eye can be performed easily and quickly with a minimum of equipment (see above). By far the most important single examination is visual acuity testing in each eye. This should be done on all patients and the results noted in the clinical record. Visual acuity is tested at a distance of 6 meters (20 feet) using the Snellen chart. It is usually noted with and without glasses. However, corrected visual acuity has greater significance, since it is presumably the best possible visual acuity.

Inspection is facilitated by adequate illumination and should include a mental note of the patient's age, body build, and the structure of the head, face, and eyelids (eg, a patient with Marfan's syndrome is tall and thin and has long fingers). Bell's palsy and acromegaly may also be noted. Observe the eyes grossly for evidence of exophthalmos or enophthalmos.

Using a hand flashlight, examine the lids, conjunctivas, and corneas to rule out inflammation. Observe for icteric scleras (eg, hepatitis), pale conjunctivas (anemia), tumors, and scars. The pupillary light response should also be noted at this time. Gross disorders of ocular movements can be observed by having the patient follow the light of a moving flashlight by moving the eyes to the right, left, up, down, and inward while holding the head in fixed position.

Pressure over the tear sac will produce a mucoid or purulent discharge if significant infection is present.

With the ophthalmoscope, one can judge the clarity of the aqueous, lens, and vitreous as well as the appearance of the optic nerve, macula, retina, retinal blood vessels, and choroid. The ophthalmoscopic examination is facilitated by dim illumination in the examining room and a strong, well-focused light in the ophthalmoscope. If the ocular fundi cannot be easily inspected through the normal pupil, the pupil should be dilated. *Caution:* Before instilling the mydriatic, examine the anterior chamber by oblique illumination with a hand light (see p 166). If the anterior chamber is shallow (iris and lens quite close to the cornea), dilatation of the pupils should be performed only by an ophthalmologist, since in these cases dilatation may precipitate an attack of acute glaucoma.

In any patient over 20 years of age, tonometry should be performed as a screening test for glaucoma. Determining the intraocular pressure by finger palpation of the eyes (tactile tension) is not a reliable procedure.

BACTERIOLOGIC & MICROSCOPIC EXAMINATION

In the management of all serious external eye infections, the first step is to obtain a stained smear of the exudate. In conjunctivitis, for example, the scraping is taken directly from the conjunctival surface, and in corneal ulcer the scraping is taken directly from the advancing border of the lesion. The equipment necessary for the study of stained smears is as follows: sterile spatula, glass slides, stains (methylene blue, Wright's, Gram's, and Giemsa's), and microscope, light, and immersion oil. Pull down on the patient's lower lid to expose the conjunctiva, make 3–4 horizontal scrapings, and smear on a clean glass slide. Fix with heat, stain, and dry in air. Prior instillation of local anesthetic drops minimizes discomfort from the scraping.

Cultures and antibiotic sensitivity studies should be done in *all* cases of corneal ulcer and in severe cases of bacterial conjunctivitis.

Study of the stained smear is far more important than culturing in the average ocular infection, since by this means one can immediately determine whether the causative agent is bacterial, viral, fungal, or allergic and because in some instances the exact cause can be determined on the spot. This information serves as a guide to treatment. For example, if pneumococci are found, almost any type of antibiotic will be effective, whereas staphylococcal infection will require more specific measures. If there is considerable inflammation of the conjunctiva, if no bacteria are found, and if monocytes are present in increased numbers in the smear, a diagnosis of viral conjunctivitis can be made, and the physician knows that the condition will probably last 10–14 days with or without treatment. If many eosinophils are noted in the stained conjunctival smear, the conjunctivitis is probably due to allergy.

TREATMENT OF SPECIFIC EYE CONDITIONS

LIDS

Marginal Blepharitis

Marginal blepharitis is the most common disorder of the lids. The most important factor in its treatment is cleanliness, which is best maintained by rubbing the scales from the eyelid margins daily with a wet cotton applicator or clean washcloth or by scrubbing the lid margin and the base of the eyelashes with baby shampoo. Since this disorder is frequently associated with dandruff, vigorous efforts to keep the scalp clean are warranted. Specific antibiotic ointment should be applied to the lid margins once daily at bedtime when the condition is associated with microbial infection.

Internal Hordeolum

This common condition is essentially a meibomian gland abscess caused by infection with *Staphylococcus aureus*. The treatment is similar to that of a boil elsewhere on the body. Warm compresses should be applied for 15 minutes 3–4 times daily, followed by the instillation of sulfonamide or antibiotic ointment. Incision or expression is required when the hordeolum is pointing. If the hordeolum points toward the conjunctival surface, the incision should be a vertical one on the conjunctival side to avoid cutting across the meibomian glands. If the hordeolum is pointing on the lid side, a horizontal incision is made through the skin, since most of the lines of the skin in this region are horizontal.

External Hordeolum (Sty)

Infection of Zeis's or Moll's glands (sty) is smaller and more superficial than internal hordeolum (meibomian gland abscess). Pain and redness are the principal symptoms. Treatment is similar to that outlined for internal hordeolum.

Chalazion

A chalazion is a nontender lipogranulomatous inflammation of a meibomian gland. It should be excised by an ophthalmologist.

Dacryocystitis

A. In Adults: Acute dacryocystitis in adults usually implies that the nasolacrimal duct is completely blocked. Systemic administration of penicillin is effective treatment. Local treatment is generally ineffective. Operation is indicated if the infection does not respond to medical treatment. Dacryocystorhinostomy is the operation of choice for the prevention of recurrences of dacryocystitis.

B. In Infants: In infantile dacryocystitis, the tear sac should be massaged 3–4 times daily. Following the massage, instill sulfonamide or antibiotic drops into the conjunctival sac. If this is not successful, probing of the nasolacrimal duct by an ophthalmologist is indicated.

Tumors

Verrucae and papillomas are common and can usually be easily excised as well by the general physician as by the ophthalmologist as long as they are not near the lid margin. All lid tumors should be examined microscopically to rule out malignancy. Improper excision of tumors near the lid margin may result in lid abnormalities.

CONJUNCTIVA

Hyperemia of the conjunctival vessels is the most common cause of red eyes. Smog, smoke, and other irritants found in the environment may cause hyperemia of the conjunctival vessels. Local vasoconstrictors or cold compresses may be helpful in alleviating the symptoms and the redness.

Conjunctivitis caused by allergy can be helped by local vasoconstrictors and cold compresses. Topical corticosteroid drops may be used in severe cases under ophthalmologic supervision.

Conjunctivitis due to microbial agents — bacterial, viral, fungal, chlamydial, or parasitic — may be treated specifically after proper identification of the agent. Because treatment with ointments may cause blurring of vision for half an hour after instillation, eye drops are prescribed if it is necessary to use the eyes during the day; ointment can be used at bedtime to ensure prolonged effect during the sleeping hours. Patients are cautioned to wash their hands frequently and not to touch their eyes. This is to prevent spread of infection to the other eye as well as to other people. Individual washcloths and towels should be used. Systemic therapy may be indicated in certain forms of conjunctivitis, eg, chlamydial conjunctivitis.

CORNEA*

Corneal Foreign Bodies

Note the time and place of the accident and what the patient was doing when it occurred. Visual acuity testing — if possible, before treatment is instituted — is important for legal as well as medical reasons in all cases.

If the patient complains of a foreign body sensation and gives a consistent history, there usually is one even though it may not be readily visible on the initial examination. However, if oblique illumination is used with the hand flashlight, almost all foreign bodies can be detected. If no corneal foreign bodies are seen and the patient continues to have a foreign body sensation, instill a local anesthetic and turn the upper lid to exclude the possibility of an upper tarsal conjunctival foreign body. If there is no conjunctival foreign body, stain the cornea with fluorescein paper. When the corneal foreign body is found, remove it with a wet cotton applicator or spud under good illumination, using an ocular loupe if one is available. Instill gentamicin ointment to prevent contamination with a gram-negative or gram-positive organism. It is not necessary to patch the eye, but it is essential that the patient be observed on the following day to exclude the possibility of secondary infection of the crater. If no infection occurs, the corneal wound will heal by epithelial regeneration. If infection occurs, the wound area may take weeks or months to heal.

Untreated infection may cause severe corneal ulceration with consequent marked visual loss. Early infection is manifested by a white necrotic area around the foreign body crater and a slight gray exudate. *Note:* These patients should be referred immediately to an ophthalmologist.

Corneal Abrasions

The history should be taken and visual acuity tested before treatment. A patient with a corneal abrasion complains of severe pain, especially with movement of the lid over the cornea. The surface of the cornea may be examined with a light and loupe. If an abrasion is suspected but cannot be seen, stain the cornea with sterile 2% fluorescein solution. The area of corneal abrasion will have a deeper green stain than the surrounding cornea.

Instill gentamicin ophthalmic ointment. Apply a tight pressure bandage to prevent movement of the lid and resultant irritation of the abraded corneal area. Bed rest may be necessary. The patient should be observed on the following day to be certain that the cornea is healing. Corneal abrasions heal in 24–72 hours if a pressure bandage is properly applied. In contrast to corneal foreign body wounds, there is little chance of infection. The main dangers are delayed healing and recurrent corneal erosion due to imperfect healing. Do not use corticosteroids or topical anesthetics in any

*All corneal conditions except superficial foreign bodies should be treated by an ophthalmologist.

form of physical injury of the cornea. Systemic analgesics may be necessary in certain cases.

UVEAL TRACT

Any uveal tract disorder may lead to permanent visual impairment. Therefore, the treatment should be supervised by an ophthalmologist.

Acute Anterior Uveitis (Iritis)

This is the most common disorder of the uveal tract and can easily be confused with both conjunctivitis and acute glaucoma. Treatment with local cycloplegics and steroids is usually effective within 10 days. However, recurrences are common.

Posterior Uveitis

This disorder is more difficult to diagnose than anterior uveitis, and treatment is much less effective.

Neoplasms of the Uveal Tract

Melanoma is a primary tumor of the uveal tract. Its usual location is in the posterior choroid, where it can be seen with the ophthalmoscope. The treatment is enucleation. If a melanoma is situated in the iris, iridectomy is usually successful in removing the growth.

VITREOUS

One of the most common of eye complaints is "spots before the eyes." These are usually due to vitreous opacities (visible upon ophthalmoscopic examination). If the spots move about in the field of vision, as is usually the case, the patient may be reassured that they are not serious, only "little spots floating in the jellylike fluid [vitreous] inside the eye."

There is no treatment. With time, the opacities tend to fall inferiorly in the vitreous and thus out of the patient's line of sight. The examiner must bear in mind that vitreous floaters are occasionally the forerunners of retinal detachment.

RETINA

Retinal Detachment

This is an extremely important condition to keep in mind, since the diagnosis is fairly simple, and surgery is often effective if undertaken soon after onset. A complaint of sudden loss of vision, a shower of floaters, "soot," "lightning flashes," or "a curtain coming up [or down] in front of my eye," is an indication for examination with the ophthalmoscope through a dilated pupil for the presence of retinal detachment. This is particularly true if the patient is myopic, has undergone cataract surgery, or has sustained recent trauma.

A patient with retinal detachment should be hospitalized without delay and prepared for surgery. During transportation, a patient with retinal detachment should keep both eyes closed to avoid undue ocular movement. The area of the detachment should be in the dependent position. For example, the patient with a superior temporal retinal detachment of the right eye should be supine with the head turned to the right; if the right inferior nasal retina is detached, the patient should be transported sitting up with the head turned to the left.

Retinoblastoma

Retinoblastoma is the most common intraocular tumor in childhood. Any child with a suspected retinoblastoma should be referred to the ophthalmologist for prompt treatment.

LENS

Cataract

There is no medical treatment for cataract. The only treatment is lens extraction, which is indicated when visual acuity decreases to the point where the patient can no longer lead a normal life. Congenital cataracts should be removed as early as possible to prevent amblyopia.

Dislocated Lens

Lens dislocation may be genetically determined (eg, as one component of Marfan's syndrome) or may be caused by trauma. Visual impairment and secondary glaucoma are the principal indications for lens removal.

OPTIC NERVE

Optic Neuritis

Optic neuritis occurs as a manifestation of several neurologic diseases. It may be the first sign of multiple sclerosis. The presenting complaint is sudden loss of central vision with pain on moving the globe. On ophthalmoscopic examination, the optic disk may appear normal or may be slightly elevated, with increased vascularity. Systemic corticosteroid treatment has not been effective.

The vision ordinarily returns to normal in a matter of weeks.

Papilledema

Papilledema is most commonly caused by increased intracranial pressure, malignant hypertension, or thrombosis of the central retinal vein. It is manifested as an elevation of the optic disk and dilatation of the veins in the optic disk area. Parapapillary hemorrhages may occur. Papilledema can be observed easily with the ophthalmoscope through an undilated pupil. Intracranial tumors in the posterior fossa characteristically produce papilledema because of their blocking effect on the cerebrospinal fluid. Conversely, frontal lobe tumors usually do not produce papilledema. The rate of onset of papilledema after increased intracranial pressure produced by trauma (eg, subdural hematoma) is extremely variable and is of course related to the magnitude of the process. Moderate degrees of papilledema will not affect visual acuity, but the blind spots will be enlarged as shown by central visual field testing.

Optic Atrophy

In this condition, the disk is pale or white. Optic atrophy is usually an end-stage process for which no treatment is available. (See fuller discussion on p 210.).

Visual Field Loss in Intracranial Diseases

Some tumors of the central nervous system that produce gross visual defects in moderately advanced but still treatable stages can be suspected by the general physician on the basis of confrontation field tests. These include pituitary tumors, meningiomas, and posterior fossa tumors. These patients should be referred to a neurosurgeon for treatment.

STRABISMUS

There are 3 principal objectives in the treatment of strabismus: (1) to develop good visual acuity in each eye; (2) to straighten the eyes, for cosmetic purposes; and (3) to develop coordinate function of the 2 eyes (binocular vision). The best time to initiate nonsurgical treatment of a strabismus patient is by age 6 months. If treatment is delayed beyond this time, the child will favor the straight eye and suppress the image in the other eye; this results in failure of visual development (amblyopia) in the deviating eye. In such a case, patching of the good eye should be instituted without delay.

If the child is under 6 years of age and has an amblyopic eye, the amblyopia can be cured by patching the good eye. At 1 year of age, patching may be successful within 1 week; at 6 years, it may take a year to achieve the same result, ie, to equalize the visual acuity in the 2 eyes.

There is no firm rule about the proper time for surgery. Some surgeons operate as early as age 6 months; in some cases, there may be valid reasons for deferring strabismus surgery. If the visual acuity is equal and the eyes are made reasonably straight with surgery (or with glasses, as in the case of accommodative esotropia), eye exercises (orthoptics) may assist the patient in learning to use the eyes together. This is the seldom achieved ideal result in strabismus therapy. The prognosis is more favorable for strabismus with onset at age 2 or 3 than for strabismus present at birth; better for divergent (outward deviation of the eyes) than for convergent (inward deviation) strabismus; and better for intermittent than for constant strabismus.

GLAUCOMA

Ninety to 95% of glaucoma cases are of the chronic open-angle type. There are no symptoms in the early stages of open-angle glaucoma. The best means of detection is by routine tonometry and ophthalmoscopic inspection of the optic disk in all persons over 20 years of age. Chronic glaucoma comes on insidiously and causes slowly progressive loss of peripheral vision by interference with the blood supply of the optic nerve. The response to antiglaucoma eye drops is usually good, and surgery is seldom necessary.

Acetazolamide and other carbonic anhydrase inhibitors (eg, dichlorphenamide) have been shown to be extremely effective in inhibiting the production of aqueous by the ciliary body. Consequently, they are most valuable as preoperative adjuncts in the treatment of acute glaucoma and in the management of secondary glaucoma. Because of their side-effects (particularly renal calculi), long-term therapy of open-angle glaucoma with such drugs is not always feasible.

Epinephrine, 0.5–2%, when instilled as drops into the conjunctival sac, lowers the intraocular pressure.

Timolol is a beta-adrenergic agent effective in lowering the intraocular pressure by decreasing aqueous production. It is available as drops containing 0.25% and 0.5%.

Pilocarpine continues to be the most widely used antiglaucoma drop.

It is essential to diagnose glaucoma before significant visual loss has occurred, since visual field loss is not reversible. Tonometry, ophthalmoscopy, visual field tests, and gonioscopy are the most important procedures in evaluating and treating a glaucoma patient.

Approximately 5% of cases are angle-closure glaucoma, which produces pain, injection, and blurred vision. The patient seeks treatment immediately because of the pain. Acute glaucoma is treated surgically. The surgery is preceded by intensive miotic therapy and carbonic anhydrase inhibitors over a period of hours to lower the pressure in order to minimize complications during surgery. If miotics and carbonic anhydrase inhibitors do not lower the intraocular pressure sufficiently before surgery, glycerin or isosorbide by mouth or intravenous mannitol will nearly always do so within 2 hours.

TRAUMA

Chemical Conjunctivitis & Keratitis

This is best treated with irrigation of the eyes with isotonic saline solution or water immediately after exposure. It is wise not to try to neutralize an acid or alkali by using its chemical counterpart, as the heat generated by the reaction may cause further damage. If the chemical irritant is an alkali, the irrigation should be continued for at least 1 hour; this is because alkalies are not precipitated by the proteins of the eye, as acids are, but tend to linger in the tissues, producing further damage for hours after exposure. A local anesthetic solution is instilled before the irrigation to relieve pain. The pupil should be dilated with 5% homatropine or 0.2% scopolamine solution. Collagenase inhibitors such as sodium edetate (EDTA) or acetylcysteine (Mucomyst) are now being used in the treatment of severe alkali burns. Acetylcysteine is available as 10% or 20% solution in a preparation suitable for ophthalmic use. Sodium edetate solution must be specially prepared for the purpose. The patient's own serum (full strength or diluted 2:1) may also be used for its lubricant and mild anticollagenase activity. The patient must be watched carefully for such complications as symblepharon, corneal scarring, closure of the puncta, and secondary infection. Soft contact lenses may sometimes be helpful in such patients.

Lids

Lacerations of the lids not involving the lid margins, no matter how deep, can be sutured just as any other skin laceration. If the lid margin is involved, whether the canaliculi are also involved or not, the patient should be referred for specialized care; permanent notching of the lid margin may occur if the edges are not properly sutured.

Conjunctiva

In minor lacerations of the conjunctiva, sutures are not necessary. To prevent infection, instill an antibiotic 2–3 times a day until the laceration is healed.

Cornea, Sclera; Intraocular Foreign Bodies

The best emergency treatment for a laceration of the cornea or sclera or an intraocular foreign body is to bandage the eye lightly and cover the bandage with a metal shield that rests on the orbital bones superiorly and inferiorly and is held in place with tape passing over the shield from the forehead to the cheek. Examination, manipulation, and eye movement should be kept to the absolute minimum, since any undue pressure on the eye may cause extrusion of the intraocular contents.

OCULAR EMERGENCIES

Ocular emergencies may be classified as true emergencies and urgent cases. A true emergency is defined as one in which a few hours' delay in treatment can lead to permanent ocular damage or extreme discomfort to the patient. An urgent case is one in which treatment should be started as soon as possible but in which a delay of a few days can be tolerated.

TRUE EMERGENCIES

Trauma

Corneal foreign bodies and corneal abrasions must be treated early in order to relieve the progressively more severe pain and irritation. Lacerations of the eyeball should be sutured as soon as possible in order to avoid extrusion of the internal contents of the eye. Intraocular foreign bodies should be removed without delay. It is sometimes possible to remove them through the point of entry with a magnet. Because the ocular media become cloudy if the foreign body is not removed, a foreign body that is visible with the ophthalmoscope shortly after the injury might not be visible several hours or a day later. These procedures are best undertaken by an ophthalmologist.

A foreign body beneath the upper lid is suggested by blepharospasm and a history of foreign body but no foreign body that is visible. Evert the lid by grasping the lashes gently and exerting pressure in the midportion of the outer surface of the upper lid with a cotton applicator. If a foreign body is present on the tarsal conjunctiva, it can be easily seen when the lid is everted and then removed with a wet cotton applicator.

Corneal Ulcer

Corneal tissue is a good culture medium for bacteria, particularly *Pseudomonas aeruginosa*. Specific treatment of any corneal wound or infection by an ophthalmologist should be instituted as soon as possible to avoid corneal perforation and possible loss of the eye.

Severe Conjunctivitis

Most cases of conjunctivitis are not urgent. One exception to this rule is gonococcal conjunctivitis, which has the serious complication of corneal ulceration; a delay in treatment of 1–2 days may result in corneal ulceration or perforation.

Orbital Cellulitis

Orbital cellulitis may be complicated by brain abscess. Immediate treatment with systemic antibiotics is indicated. The bacteriology of orbital cellulitis is similar to that of sinusitis. For example, pneumococci and staphylococci are common invaders and require intensive systemic antibiotic therapy.

Chemical Burns

Chemical burns of the external ocular tissues must be treated immediately by copious irrigation with sterile water or saline, if available, or tap water, for at least 5 minutes. Do not use chemical antidotes, since the heat generated by the reaction may increase the degree of injury. After irrigation, instill sterile local anesthetics as necessary to relieve pain, and dilate the pupil. Local corticosteroid therapy may limit the degree of corneal damage. These patients should be referred to an ophthalmologist as soon as possible after injury.

Acute Iritis

Severe acute iritis causes extreme pain and photophobia. The pupil should be dilated as soon as possible to prevent the formation of posterior synechiae, which further increase the possibility of secondary cataract and glaucoma. Slit lamp examination is necessary to confirm the diagnosis.

Acute Glaucoma

If the intraocular pressure is unusually high (60–100 mm Hg), permanent optic nerve damage can occur within 24–48 hours. Therefore, these patients should be referred immediately for definitive care.

Occlusion of the Central Retinal Artery

This is a true emergency because the retina is completely without blood as long as the artery is occluded, and the visual receptors in the retina will degenerate within 30–60 minutes if the flow of blood is not restored. The diagnosis is based upon a history of sudden, complete, painless loss of vision in one eye in an older person and the following ophthalmoscopic findings: pallor of the optic disk, edema of the macula, cherry-red fovea, bloodless arterioles that may be difficult to detect, and ''boxcar'' segmentation of the blood in the veins.

The best treatment (of value only when the patient is seen within 30–60 minutes of onset) is to pass a sharp instrument such as a No. 11 Bard-Parker blade or No. 25 needle with syringe (see p 139) into the anterior chamber. The knife is inserted at the limbus and passed into the anterior chamber on a plane with the iris. The objective is to permit the extrusion of some of the anterior chamber fluid (aqueous) without striking the lens with the knife. This sudden decrease in the intraocular pressure may restore the flow of blood in the central retinal artery. No treatment is required for the wound. There are some favorable reports on the use of anticoagulants in cases of partial occlusion of the central retinal artery or its branches.

Retinal Detachment

Retinal detachment is a true emergency if the macula is threatened. If the macula is detached, permanent loss of central vision usually occurs even though the retina is eventually reattached successfully by surgical means.

URGENT CASES

Strabismus or Anisometropia in a Preschool Child With Amblyopia

The sense of sight develops from birth to about 7 years of age. If a child tends to favor one eye as a result of strabismus or anisometropia, vision may fail to develop in the other eye. These children should be treated without delay with glasses and alternate patching of the eyes. Surgery is performed if indicated after visual acuity has been equalized in the 2 eyes.

Chronic Glaucoma

Antiglaucoma therapy should be instituted without delay in order to decrease the intraocular pressure and preserve the remaining visual field.

Vitreous Hemorrhage

A patient with hemorrhage into the vitreous body should be referred, as the hemorrhage may later clear to reveal a retinal detachment.

Unilateral Exophthalmos of Recent Origin

The most common cause of bilateral exophthalmos is hyperthyroidism, although it may also appear after thyroidectomy. Unilateral exophthalmos may also be due to an orbital tumor, cavernous sinus thrombosis, or carotid cavernous fistula. These disorders are treatable.

Acute Dacryocystitis

Early treatment with warm compresses and systemic antibiotics is usually effective. If not, surgery is indicated.

Ocular Tumors

Many tumors of the ocular adnexa can be completely excised if they are diagnosed in an early stage. Malignant intraocular tumors (except those of the iris) may require enucleation.

Optic Nerve Disorders

Optic nerve disorders are quite serious and may indicate accompanying intracranial or systemic disease. The patient should be examined from a neurologic as well as an ophthalmologic standpoint.

Sympathetic Ophthalmia

With the availability of effective steroid treatment, sympathetic ophthalmia is now a condition that should be referred for immediate local and systemic corticosteroid or other immunosuppressive therapy. Sympathetic ophthalmia should be suspected if the patient has inflammation in both eyes and a history of penetrating injury to one eye.

•   •   •

PRINCIPLES OF ANTIBIOTIC & CHEMOTHERAPEUTIC TREATMENT OF OCULAR INFECTIONS

In the treatment of infectious eye disease, eg, conjunctivitis, one should always use the drug that is most effective, least likely to cause complications, least likely to be used systemically at a later date, and least expensive. Of the available antibacterial agents, the sulfonamides come closest to meeting these specifications. Two reliable sulfonamides are sulfisoxazole and sodium sulfacetamide. The sulfonamides have the added advantage of low allergenicity. They are available in ointment or solution form.

If sulfonamides are not effective, the antibiotics can be used. One of the most effective broad-spectrum antibiotics for ophthalmic use is gentamicin. It has some effect against gram-negative as well as gram-positive organisms. Other antibiotics frequently used are erythromycin, tetracycline, bacitracin, and polymyxin. Combined bacitracin-polymyxin ointment is often used prophylactically for the protection it affords against both gram-positive (bacitracin) and gram-negative (polymyxin) organisms.

The great majority of antibiotic and chemotherapeutic medications for eye infections are administered locally. Systemic administration is required for all intraocular infections, corneal ulcer, chlamydial conjunctivitis (trachoma and inclusion blennorrhea), orbital cellulitis, dacryocystitis, and any serious external infection that does not respond to local treatment.

Ointments have greater therapeutic effectiveness than solutions, since in this way contact can be maintained for at least 1 hour. However, they do have the disadvantage of causing blurred vision; where this must be avoided, solutions should be used.

Before one can determine the drug of choice, the causative organisms must be known. For example, a pneumococcal corneal ulcer will respond to treatment with a sulfonamide or any broad-spectrum antibiotic, but this is not true in the case of corneal ulcer due to *P aeruginosa*, which responds only to vigorous treatment with polymyxin, colistin, or gentamicin. Another example is staphylococcal dacryocystitis; staphylococci not sensitive to penicillin are most likely to be susceptible to erythromycin or methicillin.

Caution: It is well to keep in mind that the antibiotics, like the steroids, when used over a prolonged period of time in bacterial corneal ulcers, favor the development of secondary fungal infection of the cornea. This is another reason for using the sulfonamides whenever they are adequate for the purpose.

COMMON TECHNIQUES USED IN THE TREATMENT OF OCULAR DISORDERS

Liquid Medications

Place the patient in a sitting position with both eyes open and looking up. Pull down slightly on the lower lid and instill 2 drops in the lower cul-de-sac. The patient is then asked to look down while finger contact on the lower lid is maintained. Do not let the patient squeeze the eye shut.

Ointments

Ointments are instilled in the same way as liquids. While the patient is looking down, lift out the lower lid to trap the medication in the conjunctival sac. The lids should be kept closed for at least 1 minute to allow the ointment to melt.

Eye Bandages

Eye bandages should be applied firmly enough to hold the lid fairly securely against the cornea. A single patch consisting of gauze-covered cotton is usually sufficient. A wraparound head bandage is seldom necessary. Tape is passed from the cheek to the forehead. If more pressure is desired, use 2 or 3 patches.

Warm Compresses

Use a clean towel or washcloth soaked in hot tap water well below the temperature that will burn the thin skin covering the eyelids. Warm compresses are usually applied for 15 minutes 4 times a day. The therapeutic rationale is to increase blood flow to the affected area and decrease pain and inflammation.

Removal of Superficial Corneal Foreign Body

The main considerations are good illumination, magnification, anesthesia, position of the patient, and sterile technique. If possible, the patient's visual acuity is always recorded first.

The patient may be in the sitting or supine position. The examiner should use a loupe unless a slit lamp is available. An assistant should direct a strong flashlight into the eye with the rays of light striking the cornea at an oblique angle. The examiner may then see the corneal foreign body and remove it with a wet cotton applicator. If this is not successful, the foreign body may be removed with a metal spud while the lids are held apart with the other hand to prevent blinking. An antibacterial ointment is instilled after the foreign body has been removed.

Most patients are more comfortable without a patch on the eye after removal of a foreign body.

Note: It is essential to see the patient the next day to be certain that no infection has occurred and that healing is under way.

Home Medication

At home, the same techniques should be used as described above except that drops should be instilled with the patient in the supine position. Experienced patients (eg, those with glaucoma) are usually quite skillful in self-administration of eye drops.

COMMON PITFALLS TO BE AVOIDED IN THE MANAGEMENT OF OCULAR DISORDERS

Dangers in the Use of Local Anesthetics

Unsupervised self-administration of local anesthetics is dangerous because the patient may further injure an anesthetized eye without knowing it. Furthermore, most anesthetics delay healing. *Caution:* Do not give patients local anesthetics to take home with them. Eye pain should be controlled by systemic analgesics.

Errors in Diagnosis

Of these the most common is a diagnosis of conjunctivitis when the correct diagnosis is iritis (anterior uveitis), glaucoma, or corneal ulcer (especially herpes simplex). The differentiation between iritis and acute glaucoma may be difficult also.

Misuse of Atropine

Atropine must never be used in routine diagnosis or treatment. It causes cycloplegia (paralysis of the ciliary muscle) of about 14 days' duration and can precipitate an attack of glaucoma if the patient has a narrow anterior chamber angle (see p 372).

Dangers of Local Corticosteroid Therapy

Local ophthalmologic corticosteroid preparations, eg, prednisolone, are often used for their anti-inflammatory effect on the conjunctiva, cornea, and iris. Although it is true that a patient with conjunctivitis, corneal inflammation, or iritis can be made more comfortable with local corticosteroids, it must be stressed that the corticosteroids are associated with 4 very serious complications when used in the eye over a long period of time: herpes simplex keratitis, open-angle glaucoma, cataract formation, and fungal infection. The most common complications are herpes simplex keratitis and glaucoma. Corticosteroids enhance the activity of the herpes simplex virus, apparently by increasing the destructive effect of collagenase on the collagen of the cornea. This is evidenced by the fact that perforation of the cornea occasionally occurs when the corticosteroids are used during the more active stage of a herpes simplex corneal infection. Corneal perforation was a very rare complication of dendritic keratitis before the corticosteroids came into general use. In the treatment of any corneal inflammation, particularly if the corneal epithelium is not intact, the prolonged use of corticosteroids is sometimes complicated by fungal infection

(eg, *Candida albicans*), and this may lead to loss of the eye. Topical corticosteroids can cause or aggravate open-angle glaucoma and, less commonly, can produce cataracts.

For these reasons, although the corticosteroids are valuable in the treatment of ocular disease, any patient on whom they are being used should be watched carefully for the development of complications. The corticosteroids should not be used unless specifically indicated, eg, in iritis, certain types of keratitis, and acute allergic disorders.

Use of Contaminated Eye Medications

The external coats of the eye, including the sclera and the corneal epithelium, are resistant to infection. However, once the corneal epithelium or sclera is broken by trauma, the tissues become markedly susceptible to bacterial infection. For this reason, ophthalmic solutions that may be used in injured eyes must be prepared with the same degree of caution as fluids intended for intravenous administration.

Sterile, single-use disposable units of the common ophthalmic solutions should be used whenever liquid medication is instilled into an injured eye. For routine use in intact eyes, nearly all eye medications are now available in small plastic containers. It is perfectly safe to use these provided they are not kept a long time after opening and are not contaminated accidentally.

Overtreatment

Some patients with chronic conjunctivitis or keratitis may be made worse by overtreatment with topical medications. If a patient is not improving as expected, make certain the preservative in the local medication is not the cause.

•   •   •

References

Cogan DG: *Ophthalmic Manifestations of Systemic Vascular Disease.* Saunders, 1974.

Ellis PP, Smith DL: *Ocular Therapeutics and Pharmacology,* 6th ed. Mosby, 1981.

Fraunfelder FT: *Drug-Induced Ocular Side Effects and Drug Interactions.* Lea & Febiger, 1976.

Gardiner PA: ABC of ophthalmology: Accidents and first aid. (ABC of Ophthalmology Series.) Br Med J 1978;**2:**1347.

Gombos GM: *Handbook of Ophthalmologic Emergencies,* 2nd ed. Medical Examination Publishing Co, 1977.

Harrington DO: *The Visual Fields: A Textbook and Atlas of Clinical Perimetry,* 5th ed. Mosby, 1981.

Havener WH: *Ocular Pharmacology,* 4th ed. Mosby, 1978.

Henkind P et al (editorial consultants): *Physicians' Desk Reference (PDR) for Ophthalmology.* 11th ed. Medical Economics, 1983.

Hughes WF (editor): *Year Book of Ophthalmology.* Year Book, 1981.

Keeney AH: *Ocular Examination: Basis and Techniques,* 2nd ed. Mosby, 1976.

Kolker AE, Hetherington J: *Becker-Shaffer's Diagnosis and Therapy of the Glaucomas.* 5th ed. Mosby, 1982.

Miller NR (editor): *Walsh & Hoyt's Clinical Neuro-ophthalmology,* 4th ed. Vol 1. Williams & Wilkins, 1982.

Miller SJ: *Parson's Diseases of the Eye,* 16th ed. Churchill Livingstone, 1978.

Newell FW: *Ophthalmology: Principles and Concepts.* 5th ed. Mosby, 1982.

Paton D, Goldberg MF: *Management of Ocular Injuries.* Saunders, 1976.

Thygeson P: The unfavorable role of corticosteroids in herpetic keratitis. Page 450 in: *Controversy in Ophthalmology.* Brockhurst RJ et al (editors). Saunders, 1977.

Von Noorden GK: *Von Noorden-Maumenee's Atlas of Strabismus,* 3rd ed. Mosby, 1977.

Lids & Lacrimal Apparatus | 5

I. THE LIDS

Anatomy (Fig 5–1)

The eyelids are movable folds of tissue that serve to protect the eye. The skin of the lids, the thinnest in the body, is loose and elastic, permitting extreme swelling and subsequent return to normal shape and size. The tarsal plates consist of dense fibrous tissue with some elastic tissue. They are lined posteriorly by conjunctiva. The **orbital septum** is the fascia lying posterior to the portion of the orbicularis muscle between the orbital rim and the tarsi and serves as a barrier between the lid and the orbit.

The **orbicularis oculi** muscle, which receives its innervation from the seventh cranial nerve, is roughly circular. Its function is to close the lids. The muscle is divided into **orbital, preseptal,** and **pretarsal** portions. The preseptal and pretarsal muscles have deep points of origin over the fascia of the lacrimal sac. Contraction causes lacrimal secretions to be pumped into the nasolacrimal duct.

The **levator palpebrae** muscle is supplied by the third nerve; its aponeurosis inserts into the anterior surface of the tarsal plate and the skin and serves to elevate the lid. The superior tarsal muscle (of Müller), supplied by sympathetic nerves, originates in the levator muscle and inserts at the superior edge of the tarsus, coursing deep to the levator aponeurosis.

The 4 types of glands in the lid are the meibomian glands, the glands of Moll and Zeis, and the accessory lacrimal glands (of Krause and Wolfring). The

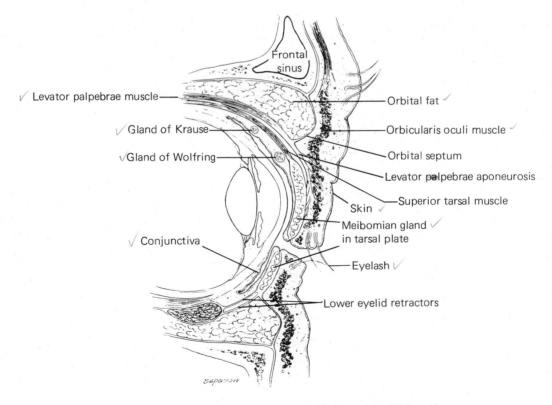

Levator palpebrae muscle

Gland of Krause

Gland of Wolfring

Conjunctiva

Frontal sinus

Orbital fat

Orbicularis oculi muscle

Orbital septum

Levator palpebrae aponeurosis

Superior tarsal muscle

Skin

Meibomian gland in tarsal plate

Eyelash

Lower eyelid retractors

Figure 5–1 Cross section of the upper lid. (Courtesy of C Beard.)

meibomian glands are long sebaceous glands in the tarsal plate. They do not communicate with the hair follicles. There are about 25 in the upper lid and 20 in the lower lid, and they appear as yellow vertical streaks deep to the conjunctiva. The meibomian glands produce a sebaceous substance that creates an oily layer on the surface of the tear film. This helps to prevent rapid evaporation of the normal tear layer. The glands of Zeis are smaller, modified sebaceous glands that are connected with the follicles of the eyelashes. The sweat glands of Moll are unbranched sinuous tubules that begin in a simple spiral and not in a glomerulus, as do ordinary sweat glands. Accessory lacrimal glands (Krause and Wolfring) are formed beneath the palpebral conjunctiva. They supply most of the needed moisture to the conjunctival sac and cornea.

There is a **gray line** (mucocutaneous border) on the margins of both the upper and lower eyelids. If an incision is made along this line, the lid can be cleanly split into a posterior portion, containing the tarsal plate and conjunctiva, and an anterior portion, containing the orbicularis oculi muscle, skin, and hair follicles.

The blood supply to the lids is derived mainly from the ophthalmic, zygomatic, and angular arteries. The lymphatics drain into the preauricular, parotid, and submaxillary lymph glands.

PHYSIOLOGY OF SYMPTOMS

Lid disorders are among the most common of all ocular problems. The patient with disorders of the eyelids will have varied complaints. There are many pain fibers in the tissues near the lid margins. Consequently, if there is inflammation with stretching of tissues, as in hordeolum, the patient complains of moderately severe pain. In marginal blepharitis there is no pain but the patient complains of red-rimmed eyes; because of the proximity of the lid margins to the conjunctiva, frequent attacks of conjunctivitis are a common complaint.

If the patient has a foreign body sensation, entropion, with eyelashes rubbing on the cornea, should be ruled out. If the diagnosis is not immediately apparent, entropion will be produced by asking the patient to close the eyelids tightly. If the lid falls away from the eyeball, as in ectropion, tearing will be the chief complaint, since the tears do not have access to the lower punctum. Exposure keratitis may also occur with ectropion.

TECHNIQUE OF UPPER LID EVERSION

Have the patient look down. Grasp the lashes gently and exert pressure posteriorly and medially on the upper lid at the upper tarsal border with a cotton applicator.

INFECTIONS & INFLAMMATIONS OF THE LIDS

HORDEOLUM

Hordeolum is a common staphylococcal infection of the lid glands that is characterized by a localized red, swollen, and acutely tender area. It is essentially an abscess, as there is pus formation within the lumen of the affected gland. When it affects the meibomian glands it is relatively large and is known as an **internal hordeolum** (Fig 5–2). The smaller and more superficial **external hordeolum** (sty) is an infection of Zeis's or Moll's glands. Pain is the primary symptom, and the intensity of the pain is in direct proportion to the amount of lid swelling. An internal hordeolum may point to the skin or to the conjunctival side of the lid; external hordeolum always points to the skin side of the lid margin.

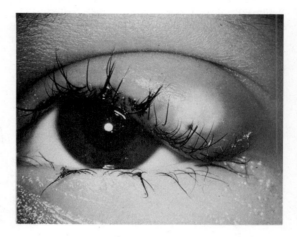

Figure 5–2. Internal hordeolum, left upper eyelid, pointing on skin side. This should be opened by a horizontal skin incision. (Courtesy of A Rosenberg.)

Treatment of both internal and external hordeolum is with warm compresses for 10–15 minutes 3–4 times a day, and incision and drainage of the purulent material if the process does not begin to resolve within 48 hours. An antibacterial ophthalmic ointment instilled into the conjunctival sac every 3 hours is beneficial. A large internal hordeolum can be complicated by cellulitis of the entire lid.

CHALAZION

Chalazion (Fig 5–3) is a sterile granulomatous inflammation of a meibomian gland, of unknown cause, characterized by localized swelling in the upper or lower eyelid. It may begin with inflammation and

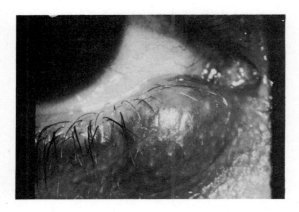

Figure 5–3. Chalazion, right lower eyelid. (Courtesy of K Tabbara.)

tenderness similar to a hordeolum and develop over a period of weeks. The majority point toward the conjunctival side of the lid. When the lid is everted, the conjunctiva over the chalazion is seen to be reddened and elevated.

If sufficiently large, a chalazion may press upon the eyeball and cause astigmatism.

In general, a fully developed chalazion is differentiated from hordeolum by the absence of acute inflammatory signs.

Chalazion seldom subsides spontaneously; if it is large enough to distort vision or to be a cosmetic blemish, excision is indicated. Pathologically, there is proliferation of the endothelium of the acinus and a granulomatous inflammatory response, including some Langhans type giant cells.

If chalazions are recurrent in the same area, biopsy should be performed to rule out malignancy.

MARGINAL BLEPHARITIS
(Granulated Eyelids)

Blepharitis is a common chronic bilateral inflammation of the lid margins. There are 2 main types: staphylococcal and seborrheic. Staphylococcal blepharitis is usually ulcerative. Seborrheic blepharitis (nonulcerative) is usually associated with the presence of *Pityrosporum ovale*, although this organism has not been shown to be the etiologic factor. Often, both types are present (mixed infection). Seborrhea of the scalp, brows, and ears is frequently associated with seborrheic blepharitis.

The chief symptoms are irritation, burning, and itching of the lid margins. The eyes are "red-rimmed." Many scales or "granulations" can be seen clinging to the lashes of both the upper and lower lids. In the staphylococcal type, the scales are dry, the lids are red, tiny ulcerated areas are found along the lid margins, and the lashes tend to fall out. In the seborrheic type, the scales are greasy, ulceration does not occur, and the lid margins are less red. In the more

common mixed type, both dry and greasy scales are present and the lid margins are red and may be ulcerated. *Staphylococcus aureus* and *P ovale* can be seen together or singly in stained material scraped from the lid margins.

Conjunctivitis, superficial keratitis of the lower third of the cornea, and chronic meibomianitis are the main complaints in the early morning hours. Seborrheic blepharitis is occasionally complicated by a mild keratitis. Persons with staphylococcal blepharitis are prone to develop chalazions and hordeola.

The scalp, eyebrows, and lid margins must be kept clean, particularly in the seborrheic type of blepharitis, by means of soap and water shampoo. Scales must be removed from the lid margins daily with a damp cotton applicator.

Staphylococcal blepharitis is treated with antistaphylococcal antibiotic or sulfonamide eye ointment applied on a cotton applicator once daily to the lid margins.

Meibomianitis is very resistant to treatment and requires repeated expression of the glands. It may be complicated by secondary infection with one of the prominent gram-negative organisms (eg, *Pseudomonas aeruginosa*).

The seborrheic and staphylococcal types usually become mixed and may run a chronic course over a period of months or years if not treated adequately; associated staphylococcal conjunctivitis or keratitis usually disappears promptly following local antistaphylococcal medication.

MEIBOMIANITIS

Bilateral, chronic inflammation of the meibomian glands is an uncommon disease of unknown cause that occurs during or after the middle years of life. It is generally preceded by or associated with blepharitis.

The patient complains of chronically red and irritated eyes and a slight but continuous discharge. The meibomian glands are prominent, the lid margins are red, and there is a frothy conjunctival discharge. A soft, cheesy, yellow material that contains no organisms can be expressed from the glands. An irritative conjunctivitis due to contact with meibomian secretion is a frequent complication, especially in the morning upon awakening.

The only treatment is repeated expression of the meibomian glands. However, because this treatment never produces dramatic results, the patient usually neglects to do it or have it done, and the disease process continues indefinitely with a slight tendency to become worse.

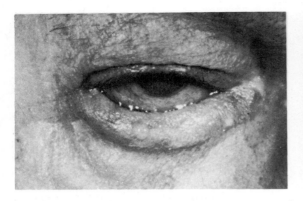

Figure 5–4. Entropion. (Courtesy of M Quickert.)

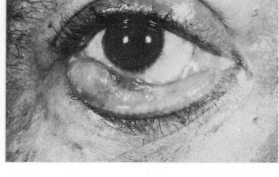

Figure 5–5. Ectropion. (Courtesy of M Quickert.)

POSITIONAL DEFECTS OF THE LIDS

ENTROPION

Entropion (turning inward of the lid) (Fig 5–4) usually affects the lower lid but may affect the upper lid. It seldom occurs in persons under 40 years of age. The common types are senile (spastic) and cicatricial. Senile entropion is due to a degeneration of fascial attachments in the lower eyelid, including a dehiscence of the lower eyelid aponeurosis (retractors) from the lower eyelid tarsus. This allows preseptal orbicularis to override pretarsal orbicularis and rotate the lid margin inward. Cicatricial entropion is due to scarring of the palpebral conjunctiva and the tarsus and is therefore common in trachoma. Trichiasis (turning inward of the lashes so that they rub on the cornea) results from entropion. It causes corneal irritation and may encourage corneal ulceration.

Surgery to evert the lid is effective in the treatment of both types of entropion. A useful temporary measure is to tape the lower lid to the cheek with tension temporally and inferiorly.

ECTROPION

Ectropion (sagging and eversion of the lower lid) (Fig 5–5), usually bilateral, is a frequent finding in older persons. Ectropion may be caused by relaxation of the orbicularis oculi muscle, either as part of the aging process or following seventh nerve palsy. The symptoms are tearing and irritation. Exposure keratitis may occur.

Marked ectropion is treated by surgical shortening of the lower lid in a horizontal direction. Cicatricial ectropion is caused by contracture of the anterior lamella of the lid. It requires surgical revision of the scar and often skin grafting for relief. Minor degrees of ectropion can be treated by several fairly deep electrocautery penetrations through the conjunctiva 4–5 mm from the lid margins at the inferior aspect of the tarsal plate. The fibrotic reaction that follows will frequently draw the lid up to its normal position.

ANATOMIC DEFORMITIES OF THE LIDS

DERMATOCHALASIS & BLEPHAROCHALASIS

Dermatochalasis (Fig 5–6) is redundancy and loss of elasticity of skin such that a skin fold covers the tarsal portion of the eyelid. It is a common condition that is most often a function of aging, although occasionally it may be the result of repeated episodes of lid edema. When severe, pseudoptosis may result. Excision of a portion of the skin is required if vision is affected or for cosmetic reasons.

Blepharochalasis (Fig 5–7) is a rare condition caused by recurrent episodes of edema, resulting in thin, wrinkled, and redundant eyelid skin sometimes described as resembling cigarette paper. Atrophic changes of all eyelid tissues frequently produce ptosis and a sunken appearance in the location of the medial fat pads. Symptoms of edema begin around puberty and diminish with age. Surgery consists of removal of the redundant skin and repair of the levator aponeurosis.

EPICANTHUS

Epicanthus (Fig 5–8) is characterized by vertical folds of skin over the medial canthi. It is characteristic of Asians and is present to some degree in most children of all races. The skin fold is often large enough to cover part of the nasal sclera and cause "pseudoesotropia," as the eyes appear to be crossed when a normal amount of medial sclera is not visible. Prominent epicanthal folds in children gradually decrease as the child grows older and are seldom apparent by school age.

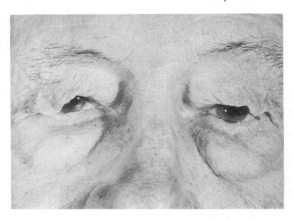

Figure 5–6. Dermatochalasis of upper lids and herniation of orbital fat of lower lids. (Courtesy of M Quickert.)

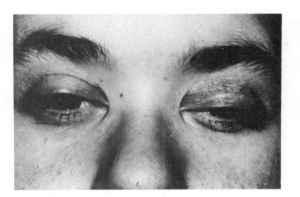

Figure 5–7. Blepharochalasis.

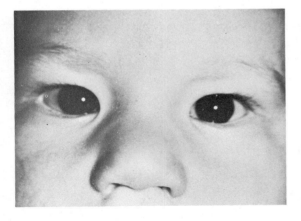

Figure 5–8. Epicanthus.

BLEPHAROSPASM
(Tic)

Blepharospasm is persistent or repetitive involuntary contraction of the orbicularis oculi muscle. It is usually bilateral and is more common in older persons. The cause is not known. It may be due to irritative lesions of the cornea and conjunctiva or of the seventh cranial nerve. Emotional stress and fatigue make it worse. The eyes should be examined carefully to rule out irritative lesions such as corneal foreign body, meibomianitis, and trichiasis.

Treatment consists of removal of the causative factor if possible. If the specific cause is not known, explanation and reassurance are in order. Intractable cases may require alcohol injection of the orbicularis oculi muscle to produce temporary paralysis. Seventh nerve block with a long-acting local anesthetic should be tried before alcohol injection is resorted to. Plastic surgery designed to weaken orbicularis function and selective removal of seventh nerve branches have been successful in some cases.

If the condition has been present for only a short time, the prognosis for cessation of the blepharospasm is good. Long-standing cases tend to persist regardless of treatment.

PTOSIS

Drooping of the upper lids when the eyes are open may be unilateral or bilateral and constant or intermittent.

Etiology
A. Congenital: Congenital ptosis is usually the result of developmental failure of the levator muscle of the lid, alone or in association with anomalies of the superior rectus muscle (most frequent) or complete external ophthalmoplegia (rare). It may be transmitted as a dominant characteristic.

B. Acquired: Acquired ptosis can be considered in 3 main categories:

1. Mechanical factors–Abnormal weight of the lids may make it difficult for a normal levator muscle to elevate fully. This may be due to acute or chronic inflammatory edema or swelling, tumor, or an extra fold of fatty material, as in xanthelasma.

2. Myogenic factors (eg, muscular dystrophy, myasthenia gravis)–Ptosis of one or both lids is often the first sign of myasthenia gravis and occurs eventually in over 95% of cases. The essential defect in myasthenia gravis seems to be in the humoral transmission at the myoneural junction.

3. Neurogenic (paralytic) factors–There is interference with the pathways of the portion of the third cranial nerve supplying the levator muscle at any level from the oculomotor nucleus (midbrain) to the

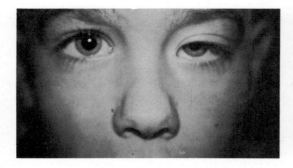 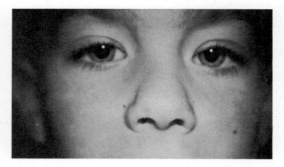

Figure 5–9. Surgical correction of ptosis. *Left:* Before operation, ptosis of the upper lid was present. *Right:* After the operation (levator resection), the ptosis was well corrected and a natural-appearing upper lid fold produced. (Courtesy of C Beard.)

myoneural junction (discussed in greater detail in Chapter 7).

Clinical Findings

Congenital ptosis is immediately evident and is occasionally observed to be associated with weakness of other extraocular muscles. The affected lid has a smooth, flat appearance, and the tarsal fold caused by the pull of a normal levator muscle is absent. This is more noticeable on upward gaze, when the lid fails to retract as the eye moves upward.

If the lid droops enough to partially occlude the pupil, the child usually attempts to compensate by elevating the brow with the frontalis muscle. This produces a marked wrinkling of the forehead, most evident when the condition is bilateral.

If one pupil is completely occluded, amblyopia may occur.

The ptosis of muscular dystrophy progresses very slowly and insidiously but finally becomes complete.

Ptosis in myasthenia gravis is gradual in onset, characteristically appearing in the evening with fatigue, and improving overnight. Later it becomes permanent. In over 80% of cases, some degree of transient or permanent ophthalmoplegia follows and produces diplopia. A diagnostic test of injection of edrophonium usually gives a dramatic response by temporarily abolishing the ptosis.

Neurogenic ptosis presents different clinical pictures according to the level of the pathway affected. The finding of other portions of a neurologic syndrome usually helps establish the diagnosis.

Treatment

If the condition is so slight that no cosmetic deformity is present and there is no interference with visual acuity, it is best left alone.

Myasthenia gravis should be treated as indicated (with neostigmine or a similar drug).

Some relief may be obtained by wearing special spectacle frames which have a posteriorly attached wire crutch that suspends or elevates the lid by traction. This may be indicated in temporary paresis or in those who are not good candidates for surgery.

Surgery (Fig 5–9) is the treatment of choice for cosmetic reasons. The type of surgery varies with the cause:

(1) If the levator muscle is not completely paralyzed, resection or shortening of the muscle is the procedure of choice.

(2) If the levator muscle has no action, the elevating effect of the frontalis muscle may be utilized by passing some type of traction device (wire, fascia, cotton or silk suture) subcutaneously from the frontalis to the tissue of the eyelid (tarsus), so that when the brow is raised the lid will be elevated. Using the patient's own fascia lata decreases the risk of infection.

PSEUDOPTOSIS

Pseudoptosis may occur when the upper lid lacks its normal support, as with a shrunken or absent eye or an inadequate prosthesis. Pseudoptosis can also result from hypotropia and dermatochalasis.

II. THE LACRIMAL APPARATUS*

Anatomy (Fig 5–10)

The lacrimal apparatus consists of the lacrimal gland, accessory glands, puncta, canaliculi, tear sac, and nasolacrimal duct. The lacrimal gland is a tear-secreting gland located in the anterior superior temporal portion of the orbit. Several secretory ducts connect the gland to the superior conjunctival fornix. The tears pass down over the cornea and the bulbar and palpebral conjunctiva, moistening the surfaces of these structures. They drain into the lacrimal canaliculi through the lacrimal puncta, round apertures about 0.5 mm in diameter on the medial aspect of both the upper and lower lid margins. The canaliculi are about 1 mm in diameter and 8 mm long and join to form a common

*See also Chapter 6.

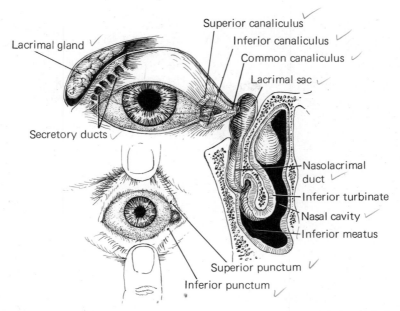

Figure 5–10. The lacrimal drainage system. (Redrawn with modifications and reproduced, with permission, from Thompson J, Elstrom ER: Radiography of the nasolacrimal passageways. *Med Radiogr Photogr* 1949;**25(3)**:66.)

canaliculus just before opening into the lacrimal sac. Diverticula may be a part of the normal structure and are susceptible to higher bacteria *(Actinomyces)* or fungal infection.

The lacrimal sac is the dilated portion of the lacrimal drainage system that lies in the bony lacrimal fossa.

The nasolacrimal duct is the downward continuation of the lacrimal sac. It opens into the inferior meatus lateral to the inferior turbinate.

All of the passages of the lacrimal drainage system are lined with epithelium. The tears pass into the puncta by capillary attraction. The combined forces of the capillary attraction in the canaliculi, gravity, and the pumping action of the orbicularis oculi muscle on the lacrimal sac tend to continue the flow of tears down the nasolacrimal duct into the nose and nasopharynx.

Physiology of Symptoms

Patients with disorders of the lacrimal apparatus complain of tearing or "dry eyes." In the event of "tearing" without associated symptoms, the disorder is usually in the lacrimal drainage system or (rarely) the result of hypersecretion. Paradoxic lacrimation (an occasional late complication of seventh nerve palsy) is a condition in which salivary gland fibers innervate the lacrimal gland. If the eyes are dry, there is faulty production of tears. The symptoms are investigated by irrigation to test the patency of the canaliculi and the nasolacrimal ducts and by palpation of the lacrimal gland. If the complaint is of "dry eyes," the quantity of tear production should be assessed (Schirmer test) and the appearance of the tear film studied with the aid of the slit lamp.

There are many causes of tearing, eg, conjunctivitis, keratitis, iritis, and foreign bodies. However, if tearing is the only symptom, the cause in the great majority of cases will be found in the lacrimal drainage apparatus.

INFECTIONS OF THE LACRIMAL APPARATUS

DACRYOCYSTITIS
(Fig 5–11)

Infection of the lacrimal sac is a common acute or chronic disease that usually occurs in infants or in persons over 40 (about 9 out of 10 chronic adult cases occur in menopausal women); it is uncommon in the intermediate age groups unless it follows trauma or is caused by a fungal infection. It is most often unilateral and is always secondary to obstruction of the nasolacrimal duct. In many adult cases the cause of the obstruction remains unknown, but there may be a history of severe trauma to the mid face. Acute cases are often preceded by chronic dacryocystitis; some cases are preceded by chronic conjunctiva (eg, trachoma). In acute dacryocystitis the usual infectious agent is *S aureus* or, occasionally, beta-hemolytic *Streptococcus*. In chronic dacryocystitis, *Streptococcus pneumoniae* is the predominant organism (rarely, *Candida albicans*). (Mixed infections do not occur.)

In fungal dacryocystitis, obstruction of the nasolacrimal duct by a dacryolith sometimes occurs.

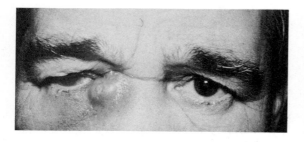

Figure 5-11. Acute dacryocystitis.

Spontaneous improvement follows passage of the stone, but recurrence is the rule.

It is curious that dacryocystitis is seldom complicated by conjunctivitis even though the conjunctival sac is constantly being bathed with pus exuding through the lacrimal puncta.

Clinical Findings

The chief symptoms are tearing and discharge. In the acute form, inflammation, pain, swelling, and tenderness are present in the tear sac area; purulent material can be expressed from the tear sac. In the chronic form, tearing is usually the only sign; mucoid material can usually be expressed from the tear sac.

The infectious agent can be identified microscopically by staining a conjunctival smear taken after expression of the tear sac.

Corneal ulcer occasionally occurs following minor corneal trauma in the presence of pneumococcal dacryocystitis. Perforation of the skin and fistula formation may also occur. If a corneal ulcer occurs, vigorous local and systemic treatment is indicated and a dacryocystectomy or dacryocystorhinostomy should be done without delay.

Treatment

A. Adult Dacryocystitis: Warm compresses to the affected eye at frequent intervals during the acute stage.

1. Acute—Specific treatment for acute staphylococcal or pneumococcal dacryocystitis consists of penicillin or other antibiotic until the inflammation subsides.

2. Chronic—Since an obstruction of the nasolacrimal duct is the basic cause of dacryocystitis, the disease is usually persistent until the obstruction is relieved. However, probing is notably unsuccessful in adults, and dacryocystorhinostomy is usually necessary if symptoms are severe. If chronic tearing is the only symptom, many patients prefer the tearing to surgery.

B. Infantile Dacryocystitis: Normally, the nasolacrimal ducts open spontaneously before birth or during the first month of life. Occasionally, one of the ducts fails to canalize and a secondary *Haemophilus influenzae* dacryocystitis develops. When this happens, forceful massage of the tear sac is indicated, and

antibiotic or sulfonamide drops should be instilled in the conjunctival sac 4–5 times daily. If this is not successful after a few weeks, probing of the nasolacrimal duct is indicated regardless of the infant's age. The tear sac is irrigated freely just before probing. One probing is effective in about 75% of cases; in the remainder, cure can almost always be achieved by repeated probings or by a temporary silicone lacrimal drainage splint.

Course & Prognosis

Acute adult dacryocystitis responds well to systemic antibiotic therapy. Recurrences are common if the nasolacrimal duct obstruction is not removed. The chronic form can be kept latent by using antibiotic eye drops, but relief of the obstruction is the only cure.

CANALICULITIS

Canaliculitis is an uncommon chronic unilateral condition caused by infection with *Actinomyces israelii, C albicans,* or *Aspergillus* species (Fig 5–12). It affects the lower canaliculus more often than the upper, occurs exclusively in adults, and causes a secondary purulent unilateral conjunctivitis that frequently escapes etiologic diagnosis.

The patient complains of a mildly red and irritated eye with a slight discharge. The punctum usually pouts; material can be readily expressed from the canaliculus. The organism can be seen microscopically on a direct smear taken from the canaliculus.

Curettage of the necrotic material in the involved canaliculus, followed by forceful irrigation, is usually effective. Canaliculotomy is sometimes necessary. Tincture of iodine should be applied to the lining of the canaliculus after canaliculotomy.

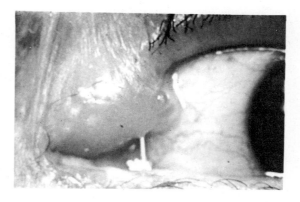

Figure 5-12. *Actinomyces israelii* canaliculitis, left eye. (Courtesy of P Thygeson.)

DACRYOADENITIS

Acute inflammation of the lacrimal gland is a rare unilateral condition that may be seen in children as a complication of mumps, measles, or influenza, and in adults in association with gonorrhea. It may also develop following a perforating injury to the lacrimal gland or as a retrograde infection from a bacterial conjunctivitis.

In the acute type, considerable swelling, pain, and injection occur over the upper temporal aspect of the eye. The lid has an S-shaped curve.

If bacterial infection is present, antibiotics are given systemically. Incision may be necessary if pus collects in the gland under tension.

Chronic dacryoadenitis is occasionally seen bilaterally as one manifestation of sarcoidosis. This condition (which, with lacrimal gland swelling, is called Mikulicz's syndrome) usually occurs in blacks and is self-limited. The prognosis is good. Chronic dacryoadenitis may also occur in tuberculosis, lymphatic leukemia, and lymphosarcoma.

• • •

References

Beard C: Malignancy of the eyelids. *Am J Ophthalmol* 1981;**92**:1.

Beard C: *Ptosis,* 2nd ed. Mosby, 1981.

Callahan A et al: Lid cancer: Operate or radiate? Pages 381–398 in: *Controversy in Ophthalmology.* Brockhurst RJ et al (editors). Saunders, 1977.

Callahan MA: Surgically mismanaged ptosis associated with double elevator palsy. *Arch Ophthalmol* 1981;**99**:108.

Char D: Therapeutic review: The management of lid and conjunctival malignancies. *Surv Ophthalmol* 1980;**24**:679.

Collin JRO, Rathbun JE: Involutional entropion. *Arch Ophthalmol* 1978;**96**:1058.

Collin JRO et al: Blepharochalasis. *Br J Ophthalmol* 1979; **63**:542.

Dawson CR: Annual review: Lids, conjunctiva and lacrimal apparatus. *Arch Ophthalmol* 1975;**93**:854.

Fraunfelder FT et al: Role of cryosurgery in external ocular and periocular disease. *Trans Am Acad Ophthalmol Otolaryngol* 1977;**83**:713.

Jones LT: The lacrimal secretory system and its treatment. *Am J Ophthalmol* 1966;**62**:47.

Jones LT, Wobig JL: *Surgery of the Eyelids and Lacrimal Apparatus.* Aesculapius, 1976.

Quickert MH: The eyelids. Pages 937–954 in: *Modern Ophthalmology.* Vols 3 and 4. Sorsby A (editor). Butterworth, 1972.

Reeh MJ, Beyer CK, Shannon GM: *Practical Ophthalmic Plastic and Reconstructive Surgery.* Lea & Febiger, 1976.

Richards WW: Actinomycotic lacrimal canaliculitis. *Am J Ophthalmol* 1973;**75**:155.

Salvaggio JE (editor): Primer on allergic and immunologic diseases. *JAMA* 1982;**248**:2579. [Special issue.]

Sullivan JH, Beard C, Bullock JD: Cryosurgery for treatment of trichiasis. *Am J Ophthalmol* 1976;**82**:117.

Thygeson P: Complications of staphylococcic blepharitis. *Am J Ophthalmol* 1969;**68**:446.

6 | Tears

SOURCE & FUNCTION OF THE TEARS

The tears are a mixture of secretions from the major and minor (accessory) lacrimal glands, the goblet cells, and the meibomian glands. Under normal circumstances, the tear fluid forms a thin layer approximately 7–10 μm thick that covers the corneal and conjunctival epithelium. The functions of this ultrathin layer are (1) to make the cornea a smooth optical surface by abolishing minute surface irregularities of its epithelium; (2) to wet the surface of the corneal and conjunctival epithelium, preventing damage to the epithelial cells; and (3) to inhibit the growth of microorganisms on the conjunctiva and cornea by mechanical flushing and the antimicrobial action of the tear fluid.

The total mass of the accessory lacrimal glands has been estimated to be approximately one-tenth that of the lacrimal gland mass.

COMPOSITION OF THE TEARS

The normal tear volume is estimated to be about 6 μL in each eye, and the average rate of turnover about 1.2 μL/min. When collected with minimal trauma, tear fluid contains a high concentration of proteins. Three fractions are demonstrable by paper electrophoresis: albumin, globulins, and lysozyme. The antimicrobial activity of the tears is in the gamma globulin and lysozyme fractions.

The gamma globulins found in the normal tear fluid are IgA, IgG, and IgE. The IgA predominates and is similar to the IgA found in other body secretions bathing mucous membrane surfaces such as saliva and the bronchial, nasal, and gastrointestinal secretions. The IgA found in tears differs from serum IgA, however, and is more concentrated. In certain allergic conditions such as vernal conjunctivitis, the IgE concentration of tear fluid increases. Lysozyme may act synergistically with IgA in causing lysis of bacteria.

Although lysozyme is known to have a lytic effect on certain bacteria, its absence does not necessarily increase the risk of infection. Reduction in tear lysozyme concentration usually occurs early in the course of Sjögren's syndrome and is considered helpful in the diagnosis of that disorder. Lysozyme in tears can be measured by turbidimetric assays utilizing the microorganism *Micrococcus lysodeikticus* (heat-killed) as the substrate. This can be performed on tear samples collected on regular Schirmer strips. More recently, an antibacterial factor that is closely related to betalysin was identified and measured in human tears. It appears that betalysin is a normal constituent of human tears and complements the antibacterial action of lysozyme.

The average glucose concentration of the tears is 2.5 mg/dL. An approximate determination of the amount in patients with hyperglycemia can be made with a commercially available colorimetric paper test strip (Clinistix) that has been moistened with tears. This is a useful test in comatose patients.

The average tear urea level is 0.04 mg/dL.

Changes in the blood concentrations of both glucose and urea parallel changes in the tear glucose and tear urea levels.

K^+, Na^+, and Cl^- occur in higher concentrations in tears than in plasma. The average pH of tears is 7.35. Under normal conditions, tear fluid is isotonic. Tear film osmolarity ranges from 295 to 309 mosm/L. In keratoconjunctivitis sicca, there is hyperosmolarity of the tear film.

If collection of the tear fluid is traumatic, the normal constituents of the tears may be altered and there may be transudation of substances from the conjunctival blood vessels. In certain inflammatory conditions of the conjunctiva, there is marked transudation of immunoglobulins directly from the blood to the tear fluid.

LAYERS OF THE PREOCULAR TEAR FILM

The tear film covering the corneal and conjunctival epithelium (preocular tear film) is composed of 3 layers (Fig 6–1): (1) The superficial lipid layer is a monomolecular layer derived from the secretions of the meibomian glands and thought to retard evaporation of the aqueous layer. (2) The middle aqueous layer is elaborated by the major and minor lacrimal glands and contains water-soluble substances (salts and proteins). (3) The deep mucinous layer is composed of glycoprotein mucin and overlies the corneal and con-

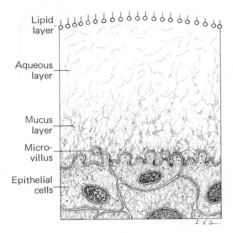

Lipid layer
Aqueous layer
Mucus layer
Micro-villus
Epithelial cells

Figure 6–1. The 3 layers of the tear film covering the superficial epithelial layer of the cornea.

junctival epithelial cells. The epithelial cell membranes are composed of lipoproteins and are therefore relatively hydrophobic. Such a surface cannot be wetted with an aqueous solution alone. Mucin (glycoprotein) plays an important role in wetting this surface. It is partly adsorbed onto the corneal epithelial cell membranes and is anchored by the microvilli of the surface epithelial cells. This provides a new hydrophilic surface for the aqueous tears to spread on, and the surface is wetted by a lowering of the tears' surface tension. Mucin is elaborated by the goblet cells of the conjunctiva, and recent studies have shown that the lacrimal gland contributes to its production.

Periodic resurfacing of the tear film is important to prevent dry spots and is accomplished by blinking. In the normal eye, blinking maintains a continuous tear film over the ocular surface.

DRY EYE SYNDROME
(Keratoconjunctivitis Sicca)

Deficiency in any of the tear film components may lead to loss of the film's stability. This will cause rapid break-up of the tear film, and dry spots will appear on the corneal and conjunctival epithelium. Dryness of the eye may therefore result from any disease associated with deficiency of the tear film components (aqueous, mucin, or lipid). Although there are many forms of keratoconjunctivitis sicca, those connected with rheumatoid arthritis or other connective tissue diseases are commonly referred to as **Sjögren's syndrome.** The etiology, diagnosis, and therapy of keratoconjunctivitis sicca are summarized in Table 6–1.

Clinical Findings
A. Symptoms and Signs: Patients with dry eyes complain most frequently of a scratchy or sandy (foreign body) sensation. Other common symptoms

Table 6–1. Dry eye syndrome: Etiology, diagnosis, and treatment.

I. Etiology:
  A. Conditions Characterized by Hypofunction of the Lacrimal Gland:
   1. Congenital—
     a. Familial dysautonomia (Riley-Day syndrome).
     b. Aplasia of the lacrimal gland (congenital alacrima).
     c. Trigeminal nerve aplasia.
     d. Ectodermal dysplasia.
   2. Acquired—
     a. Systemic diseases—
       (1) Sjögren's syndrome.
       (2) Progressive systemic sclerosis.
       (3) Sarcoidosis.
       (4) Leukemia, lymphoma.
       (5) Amyloidosis.
       (6) Hemochromatosis.
     b. Infection—
       (1) Trachoma.
       (2) Mumps.
     c. Injury—
       (1) Surgical removal of lacrimal gland.
       (2) Irradiation.
       (3) Chemical burn.
     d. Medications—
       (1) Antihistamines.
       (2) Antimuscarinics: atropine, scopolamine.
       (3) General anesthetics: halothane, nitrous oxide.
       (4) Beta-adrenergic blockers: timolol, practolol.
     e. Neurogenic—Neuroparalytic (facial nerve palsy).
  B. Conditions Characterized by Mucin Deficiency:
   1. Avitaminosis A.
   2. Stevens-Johnson syndrome.
   3. Ocular pemphigoid.
   4. Chronic conjunctivitis, eg, trachoma.
   5. Chemical burns.
   6. Medications—Antihistamines, antimuscarinic agents, beta-adrenergic blocking agents (eg, practolol).
  C. Defective Spreading of Tear Film Caused by the Following:
   1. Eyelid abnormalities—
     a. Defects, coloboma.
     b. Ectropion or entropion.
     c. Keratinization of lid margin.
     d. Decreased or absent blinking.
       (1) Neurologic disorders.
       (2) Hyperthyroidism.
       (3) Contact lens.
       (4) Drugs.
     e. Lagophthalmos—
       (1) Nocturnal lagophthalmos.
       (2) Hyperthyroidism.
   2. Conjunctival abnormalities—
     a. Pterygium.
     b. Symblepharon.
   3. Proptosis.
II. Diagnostic Tests:
  A. Biomicroscopy.
  B. Rose Bengal Staining.
  C. Fluorescein Staining.
  D. Tear Break-Up Time.
  E. Tear Film Osmolarity.
  F. Tear Lysozyme.
  G. Schirmer Test Without Anesthesia.

Table 6—1 (cont'd). Dry eye syndrome: Etiology, diagnosis, and treatment.

III. **Local Therapy of Keratoconjunctivitis Sicca:**
   A. Mild:
     1. Artificial tears 4—5 times daily.
     2. Lubricating ointment at bedtime.
   B. Moderate:
     1. Artificial tears every 2 hours.
     2. Lubricating ointment at bedtime.
     3. Consider sustained-release tear insert (Lacrisert), one insert in each eye once daily.
     4. Mucolytic agent (acetylcysteine, 10%, 4 times daily).
   C. Severe:
     1. Artificial tears (or gum cellulose, 0.625%) every hour. Avoid benzalkonium chloride.
     2. Tight goggles.
     3. Punctal occlusion.
     4. Lubricating ointment at bedtime.
     5. Change environment; use humidifier.

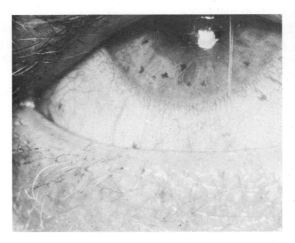

Figure 6—2. Rose bengal staining of corneal and conjunctival cells in a 54-year-old woman with keratoconjunctivitis sicca. (Courtesy of K Tabbara.)

are itching, excessive mucus secretion, inability to produce tears, a burning sensation, photosensitivity, redness, pain, and difficulty in moving the lids. In most patients, the most remarkable feature of the eye examination is the grossly normal appearance of the eye.

Lacrimal gland enlargement occurs uncommonly in patients with Sjögren's syndrome. The most characteristic feature on slit lamp examination is the interrupted or absent tear meniscus at the lower lid margin. Tenacious yellowish mucous strands are sometimes seen in the lower conjunctival fornix. The bulbar conjunctiva loses its normal luster and may be thickened, edematous, and hyperemic.

The damaged corneal and conjunctival epithelial cells stain with 1% rose bengal (Fig 6–2), and defects in the corneal epithelium stain with fluorescein. The corneal epithelium shows varying degrees of fine punctate stippling in the interpalpebral fissure.

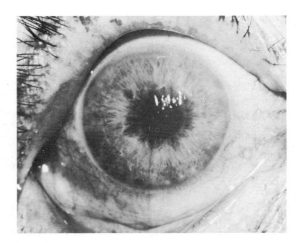

Figure 6–3. Corneal filaments in a 56-year-old patient with keratoconjunctivitis sicca. (Courtesy of K Tabbara.)

In the late stages of keratoconjunctivitis sicca, filaments may be seen—one end of each filament attached to the corneal epithelium and the other end moving freely (Figs 6–3 and 6–4). Three types of corneal filaments have been recognized: (1) filaments consisting entirely of mucus, (2) filaments consisting entirely of epithelial cells, and (3) filaments consisting of epithelial cells and mucus.

In patients with Sjögren's syndrome, conjunctival scrapings may show increased numbers of goblet cells (Fig 6–5).

B. Schirmer Test: The use of wettable filter paper strips as a device for measuring tear secretion was first described by Köster in 1900 in connection with a study of facial nerve paralysis. Köster placed one end of a filter paper strip 1 cm wide and 20 cm long in the conjunctival sac in each eye and noted the extent of wetting by the tear fluid. In 1903, Otto Schirmer modified Köster's method by reducing the width of the strips to 0.5 cm and their length to 3.5 cm.

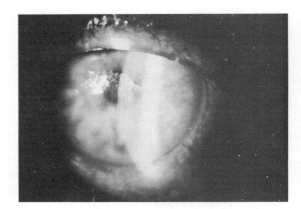

Figure 6–4. Slit lamp picture of a 48-year-old patient with keratoconjunctivitis sicca and corneal filaments. (Courtesy of K Tabbara.)

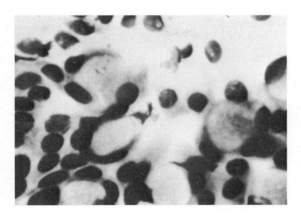

Figure 6–5. Goblet cells in conjunctival scrapings from a patient with Sjögren's syndrome. (Stained with Giemsa's stain.) (Courtesy of K Tabbara.)

The accessory lacrimal glands of Wolfring and Krause secrete enough tears to keep the cornea adequately wetted under most circumstances, and the major lacrimal glands secrete enough to help cover stressful circumstances such as drying from exposure to hot air, irritation from corneal injury, foreign bodies, emotional upsets, and various noxious stimuli. Schirmer tests performed without topical anesthesia measure the function of the lacrimal gland, whose secretory activity is stimulated by the irritating nature of the filter paper. Schirmer tests performed after topical anesthesia (instillation of 0.5% tetracaine) measure the function of the accessory lacrimal glands (the basic secretors).

The Schirmer test is a good screening test—and definitely the simplest test—for the assessment of tear production. However, false-positive and false-negative results occur in 15% of eyes tested; a positive result (decreased wetting of the filter paper strip) should be confirmed and a negative result should by no means rule out dryness of the eyes, particularly if it is secondary to mucin deficiency.

A Schirmer test showing less than 10 mm of wetting in 5 minutes is considered abnormal.

C. Tear Film Break-Up Time: At present there is no practical method of measuring the mucin content of the tear fluid, but measurement of the tear film break-up time may sometimes be very useful. Deficiency in mucin may not affect the Schirmer test but may lead to instability of the tear film. This causes the film's rapid break-up. "Dry holes" (Fig 6–6) are formed in the tear film, and a baring of the corneal or conjunctival epithelium follows. This process ultimately damages the epithelial cells, which can then be stained with rose bengal. Damaged epithelial cells may be shed from the cornea, leaving areas susceptible to punctate staining when the corneal surface is flooded with fluorescein.

The tear film break-up time can be measured by applying a slightly moistened fluorescein strip to the bulbar conjunctiva and asking the patient to blink. The tear film is then scanned with the aid of a slit lamp while the patient refrains from blinking. A cobalt blue filter and a broad light beam are used for this purpose. The time that elapses before the first hole (dry spot) appears in the corneal fluorescein layer is the tear film break-up time. Normally, the break-up time is over 15 seconds, but it can be reduced appreciably by the use of local anesthetics, by manipulating the eye, or by holding the lids open. The break-up time is shorter in eyes with aqueous tear deficiency and is always shorter than normal in eyes with mucin deficiency.

D. Ocular Ferning Test: A simple and inexpensive qualitative test for the study of conjunctival mucus has been described. The test is performed by spreading conjunctival scrapings on a clean glass slide and letting them dry. Microscopic arborization (ferning) is observed in normal eyes. In patients with cicatrizing conjunctivitis (ocular pemphigoid, Stevens-Johnson syndrome, diffuse conjunctival cicatrization), ferning of the mucus is either reduced or absent.

Complications

Early in the course of keratoconjunctivitis sicca, vision is slightly impaired and a few patients develop corneal ulceration, corneal thinning, and perforation. Secondary bacterial infection occasionally occurs, and corneal scarring and vascularization may result in marked reduction in vision. Early treatment may prevent these complications.

Treatment

Treatment depends upon the cause. In most early cases, the corneal and conjunctival epithelial changes are reversible.

Aqueous deficiency can be treated by replacement of the aqueous with various types of artificial

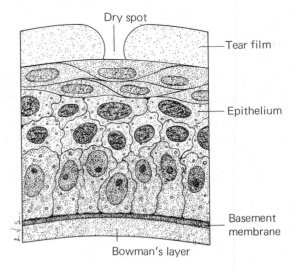

Figure 6–6. Baring of the corneal epithelium following formation of a dry spot in the tear film. (Modified and redrawn from Dohlman CH: The function of the corneal epithelium in health and disease. *Invest Ophthalmol* 1971;**10**:383.)

tears. Mucin deficiency can be partially compensated for by the use of ophthalmic vehicles of high molecular weight—eg, water-soluble polymers—or by the use of the patient's own serum as local eye drops. Serum used for this purpose must be kept refrigerated at all times. It acts by lowering the surface tension of the tears, assisting in the spreading of the tears, and wetting the epithelium. If the mucus is tenacious, as in Sjögren's syndrome, mucolytic agents (eg, acetylcysteine, 10%) may give some relief.

Recently, a slow-release artificial tear insert (Lacrisert) has been developed and made commercially available for clinical use. The insert is a solid 5-mg rod made of hydroxypropylcellulose. When inserted into the inferior cul-de-sac, the rod swells up to 10 times its original size by imbibition of fluid from the capillary bed, and the hydroxypropylcellulose is slowly released over a period of 12 hours. About half of patients with keratoconjunctivitis sicca have good relief with one insert in each eye once in the morning. Some patients complain of irritation or blurring of vision. Topical artificial tears may be used simultaneously with these preservative-free inserts.

OTHER DISORDERS OF THE LACRIMAL SYSTEM

Lacrimal Hypersecretion

The causes of excessive tearing are varied but are due to stimulation of the lacrimal gland.

Psychic lacrimation is normally associated with pain or emotional upsets. The fact that this type of lacrimation appears after the first few months of life explains why newborns do not produce tears when they cry.

Neurogenic lacrimation is brought about by reflex stimulation. Eyestrain, corneal injury, a blast of hot air, dry wind, or foreign body in the cornea or conjunctiva may cause reflex trigeminal irritation that excites lacrimation. Strong light causes reflex visual irritation and copious lacrimation. Irritation of the facial nerve, yawning, vomiting, and laughing are also associated with reflex lacrimation.

Epiphora may follow obstruction of the lacrimal drainage system. This can be caused by punctal eversion or occlusion or by canalicular or nasolacrimal duct obstruction. Most cases of nasolacrimal duct obstruction can be corrected surgically.

Paradoxic Lacrimation ("Crocodile Tears")

This is an acquired unilateral (very rarely bilateral) condition characterized by excessive tearing while eating. It occurs as a sequel to Bell's palsy (facial nerve palsy) and is the result of aberrant regeneration of the facial nerve fibers.

Bloody Tears

This is a rare clinical entity attributed to a variety of causes. It has been associated with menstruation ("vicarious menses"). Blood-tinged tears may be secondary to conjunctival hemorrhage due to any cause (trauma, blood dyscrasia, etc) or to tumors of the lacrimal sac. They have also recently been reported in a hypertensive patient suffering from epistaxis with extension through the nasolacrimal duct.

•   •   •

References

Allansmith MR, O'Connor GR: Immunoglobulins: Structure, function, and relation to the eye. *Surv Ophthalmol* 1970;**14**:367.

Allansmith MR et al: Plasma cell content of main and accessory lacrimal glands and conjunctiva. *Am J Ophthalmol* 1976;**82**:70.

Allen M, Wright P, Reid L: The human lacrimal gland: A histochemical and organ culture study of the secretory cells. *Arch Ophthalmol* 1972;**88**:493.

Banta RG, Seltzer JL: Blood tears from epistaxis through the nasolacrimal duct. *Am J Ophthalmol* 1973;**75**:726.

Brauninger GE, Centifanto YM: Immunoglobulin E in human tears. *Am J Ophthalmol* 1971;**72**:558.

Crandall DC, Leopold IH: The influence of systemic drugs on tear constituents. *Ophthalmology* 1979;**86**:115.

Dohlman CH: The function of the corneal epithelium in health and disease. *Invest Ophthalmol* 1971;**10**:383.

Dohlman CH: Punctal occlusion in keratoconjunctivitis sicca. *Ophthalmology* 1978;**85**:1277.

Ford LC, DeLange RJ, Petty RW: Identification of a non-lysozymal bactericidal factor (beta lysin) in human tears and aqueous humor. *Am J Ophthalmol* 1976;**81**:30.

François J: The Riley-Day syndrome. *Ophthalmologica* 1977;**174**:20.

Frayha RA, Tabbara KF, Geha RS: Familial CRST syndrome with sicca complex. *J Rheumatol* 1977;**4**:53.

Gilbard JP, Farris RL, Santamaria J II: Osmolarity of tear microvolumes in keratoconjunctivitis sicca. *Arch Ophthalmol* 1978;**96**:677.

Gillette TE, Greiner JV, Allansmith MR: Immunohistochemical localization of human tear lysozyme. *Arch Ophthalmol* 1981;**99**:298.

Holly FJ, Lemp MA: Tear physiology and dry eyes. *Surv Ophthalmol* 1977;**22**:69.

Huth SW, Miller MJ, Leopold HI: Calcium and proteins in tears. *Arch Ophthalmol* 1981;**99**:1628.

Hypher TJ: Uptake and loss of tears from filter paper discs employed in lysozyme tests. *Br J Ophthalmol* 1979;**63**:251.

Jones DB: Prospects in the management of tear-deficiency states. *Trans Am Acad Ophthalmol Otolaryngol* 1977;**83**:693.

Katz JI, Blackman WM: A soluble sustained-release ophthalmic delivery unit. *Am J Ophthalmol* 1977;**83**:728.

Lamberts DW, Langston DP, Chu W: A clinical study of slow-releasing artificial tears. *Ophthalmology* 1978;**85**:794.

Lemp MA, Hamill JR: Factors affecting tear film break-up in normal eyes. *Arch Ophthalmol* 1973;**89**:103.

Lemp MA et al: The precorneal tear film. *Excerpta Med Int Cong* 1970;**222**:1602.

Mackie IA, Seal DV: Quantitative tear lysozyme assay in units of activity per microlitre. *Br J Ophthalmol* 1976;**60**:70.

Mackie IA, Seal DV, Pescod JM: Beta-adrenergic receptor blocking drugs: Tear lysozyme and immunological screening for adverse reaction. *Br J Ophthalmol* 1977;**61**:354.

McClellan BH et al: Immunoglobulins in tears. *Am J Ophthalmol* 1973;**76**:89.

Mishima S et al: Determination of tear volume and tear flow. *Invest Ophthalmol* 1966;**5**:264.

Moses RA: *Adler's Physiology of the Eye: Clinical Application,* 7th ed. Mosby, 1981.

Nielsen NV, Eriksen JS: Timolol transitory manifestations of dry eyes in long-term treatment. *Acta Ophthalmol* 1979;**57**:418.

Norn MS: The conjunctival fluid, its height, volume, density of cells, and flow. *Acta Ophthalmol* 1966;**44**:212.

Norn MS: Tear secretion in normal and diseased eyes, estimated by a new method. *Excerpta Med Int Cong* 1966;**146**:1164.

Spiers ASD: Syndrome of "crocodile tears": Pharmacologic study of a bilateral case. *Br J Ophthalmol* 1970;**54**:330.

Tabbara KF, Okumoto M: Ocular ferning test: A qualitative test for mucus deficiency. *Ophthalmology* 1982;**89**:712.

Tabbara KF et al: Sjögren's syndrome: A correlation between ocular findings and labial salivary gland histology. *Trans Am Acad Ophthalmol Otolaryngol* 1974;**78**:467.

Terry JE, Hill RM: Human tear osmotic pressure. *Arch Ophthalmol* 1978;**96**:120.

Warwick R: *Eugene Wolff's Anatomy of the Eye and Orbit,* 7th ed. Saunders, 1976.

Werblin TP, Rheinstrom SD, Kaufman HE: The use of slow-release artificial tears in the long-term management of keratitis sicca. *Ophthalmology* 1981;**88**:78.

7 | Conjunctiva

ANATOMY & PHYSIOLOGY

The conjunctiva is the thin, transparent mucous membrane that covers the posterior surface of the lids (the palpebral conjunctiva) and the anterior surface of the sclera (the bulbar conjunctiva). It is continuous with the skin at the lid margin (a mucocutaneous junction) and with the corneal epithelium at the limbus.

The **palpebral conjunctiva** lines the posterior surface of the lids and is firmly adherent to the tarsus. At the superior and inferior margins of the tarsus, the conjunctiva is reflected posteriorly (at the superior and inferior fornices) and attaches to the sclera to become the bulbar conjunctiva.

The **bulbar conjunctiva** is loosely attached to the orbital septum in the fornices and is folded many times. This allows the eye to move and enlarges the secretory conjunctival surface. (The ducts of the lacrimal gland open into the superior temporal fornix.) Except at the limbus (where Tenon's capsule and the conjunctiva are fused for about 3 mm), the bulbar conjunctiva is loosely attached to Tenon's capsule and the underlying sclera.

A soft, movable, thickened fold of bulbar conjunctiva (the **semilunar fold**) is located at the inner canthus and corresponds to the nictitating membrane of some lower animals. A small, fleshy, epidermoid structure (the **caruncle**) is attached superficially to the inner portion of the semilunar fold and is a transition zone containing both cutaneous and mucous membrane elements.

Histology

The **conjunctival epithelium** consists of 2 or more layers of cylindric epithelial cells, superficial and basal. Conjunctival epithelium near the limbus and over the caruncle consists of stratified squamous epithelial cells. The **superficial epithelial cells** contain round or oval mucus-secreting goblet cells. The mucus, as it forms, pushes aside the goblet cell nucleus and is necessary for proper dispersion of the precorneal tear film. The **basal epithelial cells** stain more deeply than the superficial cells and near the limbus may contain pigment.

The **conjunctival stroma** is divided into an adenoid (superficial) layer and a fibrous (deep) layer.

The **adenoid layer** contains lymphoid tissue and in some areas may contain "folliclelike" structures without germinal centers. The adenoid layer does not develop until after the first 2 or 3 months of life. This explains why inclusion conjunctivitis of the newborn is papillary in nature rather than follicular and why it later becomes follicular. The **fibrous layer** is composed of connective tissue and is compact over the tarsus and loosely arranged in other areas.

The **accessory lacrimal glands** (glands of Krause and Wolfring), which resemble the lacrimal gland in structure and function, are located in the stroma. Most of the glands of Krause are in the upper fornix, the remaining few in the lower fornix. The glands of Wolfring lie at the superior margin of the upper tarsus.

The conjunctival blood vessels are derived from the anterior ciliary and palpebral arteries. The nerves arise from the ophthalmic division of the fifth cranial nerve. There are only a few pain fibers. The conjunctiva is rich in lymphatics.

CONJUNCTIVITIS

Inflammation of the conjunctiva (conjunctivitis) is the most common eye disease in the western hemisphere. It varies in severity from a mild hyperemia with tearing (hay fever conjunctivitis) to a severe necrotic process (membranous conjunctivitis). The source is usually exogenous, sometimes endogenous.

Etiologic Classification of Conjunctivitis

The types of conjunctivitis and their commonest causes are as follows:

A. Bacterial:
1. Purulent–
   Neisseria gonorrhoeae
   Neisseria meningitidis
2. Acute catarrhal (pinkeye)–
   Pneumococcus *(Streptococcus pneumoniae)* (temperate climates)
   Haemophilus aegyptius (Koch-Weeks bacillus) (tropical climates)

3. Subacute catarrhal—*Haemophilus influenzae* (temperate climates)
4. Chronic, including blepharoconjunctivitis—
   Staphylococcus aureus
   Moraxella lacunata (diplobacillus of Morax-Axenfeld)
5. Rare types—(Acute, subacute, chronic)
   Streptococci
   Neisseria (Branhamella) catarrhalis
   Coliforms
   Proteus
   Corynebacterium diphtheriae

B. Chlamydial:*
1. Trachoma *(Chlamydia trachomatis)*
2. Inclusion conjunctivitis *(Chlamydia oculogenitalis)*
3. Lymphogranuloma venereum (LGV) *(Chlamydia lymphogranulomatis)*
4. Psittacosis *(Chlamydia psittaci)*
5. Rare types—Agents of parakeet psittacosis, feline pneumonitis, and ovine abortion

C. Viral:
1. Acute viral follicular conjunctivitis—
   Pharyngoconjunctival fever due to adenoviruses types 3 and 7
   Epidemic keratoconjunctivitis due to adenovirus types 8 and 19
   Herpes simplex virus
   Newcastle disease
   Acute hemorrhagic conjunctivitis due to enterovirus type 70; rarely, coxsackievirus type A28
2. Chronic viral follicular conjunctivitis—
   Molluscum contagiosum virus
3. Viral blepharoconjunctivitis—
   Vaccinia due to vaccinia-variola viruses
   Varicella, zoster due to varicella-zoster virus
   Measles virus

D. Rickettsial: Nonpurulent conjunctivitis with hyperemia and minimal infiltration, often a feature of rickettsial diseases:
   Typhus
   Murine typhus
   Scrub typhus
   Rocky Mountain spotted fever
   Mediterranean fever
   Q fever

E. Fungal: (Rare.)
1. Catarrhal, complicating blepharitis—
   Candida
2. Granulomatous—
   Rhinosporidium seeberi
   Coccidioides immitis (San Joaquin Valley fever)
   Sporothrix schenckii

F. Parasitic: (Rare but important.) Chronic conjunctivitis and blepharoconjunctivitis due to—
   Onchocerca volvulus (Central America, Africa)
   Thelazia californiensis
   Loa loa
   Ascaris lumbricoides
   Trichinella spiralis
   Schistosoma haematobium (bladder fluke)
   Taenia solium (cysticercus)
   Pthirus pubis (Pediculus pubis, pubic louse)
   Fly larvae *(Oestrus ovis,* etc) (ocular myiasis)
   Caterpillar hair

G. Atopic (Allergic):
1. Immediate (humoral) hypersensitivity reactions—
   Hay fever conjunctivitis (pollens, grasses, animal dander, etc)
   Vernal keratoconjunctivitis
   Atopic keratoconjunctivitis
   Giant papillary conjunctivitis
2. Delayed (cellular) hypersensitivity reactions—
   Phlyctenulosis
   Mild conjunctivitis secondary to contact blepharitis
3. Autoimmune disease—
   Keratoconjunctivitis sicca associated with Sjögren's syndrome
   Psoriasis
   Mucous membrane pemphigoid
   Midline lethal granuloma and Wegener's granulomatosis

H. Chemical or Irritative:
1. Iatrogenic—Miotics, idoxuridine, other topically applied drugs
2. Occupational—Acids, alkalies, smoke, wind, ultraviolet light

I. Etiology Unknown:
1. Folliculosis
2. Chronic follicular conjunctivitis (orphan's conjunctivitis, Axenfeld's conjunctivitis)
3. Ocular rosacea
4. Erythema multiforme major (Stevens-Johnson syndrome) and minor
5. Dermatitis herpetiformis
6. Epidermolysis bullosa
7. Superior limbic keratoconjunctivitis
8. Ligneous conjunctivitis
9. Reiter's syndrome

J. Associated With Systemic Disease:
1. Conjunctivitis in thyroid disease
2. Gouty conjunctivitis
3. Carcinoid conjunctivitis

K. Secondary to Dacryocystitis or Canaliculitis:
1. Conjunctivitis secondary to dacryocystitis—

---

*See box on p 64 for a note on the taxonomic status of these organisms.

Pneumococci or beta-hemolytic streptococci

2. Conjunctivitis secondary to canaliculitis—
   Actinomyces israelii, Candida sp, *Aspergillus* sp (rarely)
3. Conjunctivitis secondary to tumors of conjunctiva or lid margins

GENERAL CONSIDERATIONS

Because of its location, the conjunctiva is exposed to many microorganisms and other noxious substances. Resisting this bombardment are the tears. By diluting the infectious material and sluicing the conjunctival debris and organisms into the nasal passages for excretion, they greatly reduce the conjunctiva's vulnerability. They also contain lysozyme, betalysin, IgA, and IgG, all of which can inhibit bacterial growth.

The following factors make established conjunctivitis a self-limiting disease: tears, abundant lymphoid elements, constant epithelial exfoliation, a cool conjunctival sac due to tear evaporation, the pumping action of the tear drainage system (unimpeded when the lids are open), and the fact that bacteria are caught in the conjunctival mucus and then excreted.

Although organisms pathogenic for the genitourinary tract are also pathogenic for the conjunctiva, those that grow abundantly on the nasal mucosa tend to grow less well in the conjunctival sac, and vice versa. For example, whereas the conjunctiva is usually resistant to the viruses of the common cold, it is highly susceptible to the gonococcus and inclusion conjunctivitis agents, both of which are infectious for the genitourinary tract. Moreover, when these organisms are established on the conjunctiva, they are constantly washed down the nasolacrimal duct into the nose by the tears, yet they grow in the nose only rarely and with difficulty.

In the differential diagnosis of conjunctivitis as the cause of a red, painful, or irritated eye, it is important to rule out keratitis, iritis, and acute glaucoma. The causal organisms can then be identified by the microscopic examination of stained conjunctival material. Before treatment is started, culture studies should be made and antibiotic sensitivity tests performed.

Cytology of Conjunctivitis

Damage to the conjunctival epithelium by a noxious agent may be followed by epithelial edema, cellular death and exfoliation, epithelial hypertrophy, or granulomas. There may also be edema of the conjunctival stroma (chemosis) and hypertrophy of the adenoid layer of the stroma (follicle formation). Inflammatory cells, including neutrophils, eosinophils, basophils, lymphocytes, and plasma cells, may be seen and often indicate the nature of the damaging agent. The inflammatory cells migrate from the conjunctival stroma through the epithelium to the surface. They then combine with fibrin and with the mucus

produced by the conjunctival goblet cells to form the conjunctival exudate, which accounts for the gumming of the eyelids noted on waking.

The inflammatory cells appear in the exudate or in scrapings taken with a sterile platinum spatula from the anesthetized conjunctival surface. The material is stained with Gram's stain (to identify the bacterial organisms) and with Giemsa's stain (to identify the cell types). A predominance of polymorphonuclear leukocytes is characteristic of both bacterial and chlamydial conjunctivitis. (Infections with *N catarrhalis* and *M lacunata* are exceptions; in a conjunctivitis arising from either of these bacteria, the inflammatory response is minimal, and mononuclear cells predominate.) As a rule, a predominance of mononuclear cells, especially lymphocytes, is characteristic of viral conjunctivitis except when a pseudomembrane forms, as it may in epidemic keratoconjunctivitis or herpes simplex virus conjunctivitis. Polymorphonuclear cells then predominate because of necrosis.

Eosinophils and basophils are found in allergic conjunctivitis, and scattered eosinophil granules and eosinophils are found in vernal keratoconjunctivitis. In all types of conjunctivitis there are plasma cells in the conjunctival stroma. They do not migrate through the epithelium, however, and are therefore not seen in smears of exudate or of scrapings from the conjunctival surface unless the epithelium has become necrosed, as it may in trachoma; in this event, the rupturing of a follicle allows the plasma cells to reach the epithelial surface. Since the mature follicles of trachoma rupture easily, the finding of large, palely staining, lymphoblastic (germinal center) cells in scrapings strongly suggests trachoma.

Symptoms of Conjunctivitis

The important symptoms of conjunctivitis are a foreign body sensation, a scratching or burning sensation, a sensation of fullness around the eyes, itching, and (when the cornea is also affected) photophobia.

Foreign body sensation and a scratching or burning sensation are often associated with the swelling and papillary hypertrophy that normally accompany conjunctival hyperemia. If there is pain, the cornea is probably also affected. Pain that is more severe on waking and improves during the day suggests staphylococcal infection, and pain that is severe during the day and better on waking suggests keratoconjunctivitis sicca. Itching, if complained of spontaneously rather than in response to questioning, usually indicates that the patient has an allergic conjunctivitis of the immediate hypersensitivity type.

Signs of Conjunctivitis

The important signs of conjunctivitis are hyperemia, tearing, exudation, pseudoptosis, papillary hypertrophy, chemosis, follicles, pseudomembranes and membranes, granulomas, and preauricular adenopathy.

Hyperemia is the most conspicuous clinical sign of acute conjunctivitis. The redness is most marked in the fornix and diminishes toward the limbus by virtue of the dilatation of the posterior conjunctival vessels. (A perilimbal dilatation suggests inflammation of the cornea or deeper structures.) A brilliant red suggests bacterial conjunctivitis, and a milky appearance suggests allergic conjunctivitis. Hyperemia without cellular infiltration suggests irritation from physical causes such as wind, sun, smoke, etc, and also occurs occasionally as part of a general vascular dilatation, eg, acne rosacea or carcinoid.

Tearing is often prominent in conjunctivitis, the tears resulting from the foreign body sensation, the burning or scratching sensation, or the itching. Mild transudation also arises from the hyperemic vessels and adds to the tearing. An abnormally scant secretion of tears suggests granulomatous conjunctivitis or keratoconjunctivitis sicca.

Exudation is a feature of all types of acute conjunctivitis. The exudate is flaky and amorphous in bacterial conjunctivitis and stringy in allergic conjunctivitis. A mild gumming of the lids on waking occurs in almost all types of conjunctivitis, and if the exudate is copious and the lids are firmly stuck together the conjunctivitis is probably bacterial or chlamydial.

Pseudoptosis is a drooping of the upper lid due to its increased weight from cellular infiltration. This sign is typical of several types of conjunctivitis (trachoma, epidemic keratoconjunctivitis, etc).

Papillary hypertrophy is a nonspecific conjunctival reaction that occurs only when the conjunctiva is bound down to the underlying tarsus or limbus by fine fibrils. When the tuft of vessels that forms the substance of the papilla (along with cellular elements and exudates) reaches the basement membrane of the epithelium, it branches over the papilla like the spokes in the frame of an umbrella. An inflammatory exudate accumulates between the fibrils, heaping the conjunctiva into mounds. In necrotizing disease (eg, trachoma), the exudate may be replaced by granulation tissue or connective tissue.

When the papillae are small, the conjunctiva usually has a smooth, velvety appearance. A red papillary conjunctiva suggests bacterial or chlamydial disease (eg, a velvety red tarsal conjunctiva is characteristic of stage IIb trachoma). When the papillae are large they are flat-topped, polygonal, and milky in color. On the upper tarsus they suggest vernal keratoconjunctivitis, and on the lower tarsus they suggest atopic keratoconjunctivitis. Giant papillae may also occur at the limbus, especially in the area that is normally exposed when the eyes are open (between 2 and 4 o'clock and between 8 and 10 o'clock). Here they appear as gelatinous infiltrates that may encroach on the cornea. Limbal papillae are characteristic of vernal keratoconjunctivitis, rare in atopic keratoconjunctivitis.

Chemosis of the conjunctiva strongly suggests acute hay fever conjunctivitis but may also occur in acute gonococcal or meningococcal conjunctivitis and in epidemic keratoconjunctivitis. Chemosis of the bulbar conjunctiva is a conspicuous sign in trichinosis.

Occasionally, chemosis may appear before there is any gross cellular infiltration or exudation.

Follicles are seen in most cases of viral conjunctivitis, in all cases of chlamydial conjunctivitis, and in all cases of toxic conjunctivitis induced by topical medications such as idoxuridine and miotics. Follicles in the fornix and at the tarsal margins have limited diagnostic value, but when they are located on the tarsi (especially the upper tarsus) a chlamydial, viral, or toxic conjunctivitis following topical medication should be suspected.

The follicle is a focal lymphoid hyperplasia within the adenoid layer of the conjunctiva and usually contains a germinal center. Clinically, it can be recognized as an avascular white or gray, round structure. On slit lamp examination, small vessels can be seen arising at the border of the follicle and encircling it.

Pseudomembranes and membranes—the result of a coagulating process and differing only in degree—are produced by infectious or toxic agents. A pseudomembrane is a coagulum on the *surface* of the epithelium, and when it is removed the epithelium remains intact. A membrane is a coagulum involving the *entire* epithelium, and when it is removed a raw, bleeding surface remains. Pseudomembranes or membranes may accompany epidemic keratoconjunctivitis, primary herpes simplex virus conjunctivitis, streptococcal conjunctivitis, diphtheria, and erythema multiforme major. They may also be an aftermath of chemical burns, especially alkali burns.

In a peculiar form of chronic conjunctivitis (ligneous), bilateral membranes or pseudomembranes form repeatedly on the upper and lower tarsal conjunctivas and often spread out from a granulomatous area. Sometimes simulating pseudomembranes are conjunctival mucous patches—minimally elevated, whitish, and surrounded by a narrow border of erythema—seen in secondary syphilis.

Granulomas of the conjunctiva always affect the stroma. Although they usually arise endogenously (eg, from tuberculosis, syphilis, coccidioidomycosis), there are also many exogenous causes (eg, leptotrichosis, lymphogranuloma venereum conjunctivitis, tularemia). Both chalazions (lipogranulomas) and the lesions of Parinaud's oculoglandular syndrome are granulomas, and biopsies are often necessary to determine their causes.

Phlyctenules are localized manifestations of microbial allergy (like tuberculids of the skin).

Preauricular adenopathy is an important sign. A grossly visible preauricular node is seen in Parinaud's oculoglandular syndrome and, rarely, in epidemic keratoconjunctivitis. A large or small preauricular node, sometimes slightly tender, occurs in primary herpes simplex conjunctivitis, epidemic keratoconjunctivitis, inclusion conjunctivitis, and trachoma. Small but nontender preauricular nodes occur in pharyngoconjunctival fever, Newcastle disease conjunctivitis, and acute hemorrhagic conjunctivitis. There is no preauricular adenopathy in bacterial conjunctivitis.

BACTERIAL CONJUNCTIVITIS

The acute and chronic bacterial conjunctivitides are the commonest types of conjunctivitis. The acute types occasionally become chronic but are usually self-limited, lasting a maximum of 2 weeks if untreated. Treatment with one of the many available antibacterial agents usually cures them in a few days.

Clinical Findings

A. Symptoms and Signs: The organisms listed on p 58 account for most cases of bacterial conjunctivitis. They produce bilateral irritation and injection, a purulent exudate with agglutination of the lids on waking, and occasionally lid edema. The infection usually starts in one eye and is spread to the other by the hands. It may spread from one person to another by fomites.

Purulent conjunctivitis (caused by *N gonorrhoeae* and *N meningitidis*) is marked by a profuse purulent exudate (Fig 7–1). Meningococcal conjunctivitis is usually milder than gonococcal conjunctivitis and has fewer sequelae, but any severe, profusely exudative conjunctivitis demands immediate laboratory investigation and immediate treatment. If there is any delay, there may be severe corneal damage and the conjunctiva may become the portal of entry of the meningococcus to the bloodstream and meninges.

Acute catarrhal conjunctivitis often occurs in epidemic form and is called "pinkeye" by most laymen (Fig 7–2). It is characterized by an acute onset of conjunctival hyperemia and a moderate amount of mucopurulent discharge. The commonest causes are the pneumococcus in temperate climates and *H aegyptius* in warm climates. Rare causes are staphylococci and streptococci. The types caused by the pneumococ-

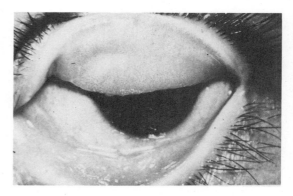

Figure 7–2. Acute catarrhal conjunctivitis caused by Koch-Weeks bacillus *(Haemophilus aegyptius)*. (Courtesy of HB Ostler.)

cus (Fig 7–3) and *H aegyptius* may be accompanied by subconjunctival hemorrhages.

Subacute catarrhal conjunctivitis is caused most often by *H influenzae* and occasionally by *Escherichia coli* and *Proteus* sp. *H influenzae* infection is characterized by a thin, watery, or flocculent exudate.

Chronic catarrhal conjunctivitis is usually

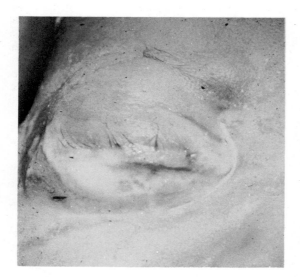

Figure 7–1. Gonorrheal conjunctivitis. Profuse purulent exudate. (Courtesy of P Thygeson.)

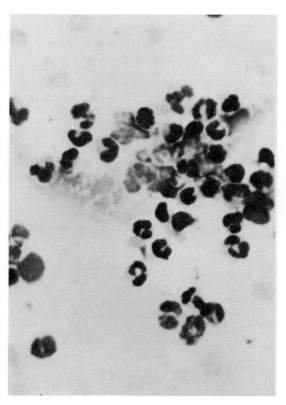

Figure 7–3. Polymorphonuclear reaction in Giemsa-stained scrapings from a patient with bacterial conjunctivitis. (Courtesy of M Okumoto.)

caused by *S aureus,* but *M lacunata* is also a frequent cause in warm climates. *M lacunata*—and occasionally the staphylococcus—produce a localized angular conjunctivitis that is commonly associated with dermatitis, fissuring of the external or internal canthi, and a scant conjunctival discharge.

Rare bacterial conjunctivitides may be caused by *C diphtheriae* and *Streptococcus pyogenes.* Pseudomembranes or membranes caused by these organisms may form on the palpebral conjunctiva. The rare cases of chronic conjunctivitis produced by *N catarrhalis,* the coliform bacilli, *Proteus* sp, etc are as a rule indistinguishable clinically. *Mycobacterium tuberculosis* and *Treponema pallidum,* both of which produce granulomatous conjunctival disease associated with large, grossly visible preauricular nodes, will be discussed in the section on oculoglandular syndromes.

B. Laboratory Findings: In most cases of bacterial conjunctivitis, the organisms can be identified by the microscopic examination of stained conjunctival scrapings, which reveals numerous polymorphonuclear neutrophils (Fig 7–3). Direct examination and culture study are recommended for all cases and are mandatory if the disease is purulent, membranous, or pseudomembranous. Antibiotic sensitivity studies are also highly desirable, so that an appropriate drug can be started at once.

Complications & Sequelae

A chronic marginal blepharitis may complicate an untreated staphylococcal conjunctivitis except in very young patients who are not subject to blepharitis. Conjunctival scarring follows both pseudomembranous and membranous conjunctivitis, and in some cases the corneal nutrition may be so compromised that corneal ulceration and perforation supervene.

Marginal corneal ulceration may follow infection with *N gonorrhoeae, H aegyptius,* or *S aureus,* and if the toxic products of *N gonorrhoeae* diffuse through the cornea into the anterior chamber, they may cause toxic iritis.

Treatment

Specific therapy of bacterial conjunctivitis depends on the identification of the etiologic agent. While waiting for the laboratory results, the physician can start topical therapy with a sulfonamide or an antibiotic. In any purulent conjunctivitis, an antibiotic suitable for treating *N gonorrhoeae* and *N meningitidis* infection should be selected, and both systemic and topical therapy should be started immediately after material for laboratory study has been collected.

In both purulent and acute catarrhal conjunctivitis, the conjunctival sac should be irrigated with saline solution as necessary to remove the conjunctival secretions. To prevent spread of the disease, the patient and family should be instructed to give special attention to their personal hygiene.

Course & Prognosis

Acute bacterial conjunctivitis is almost always self-limited. Untreated, it usually lasts 10–14 days; if properly treated, 1–3 days. The exceptions are staphylococcal conjunctivitis (which may progress to blepharoconjunctivitis and enter a chronic phase) and gonococcal conjunctivitis (which when untreated can lead to corneal perforation and endophthalmitis). Since the conjunctiva may be the portal of entry for the meningococcus to the bloodstream and meninges, systemic meningitis may be the end result of meningococcal conjunctivitis.

Chronic bacterial conjunctivitis may not be self-limited and may become a troublesome therapeutic problem.

CHLAMYDIAL CONJUNCTIVITIS

1. TRACHOMA

Trachoma is one of the most ancient of known diseases. It was recognized as a cause of trichiasis as early as the 27th century BC and affects all races. With over 400 million of the world's population afflicted, it is one of the most common of all chronic human diseases. Its regional variations in prevalence and severity can be explained on the basis of variations in the personal hygiene and standards of living of the world's peoples, the climatic conditions under which they live,

Table 7–1. Differentiation of the common types of conjunctivitis.

Clinical Findings and Cytology	Viral	Bacterial	Chlamydial	Atopic (Allergic)
Itching	Minimal	Minimal	Minimal	Severe
Hyperemia	Generalized	Generalized	Generalized	Generalized
Tearing	Profuse	Moderate	Moderate	Moderate
Exudation	Minimal	Profuse	Profuse	Minimal
Preauricular adenopathy	Common	Uncommon	Common only in inclusion conjunctivitis	None
In stained scrapings and exudates	Monocytes	Bacteria, PMNs*	PMNs,* plasma cells, inclusion bodies	Eosinophils
Associated sore throat and fever	Occasionally	Occasionally	Never	Never

*Polymorphonuclear cells.

the prevailing age at onset, and the frequency and type of the prevailing concomitant bacterial eye infections. Although sporadic cases occur in the white population of the USA, trachoma is rare here except among the American Indians of the southwestern states, where it is now mild and relatively uncomplicated.

Trachoma has a special affinity for the eye and is usually bilateral. Spread is by direct contact or fomites, usually from mother to child or grandmother to grandchild. Family members in contact with a child with trachoma should always be investigated and should be treated when found to harbor the disease. Insect vectors, especially flies and gnats, may play a role in transmission. The acute forms of the disease are more infectious than the cicatricial forms, and the larger the inoculum the more severe the onset. Spread is often associated with epidemics of bacterial conjunctivitis and with the dry seasons in tropical and semitropical countries.

Clinical Findings

A. Symptoms and Signs: The incubation period of trachoma averages 7 days but varies from 5 to 14 days. In an infant or child the onset is usually insidious, and the disease may resolve with minimal or no complications. In the adult the onset is often subacute or acute, and complications may develop early. At onset, trachoma often resembles bacterial conjunctivitis, the signs and symptoms usually consisting of tearing, photophobia, pain, exudation, edema of the eyelids, chemosis of the bulbar conjunctiva, hyperemia, papillary hypertrophy, tarsal and limbal follicles, superior keratitis, pannus formation, and a small, tender preauricular node.

According to MacCallan's classification, the disease passes through the following 4 clinical stages:

Stage I (early lymphoid hyperplasia): Papillary

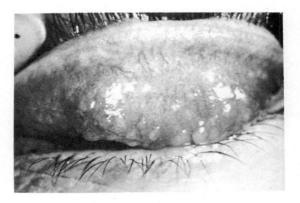

Figure 7–4. Trachoma, stage IIb. Papillae and follicles in upper tarsal conjunctiva. (Courtesy of P Thygeson.)

hypertrophy and immature (small) follicles on the upper tarsus.

Stage IIa (established trachoma): Papillary hypertrophy and mature (large) follicles on the upper tarsus.

Stage IIb (established trachoma): Papillary hypertrophy predominating and masking the follicles on the upper tarsus (Fig 7–4).

Stage III (cicatricial trachoma): Early conjunctival scarring, shown by fine white lines in the subepithelial conjunctiva and associated with persistent follicles and papillary hypertrophy of the upper tarsal conjunctiva. (Since the agent of trachoma is epitheliotropic, the subepithelial scarring of the tarsal conjunctiva and the cornea may be due to a diffusible toxin.)

Stage IV (healed trachoma): Conjunctival stellate and linear cicatrization without inflammation of the upper tarsus.

Note on the Taxonomic Status of the Chlamydiae

The classification of the chlamydiae (formerly the bedsoniae) is currently the subject of a dispute reminiscent of one that arose over the classification of another group of small intracellular microorganisms: the rickettsiae. Officially, there are at present only 2 species: *C trachomatis* (also known as "subgroup A") and *C psittaci* (also known as "subgroup B"). This grouping is based on the sulfonamide susceptibility of *C trachomatis* and the iodine-staining properties of its inclusions—2 important properties not shared by *C psittaci*. But the lack of official speciation of the agents of trachoma, inclusion disease (conjunctivitis, urethritis, and cervicitis), and lymphogranuloma venereum has led to serious confusion and some startling misconceptions. For example, headlines in a recent issue of *Sight-Saving Review* stated that trachoma was the commonest cause of venereal disease in the USA!

An excellent speciation was made by Rake in 1957, who designated the agent of trachoma as *C trachomatis;* the agent of inclusion conjunctivitis, urethritis, and cervicitis as *C oculogenitalis;* and the agent of lymphogranuloma venereum as *C lymphogranulomatis.** Speciation based on biologic properties is difficult with the chlamydiae because of the many shared properties; but speciation based on immunologic typing, pathogenicity patterns in primates, tissue tropism, and disease manifestations in humans is both reasonable and inevitable. Most ophthalmic microbiologists still use the Rake classification, and we can only hope that with some slight modification it will soon become the official one.

*Breed RS et al: *Bergey's Manual of Determinative Bacteriology.* Williams & Wilkins, 1957.

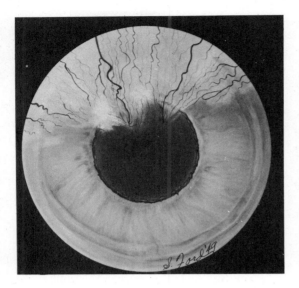

Figure 7–5. Trachomatous pannus. (Courtesy of P Thygeson.)

In established trachoma there may also be superior epithelial keratitis, subepithelial keratitis, pannus, superior limbal follicles, and ultimately the cicatricial remains of these follicles, known as **Herbert's peripheral pits.** Both the limbal follicles and Herbert's pits are pathognomonic of trachoma; the follicles are gelatinous, semiopaque, dome-shaped elevations surrounded by the pannus, and the pits are small depressions in the connective tissue of the limbocorneal junction. They are filled with epithelium and look like small, lucid circles or semicircles in a fibrovascular membrane arising at the limbus, from which vascular loops encroach on the cornea from above (Fig 7–5). All of the signs of trachoma are more severe in the upper than in the lower conjunctiva and cornea.

B. Laboratory Findings: Giemsa-stained conjunctival scrapings show a predominantly polymorphonuclear reaction, but plasma cells, Leber cells (large macrophages containing phagocytosed debris), and follicle cells (lymphoblasts) may also be seen. Plasma cells and Leber cells suggest trachoma, but follicle cells are diagnostic. Unfortunately, they are not always present. When inclusion bodies, which cannot always be found in chronic active trachoma, appear in the Giemsa-stained preparations, they are dark purple, purplish-blue, or blue inclusions that cap the nucleus of the epithelial cell (Fig 7–6).

The agent of trachoma resembles the agent of inclusion conjunctivitis morphologically, but the 2 can be differentiated serologically by microimmunofluorescence and by their pathogenicity patterns in monkeys and apes. Trachoma is caused by serotypes A, B, or C. Both agents can be isolated in the yolk sac of embryonated hen eggs or in tissue cultures (irradiated with diethylaminoethyl dextran) if the agent is centrifuged onto the monolayer.

Differential Diagnosis

In the differentiation of trachoma from viral infections, 2 differences are important: (1) With one exception (the follicular conjunctivitis associated with a molluscum contagiosum nodule on the lid margin), all viral conjunctivitides are of less than 3 weeks' duration; and (2) unless there is a pseudomembrane, all viral infections are associated with a predominantly mononuclear inflammatory reaction. Follicular conjunctivitis following treatment with idoxuridine or miotics may simulate trachoma, but the drug-induced follicular reaction subsides when the drug is withdrawn, and a conjunctival scraping contains a limited and approximately equal number of polymorphonuclear and mononuclear cells. Long-standing dacryocystitis or chronic canaliculitis in children may occasionally be complicated by chronic follicular conjunctivitis, but there are no corneal changes in these conditions, and as soon as the underlying infections are eradicated the conjunctivitis clears and leaves no scars. In children, folliculosis of the adenoid type may simulate trachoma grossly, but there are no associated corneal changes and no papillary hypertrophy, and the conjunctiva between follicles is normal.

The agents of inclusion conjunctivitis, feline pneumonitis, and psittacosis (all chlamydial infections) may produce follicular conjunctivitis, but except for the flat scars associated with the pseudomembranes that occasionally form in neonatal inclusion conjunctivitis, there is no scarring.

Parinaud's oculoglandular syndrome in children may have an associated follicular conjunctivitis, but a prominent feature of Parinaud's syndrome, never seen in trachoma, is a grossly visible preauricular node.

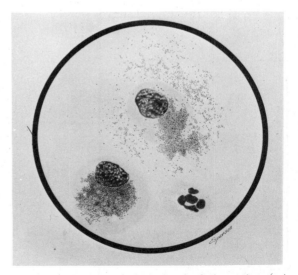

Figure 7–6. Cytoplasmic inclusion body in conjunctival epithelial cells in trachoma. Ruptured inclusion at right. Polymorphonuclear neutrophil (typical in conjunctival scrapings of trachoma) below. (Courtesy of P Thygeson and C Dawson.)

Vernal keratoconjunctivitis is occasionally mistaken for trachoma because of its upper tarsal lesions, but the conjunctiva in vernal keratoconjunctivitis has a milky appearance, polygonal, flat-topped giant papillae, and numerous eosinophils and eosinophil granules in conjunctival scrapings.

Complications & Sequelae

Conjunctival scarring is a frequent complication of trachoma and can shut off the ductules of the accessory lacrimal glands and obliterate the orifices of the lacrimal gland. These effects may drastically reduce the aqueous component of the precorneal tear film, and the film's mucous components may be reduced by loss of goblet cells. The scars may also cause entropion of the upper lid, and if there is an associated trichiasis the aberrant lashes may abrade the cornea. This often leads to corneal ulceration, bacterial corneal infections, and corneal scarring (Fig 7–7).

Ptosis (Fig 7–8), nasolacrimal duct obstruction, and dacryocystitis are other common complications of trachoma.

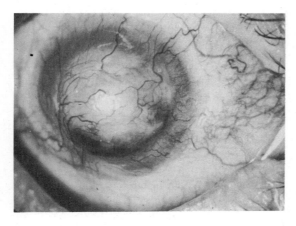

Figure 7–7. Advanced trachoma following corneal ulceration and scarring. (Courtesy of P Thygeson.)

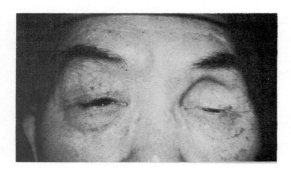

Figure 7–8. Ptosis with an "S"-shaped curve of lids associated with chronic trachoma. (Courtesy of P Thygeson.)

Treatment

Tetracycline, 1–1.5 g/d orally in 4 divided doses for 3–4 weeks, or erythromycin, 1 g/d orally in 4 divided doses for 3–4 weeks, will usually result in striking clinical improvement. Several courses are sometimes necessary for actual cure. Systemic tetracyclines should not be given to a child under 7 years of age or to a pregnant woman since they may cause staining of the developing child's incisors and may produce epiphyseal problems in the fetus.

Topical ointments or drops, including preparations of sulfonamides, tetracyclines, erythromycin, and rifampin, used 4 times daily for 6 weeks, have had some success.

From the time therapy is begun, its maximum effect is usually not achieved for 10–12 weeks. The persistence of follicles on the upper tarsus for some weeks after a course of therapy should therefore not be construed as evidence of therapeutic failure.

Course & Prognosis

Characteristically, trachoma is a chronic disease of long duration. In an ideal environment, however, about 20% of cases detected in any one year heal spontaneously; and when treatment is given early the prognosis is excellent. Unfortunately, however, because of unfavorable conditions and lack of treatment, about 20,000,000 people in the world today have major visual loss from trachoma.

2. INCLUSION CONJUNCTIVITIS
(Inclusion Blennorrhea)

Inclusion conjunctivitis, usually bilateral, is a common disease, especially in sexually active young people. Characteristically, the chlamydial agent infects the urethra of the male and the cervix of the female. Transmission to the eyes of adults is usually from the genitourinary tract to the eye. Indirect transmission in inadequately chlorinated swimming pools can also occur, and in the newborn the agent is transmitted during birth by direct contamination of the conjunctiva with cervical secretions. The Credé prophylaxis does not protect against inclusion conjunctivitis.

Clinical Findings

A. Symptoms and Signs: Inclusion conjunctivitis may have an acute or a subacute onset. The patient frequently complains of redness of the eyes, pseudoptosis, and discharge, especially in the mornings. The newborn has a papillary conjunctivitis and a moderate amount of exudate, and in hyperacute cases pseudomembranes occasionally form and can lead to scarring. Since the newborn has no adenoid tissue in the stroma of the conjunctiva (see p 58), there is no follicle formation; but if the conjunctivitis persists for 2–3 months, follicles appear and the conjunctival picture is like that in older children and adults.

In adults the conjunctivas of both tarsi, and espe-

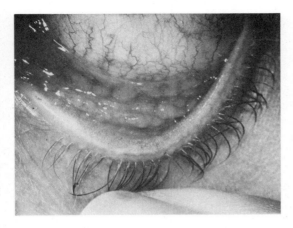

Figure 7–9. Acute follicular conjunctivitis caused by inclusion conjunctivitis in a 22-year-old male with urethritis. (Courtesy of K Tabbara.)

cially of the lower tarsus, are loaded with both papillae and follicles (Fig 7–9). Since pseudomembranes never form in the adult, scarring does not occur. A superficial keratitis may be noted superiorly and, less often, a small superior micropannus (less than 1–2 mm). Rarely, subepithelial opacities, usually marginal, may develop. A complicating otitis media may arise from infection of the eustachian tube.

B. Laboratory Findings: The examination of conjunctival scrapings shows (1) a predominantly polymorphonuclear neutrophil reaction, (2) no bacteria, and (3) basophilic cytoplasmic inclusion bodies (identical to those seen in trachoma and often numerous) in epithelial cells. Bacterial cultures are negative. Inclusion conjunctivitis may be caused by serotypes D–K.

Differential Diagnosis

Inclusion conjunctivitis can be clinically differentiated from trachoma on the following grounds: (1) Inclusion conjunctivitis is transmitted venereally; trachoma from eye to eye. (2) Conjunctival scarring, which is common in trachoma, occurs in inclusion conjunctivitis only in the newborn and only after the formation of a pseudomembrane. If scars develop under these circumstances, they are flat and diffuse rather than linear or stellate, as in trachoma. (3) Inclusion conjunctivitis sometimes causes a micropannus but never the gross pannus seen regularly in trachoma. (4) The corneal scarring and Herbert's pits (limbal scars) that occur in trachoma are never seen in inclusion conjunctivitis.

Treatment

In infants, 1% tetracycline in oil or ointment, erythromycin ophthalmic ointment, or a sulfonamide drop (instilled 5–6 times daily for 14 days) is very effective. In adults, a 3-week course of oral tetracycline, 1–1.5 g/d, or of erythromycin, 1 g/d, is curative. (Systemic tetracyclines should not be given to a preg-

nant woman or a child under 7 years of age since they cause epiphyseal problems in the fetus or staining of the young child's incisors.) The patient's sexual partners should be examined and treated if infected.

When one of the standard therapeutic regimens is followed, recurrences are rare. If untreated, inclusion conjunctivitis runs a course of 3–9 months or longer. The average duration is 5 months.

3. LYMPHOGRANULOMA VENEREUM CONJUNCTIVITIS

Lymphogranuloma venereum infections of the conjunctiva, which can result from accidental laboratory accidents or venereal transmission, are rare. The conjunctival reaction is nonfollicular and largely granulomatous, and there is a grossly visible preauricular node (bubo). Elephantiasis of the eyelids may occur because of lymph blockage and has been compared to the esthiomene of the female genitalia. The conjunctiva and cornea become diffusely scarred. In endogenous disease secondary to a genitourinary focus, optic neuritis, uveitis, episcleritis, and phlyctenulosis have all been reported.

The causal organism, *C lymphogranulomatis,** may be recovered by inoculating mouse brains or tissue cultures with scrapings from an infected conjunctiva. Examination of the scrapings may show typical inclusions within monocytes and macrophages but not in epithelial cells. In more than 50% of patients, the Frei test is positive, and a high titer of complement-fixing antibodies is the rule. Lymphogranuloma venereum conjunctivitis is caused by chlamydia of serotypes L1, L2, and L3.

A sulfonamide or broad-spectrum antibiotic, given systemically for 3–4 weeks, is curative.

4. PSITTACOSIS

One reported case of conjunctivitis due to an accidental laboratory infection with *C psittaci** of parakeet origin was characterized by chronic conjunctival infiltration and papillary hypertrophy of the upper tarsus and by epithelial keratitis. No inclusions were seen in epithelial cells, but cultures were positive for chlamydia. The conjunctivitis and keratitis responded only after prolonged treatment with systemic tetracycline.

5. FELINE PNEUMONITIS

Two cases have been reported of follicular conjunctivitis associated with intimate exposure to domestic cats with feline pneumonitis (a chlamydial infection caused by *C psittaci*). In both cases the conjunctivitis was associated with central epithelial keratitis and

*See box on p 64.

cleared after 4 weeks of therapy with systemic tetracycline. There were no sequelae. Cytoplasmic epithelial cell inclusions were seen in Giemsa-stained scrapings from the conjunctiva. This was in sharp contrast to the absence of inclusions in the parakeet-derived disease.

VIRAL CONJUNCTIVITIS

Viral conjunctivitis, a common affliction, can be caused by a wide variety of viruses. Some of these produce severe, disabling disease; others only mild, rapidly self-limited disease.

I. Acute Viral Follicular Conjunctivitis

1. PHARYNGOCONJUNCTIVAL FEVER

Pharyngoconjunctival fever is characterized by fever of 38.5–40 °C (101–104 °F), sore throat, and a follicular conjunctivitis in one or both eyes. The follicles are often very prominent on both the conjunctiva (Fig 7–10) and the pharyngeal mucosa. Bilateral and, less commonly, unilateral injection and tearing occur, and there may be transient superficial epithelial keratitis and occasionally some subepithelial opacities. Preauricular lymphadenopathy (nontender) is characteristic. The syndrome may be incomplete, consisting of only one or 2 or the cardinal signs (fever, pharyngitis, and conjunctivitis).

Pharyngoconjunctival fever is caused regularly by adenovirus type 3 and occasionally by types 4 and 7. The virus can be grown on HeLa cells and identified by neutralization tests. As the disease progresses, it can also be diagnosed serologically by a rising titer of neutralizing antibody to the virus. Clinical diagnosis is a simple matter, however, and clearly more practical.

Conjunctival scrapings contain predominantly mononuclear cells, and no bacteria grow in cultures. The condition is more common in children than in adults and can be transmitted in chlorinated swimming pools. There is no specific treatment, but the conjunctivitis is self-limited, usually lasting about 10 days.

2. EPIDEMIC KERATOCONJUNCTIVITIS

Epidemic keratoconjunctivitis is usually bilateral. The onset is often in one eye only, however, and as a rule the first eye is more severely affected. At onset the patient notes injection, moderate pain, and tearing, followed in 5–14 days by photophobia, epithelial keratitis, and round subepithelial opacities. Corneal sensation is normal. A large, tender preauricular node, rarely grossly visible, is characteristic. Edema of the eyelids, chemosis, and conjunctival hyperemia mark the acute phase, with follicles and subconjunctival hemorrhages often appearing within 48 hours. Pseudomembranes (and occasionally true membranes) may occur and may be followed by flat scars or symblepharons (Fig 7–11).

The conjunctivitis lasts for 3–4 weeks at most. The subepithelial opacities are concentrated in the central cornea, sparing the periphery, and may persist for months but heal without scars.

Epidemic keratoconjunctivitis is caused by adenovirus types 8 and 19, which can be cultivated on HeLa cells and identified by neutralization tests. Rising neutralizing antibody titers during the course of the disease are diagnostic. Scrapings from the conjunctiva show a primarily mononuclear inflammatory reaction (Fig 7–12); when pseudomembranes occur, neutrophils may also be prominent.

Epidemic keratoconjunctivitis in adults is confined to the external eye, but in children there may be such systemic symptoms of viral infection as fever, sore throat, and diarrhea. Spread takes place all too often by way of the physician's fingers or use of improperly sterilized ophthalmic instruments or contaminated solutions. Eye solutions, particularly topical

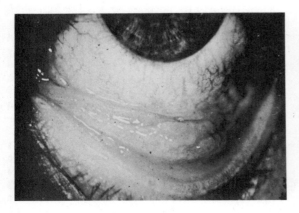

Figure 7–10. Acute follicular conjunctivitis due to adenovirus type 3. (Courtesy of P Thygeson.)

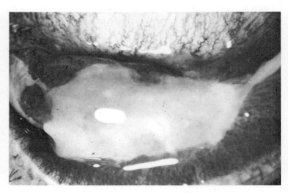

Figure 7–11. Epidemic keratoconjunctivitis. Thick white membrane in lower palpebral conjunctiva. (Courtesy of P Thygeson.)

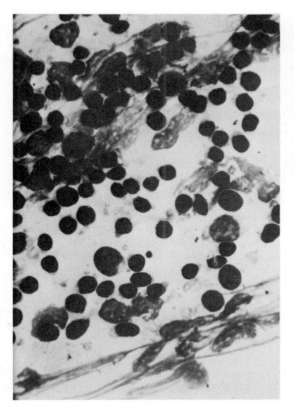

Figure 7–12. Mononuclear cell reaction in conjunctival scrapings of a patient with viral conjunctivitis caused by adenovirus type 8. (Courtesy of M Okumoto.)

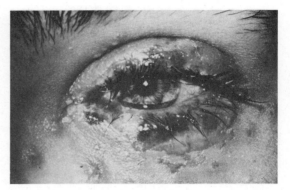

Figure 7–13. Primary ocular herpes. (Courtesy of HB Ostler.)

anesthetics, can be contaminated when a dropper tip rubs the conjunctiva or cilia. There the virus may persist, and the solution becomes a source of spread.

The danger of contaminated solution bottles can be averted by the use of individual sterile droppers for each patient. Handwashing between examinations and meticulous sterilization, especially of tonometers, are also mandatory. The tonometer footplate should be cleansed carefully with a sterile solution after each use, and the instrument should be sterilized by flame or in a hot air tonometer sterilizer after use on an inflamed eye. Applanation tonometers should be cleaned by rinsing with a sterile nonirritating solution and careful wiping several times with a facial tissue. (Epidemic keratoconjunctivitis is the only serious eye disease known to be transmissible by tonometry.)

3. HERPES SIMPLEX VIRUS CONJUNCTIVITIS

Herpes simplex virus conjunctivitis, a disease of young children, is an uncommon entity characterized by unilateral injection, irritation, mucoid discharge, pain, and mild photophobia. It occurs only in first attacks of herpes simplex virus infection, ie, in primary infections (Fig 7–13), and is often associated with herpes simplex virus keratitis, in which the cornea shows discrete epithelial lesions that usually coalesce to form single or multiple dendrites. The conjunctivitis is follicular or, less often, pseudomembranous. (Patients receiving idoxuridine may develop follicular conjunctivitis that is not to be confused with primary herpes simplex virus conjunctivitis.) Herpetic vesicles often appear on the eyelids and lid margins, usually associated with severe edema of the eyelids. Typically, there is a large or small tender preauricular node.

No bacteria are found in scrapings or recovered in cultures. If the conjunctivitis is follicular, the predominant inflammatory reaction is mononuclear, but if it is pseudomembranous the predominant reaction is polymorphonuclear due to the chemotaxis of necrosis. Intranuclear inclusions cannot be seen in Giemsa-stained preparations (because of the margination of the chromatin), but they appear if Bouin fixation and the Papanicolaou stain are used. The finding of multinucleated giant epithelial cells has diagnostic value.

The virus can be isolated readily by gently rubbing a dry cotton-tipped applicator over an infected conjunctiva and then transferring the infected cells on the applicator directly to either an abraded rabbit cornea or a susceptible tissue culture.

Herpes simplex virus conjunctivitis may persist for 2–3 weeks, and if it is pseudomembranous it may leave fine linear or flat scars. Complications include corneal dendrites and vesicles on the skin. Although type 1 herpesvirus causes the overwhelming majority of cases, type 2 can be a rare cause in both the newborn and adult. In the newborn there may be generalized disease with encephalitis, chorioretinitis, hepatitis, etc. In the newborn there may be generalized disease with encephalitis, chorioretinitis, hepatitis, etc.

Since the conjunctivitis is self-limited, therapy is usually not necessary. Corneal debridement may be performed, or idoxuridine ointment may be applied 4 times daily for 7–10 days. (Treatment with acyclovir is investigational for ophthalmic use in the USA.) The use of steroids is contraindicated since they aggravate herpes simplex infections and convert the disease from a short, self-limited process to a severe, greatly prolonged process.

4. NEWCASTLE DISEASE CONJUNCTIVITIS

Newcastle disease conjunctivitis is a rare disorder characterized by burning, itching, pain, redness, tearing, and (rarely) blurring of vision. It often occurs in small epidemics among poultry workers handling infected birds, or among veterinarians or laboratory helpers working with live vaccines or virus.

The disease often presents as chemosis and mild lid edema, and, although usually unilateral, it may sometimes affect both eyes at onset or within the first few days. There is a small nontender preauricular node, minimal discharge, and follicles that are more prominent on the lower tarsus than elsewhere. Rarely, there is corneal involvement in the form of fine epithelial keratitis or round, central subepithelial opacities. An influenzalike syndrome with mild fever, headaches, and mild arthralgia may develop. The disease subsides in less than a week, and there is no specific treatment.

No bacteria appear in scrapings or grow in cultures, and the inflammatory reaction is predominantly mononuclear. The virus can be isolated readily in embryonated hen eggs or tissue cultures, and complement-fixing, neutralizing, and hemagglutination-inhibiting antibodies can be found in the patient's serum.

5. ACUTE HEMORRHAGIC CONJUNCTIVITIS

Except for North and South America, all of the continents and most of the islands of the world have had major epidemics of acute hemorrhagic conjunctivitis. Because it was first recognized in Ghana in 1969 at the time of the Apollo XI moon trip, the disease has often been called Apollo XI conjunctivitis. It is caused by enterovirus type 70. Coxsackievirus type A24 has been found in some cases.

Characteristically, the disease has a short incubation period (8–48 hours) and course (5–7 days). The usual signs and symptoms are pain, photophobia, foreign body sensation, copious tearing, redness, lid edema, and subconjunctival hemorrhages (Fig 7–14). Chemosis sometimes also occurs. The subconjunctival hemorrhages are usually diffuse but may be punctate at onset, beginning in the upper bulbar conjunctiva and spreading to the lower. Most patients have preauricular lymphadenopathy, conjunctival follicles, and epithelial keratitis. Anterior uveitis has been reported; fever, malaise, and generalized myalgia have been observed in 25% of cases; and motor paralysis of the lower extremities has occurred in rare cases in India and Japan.

The virus is transmitted by close person-to-person contact and by such fomites as common linens, contaminated optical instruments, and water. Recovery occurs within 5–7 days, and there is no known treatment.

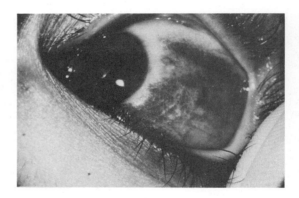

Figure 7–14. Acute hemorrhagic conjunctivitis. (Courtesy of K Tabbara.)

6. COXSACKIEVIRUS CONJUNCTIVITIS

Various coxsackieviruses have caused acute conjunctivitis accidentally in laboratory workers and in children with hand-foot-and-mouth disease.

II. Chronic Viral Conjunctivitis

1. MOLLUSCUM CONTAGIOSUM BLEPHAROCONJUNCTIVITIS

A molluscum nodule on the lid margin, especially if it is on the upper lid, may produce unilateral chronic conjunctivitis, superior keratitis, and superior pannus, all of which are also typical of trachoma. The inflammatory reaction is predominantly mononuclear (unlike the reaction in trachoma), and the round, waxy, pearl-white, noninflammatory lesion with an umbilicated center is typical of molluscum contagiosum (Fig 7–15). Prolonged (24-hour) Giemsa staining of scrapings from the lid nodule shows small red elementary bodies, and biopsy shows eosinophilic cytoplasmic

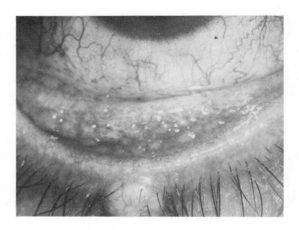

Figure 7–15. Molluscum contagiosum of lid margin with follicular conjunctivitis. (Courtesy of HB Ostler.)

inclusions that fill the entire cytoplasm of the enlarged cell, pushing its nucleus to one side.

Excision or simple incision of the nodule to allow peripheral blood to permeate it cures the conjunctivitis. On very rare occasions (reports of only 2 cases have appeared in the literature), molluscum nodules have occurred on the conjunctiva. In these cases, excision of the nodule has also relieved the conjunctivitis.

2. VACCINIAL BLEPHAROCONJUNCTIVITIS

This was an important complication of smallpox vaccination at one time but is now of historical interest only.

3. VARICELLA-ZOSTER BLEPHAROCONJUNCTIVITIS

Hyperemia and an infiltrative conjunctivitis, associated with the typical vesicular eruption along the dermatomal distribution of the ophthalmic branch of the trigeminal nerve, are characteristic of herpes zoster (preferably called simply zoster). The conjunctivitis is usually papillary, but follicles, pseudomembranes, and transitory vesicles that later ulcerate have all been noted. A tender preauricular lymph node occurs early in the disease. Scarring of the lid, entropion, and the misdirection of individual lashes are rare sequelae.

The lid lesions of varicella, which are like the skin lesions (pox) elsewhere, may appear on both the lid margins and the lids and may leave scars on the lid margins. A mild catarrhal type of conjunctivitis often occurs, but discrete conjunctival lesions (except at the limbus) are very rare. Limbal lesions resemble phlyctenules and may go through all the stages of vesicle, papule, and ulcer. The adjacent cornea becomes infiltrated and may vascularize.

In both zoster and varicella, scrapings from lid vesicles contain giant cells and a predominance of polymorphonuclear neutrophil cells; scrapings from the conjunctiva in varicella and from conjunctival vesicles in zoster contain giant cells and monocytes. The virus can be recovered in tissue cultures of human embryo cells.

There is no satisfactory treatment, but studies with interferon and acyclovir are promising.

4. MEASLES KERATOCONJUNCTIVITIS

The characteristic enanthem of measles frequently precedes the skin eruption. At this early stage the conjunctiva may have a peculiar glassy appearance, followed within a few days by swelling of the semilunar fold (Meyer's sign). Several days before the skin eruption, a catarrhal conjunctivitis with a mucopurulent discharge develops, and at the time of the skin eruption Koplik's spots appear on the conjunctiva and occasionally on the caruncle. At some time (early in children, late in adults), epithelial keratitis supervenes.

In the immunocompetent patient, measles keratoconjunctivitis has few or no sequelae, but in malnourished or otherwise immunoincompetent patients the ocular disease is frequently associated with a secondary bacterial infection due to the pneumococcus, *H influenzae,* and other organisms. In this event there is often a severe purulent or even pseudomembranous conjunctivitis with associated corneal ulceration and perforation. In many developing countries, measles and the folk remedies used to treat measles-associated eye disease are major causes of blindness.

Conjunctival scrapings show a mononuclear cell reaction unless there are pseudomembranes or secondary infection. Giemsa-stained preparations contain giant cells. Since there is no specific therapy, only supportive measures are indicated unless there is secondary infection.

RICKETTSIAL CONJUNCTIVITIS

All rickettsiae recognized as pathogenic for humans are likely to attack the conjunctiva. The conjunctiva is in fact often their portal of entry, eg, in Q fever, Marseilles fever (boutonneuse fever), endemic (murine) typhus, scrub typhus, Rocky Mountain spotted fever, and epidemic typhus.

1. Q FEVER

In Q fever there is usually severe conjunctival hyperemia. Rarely there may also be severe inflammation followed by gangrene of the lids.

Conjunctival scrapings, in which neither bacteria nor inclusions are seen, show a predominantly polymorphonuclear cell response. Diagnosis can be verified serologically by complement fixation and the Weil-Felix reaction.

Treatment with systemic tetracyclines or chloramphenicol is curative.

2. MARSEILLES FEVER (Boutonneuse Fever)

The conjunctivitis associated with Marseilles fever is ulcerative or granulomatous and associated with a grossly visible preauricular lymph node (Parinaud's oculoglandular syndrome). The conjunctivitis usually precedes the systemic signs and symptoms by 5 or 6 days.

3. ENDEMIC (MURINE) TYPHUS, SCRUB TYPHUS, ROCKY MOUNTAIN SPOTTED FEVER

The conjunctivitis associated with these rickettsial diseases is usually mild, varying from a conjunctival hyperemia with photophobia to a mild catarrhal conjunctivitis.

4. EPIDEMIC TYPHUS

The signs of conjunctivitis in epidemic typhus vary from hyperemia alone to subconjunctival hemorrhages and a low-grade conjunctival inflammation. Small, purplish oval spots appear on the conjunctiva concurrently with the cutaneous manifestations of the disease.

FUNGAL CONJUNCTIVITIS

1. CANDIDAL CONJUNCTIVITIS

Candidal conjunctivitis of the newborn, a rare phenomenon, appears as a white conjunctival plaque that can be mistaken for a pseudomembrane. There is often some exudate. In adults, candidal blepharitis may be accompanied by ulcerative or granulomatous conjunctivitis, which in rare cases may be followed by conjunctival scarring.

Scrapings show a polymorphonuclear cell inflammatory reaction. The organism grows readily on blood agar or Sabouraud's medium and can be readily identified as a budding yeast or, rarely, as pseudohyphae.

The fungus responds to amphotericin B (3–8 mg/mL) in aqueous (not saline) solution, or to applications of nystatin dermatologic cream (100,000 units/g) 4–6 times daily. The ointment must be applied carefully to be sure that it reaches the conjunctival sac and does not just build up on the lid margins.

2. *SPOROTHRIX SCHENCKII* CONJUNCTIVITIS

Occasionally, *S schenckii* invades the conjunctiva alone or in conjunction with granulomatous lesions on the lids. The conjunctival lesion is typically a small, yellow granuloma that may ulcerate. It is associated with a grossly visible preauricular node (Parinaud's oculoglandular syndrome). The lid lesions proceed along the lymphatic chain and gradually ulcerate. The infection usually follows injury or an abrasion with thorns, often barberry bush thorns.

Microscopic examination of a biopsy of the granuloma reveals gram-positive, cigar-shaped conidia (spores). The lesions respond readily to systemic iodides, although in vitro the organism is not iodide-sensitive.

3. *RHINOSPORIDIUM SEEBERI* CONJUNCTIVITIS

R seeberi has many of the characteristics of a fungus but never has been cultivated. The ocular disease it causes may affect the conjunctiva, lacrimal sac, lids, canaliculi, and sclera.

The typical lesion is a polypoid granuloma arising from the upper or lower palpebral or bulbar conjunctiva. It is a painless, soft, pink lesion that sometimes has white spots on its surface. The patient often complains of a small mass that bleeds after minimal trauma. The rest of the conjunctiva appears to be normal, and there is no regional lymphadenopathy.

Histologic examination discloses a granuloma in which there are large spherules that contain myriads of endospores. Treatment is by simple excision of the lesion with cauterization of its base.

4. COCCIDIOIDOMYCOSIS
(San Joaquin Valley Fever)

C immitis may on rare occasions cause a granulomatous conjunctivitis associated with a grossly visible preauricular node (Parinaud's oculoglandular syndrome). There is often a mucopurulent discharge and occasionally a thin, transparent pseudomembrane. The granulomas are raised, indolent, discrete or diffuse, reddish lesions showing tiny areas of focal necrosis. Primary ocular disease has not been recognized; the conjunctivitis is usually only a metastasis from the primary pulmonary infection. In disseminated coccidioidomycosis, the skin (including the skin of the lids) is more frequently affected than the conjunctiva.

The primary disease is an influenzalike illness with fever, malaise, cough, aches and pains, and night sweats. It is more common among dark-skinned than among light-skinned races, with Filipinos especially susceptible. Dissemination follows the rare failure of the body to limit the organism to its primary site.

Low titers of complement-fixing antibodies (less than 1:16) indicate the usually limited spread of the disease; titers over 1:16 suggest widespread dissemination and a poor prognosis.

Histologic examination shows granulomatous lesions with spherules that are thick, doubly refractile, and filled with endospores. A fluffy, cotton-white colony grows on Sabouraud's medium.

Treatment with systemically administered amphotericin B yields the best results in disseminated cases, but transfer factor is now offering promise. In mild cases, only supportive therapy is needed.

PARASITIC CONJUNCTIVITIS

1. ONCHOCERCIASIS

Onchocerciasis is a common cause of blindness in the world today, only less common than such scourges as trachoma and vitamin A deficiency. The disease is a chronic infection with the parasite *O volvulus*. It is endemic in most of tropical Africa and in several countries of Central and South America (Mexico, Guatemala, Venezuela, Colombia). The parasites are transmitted by the bites of infected blackflies of the genus *Simulium,* which breed only in rapidly flowing streams (hence the term "river blindness").

The microfilariae present in the dermis of a human host are ingested by the female *Simulium* when she bites the host in the feeding process. The larvae develop in the fly for 6–12 days. Infective by then, they migrate to the labium and, again in the feeding process, are injected into another human host. In humans, the larvae mature for 12–18 months to form filarial adults that collect in subcutaneous nodules and may live as long as 15 years.

The adult female filaria discharges large numbers of microfilariae, which may migrate to the eye and cause a variety of anterior segment ocular lesions. Live microfilariae have been seen in the anterior chamber, and the eye lesions include conjunctivitis, keratitis, chronic uveitis, cataract, and, rarely, chorioretinitis and optic neuritis. The ocular changes are caused by local invasion of the microfilariae and by the tissue reactions that follow their death.

The disease can be diagnosed by teasing a snip of skin or conjunctiva in saline solution, or by aspirating a nodule and then examining the material for microfilariae.

Treatment with diethylcarbamazine citrate (Hetrazan) can eradicate the filaria, but allergic reactions to the drug and allergic and febrile reactions to the disintegration of the worms often occur and may require use of corticosteroids. Nodulectomy may be of some prophylactic value.

2. *THELAZIA CALIFORNIENSIS* INFECTION

The natural habitat of this roundworm is the eye of the dog, but it can also infest the eyes of cats, sheep, black bears, horses, and deer. Accidental infection of the human conjunctival sac has occurred.

In the dog, the worms usually remain on the surface of the conjunctiva, causing irritation or tearing, but occasionally the corneal epithelium may be abraded. The eggs are laid in the lacrimal duct, conjunctival sac, or nictitating membrane, and the full life cycle may take place in the conjunctival sac and lacrimal apparatus. Transmission to other animals probably requires an intermediate arthropod host such as a fly (eg, *Fannia canicularis* or *Fannia benjamini*).

The disease can be treated effectively by removing the worms from the conjunctival sac with forceps or a cotton-tipped applicator.

3. *LOA LOA* INFECTION

L loa is the eye worm of Africa. It lives in the connective tissue of humans and monkeys, and the monkey may be its reservoir. The adult worm measures up to 55 mm in length. The female deposits the sheathed embryo (microfilaria) in its host's connective tissue, whence it migrates to the bloodstream and is taken up by the horse fly or mango fly as the fly bites its host. After 10 days the filariform larvae have developed, are infective, and are transferred to humans by the bite of the fly. (The fly feeds during the daylight hours only and especially in the middle of the day.)

The worm wanders in the connective tissue of humans for a year while it matures. During this time it may wander into the orbit or under the conjunctiva, sometimes giving pain or a feeling of vermiculation. Subcutaneous migration to the lid has also been seen, and the worm has been found in the anterior chamber, the vitreous, and (rarely) the retina.

Infestation with *L loa* is accompanied by a 60–80% eosinophilia, but diagnosis is made by identifying the worm on removal or by finding microfilariae in blood examined at midday.

Systemic diethylcarbamazine citrate (Hetrazan) is the treatment of choice.

4. *ASCARIS LUMBRICOIDES* INFECTION
(Butcher's Conjunctivitis)

Ascaris may cause a rare type of violent conjunctivitis. When butchers or persons performing postmortem examinations cut tissue containing *Ascaris,* the tissue juice of some of the organisms may hit them in the eye. This can be followed by a violent, toxic, painful conjunctivitis marked by extreme chemosis and lid edema. Treatment consists of rapid and thorough irrigation of the conjunctival sac.

5. *TRICHINELLA SPIRALIS* INFECTION

This parasite does not cause a true conjunctivitis, but in the course of its general dissemination there is often a doughy edema of the upper and lower eyelids, and over 50% of patients have chemosis—a pale, lemon-yellow swelling most marked over the lateral and medial rectus muscles and fading toward the limbus. The chemosis may last a week or more, and there is often pain on movement of the eyes.

The diagnosis is verified by a positive serologic test, a positive skin test, or a positive muscle biopsy. There is always eosinophilia of 10–50%.

The conjunctival aspect of the infection does not require therapy, but thiabendazole may be of value in allaying symptoms and reducing the eosinophilia.

Whether or not systemic corticosteroids should be used is controversial.

6. *SCHISTOSOMA HAEMATOBIUM* INFECTION

This parasitic disease (schistosomiasis, bilharziasis) is endemic in Egypt, especially in the region irrigated by the Nile. Granulomatous conjunctival lesions appearing as small, soft, smooth, pinkish-yellow tumors occur, especially in males. The symptoms are minimal. Diagnosis depends on the microscopic examination of biopsy material, which shows a granuloma containing lymphocytes, plasma cells, giant cells, and eosinophils surrounding the bilharzial ova in various stages of disintegration.

Treatment consists of excision of the conjunctival granuloma and systemic therapy with antimonials such as niridazole.

7. *TAENIA SOLIUM* INFECTION

This parasite occasionally causes conjunctivitis but more often invades the retina, choroid, or vitreous to produce ocular cysticercosis. As a rule, the affected conjunctiva shows a subconjunctival cyst in the form of a localized hemispherical swelling, usually at the inner angle of the lower fornix, which is adherent to the underlying sclera and painful on pressure. The conjunctiva and lid may be inflamed and edematous.

Diagnosis is based on a positive complement fixation or precipitin test or on the demonstration of the organism in the gastrointestinal tract. Eosinophilia is a constant feature.

The best treatment is to excise the lesion. The intestinal condition can be treated by niclosamide.

8. *PTHIRUS PUBIS* INFECTION (Pubic Louse Infection)

P pubis may infest the cilia and margins of the eyelids. Because of its size, the pubic louse seems to require widely spaced hair. For this reason it has a predilection for the widely spaced cilia as well as for pubic hair. The parasites apparently release an irritating substance (probably feces) that produces a toxic follicular conjunctivitis in children and an irritating papillary conjunctivitis in adults. The lid margin is usually red, and the patient may complain of intense itching.

Finding the adult organism or the ova-shaped nits cemented to the eyelashes is diagnostic.

Lindane (gamma benzene hexachloride [Kwell]), 1%, applied to the pubic area and lash margins after mechanical removal of the nits, is usually curative, although any ointment applied to the lid margin tends to smother the adult organisms. The patient's family and close contacts should be examined and treated.

9. FLY LARVA CONJUNCTIVITIS (Ocular Myiasis)

Conjunctival infestation with the larvae of flies (*O ovis,* etc) occurs frequently in the tropics but rarely in the USA. Several species of flies have been incriminated. There is a mild type of larval conjunctivitis (ocular myiasis) in which the larvae are deposited in the conjunctival sac, the fly depositing them by alighting or while in flight. The symptoms are extreme itching, irritation, burning, and lacrimation. The conjunctiva is red and is infested with numerous elongated white larvae, especially in the fornices. The larvae tend to become buried in the depths of the conjunctiva and may escape detection.

Myiasis can also be destructive if the larvae are present in large numbers in compromised patients. If the larvae are numerous enough to convert the orbital tissues into a destructive mass, death may ensue as a result of meningeal involvement, often within 24–48 hours.

Treatment consists of paralyzing the larvae with instillations of 10% cocaine and then removing them mechanically.

10. CATERPILLAR HAIR CONJUNCTIVITIS (Ophthalmia Nodosum)

On rare occasions, caterpillar hairs are introduced into the conjunctival sac, where they produce one or many granulomas (ophthalmia nodosum). Under magnification, each granuloma is seen to contain a small foreign body.

Treatment by removal of each hair individually is effective. If a hair is retained, invasion of the sclera and uveal tract usually occurs.

ATOPIC (ALLERGIC) CONJUNCTIVITIS

I. Immediate (Humoral) Hypersensitivity Reactions

1. HAY FEVER CONJUNCTIVITIS

A mild, nonspecific conjunctival inflammation is commonly associated with hay fever (allergic rhinitis). There is usually a history of allergy to pollens, grasses, animal dander, etc. The patient complains of itching, tearing, and redness of the eyes and often states that his or her eyes seem to be sinking into the surrounding tissue. There is mild injection of the palpebral and bulbar conjunctiva, and during acute attacks there is often severe chemosis (which no doubt explains the concept that the eyes are "sinking into the surrounding tissue"). There may be a small amount of ropy discharge, especially if the patient has been rubbing the eyes. A few eosinophils are found in conjunctival scrapings. There are no conjunctival papillae or follicles.

Treatment consists of the instillation of local vasoconstrictors during the acute phase (epinephrine, 1:1000 solution applied topically, will relieve the chemosis and symptoms within 30 minutes). Cold compresses are helpful to relieve itching, and antihistamines by mouth are of some value. The immediate response to treatment is satisfactory, but recurrences are common unless the antigen is eliminated. Fortunately, the frequency of the attacks and the severity of the symptoms tend to moderate as the patient ages.

2. VERNAL KERATOCONJUNCTIVITIS

This disease, also known as seasonal or warm weather conjunctivitis, is an uncommon bilateral allergic disease that usually begins in the prepubertal years and lasts for 5–10 years. It occurs much oftener in boys than in girls. The identity of the specific allergen or allergens is still a mystery, but patients with vernal keratoconjunctivitis sometimes show other manifestations of allergy known to be related to grass pollen sensitivity. The disease is less common in temperate than in warm climates and is almost nonexistent in cold climates. It is almost always more severe during the spring, summer, and fall than in the winter.

The patient usually complains of extreme itching and a ropy discharge. There is often a family history of allergy (hay fever, eczema, etc) and sometimes in the young patient as well. The conjunctiva has a milky appearance, and there are many fine papillae in the lower tarsal conjunctiva. In "palpebral vernal keratoconjunctivitis," the upper tarsal conjunctiva often has giant papillae that give the conjunctiva a cobblestone appearance (Fig 7–16). Each giant papilla is polygonal, has a flat top, and contains tufts of capillaries.

A stringy conjunctival discharge and a fine, fibrinous pseudomembrane (Maxwell-Lyons sign) may be noted. In some cases, especially in the black race, the most prominent lesions are located at the limbus, where gelatinous swellings (papillae) are noted. The disease is then called **limbal vernal keratoconjunctivitis.** A pseudogerontoxon (arcus) is often noted

in the cornea adjacent to the limbal papillae. Many eosinophils and free eosinophil granules are found in Giemsa-stained smears of the conjunctival exudate.

Micropannus is often seen in both palpebral and limbal vernal keratoconjunctivitis, but total pannus is extremely rare. Conjunctival scarring does not occur unless the patient has been treated with cryotherapy, surgical removal of the papillae, irradiation, or other damaging procedure. Superficial corneal ulcers (oval and located superiorly) may form and may be followed by mild corneal scarring. A characteristic diffuse epithelial keratitis frequently occurs. None of the corneal lesions responds well to standard treatment.

Treatment

Since vernal keratoconjunctivitis is a self-limited disease, it must be recognized that the medication used to treat the symptoms may provide short-term benefit but do long-term harm. Topical and systemic steroids, which relieve the itching, affect the corneal disease only minimally and their side-effects (glaucoma, cataract, and other complications) can be severely damaging. Vasoconstrictors, cold compresses, and ice packs are helpful, and sleeping (if possible, also working) in cool, air-conditioned rooms can keep the patient reasonably comfortable. Probably the best remedy of all is to move to a cool, moist climate. Patients able to do so are benefited if not completely cured.

The severe symptoms of an extremely photophobic patient who is unable to function can often be relieved by a short course of topical or systemic steroids followed by vasoconstrictors and cold packs. As has already been indicated, the prolonged use of steroids must be avoided since it is all too often followed by herpes simplex keratitis, cataract, glaucoma, and fungal and other opportunistic corneal ulcers.

Desensitization to grass pollens and other antigens has not been rewarding. Staphylococcal blepharitis and conjunctivitis are frequent complications and should be treated. Recurrences are the rule, particularly in the spring and summer; but after a number of recurrences the papillae disappear completely, leaving no scars.

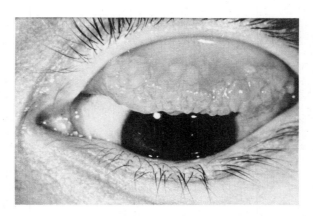

Figure 7–16. Vernal conjunctivitis. "Cobblestone" papillae in superior tarsal conjunctiva. (Courtesy of P Thygeson.)

3. ATOPIC KERATOCONJUNCTIVITIS

Patients with atopic dermatitis (eczema) often also have atopic keratoconjunctivitis. The symptoms and signs are a burning sensation, mucoid discharge, redness, and photophobia. The lid margins are erythematous, and the conjunctiva has a milky appearance. There are fine papillae, but giant papillae are rare; when they occur they are on the lower tarsus (unlike the giant papillae of vernal keratoconjunctivitis, which are on the upper tarsus). Severe corneal signs appear late in the disease after repeated exacerbations of the conjunctivitis. Superficial peripheral keratitis develops and is followed by vascularization. In severe cases, the entire cornea becomes hazy and vascularized, and visual acuity is reduced.

There is usually a history of allergy (hay fever, asthma, or eczema) in the patient or the patient's family. Most patients have had atopic dermatitis since 1 or 2 years of age. Scarring of the flexure creases of the antecubital folds and of the wrists and knees is common. Like the dermatitis with which it is associated, atopic keratoconjunctivitis has a protracted course and is subject to exacerbations and remissions. Like vernal keratoconjunctivitis, it tends to become inactive when the patient reaches the fifth decade.

Scrapings of the conjunctiva show eosinophils, although not nearly so many as are seen in vernal keratoconjunctivitis. Scarring of both the conjunctiva and cornea is often seen, and an atopic cataract, a posterior subcapsular plaque, or an anterior shieldlike cataract may develop. Keratoconus, retinal detachment, and herpes simplex keratitis are all more than usually frequent in patients with atopic keratoconjunctivitis, and there are many cases of secondary bacterial blepharitis and conjunctivitis, usually staphylococcal.

The management of atopic keratoconjunctivitis is often discouraging. Any secondary infection must of course be treated. A short course of topical steroids may relieve symptoms. In advanced cases with severe corneal complications, corneal transplantation may be needed to improve the visual acuity.

4. GIANT PAPILLARY CONJUNCTIVITIS
(Pseudo-Vernal)

A type of giant papillary conjunctivitis with signs and symptoms closely resembling those of vernal conjunctivitis may develop rarely in patients wearing plastic artificial eyes or contact lenses. It is a sensitivity reaction, possibly to components of the plastic leached out by the action of the tears. Use of glass instead of plastic for prostheses and spectacle lenses instead of contact lenses is curative.

II. Delayed (Cellular) Hypersensitivity Reactions

1. PHLYCTENULOSIS

Phlyctenular keratoconjunctivitis is a delayed hypersensitivity response to microbial proteins, including the proteins of the tubercle bacillus, staphylococcus, *Candida albicans, C immitis,* and *C lymphogranulomatis.* Until recently, by far the most frequent cause of phlyctenulosis in the USA was delayed hypersensitivity to the protein of the human tubercle bacillus. This is still the commonest cause in developing countries where tuberculosis is still prevalent. In the USA, however, most cases are now associated with delayed hypersensitivity to *S aureus.*

The conjunctival phlyctenule begins as a small lesion (usually 1–3 mm in diameter) that is hard, red, elevated, and surrounded by a zone of hyperemia. At the limbus it is often triangular in shape, with its apex toward the cornea. In this location it develops a grayish-white center that soon ulcerates and then subsides within 10–12 days. The patient's first phlyctenule and most of the recurrences develop at the limbus, but there may also be bulbar and very rarely even tarsal phlyctenules.

Unlike the conjunctival phlyctenule, which leaves no scar, the corneal phlyctenule develops as an amorphous gray infiltrate and always leaves a scar. Consistent with this difference is the fact that scars form on the corneal side of the limbal lesion and not on the conjunctival side. The result is a triangular scar with its base at the limbus—a valuable sign of old phlyctenulosis when the limbus has been involved.

Conjunctival phlyctenules usually produce only irritation and tearing; it is the typical corneal phlyctenule that is accompanied also by photophobia—severe when the disease is tuberculoprotein-induced and mild when staphylococcus protein-induced. Phlyctenulosis is often triggered by active blepharitis, acute bacterial conjunctivitis, and dietary deficiencies. Acute bacterial conjunctivitis causes hyperemia, which facilitates transfer of the tuberculoprotein to the limbus in large amounts. Phlyctenular scarring (Fig 7–17), which may be minimal or extensive, is often followed by Salzmann's nodular degeneration.

Histologically, the phlyctenule is a focal subepithelial infiltration of small round cells, followed by a preponderance of polymorphonuclear cells when the overlying epithelium necrotizes and sloughs—a sequence of events characteristic of the delayed tuberculin type hypersensitivity reaction.

Phlyctenulosis induced by tuberculoprotein and the proteins of other systemic infections responds dramatically to topical corticosteroids. There is a major reduction of symptoms within 24 hours and disappearance of the lesion in another 24 hours. In contrast, phlyctenulosis induced by the proteins of staphylococcus (from staphylococcal blepharitis) is relatively unresponsive to the corticosteroids. Treatment should be aimed at the underlying disease, and the steroids, when effective, should be used only to

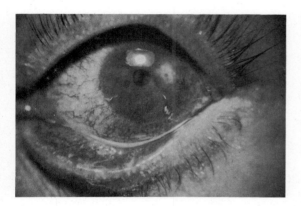

Figure 7–17. Postphlyctenulosis. Vascularized scar in temporal portion of left cornea.

control acute symptoms. A well-balanced diet is most important, and any bacterial conjunctivitis must be controlled. Severe corneal scarring may call for corneal transplantation.

2. MILD CONJUNCTIVITIS SECONDARY TO CONTACT BLEPHARITIS

Contact blepharitis caused by atropine, neomycin, broad-spectrum antibiotics, and other topically applied medications is often followed by a mild infiltrative conjunctivitis that produces hyperemia, mild papillary hypertrophy, a mild mucoid discharge, and some irritation. The examination of Giemsa-stained scrapings often shows only a few degenerated epithelial cells, a few polymorphonuclear and mononuclear cells, and no eosinophils.

Treatment should be directed toward finding the offending agent and eliminating it. The contact blepharitis may clear rapidly in response to topical corticosteroids, but their use should be limited. The long-continued use of steroids on the lids may lead to steroid glaucoma and to skin atrophy with disfiguring telangiectasis.

III. Autoimmune Disease Conjunctivitis

1. KERATOCONJUNCTIVITIS SICCA (Associated With Sjögren's Syndrome)

Sjögren's syndrome is a systemic disease characterized by a triad of disorders: keratoconjunctivitis sicca, xerostomia, and connective tissue dysfunction (arthritis). To establish the diagnosis of Sjögren's syndrome, at least 2 of the 3 disorders must be present. The disease is overwhelmingly more common in women at or beyond the menopause than in others, although men and younger women can also be affected. The lacrimal gland is infiltrated with lymphocytes and occasionally with plasma cells, and this leads to atrophy and destruction of the glandular structures.

Keratoconjunctivitis sicca is characterized by bulbar conjunctival hyperemia and symptoms of irritation that are out of proportion to the mild inflammatory signs. It often begins as a catarrhal conjunctivitis. Blotchy epithelial lesions appear on the cornea, more prominently in its lower half, and filaments may be seen. Pain builds up in the afternoon and evening but is absent or only slight in the morning. The tear film is diminished and often contains shreds of mucus (Fig 7–18).

The diagnosis is confirmed by demonstrating lymphocytic and plasma cell infiltration of the accessory salivary glands in a labial biopsy obtained by means of a simple surgical procedure (Fig 7–19).

Treatment should be directed toward preserving and replacing the tear film with artificial tears, with obliteration of the puncta, and with moisture chambers and Buller shields. As a rule, the more simple things should be tried first.

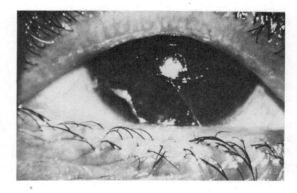

Figure 7–18. Keratoconjunctivitis sicca. (Courtesy of HB Ostler.)

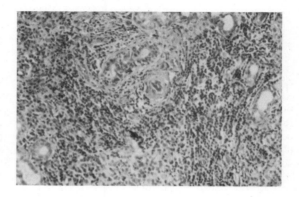

Figure 7–19. Mononuclear infiltration of the accessory salivary glands of a patient with Sjögren's syndrome. (Courtesy of K Tabbara.)

2. PSORIASIS

Psoriasis vulgaris usually affects the areas of the skin not exposed to the sun, but in about 10% of cases lesions appear on the skin of the eyelids, and the plaques may extend to the conjunctiva where they cause irritation, a foreign body sensation, and tearing. Psoriasis can also cause nonspecific chronic conjunctivitis with considerable mucoid discharge. Rarely, the cornea may show marginal ulceration or a deep, vascularized opacity.

The conjunctival and corneal lesions wax and wane with the skin lesions and are not affected by specific treatment. In rare cases, conjunctival scarring (symblepharon, trichiasis), corneal scarring, and occlusion of the nasolacrimal duct have occurred.

3. MUCOUS MEMBRANE PEMPHIGOID
(Ocular Pemphigoid, Cicatricial Pemphigoid)

This disease usually begins as a nonspecific chronic conjunctivitis that is resistant to all forms of therapy. The conjunctiva may be affected alone or in combination with the mouth, nose, esophagus, vulva, and skin. The conjunctivitis leads to progressive scarring and obliteration of the fornices, especially the lower fornix (Fig 7–20). The patient complains of pain, irritation, and blurring of vision. The cornea is affected only secondarily as a result of obliteration of the fornix and lack of the precorneal tear film. The disease is more severe in women than in men. It is typically a disease of middle life, occurring only very rarely before age 45. In women it may progress to blindness in a year or less; in men, progress is slower and spontaneous remission sometimes takes place.

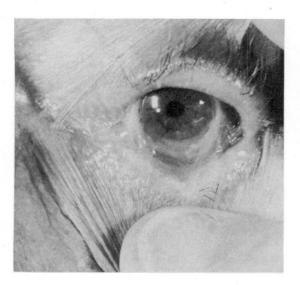

Figure 7–20. Benign mucous membrane pemphigoid. (Courtesy of M Quickert.)

Conjunctival scrapings usually contain a few eosinophils. No specific treatment is available. The course is long and the prognosis poor, with blindness due to complete symblepharon and corneal desiccation the usual outcome.

4. MIDLINE LETHAL GRANULOMA & WEGENER'S GRANULOMATOSIS

Wegener's granulomatosis is a syndrome (assumed to be autoimmune in origin) that is characterized by necrotizing granulomatous lesions, generalized arteritis, and glomerulitis. The glomerulitis differentiates it from midline lethal granuloma. In both diseases there is progressive destruction of the soft tissues and bony structures of the ethmoid region. In Wegener's granulomatosis, the lower part of the respiratory tract may also be affected, and terminally there may be uremia.

In both of these diseases there may be one or more of the following ocular manifestations: exophthalmos, chemosis, exposure keratitis, papillitis by extension of the process into the orbit, episcleritis, scleritis, marginal corneal infiltration and ulceration, uveitis, and retinitis with hemorrhages and cytoid bodies. The typical conjunctival lesions are multiple small granulomas at the limbus.

Steroids and other immunosuppressives appear to reduce the severity of the lesions.

CHEMICAL OR IRRITATIVE CONJUNCTIVITIS

1. IATROGENIC CONJUNCTIVITIS FROM TOPICALLY APPLIED DRUGS

A toxic follicular conjunctivitis or an infiltrative, nonspecific conjunctivitis, followed by scarring, is often produced by the prolonged administration of miotics, idoxuridine, neomycin, and other drugs prepared in toxic or irritating preservatives or vehicles. Silver nitrate instilled into the conjunctival sac at birth (Credé prophylaxis) is a frequent cause of mild chemical conjunctivitis. If tear production is reduced by continual irritation, the conjunctiva can be further damaged by the lack of dilution of the noxious agent as it is instilled into the conjunctival sac.

Conjunctival scrapings often contain keratinized epithelial cells, a few polymorphonuclear neutrophils, and an occasional oddly shaped cell. The treatment is to stop the offending agent and to use bland drops or none at all. Often the conjunctival reaction persists for weeks or months after its source has been eliminated.

2. OCCUPATIONAL CONJUNCTIVITIS FROM CHEMICALS & IRRITANTS

Acids, alkalies, smoke, wind, and almost any irritating substance that enters the conjunctival sac may cause conjunctivitis. Some common irritants are fertilizers, soap, deodorants, hair sprays, tobacco, makeup preparations (mascara, etc), and various acids and alkalies. In certain areas, smog has become the commonest cause of mild chemical conjunctivitis. The specific irritant in smog has not been positively identified, and treatment is nonspecific. There are no permanent ocular effects, but affected eyes are frequently chronically red and irritated.

In acid burns, the acids denature the tissue proteins and the effect is immediate. Alkalies do not denature the proteins but tend to penetrate the tissues deeply and rapidly and to linger in the conjunctival tissue. Here they continue to inflict damage for hours or days, depending on the molar concentration of the alkali and the amount of it introduced. Adhesion between the bulbar and palpebral conjunctivas (symblepharon) and corneal leukoma are more likely to occur if the offending agent is an alkali. In either event, pain, injection, photophobia, and blepharospasm are the principal symptoms of caustic burns. A history of the precipitating event can usually be elicited.

Immediate and profuse irrigation of the conjunctival sac with water or saline solution is of first importance, and any solid material should be removed mechanically. Do not use chemical antidotes. General symptomatic measures include cold compresses for 20 minutes every hour, atropine 1% drops twice daily, and systemic analgesics as necessary. Corneal scarring may require corneal transplantation, and symblepharon may require a plastic operation on the conjunctiva. Severe conjunctival and corneal burns have a poor prognosis even with surgery, but if proper treatment is started immediately, scarring may be minimized and the prognosis improved.

CONJUNCTIVITIS OF UNKNOWN CAUSE

1. FOLLICULOSIS

Folliculosis is a widespread benign, bilateral noninflammatory conjunctival disorder characterized by follicular hypertrophy. It is more common in children than in adults, and the symptoms are minimal. The follicles are more numerous in the lower than in the upper cul-de-sac and tarsal conjunctiva. There is no associated inflammation or papillary hypertrophy, and complications do not occur.

There is no treatment for folliculosis, which disappears spontaneously after a course of 2–3 years. The cause is unknown, but folliculosis may be only a manifestation of a generalized adenoidal hypertrophy.

2. CHRONIC FOLLICULAR CONJUNCTIVITIS (Orphan's Conjunctivitis, Axenfeld's Conjunctivitis)

This is a bilateral transmissible disease of children characterized by numerous follicles in the upper and lower tarsal conjunctivas. There are minimal conjunctival exudates and minimal inflammation but no complications. Treatment is ineffective, but the disease is self-limited within 2 years.

3. OCULAR ROSACEA

Ocular rosacea is an uncommon complication of acne rosacea and occurs more often in light-skinned people, especially of Irish descent, than in dark-skinned people. It is usually a blepharoconjunctivitis, but the cornea is sometimes also affected. The patient complains of mild injection and irritation. There is frequently an accompanying staphylococcal blepharitis. The blood vessels of the lid margins are dilated and the conjunctiva is hyperemic, especially in the exposed interpalpebral region. Less often, there may be a nodular conjunctivitis with small gray nodules on the bulbar conjunctiva, especially near the limbus, which may ulcerate superficially. The lesions can be differentiated from phlyctenules by the fact that even after they subside, the large dilated vessels persist.

Microscopic examination of the nodules shows lymphocytes and epithelial cells. The peripheral cornea may ulcerate and vascularize, and the keratitis may have a narrow base at the limbus and a wider infiltrate centrally. The corneal pannus is often segmented or wedge-shaped inferiorly (Figs 7–21 and 7–22).

Treatment of ocular rosacea consists of the elimination of alcohol and hot, spicy food and drink that cause dilatation of the facial vessels. Any secondary staphylococcal infection should be treated. A course of

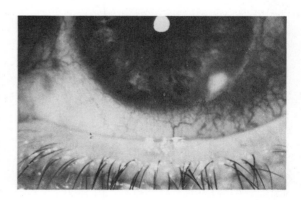

Figure 7–21. Conjunctivitis and corneal infiltrate in a patient with acne rosacea. (Courtesy of HB Ostler.)

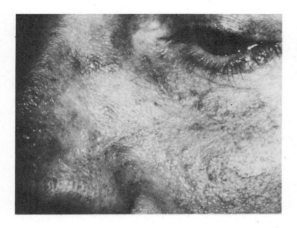

Figure 7–22. Skin lesions in acne rosacea. (Courtesy of HB Ostler.)

oral tetracycline is often helpful and a small maintenance dose may be indicated.

The disease is chronic, recurrences are common, and the response to treatment is usually poor. If the cornea is not affected, the visual prognosis is good; but corneal lesions tend to recur and progress, and the vision grows steadily worse over a period of years.

4. ERYTHEMA MULTIFORME
(Major & Minor)

Erythema multiforme major (Stevens-Johnson syndrome) is a disease of the mucous membranes and skin. The skin lesion is an erythematous, urticarial bullous eruption that appears suddenly and is often distributed symmetrically. Bilateral conjunctivitis, often pseudomembranous, is a common manifesta-

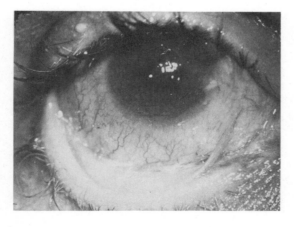

Figure 7–23. Late sequelae of Stevens-Johnson syndrome: conjunctival and corneal cicatrization and epidermalization. (Courtesy of P Thygeson.)

tion. The patient complains of pain, irritation, discharge, and photophobia. The cornea is affected secondarily, and vascularization and scarring may seriously reduce vision. Stevens-Johnson syndrome is typically a disease of young people, occurring only rarely after age 35.

Cultures are negative for bacteria; conjunctival scrapings show a preponderance of polymorphonuclear cells. Systemic steroids are thought to shorten the systemic disease but have little or no effect on the eye lesions. Careful cleansing of the conjunctiva to remove the accumulated secretion is helpful, however, and tear replacement may be indicated. If trichiasis and entropion supervene, they should be corrected. Topical steroids probably have no beneficial effect, and their protracted use can cause corneal melting and perforation.

The acute episode of Stevens-Johnson syndrome usually lasts about 6 weeks, but the conjunctival scarring, loss of tears, and complications from entropion and trichiasis may result in prolonged morbidity and progressive corneal cicatrization (Fig 7–23). Recurrences are rare.

Erythema multiforme minor sometimes complicates a catarrhal conjunctivitis associated with tearing and mucoid discharge. The patient complains of irritation, redness, and discharge. The conjunctivitis is self-limited but may recur when the skin eruption recurs (usually in the spring and fall). Conjunctival scrapings show a polymorphonuclear cell reaction. Bacterial cultures are negative.

The cause is not definitely known, but there is growing evidence that the disease is a hypersensitivity disorder mediated by the deposition of circulating immune complexes in the superficial microvasculature of the skin and mucous membranes. The disease can be triggered by herpes simplex, by antibiotics, and especially by sulfonamides.

Erythema multiforme minor is self-limited, the conjunctiva clearing as the skin lesions clear. Steroids are often used systemically for the skin eruption. In contrast to ocular erythema multiforme major, this minor conjunctivitis does not leave scars and the cornea remains clear.

5. DERMATITIS HERPETIFORMIS

This is an uncommon skin disorder characterized by grouped erythematous, papulovesicular, vesicular, or bullous lesions arranged symmetrically. The disease has a predilection for the posterior axillary fold, the sacral region, the buttocks, and the forearms. Itching is often severe. Rarely, a pseudomembranous conjunctivitis occurs and may result in cicatrization resembling that seen in benign mucous membrane pemphigoid. The skin eruption and conjunctivitis usually respond readily to systemic sulfones or sulfapyridine.

6. EPIDERMOLYSIS BULLOSA

This is a rare hereditary disease characterized by vesicles, bullae, and epidermal cysts. The lesions occur chiefly on the extensor surfaces of the joints and other areas exposed to trauma. The severe dystrophic type that leads to scarring may also produce conjunctival scars similar to those seen in dermatitis herpetiformis and benign mucous membrane pemphigoid. No known treatment is satisfactory.

7. SUPERIOR LIMBIC KERATOCONJUNCTIVITIS

Superior limbic keratoconjunctivitis is usually bilateral and limited to the upper tarsus and upper limbus. The principal complaints are irritation and hyperemia. The signs are papillary hypertrophy of the upper tarsus, redness of the superior bulbar conjunctiva, thickening and keratinization of the superior limbus, epithelial keratitis, recurrent superior filaments, and superior micropannus. Scrapings from the upper limbus show keratinizing epithelial cells.

In about 50% of cases, the condition has been associated with abnormal function of the thyroid gland. Applying 0.5% or 1% silver nitrate to the upper tarsus and allowing the tarsus to drop back onto the upper limbus usually result in shedding of the keratinizing cells and relief of symptoms for 4–6 weeks. This treatment can be repeated. There are no complications, and the disease usually runs a course of 2–4 years.

8. LIGNEOUS CONJUNCTIVITIS

This is a rare bilateral, chronic or recurrent, pseudomembranous or membranous conjunctivitis that arises early in life, most commonly in young girls, and often persists for many years. Granulomas are often associated with it, and the lids may feel very hard. There is no satisfactory treatment.

9. REITER'S SYNDROME

A triad of disease manifestations—nonspecific urethritis, arthritis, and conjunctivitis or iritis—constitutes Reiter's syndrome. The disease occurs much more often in men than in women. The conjunctivitis is papillary in type and usually bilateral. Conjunctival scrapings contain polymorphonuclear cells. No bacteria grow in cultures. The arthritis usually affects the large weight-bearing joints. There is no satisfactory treatment. The disease has been found in association with HLA-B27.

10. MUCOCUTANEOUS LYMPH NODE SYNDROME
(Kawasaki Disease)

This disease of unknown cause was first described in Japan in 1967. Conjunctivitis is one of its 6 diagnostic features. The others are (1) fever that fails to respond to antibiotics; (2) changes in the lips and oral cavity; (3) such changes in the extremities as erythema of the palms and soles, indurative edema, and membranous desquamation of the fingertips; (4) polymorphous exanthem of the trunk; and (5) acute nonpurulent swelling of the cervical lymph nodes.

The disease occurs almost exclusively in prepubertal children and carries a 1–2% mortality rate from cardiac failure. The conjunctivitis has not been severe, and no corneal lesions have been reported.

Treatment is supportive only.

CONJUNCTIVITIS ASSOCIATED WITH SYSTEMIC DISEASE

1. CONJUNCTIVITIS IN THYROID DISEASE

In both thyrotoxic exophthalmos (Graves's disease) and thyrotropic exophthalmos (exophthalmic ophthalmoplegia), the conjunctiva may be red and chemotic and the patient may complain of copious tearing. As the disease progresses the chemosis increases, and in advanced cases the chemotic conjunctiva may extrude between the lids.

Treatment is directed toward control of the thyroid disease, and every effort is made to protect the conjunctiva and cornea by bland ointment, lid adhesions if necessary, or even orbital decompression if the lids do not close enough to cover the cornea and conjunctiva.

2. GOUTY CONJUNCTIVITIS

Patients with gout often complain of a "hot eye" during their attacks. On examination, a mild conjunctivitis is found but is less severe than suggested by the symptoms. Gout may also be associated with episcleritis or scleritis, iridocyclitis, keratitis urica, vitreous opacities, and retinopathy. Treatment is aimed at controlling the gouty attack with colchicine and allopurinol.

3. CARCINOID CONJUNCTIVITIS

In carcinoid, the conjunctiva is sometimes congested and cyanotic as a result of the secretion of serotonin by the chromaffin cells of the gastrointestinal tract. The patient may complain of a "hot eye" during such attacks.

CONJUNCTIVITIS SECONDARY TO DACRYOCYSTITIS OR CANALICULITIS

1. CONJUNCTIVITIS SECONDARY TO DACRYOCYSTITIS

Both pneumococcal conjunctivitis (often unilateral and unresponsive to treatment) and beta-hemolytic streptococcal conjunctivitis (often hyperacute and purulent) may be secondary to chronic dacryocystitis. The nature and source of the conjunctivitis in both instances are often missed until the lacrimal system is investigated.

2. CONJUNCTIVITIS SECONDARY TO CANALICULITIS

Canaliculitis due to *A israelii* or *Candida* sp (or, very rarely, *Aspergillus* sp) may cause unilateral mucopurulent conjunctivitis, often chronic. The source of the condition is often missed unless the characteristic hyperemic, pouting punctum is noted. Expression of the canaliculus (upper or lower, whichever is involved) is curative provided the entire concretion is removed.

Conjunctival scrapings show a predominance of polymorphonuclear cells. Cultures (unless anaerobic) are usually negative. *Candida* grows readily on ordinary culture media, but almost all of the infections are caused by *A israelii*, which requires an anaerobic medium.

DEGENERATIVE DISEASES OF THE CONJUNCTIVA

PINGUECULA

Pinguecula is extremely common in adults. It appears as a yellow nodule on both sides of the cornea

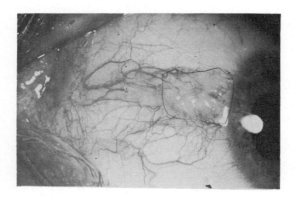

Figure 7–24. Pinguecula. (Courtesy of A Rosenberg.)

(more commonly on the nasal side) in the area of the lid fissure. The nodules, consisting of hyaline and yellow elastic tissue, rarely increase in size, but inflammation is common. No treatment is indicated (Fig 7–24).

PTERYGIUM

Pterygium is a fleshy, bilateral, triangular encroachment of a pinguecula onto the cornea, usually on the nasal side (Fig 7–25). (Pterygiums are often referred to erroneously by patients as cataracts.) It is thought to be an irritative phenomenon due to ultraviolet light since it is common in farmers and sheepherders who spend much of their lives out of doors in sunny, dusty, or sandy, windblown areas. The pathologic findings in the conjunctiva are the same as those of pinguecula. In the cornea there is replacement of Bowman's membrane by the hyaline and elastic tissue.

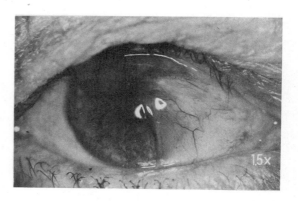

Figure 7–25. Pterygium encroaching on the cornea. (Courtesy of G Mintsioulis.)

If the pterygium is enlarging and encroaches on the pupillary area, it should be removed surgically, along with a small portion of superficial clear cornea beyond the area of corneal encroachment. To prevent recurrences, particularly in people who work out of doors, protective glasses should be prescribed.

MISCELLANEOUS DISORDERS OF THE CONJUNCTIVA

LYMPHANGIECTASIS

Lymphangiectasis is characterized by small, clear, tortuous, localized dilatations in the conjunctiva. They are merely dilated lymph vessels, and no treatment is indicated unless they are irritating or cosmetically objectionable. They can then be cauterized or excised.

CONGENITAL CONJUNCTIVAL LYMPHEDEMA

This is a rare entity, unilateral or bilateral, and characterized by pinkish, fleshy edema of the bulbar conjunctiva. Usually observed as an isolated entity at birth, the condition is thought to be due to a congenital defect in the lymphatic drainage of the conjunctiva. It has been observed in chronic hereditary lymphedema of the lower extremities (Milroy's disease) and is considered an ocular manifestation of this disease rather than an associated anomaly.

CYSTINOSIS

Cystinosis is a rare congenital disorder of amino acid metabolism characterized by a widespread intracellular deposition of cystine crystals in various body tissues, including the conjunctiva and cornea. Three types are recognized: childhood, adolescent, and adult. Life expectancy is reduced in the first 2 types.

SUBCONJUNCTIVAL HEMORRHAGE

This common disorder may occur spontaneously, usually in only one eye, in any age group. Its sudden onset and bright red appearance usually alarm the patient. The hemorrhage is caused by the rupture of a small conjunctival vessel, sometimes preceded by a bout of severe coughing or sneezing.

There is no treatment, and the hemorrhage usually absorbs in 2–3 weeks. The best treatment is reassurance.

In rare instances the hemorrhages are bilateral or recurrent; the possibility of blood dyscrasias should then be ruled out.

OPHTHALMIA NEONATORUM

Ophthalmia neonatorum in its broad sense refers to any infection of the newborn conjunctiva. In its narrow and commonly used sense, however, it refers to a conjunctival infection, chiefly gonococcal, that follows contamination of the baby's eyes during its passage through the mother's cervix and vagina. Since the newborn is a "compromised host," many opportunistic bacteria (and one virus: herpes simplex virus type 2) that are found in the female genital tract are capable of producing disease. For medicolegal reasons, the causes of all cases of ophthalmia neonatorum should be identified in smears of exudate, epithelial scrapings, and cultures.

The time of onset is important in clinical diagnosis since the 2 principal types, gonorrheal ophthalmia and inclusion blennorrhea, have widely differing incubation periods: gonococcal disease 2–3 days and chlamydial disease 5–12 days. The third important birth canal infection (herpes simplex virus type 2 keratoconjunctivitis) has a 2- to 3-day incubation period and is potentially extremely serious because of the possibility of systemic dissemination.

The Credé 1% silver nitrate prophylaxis is effective for the prevention of gonorrheal ophthalmia. (Regrettably, it is not protective against inclusion blennorrhea or herpetic infection.) The slight chemical conjunctivitis induced by silver nitrate is minor and of short duration. Accidents with concentrated solutions can be avoided by using wax ampules specially prepared for Credé prophylaxis. Silver nitrate substitutes, including penicillin and other antibiotics, are under study, and erythromycin ointment appears to be especially promising.

OCULOGLANDULAR DISEASE
(Parinaud's Oculoglandular Syndrome)

This is a group of conjunctival diseases, usually unilateral, characterized by low-grade fever, grossly visible preauricular adenopathy, and one or more conjunctival granulomas (Fig 7–26). The syndrome has a multiplicity of causes: *Mycobacterium tuberculosis, Treponema pallidum, Francisella tularensis, Leptotrichia buccalis, Pasteurella (Yersinia) pseudotuberculosis, C lymphogranulomatis,* * *C immitis,* etc. The type due to *Leptotrichia* infection is by far the most common (90% of cases).

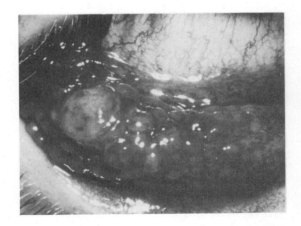

Figure 7–26. Conjunctival granuloma. (Courtesy of P Thygeson.)

Leptotrichosis Conjunctivae
(Common Parinaud's Conjunctivitis)

This protracted but benign granulomatous conjunctivitis is found most commonly in children who have been in intimate contact with cats. *Leptotrichia,* a common inhabitant of the human mouth, is constant in the mouth of the cat. Salivary contamination of the child's conjunctiva, by fingers or by cat drool on the

*See box on p 64.

child's pillow, is thought to be the usual mode of infection. The child has no systemic symptoms but runs a low-grade fever and develops a reasonably enlarged preauricular node and one or more conjunctival granulomas. These may show focal necrosis and may sometimes ulcerate. The filamentous organisms can be seen in biopsies of the necrotic areas when stained by Gram's tissue stain or other microbe stains.

Treatment consists of excision of the conjunctival nodule, which in the case of the solitary granuloma may in itself be curative. The disease is self-limited (without corneal or other complications) in 2–3 months, but systemic broad-spectrum antibiotics slightly shorten the course. The regional adenopathy does not suppurate.

Conjunctivitis Secondary to Neoplasms (Masquerade Syndrome)

When examined superficially, a neoplasm of the conjunctiva or lid margin is often misdiagnosed as a chronic infectious conjunctivitis or keratoconjunctivitis. Since the underlying lesion is often not recognized, the condition has been referred to as masquerade syndrome. The masquerading neoplasms on record are conjunctival capillary carcinoma, conjunctival carcinoma in situ, molluscum contagiosum, infectious papilloma of the conjunctiva, and verruca. Verruca and molluscum tumors of the lid margin may desquamate toxic tumor material that produces a chronic conjunctivitis, keratoconjunctivitis, or (rarely) keratitis alone.

• • •

References

Allansmith MR et al: Density of goblet cells in vernal conjunctivitis and contact lens-associated giant papillary conjunctivitis. *Arch Ophthalmol* 1981;**99**:884.

Allansmith MR et al: Giant papillary conjunctivitis in contact lens wearers. *Am J Ophthalmol* 1977;**83**:697.

Armstrong JH, Zacarias F, Rein MF: Ophthalmia neonatorum: A chart review. *Pediatrics* 1976;**57**:884.

Baker DA, Phillips A: Fatal hand-foot-and-mouth disease in an adult caused by coxsackievirus A7. *JAMA* 1979;**242**:1065.

Dawson CR: Epidemic Koch-Weeks conjunctivitis and trachoma in the Coachella Valley of California. *Am J Ophthalmol* 1960; **49**:801.

Dawson CR et al: Adenovirus type 8 keratoconjunctivitis in the United States. 3. Epidemiologic, clinical, and microbiologic features. *Am J Ophthalmol* 1970;**69**:473.

Dawson CR et al: Severe endemic trachoma in Tunisia. *Br J Ophthalmol* 1976;**60**:245.

Fahmy JA, Moller S, Bentzon MW: Bacterial flora of the normal conjunctiva. 1. Topographical distribution. *Acta Ophthalmol* 1974;**52**:786.

Forstot SL et al: Serologic studies in patients with keratoconjunctivitis sicca. *Arch Ophthalmol* 1981;**99**:888.

Friedlaender M, Allansmith MR: Ocular allergy. *Ann Ophthalmol* 1975;**7**:1171.

Hales RH, Ostler HB: Newcastle disease conjunctivitis with subepithelial infiltrates. *Br J Ophthalmol* 1973;**57**:694.

Kazmierowski JA, Wuepper KD: Erythema multiforme: Clinical spectrum and immunopathogenesis. *Springer Semin Immunopathol* 1981;**4**:45.

Kiernan JP et al: Stevens-Johnson syndrome. *Am J Ophthalmol* 1981;**92**:543.

Meisler DM et al: Giant papillary conjunctivitis. *Am J Ophthalmol* 1981;**92**:368.

Nirankari VS et al: Superoxide radical scavenging agents in treatment of alkali burns. *Arch Ophthalmol* 1981;**99**:886.

O'Day DM et al: Clinical and laboratory evaluation of epidemic keratoconjunctivitis due to adenovirus types 8 and 19. *Am J Ophthalmol* 1976;**81**:207.

Ostler HB: Acute chemotic reaction to cromolyn. *Arch Ophthalmol* 1982;**100**:412.

Ostler HB, Conant MA, Groundwater J: Lyell's disease, the Stevens-Johnson syndrome, and exfoliative dermatitis. *Trans Am Acad Ophthalmol Otolaryngol* 1970;**74**:1254.

Ostler HB, Lanier JD: Phlyctenular keratoconjunctivitis with special reference to the staphylococcal type. *Trans Pac Coast Otoophthalmol Soc* 1974;**55**:237.

Salvaggio JE (editor): Primer on allergic and immunologic diseases. *JAMA* 1982;**248**:2579. [Special issue.]

Scheie HG et al: Onchocerciasis (ocular). *Ann Ophthalmol* 1971;**3**:697.

Sjögren H: Keratoconjunctivitis sicca and the Sjögren syndrome. *Surv Ophthalmol* 1971;**16**:145.

Sommer A et al: Nutritional factors in corneal xerophthalmia and keratomalacia. *Arch Ophthalmol* 1982;**100**:399.

Stenson S, Newman R, Fedukowicz H: Conjunctivitis in the newborn: Observations on incidence, cause, and prophylaxis. *Ann Ophthalmol* 1981;**13**:329.

Tabbara KF et al: Sjögren's syndrome: A correlation between ocular findings and labial salivary gland histology. *Trans Am Acad Ophthalmol Otolaryngol* 1974;**78**:467.

Tarr KH et al: Late complications of pterygium treatment. *Br J Ophthalmol* 1980;**64**:496.

Thatcher RW, Pettit TH: Gonorrheal conjunctivitis. *JAMA* 1971;**215**:1494.

Theodore FH: Conjunctival carcinoma masquerading as chronic conjunctivitis. *Eye Ear Nose Throat Mon* (Nov) 1967; **46**:1419.

Thompson TR, Swanson RE, Wiesner PJ: Gonococcal ophthalmia neonatorum. *JAMA* 1974;**228**:186.

Thygeson P: Historical review of oculogenital disease. *Am J Ophthalmol* 1971;**71**:975.

Thygeson P: Observations on conjunctival neoplasms masquerading as chronic conjunctivitis or keratitis. *Trans Am Acad Ophthalmol Otolaryngol* 1969;**73**:969.

Thygeson P, Dawson CR: Pseudotrachoma caused by molluscum contagiosum virus and various chemical irritants. Page 1894 in: *Proceedings of the 21st International Congress of Ophthalmology, 1970.* Excerpta Medica International Series, No. 222. Elsevier, 1971.

Thygeson P, Dawson CR: Trachoma and follicular conjunctivitis in children. *Arch Ophthalmol* 1966;**75**:3.

Whitcher JP et al: Acute hemorrhagic conjunctivitis in Tunisia. *Arch Ophthalmol* 1976;**94**:51.

Zaidman GW et al: Phlyctenular keratoconjunctivitis. *Am J Ophthalmol* 1981;**92**:178.

ANATOMY

The cornea is a transparent avascular tissue comparable in size and structure to the crystal of a small wristwatch. It is inserted into the sclera at the limbus. At the scleral junction there is a circumferential depression called the scleral sulcus. The cornea functions as a refracting and protective membrane and a "window" through which light rays pass en route to the retina. It has a refractive power equavalent to a +43 diopter lens.

The average adult cornea is 0.8–1 mm thick at the periphery, 0.6 mm thick in the center, and 11.5 mm in diameter. From anterior to posterior, it has 5 distinct layers (Fig 8–1): the epithelium (which is continuous with the epithelium of the bulbar conjunctiva), Bowman's layer, the stroma, Descemet's membrane, and the endothelium. The epithelium has 5 or 6 layers of cells, the endothelium only one. Bowman's membrane is a clear acellular layer, a modified portion of the

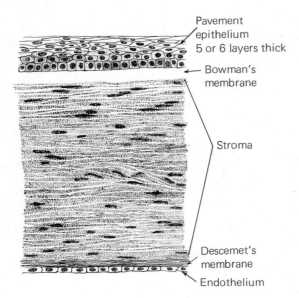

Figure 8–1. Transverse section of cornea. (Reproduced, with permission, from Wolff E: *Anatomy of the Eye and Orbit,* 4th ed. Blakiston-McGraw, 1954.)

Pavement epithelium 5 or 6 layers thick

Bowman's membrane

Stroma

Descemet's membrane

Endothelium

stroma. Descemet's membrane is a clear elastic membrane that can be seen to comprise many fine fibers when subjected to high magnification with the electron microscope. The corneal stroma accounts for about 90% of the corneal thickness. It is composed of intertwining lamellar fibers about 1 μm wide that run almost the full diameter of the cornea. They run parallel to the surface of the cornea and by virtue of their size and periodicity are optically clear. Each lamella possesses a flattened nucleus.

The source of the cornea's nutrition is the limbus, where nutritional elements pass from the vascular limbus through the avascular cornea. The superficial cornea also gets some of its oxygen from the atmosphere. The sensory nerves of the cornea are supplied by the first division of the fifth (trigeminal) cranial nerve. In the corneal epithelium there is a rich network of nerve fibers with bare ends. Whenever they are exposed, they produce a sensation of pain. The large number of nerves and the location of their endings account for the severe pain that results from even minor abrasions of the corneal epithelium.

The transparency of the cornea is due to its uniform structure, avascularity, and deturgescence. Deturgescence, or the state of relative dehydration of the corneal tissue, is maintained by the active Na^+-K^+ cell "pump" of the endothelium and epithelium and by their anatomic integrity. The endothelium is more important than the epithelium in the mechanism of dehydration, and chemical or physical damage to the endothelium is far more serious than damage to the epithelium. Destruction of the endothelial cells may cause marked swelling of the cornea and some loss of transparency. On the other hand, damage to the epithelium causes only slight transient, localized swelling of the corneal stroma that clears when the epithelial cells regenerate. Evaporation of water from the precorneal tear film produces hypertonicity of the film, which may be an important factor in drawing water from the corneal stroma and helps to maintain the state of dehydration.

The penetration of drugs into the intact cornea is biphasic. Fat-soluble substances can pass through intact epithelium, and water-soluble substances can pass through intact stroma. To pass through the cornea, drugs must therefore have both a fat-soluble and a water-soluble phase.

Corneal Resistance to Infection

The epithelium is a reliable barrier to the entrance of microorganisms into the cornea. Once the epithelium is traumatized, however, the avascular stroma and Bowman's layer become excellent culture media for a variety of organisms, particularly *Pseudomonas aeruginosa*. Descemet's membrane resists most bacteria but is not a barrier to fungi. *Streptococcus pneumoniae* (the pneumococcus) is the only true bacterial corneal pathogen; all others are opportunistic pathogens that require a heavy inoculum or a compromised host (eg, traumatized epithelium) to produce infection.

In the early days of ophthalmology, almost all bacterial ulcers were due to pneumococci and all fungal ulcers occurred in an agricultural setting. Since the advent of the corticosteroids in 1952, many bacterial ulcers are due to opportunists, and fungal ulcers are an urban as well as an agricultural disease. The misuse of local corticosteroid drops modifies the acute inflammatory reaction (the second line of defense against infection) and allows the fungal invader to flourish.

Moraxella liquefaciens, which occurs mainly in alcoholics (as a result of pyridoxine depletion), is a classic example of the bacterial opportunist, and in recent years a number of new bacterial corneal opportunists have been identified. Among them are *Serratia marcescens, Mycobacterium fortuitum, Streptococcus viridans, Staphylococcus epidermidis,* and various coliform and *Proteus* organisms.

PHYSIOLOGY OF SYMPTOMS

Since the cornea has many pain fibers, most corneal lesions, superficial or deep (corneal foreign body, corneal abrasion, phlyctenule, interstitial keratitis), cause pain and photophobia. The pain is worsened by movement of the lids (particularly the upper lid) over the cornea and usually persists until healing occurs. Since the cornea serves as the window of the eye and refracts light rays, corneal lesions usually blur vision somewhat, especially if centrally located.

Photophobia in corneal disease is the result of painful contraction of a hyperemic iris. Dilatation of iris vessels is a reflex phenomenon caused by irritation of the corneal nerve endings. Photophobia, severe in most corneal disease, is minimal in herpetic keratitis because of the hypesthesia associated with the disease, which is also a valuable diagnostic sign.

Although tearing and photophobia commonly accompany corneal disease, there is usually no discharge except in purulent bacterial ulcers.

INVESTIGATION OF CORNEAL DISEASE

Symptoms & Signs

The physician examines the cornea by inspecting it under adequate illumination. Examination is often facilitated by instillation of a local anesthetic. Fluorescein staining can outline a superficial epithelial lesion that might otherwise be impossible to see. The loupe and slit lamp are helpful but not absolutely essential aids; adequate illumination can be achieved with a hand flashlight. One should follow the course of the light reflex while moving the light carefully over the entire cornea. Rough areas indicative of epithelial defects are demonstrated in this way.

The patient's history is important in corneal disease. A history of trauma can often be elicited—in fact, foreign bodies and abrasions are the 2 most common corneal lesions. A history of corneal disease may also be of value. The keratitis of herpes simplex infection is often recurrent, but since recurrent erosion is extremely painful and herpetic keratitis is not, these disorders can be differentiated by their symptoms. The patient's use of local medications should be investigated, since corticosteroids may have been used and may have predisposed to bacterial, fungal, or viral disease, especially herpes simplex keratitis.

Laboratory Studies

To select the proper therapy for corneal infections, especially hypopyon ulceration, laboratory aid is essential. Bacterial and fungal ulcers, for example, require completely different medications. Since a few hours' delay in determining the cause may severely prejudice the ultimate visual result, scrapings from the ulcer should be stained by both Gram's and Giemsa's stains and the infecting organism identified presumptively while the patient waits. Appropriate therapy can then be instituted immediately. Cultures for bacteria and fungi should be started at the same time, but therapy should not be withheld while awaiting confirmation of the presumptive diagnosis.

Morphologic Diagnosis of Corneal Lesions

A. Subepithelial Keratitis: Table 8–1 lists a number of important types of subepithelial lesions. These are often secondary to epithelial keratitis (eg, the nummular lesions of epidemic keratoconjunctivitis, caused by adenoviruses 8 and 19). They can usually be observed grossly but may also be recog-

Table 8–1. Subepithelial keratitis.

Types of keratitis with round, discrete, subepithelial opacities:
1. Nummular keratitis (Padi keratitis of the Orient).
2. Epidemic keratoconjunctivitis.
3. Nummular opacities in wearers of soft contact lenses.
4. Nummular opacities in zoster keratitis.
5. Nummular opacities in congenital syphilitic keratitis.

nized in the course of biomicroscopic examination of epithelial keratitis.

B. Epithelial Keratitis: The corneal epithelium is involved in most types of conjunctivitis and keratitis and in rare cases may be the only tissue involved (eg, in superficial punctate keratitis). The epithelial changes vary widely from simple edema and vacuolation to minute erosions, filament formation, partial keratinization, etc. The lesions vary also in their location on the cornea. All of these variations have incalculable diagnostic significance (Table 8–2), and biomicroscopic examination with and without fluorescein staining should be a part of every external eye examination.

CORNEAL ULCERATION

Cicatrization due to corneal ulceration is a major cause of blindness and impaired vision throughout the world. Most of this visual loss is preventable, but only if an etiologic diagnosis is made early and appropriate therapy instituted. Hypopyon ulcer, the most important type, was once caused almost exclusively by the pneumococcus *(S pneumoniae),* the only true bacterial pathogen that attacks the cornea. In recent years, however, as a result of the widespread use of compromising systemic and local medications (at least in the developed countries), opportunistic bacteria, fungi, and viruses have tended to cause more cases of corneal ulcer than the pneumococcus.

CENTRAL CORNEAL ULCERS
(Hypopyon Ulcer)

Central ulcers are infectious ulcers that follow epithelial damage. The break in the epithelium may be peripheral, but the ulcer always migrates toward the center of the cornea, away from the vascularized limbus. Hypopyon usually (not always) accompanies the ulcer. It is almost always sterile in bacterial ulcers and often contains fungal elements in fungal ulcers. The pneumococcus, historically the chief cause of hypopyon ulcer, is pathogenic, even in small numbers, for an exposed corneal stroma. If the opportunists are to cause disease, one of 2 conditions must be met: The host must have been topically immunosuppressed by anesthetics, cytotoxic drugs, or a corticosteroid preparation, or must have received an overwhelming inoculum. (This would be the case, for example, if a fluorescein solution heavily contaminated with *P aeruginosa* were instilled into an eye.)

Many types of bacterial corneal ulcer look alike and vary only in severity. This is especially true of ulcers caused by opportunistic bacteria (eg, alpha-hemolytic streptococci, *Staphylococcus aureus,* *Nocardia,* and *M fortuitum*), which cause indolent corneal ulcers that tend to spread slowly and superficially.

Pneumococcal Corneal Ulcer
(Acute Serpiginous Ulcer)

The pneumococcus should still be regarded as the only microorganism that is a true corneal pathogen. In some populations (eg, the Indians of the Southwestern USA), it is almost the only bacterial cause of corneal ulcer. Before the popularization of dacryocystorhinostomy, pneumococcal ulcers often occurred in coal miners or others subjected to frequent corneal abrasions that became secondarily infected from an already infected tear sac.

Pneumococcal corneal ulcer usually occurs 24–48 hours after inoculation of an abraded cornea. It typically produces a gray, fairly well circumscribed ulcer that tends to spread erratically from the original site of infection toward the center of the cornea (Fig 8–2). The advancing border shows active ulceration and infiltration as the trailing border begins to heal. (This creeping effect suggested the term "acute serpiginous ulcer.") The superficial corneal layers become involved first and then the deep parenchyma. The cornea surrounding the ulcer is often clear.

A hypopyon of moderate size usually forms. Hypopyon is a collection of inflammatory cells, predominantly polymorphonuclear neutrophilic leukocytes with some mononuclear cells and macrophages, and is characteristic of both bacterial and fungal central corneal ulcers. Although hypopyon is sterile in bacterial corneal ulcers unless there has been a rupture of Descemet's membrane, in fungal ulcers it often contains fungal elements; this is because fungi can penetrate an intact Descemet membrane.

Scrapings from the leading edge of a pneumococcal corneal ulcer contain gram-positive lancet-shaped diplococci. Drugs recommended for use in treatment are listed in Tables 8–3 and 8–4. Concurrent dacryocystitis should also be treated.

Pseudomonas Corneal Ulcer

Pseudomonas corneal ulcer begins as a gray or yellow infiltrate at the site of break in the corneal epithelium (Fig 8–3). Severe pain usually accompanies it. The lesion tends to spread rapidly in all

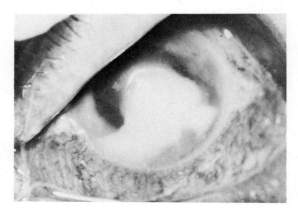

Figure 8–2. Pneumococcal corneal ulcer with hypopyon.

Table 8—2. Principal types of epithelial keratitis
(in order of frequency of occurrence).

Minute fluorescein-staining erosions; lower third of cornea affected predominantly.	Typically dendritic (occasionally round or oval) with edema and degeneration.	More diffuse than lesions of HSK; occasionally linear (pseudodendrites).
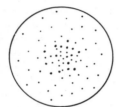	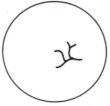	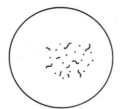
1. Staphylococcal keratitis	2. Herpetic keratitis (HSK)	3. Varicella-zoster keratitis
Minute fluorescein-staining erosions; diffuse but most conspicuous in pupillary area.	Minute pleomorphic, fluorescein-staining, damaged epithelium and erosions; epithelial and mucous filaments are typical; lower half of cornea affected predominantly.	Minute fluorescein-staining, irregular erosions; lower half of cornea affected predominantly.
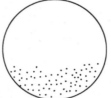	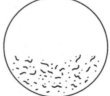	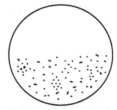
4. Adenovirus keratitis	5. Keratitis of Sjögren's syndrome	6. Exposure keratitis—due to lagophthalmos or exophthalmos
Blotchy gray, opaque, syncytiumlike lesions, most conspicuous in upper pupillary area. Sometimes a plaque of opaque epithelium forms.	Blotchy epithelial edema; diffuse but predominant in palpebral fissure, 9—3 o'clock.	Minute fluorescein-staining erosions with spotty cellular edema; highly characteristic picture.
		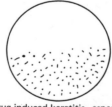
7. Vernal keratoconjunctivitis	8. Trophic keratitis—sequela of herpes simplex, herpes zoster, and gasserian ganglion destruction	9. Drug-induced keratitis—especially by broad-spectrum antibiotics
Foci of edematous epithelial cells, round or oval; elevated when disease is active.	Minute fluorescein-staining erosions of upper third of cornea; filaments during exacerbations; bulbar hyperemia, thickened limbus, micropannus.	Virus-type lesions like those of SPK; in pupillary area.
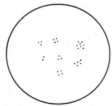	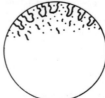	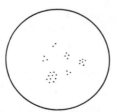
10. Superficial punctate keratitis (SPK)	11. Superior limbic keratoconjunctivitis	12. Rubeola, rubella, and mumps keratitis

Table 8—2 (cont'd). Principal types of epithelial keratitis
(in order of frequency of occurrence).

Minute fluorescein-staining epithelial erosions affecting upper third of cornea. 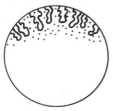 13. Trachoma	Spotty gray opacification of individual epithelial cells due to partial keratinization; associated with Bitot's spots. 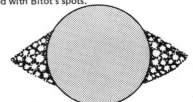 14. Vitamin A deficiency keratitis

directions because of the proteolytic enzymes produced by the organisms. Although usually superficial at first, the ulcer may affect the entire cornea. There is often a large hypopyon that tends to increase in size as the ulcer progresses. The infiltrate and exudate may have a bluish-green color. This is due to a pigment produced by the organism and is pathognomonic of *P aeruginosa* infection.

Pseudomonas ulcer often arises from the use of a contaminated fluorescein solution or from contaminated medications used either to examine or to treat a corneal abrasion or injury. Such infections must be considered iatrogenic and are to be deplored. It is mandatory that the clinician use sterile medications and a sterile technique when caring for patients with corneal injuries.

Scrapings from the ulcer contain long, thin gram-negative rods that are often few in number. Drugs recommended for use in treatment are listed in Tables 8—3 and 8—4.

Moraxella liquefaciens Corneal Ulcer

M liquefaciens (diplobacillus of Petit) causes an

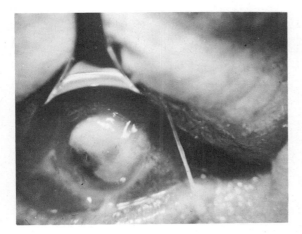

Figure 8—3. *Pseudomonas* corneal ulcer of right eye. Evisceration was done.

indolent oval ulcer that usually affects the inferior cornea and progresses into the deep stroma over a period of days. There is usually no hypopyon or only a small one, and the surrounding cornea is usually clear. *M liquefaciens* ulcer almost always occurs in a patient with alcoholism, diabetes, or other immunosuppressing disease. Scrapings contain large, square-ended gram-negative diplobacilli. Drugs recommended for use in treatment are listed in Tables 8—3 and 8—4.

Streptococcus pyogenes Corneal Ulcer

Central corneal ulcers caused by beta-hemolytic streptococci have no identifying features. The surrounding corneal stroma is often infiltrated and edematous, and there is usually a moderately large hypopyon. Scrapings contain gram-positive cocci in chains. Drugs recommended for use in treatment are listed in Tables 8—3 and 8—4.

Klebsiella pneumoniae Corneal Ulcer

The corneal ulcer caused by *K pneumoniae* is usually indolent and often without a hypopyon. There may be edema of the surrounding stroma, and scrapings contain gram-negative rods with capsules. Drugs recommended for use in treatment are listed in Tables 8—3 and 8—4.

Staphylococcus aureus, Staphylococcus epidermidis, & Streptococcus viridans Corneal Ulcers

Central corneal ulcers caused by these organisms are now being seen more often than formerly, most of them in corneas compromised by topical corticosteroids. The ulcers are often indolent but may be associated with hypopyon and some surrounding corneal infiltration. They are often superficial, and the ulcer bed feels firm when scraped. Scrapings contain gram-positive cocci—singly, in pairs, or in chains. Drugs recommended for use in treatment are listed in Tables 8—3 and 8—4.

Mycobacterium fortuitum & *Nocardia* Corneal Ulcers

Ulcers due to *M fortuitum* and *Nocardia* are rare. They often follow trauma and are often associated with

Table 8–3. Treatment of corneal ulceration.

Organisms	Drug Route	First Choice	Recommended Drugs Second Choice	Third Choice
Gram-positive cocci: lancet-shaped with capsule = pneumococcus	Topical	Erythromycin	Bacitracin	Vancomycin
	Subconjunctival[1]	Penicillin G	Cephaloridine or lincomycin	Erythromycin or methicillin
	Systemic[2]	Penicillin G	Cefazolin	Oral: Erythromycin
Other gram-positive organisms: cocci and rods	Topical	Erythromycin	Bacitracin	Gentamicin or vancomycin
	Subconjunctival	Methicillin and gentamicin	Cephaloridine and gentamicin	Vancomycin and methicillin
	Systemic	Nafcillin	Cefazolin	Oral: Erythromycin
Gram-negative cocci[3]	Topical	Erythromycin	Bacitracin	Gentamicin or vancomycin
	Subconjunctival	Methicillin and gentamicin	Gentamicin and cefazolin	Erythromycin and methicillin
	Systemic	Nafcillin	Cefazolin	Oral: Erythromycin
Gram-negative rods (thin = *Pseudomonas*)	Topical	Polymyxin B	Colistin	Gentamicin or carbenicillin
	Subconjunctival	Tobramycin	Gentamicin	Polymyxin B, colistin, or carbenicillin
	Systemic	...	...	...
Gram-negative rods: large, square-ended diplobacilli = *Moraxella*	Topical	Gentamicin	Sodium sulfacetamide	Zinc sulfate or chloramphenicol
	Subconjunctival	Rarely necessary	...	...
	Systemic	...	...	...
Other gram-negative rods	Topical	Gentamicin	Carbenicillin	Chloramphenicol and streptomycin
	Subconjunctival	Gentamicin and carbenicillin	Gentamicin and cephaloridine	Carbenicillin and cephaloridine
	Systemic	Ampicillin	Cefazolin	Carbenicillin
Gram-positive rods: slender and varying in length = *Mycobacterium fortuitum*, *Nocardia* sp, *Actinomyces* sp	Topical	Sodium sulfacetamide	Sodium sulfacetamide	Tetracycline
	Subconjunctival	Streptomycin	Streptomycin	...
	Systemic	Oral: Sulfonamides[4]	Oral: Tetracycline[4]	...
Yeastlike organisms = *Candida* sp[5]	Topical	Amphotericin B and flucytosine	Natamycin and flucytosine	Nystatin or miconazole
	Subconjunctival	Amphotericin B	Amphotericin B	...
	Systemic	Oral: Flucytosine	...	...
Hyphaelike organisms = fungal ulcer	Topical	Natamycin	Amphotericin B	Miconazole
	Subconjunctival	Amphotericin B	...	...
	Systemic	...	...	...
No organisms identified; ulcer suggestive of bacterial type	Topical	Polymyxin B and bacitracin	Gentamicin and erythromycin	Colistin and vancomycin
	Subconjunctival	Gentamicin and methicillin	Penicillin G and colistin	Cephaloridine and polymyxin B
	Systemic	Penicillin G	Nafcillin	Cefazolin
No organisms identified; ulcer suggestive of fungal type	Topical	Natamycin	Amphotericin B	Miconazole
	Subconjunctival	Rarely necessary: Amphotericin B	...	...
	Systemic	...	...	...

[1] Subconjunctival.

[2] Intravenous unless otherwise stated; only when ulcer is severe.

[3] Ulcer associated with hyperacute conjunctivitis (eg, gonococcal conjunctivitis) should be treated with same drug used to treat the conjunctivitis.

[4] These 2 drugs often act synergistically.

[5] Rarely, *Pityrosporum ovale* or *Pityrosporum orbiculare* may be confused with *Candida* sp.

Table 8–4. Drug concentrations and dosages for treatment of corneal ulceration.

Drug	Topical*	Subconjunctival*	Systemic* (intravenous unless otherwise indicated)
Amphotericin B	1.5–3.0 mg/mL	750 μg/mL/dose every other day	...
Ampicillin	...	...	150–200 mg/kg body wt/d in 4 doses
Bacitracin	10,000 units/mL		
Carbenicillin	4 mg/mL	125 mg/0.5 mL/dose	100–200 mg/kg body wt/d in 4 doses
Cefazolin	...	100 mg/0.5 mL/dose	15 mg/kg body wt/d in 4 doses
Cephaloridine	...	100 mg/0.5 mL/dose	...
Chloramphenicol	5 mg/mL	...	...
Colistin	1.5–3.0 mg/mL	25 mg/0.5 mL/dose	...
Erythromycin	5 mg/g (ointment)	100 mg/0.5 mL/dose	Oral: first dose 1 g; then 0.5 g every 6 h
Flucytosine	1% solution	...	Oral: 200 mg/kg body wt/d in 4 doses
Gentamicin	3–8 mg/mL	20 mg/0.5 mL/dose	...
Lincomycin	...	300 mg/mL; dose: 0.25–0.33 mL	...
Methicillin	...	100 mg/mL; dose: 0.5–1 mL	...
Miconazole	1% solution or 2% ointment	...	...
Nafcillin	...	...	1 g every 4–6 h
Natamycin (pimaricin)	4% or 5% suspension	...	...
Nystatin	100,000 units/g (ointment)	...	...
Penicillin G	10,000–20,000 units/mL	1 million units/mL/dose	40,000–50,000 units/kg body wt/d in 4 doses or continuously
Polymyxin B	17,000 units/mL	10 mg/mL/dose	...
Sodium sulfacetamide	10% solution	...	...
Streptomycin	50 mg/mL	40–50 mg/mL/dose	...
Sulfonamides	...	...	Oral: 70 mg/kg body wt/d in 4 doses, or 4 g, whichever is less
Tetracycline	5 mg/mL	...	Oral: 1.5 g/d in 4 doses for patients under 70 kg; 2 g/d if over 70 kg
Tobramycin	...	20 mg/0.5 mL/dose	...
Vancomycin	50 mg/mL	100 mg/mL; dose: 0.25 mL	...
Zinc sulfate	0.5 mg/mL	...	...

*Treatment schedule: Topical: Every hour during day, every 2 hours during night, for 5 days. Subconjunctival: One injection daily for 4 days unless otherwise stated; in exceptionally severe cases, initial dose sometimes repeated after 12 hours. Systemic, intravenous, or oral: One dose daily for 5 days.

contact with soil. The ulcers are indolent, and the bed of the ulcer often has radiating lines that make it look like a cracked windshield. Hypopyon may or may not be present. Scrapings may contain acid-fast slender rods *(M fortuitum)* or gram-positive filamentous, often branching organisms *(Nocardia)*. Drugs recommended for use in treatment are listed in Tables 8–3 and 8–4.

FUNGAL CORNEAL ULCERS

Fungal corneal ulcers, once seen only in agricultural workers, have become relatively common in the urban population since the introduction of the corticosteroid drugs for use in ophthalmology in 1952. Before the corticosteroid era, fungal corneal ulcers occurred only if an overwhelming inoculum of organisms was introduced into the corneal stroma—an event that can still take place in an agricultural setting. The uncompromised cornea seems to be able to handle the small inocula to which urban residents are ordinarily subjected.

Fungal ulcers are indolent and have a gray infiltrate, often a hypopyon, marked inflammation of the globe, superficial ulceration, and satellite lesions (usually infiltrates at sites distant from the main area of ulceration) (Fig 8–4). The principal lesion—and often the satellite lesions as well—is an endothelial plaque with irregular edges underlying the principal corneal lesions, associated with a severe anterior chamber reaction and a corneal abscess.

Most fungal ulcers are caused by opportunists such as *Candida, Fusarium, Aspergillus, Penicillium, Cephalosporium,* and others. There are no identifying features that help to differentiate one type of fungal ulcer from another.

Scrapings from fungal corneal ulcers, except those caused by *Candida*, contain hyphal elements; scrapings from *Candida* ulcers usually contain pseudohyphae or yeast forms that show characteristic budding. Tables 8–3 and 8–4 list the drugs recommended for the treatment of fungal ulcers.

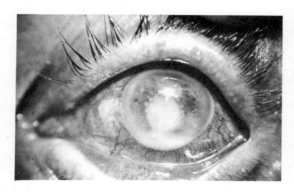

Figure 8–4. Corneal ulcer caused by *Candida albicans.* (Courtesy of P Thygeson.)

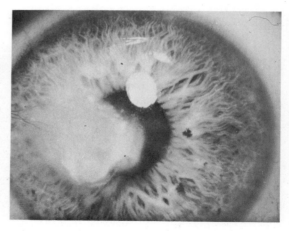

Figure 8–5. Corneal scar caused by recurrent herpes simplex keratitis. (Courtesy of A Rosenberg.)

VIRAL CORNEAL ULCERS

Herpes Simplex Keratitis

Herpes simplex virus (HSV) keratitis is the commonest cause of corneal ulceration in the USA. It occurs in 2 forms: primary and recurrent. The primary disease is a rare keratoconjunctivitis in young children, and the recurrent disease a common ulcerative keratitis, usually but not always dendritic. Formerly, all cases of herpetic keratitis were caused by HSV type 1 (the cause of labial herpes), but recently, because of a change in sexual mores, it is also caused by HSV type 2 (the cause of genital herpes).

Herpetic keratitis is the ocular counterpart of labial herpes, and the dendritic lesion resembles the fever blister immunologically, pathologically, and in clinical course. The only difference is that the clinical course of the keratitis may be slightly prolonged because of the avascularity of the corneal stroma, which retards the migration of lymphocytes and macrophages to the lesion. HSV ocular infection is self-limited and benign in the immunocompetent host, but in the immunologically compromised host its course can be chronic and damaging.

Attacks of the common recurrent type of herpetic keratitis (Fig 8–5) are triggered by fever, overexposure to ultraviolet light, trauma, psychic stress (especially anger), the onset of menstruation, or some other local or systemic source of immunosuppression. Unilaterality is the rule, but bilateral lesions develop in 4–6% of cases and are seen most often in atopic patients.

The first symptoms are usually irritation, photophobia, and tearing. When the central cornea is affected, there is also some reduction in vision. Since corneal anesthesia usually occurs early in the course of the infection, the symptoms may be minimal and the patient may not seek medical advice. There is often a history of fever blisters or other herpetic infection, but corneal ulceration can occasionally be the only sign of a recurrent herpetic infection. The most characteristic lesion is the dendritic ulcer. It occurs in the corneal epithelium, has a typical linear pattern with a tendency to branch, and has terminal bulbs at its ends (Fig 8–6). Fluorescein staining makes the dendrite very easy to identify, but unfortunately herpetic keratitis can also simulate almost any corneal infection and must be considered in the differential diagnosis of many corneal lesions.

Other corneal epithelial lesions that may be caused by HSV are a blotchy epithelial keratitis, stellate epithelial keratitis, and filamentary keratitis. All of these are usually transitory, however, and often become typical dentrites within a day or two.

Subepithelial opacities can be caused by HSV infection. A ghostlike image, corresponding in shape to the original epithelial defect but slightly larger, can be seen in the area immediately underlying the epithelial lesion. The "ghost" remains superficial but is often enlarged by the use of antiviral drugs, especially idoxuridine. As a rule, these subepithelial lesions do not persist for more than a year.

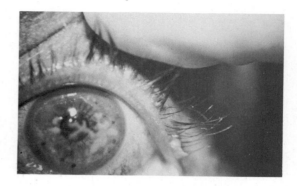

Figure 8–6. Dendritic figures seen in herpes simplex keratitis.

Disciform keratitis is the commonest complication of HSV infection. This round lesion is associated with moderate or severe edema of the affected stroma. Small or medium-sized white keratic precipitates sometimes lie directly under the lesions, and there may be folds in Descemet's membrane. Disciform keratitis is usually associated with local or systemic immunosuppression. Local immunosuppression is commonly produced by cauterization with strong iodine, by topical corticosteroids, or by prolonged use of idoxuridine.

Like all herpetic lesions in immunocompetent individuals, disciform keratitis is normally self-limited, lasting from several weeks to several months. Edema is the prominent sign, and healing occurs with minimal scarring and vascularization. But when immunosuppression, local or systemic, is severe, the lesion becomes chronic and may persist for years. In that event, the stroma often becomes necrotic, and an accompanying iridocyclitis may be severe. Hypopyon is rare and usually indicates secondary bacterial or fungal infection. In exceptional cases, however, it may be due to the pyogenic properties of necrotic tissue. Corneal perforation in disciform keratitis was virtually unknown prior to 1952, when the topical corticosteroids were first introduced; unfortunately, perforation has become less rare since that time.

If perforation has occurred or is imminent, immediate corneal transplantation should be considered. Alternative procedures are the application of a thin conjunctival flap, sealing the perforation with tissue glues, or protecting the eye with soft corneal contact lenses while healing takes place.

Focal avascular interstitial keratitis can also occur in HSV infection and—like stromal necrosis—is almost always associated with the use of corticosteroids. Small areas of focal infiltration and edema are surrounded by clear areas. There is no sign of vascularization, and the lesions may affect any level of the cornea. If they are examined by retroillumination at the slit lamp, their pattern often suggests a previous disciform lesion.

Peripheral lesions of the cornea can also be caused by HSV. They are usually linear and show a loss of epithelium before the underlying corneal stroma becomes infiltrated. (This is in sharp contrast to the marginal ulcer associated with bacterial hypersensitivity—eg, to *S aureus* in staphylococcal blepharitis, in which the infiltration precedes the loss of the overlying epithelium.) Corneal sensation is usually absent or so diminished that the patient is far less photophobic than patients with nonherpetic corneal infiltrates and ulceration usually are.

Most HSV infections of the cornea are still caused by HSV type 1, but in both infants and adults a few cases caused by HSV type 2 have been reported. The corneal lesions caused by the 2 types are indistinguishable.

Scrapings of the epithelial lesions of HSV keratitis contain multinucleated giant cells. The virus can be cultivated on the chorioallantoic membrane of embryonated hens' eggs and in many tissue cell lines—eg, HeLa cells, on which it produces characteristic plaques. In the majority of cases, however, diagnosis can be made clinically on the basis of typical dendritic or geographic ulcers and greatly reduced or absent corneal sensation.

Treatment. The treatment of HSV keratitis should be directed toward elimination of the virus from the cornea. In the immunocompetent patient, the infection is self-limited and scarring minimal. Regrettably, the clinician often immunosuppresses the patient by using corticosteroids in eagerness to reduce local inflammation. This is of course based on a misconception that reducing inflammation reduces disease.

Virus in the epithelium can be readily eliminated by debridement of the affected epithelium, which is best accomplished by removing it carefully from the anesthetized cornea with a tightly wound cotton-tipped applicator. A sterile platinum spatula or a sterile chalazion curet can also be used. The topical application of iodine or ether has no value and can produce chemical keratitis. (Unlike healthy uninfected epithelium, which adheres tightly to the cornea and is hard to remove, infected epithelium is only loosely attached to the cornea and is easy to remove.) A cycloplegic such as atropine 1% or homatropine 5% is then instilled into the conjunctival sac, and a pressure dressing is applied to promote healing. The patient should be examined daily and the dressing changed until the corneal defect has healed (usually 72 hours).

Although mechanical removal of affected epithelium is the best treatment for dendritic keratitis, topical chemotherapy with idoxuridine (IDU, Dendrid, Herplex, Stoxil) or vidarabine (Ara-A, Vira-A) is widely used. Antiviral therapy with these agents has been disappointing, and extensive research is currently under way to find more effective and less toxic preparations. The most promising of those now being tested (but not yet released) are trifluorothymidine and acyclovir (acycloguanosine). Idoxuridine and vidarabine are now useful only in epithelial disease. They are ineffective in both the stromal and uveal tract forms that are now so common because of the improper use of corticosteroids. The major toxic complications of the antivirals, particularly idoxuridine, can be avoided if treatment time is limited to less than 10 days or if the drugs are discontinued promptly when found to be ineffective after a trial of 2 or 3 days. It should be borne in mind that idoxuridine is a cytotoxic drug and can be locally immunosuppressive.

Corticosteroid therapy is contraindicated at all stages of HSV disease for the following reasons: (1) The corticosteroids increase the destructive action of collagenase (produced by the damaged corneal epithelial cells or polymorphonuclear cells) on the corneal stroma; and (2) their immunosuppressive activity increases (a) the activity of the virus and (b) the susceptibility of the HSV-infected host to secondary infections with opportunistic organisms, especially fungi and such bacteria as *S viridans* and *S epidermidis*. Unfortunately, steroids are still widely used because of their anti-inflammatory effect and their temporary but dramatically beneficial effect on symptoms.

Control of trigger mechanisms that reactivate HSV infection. Recurrent HSV infections of the eye are common, occurring in about one-third of cases within 2 years of the first attack. A trigger mechanism can often be discovered by careful questioning of the patient. Once identified, the trigger can often be avoided. Aspirin can be used to avoid fever, excessive exposure to the sun or ultraviolet light can be avoided, situations that might cause psychic stress can be minimized, and aspirin can be taken just prior to the onset of menstruation.

Varicella-Zoster Viral Keratitis

Varicella-zoster virus (VZV) infection occurs in 2 forms: primary (varicella) and recurrent (zoster). Ocular manifestations are uncommon in varicella but common in ophthalmic zoster. In varicella (chickenpox), the usual eye lesions are pocks on the lids and lid margins. Rarely, keratitis occurs (typically a phlyctenulelike lesion at the limbus), and still more rarely epithelial keratitis with or without pseudodendrites. Disciform keratitis, with uveitis of short duration, has been reported.

In contrast to the rare and benign corneal lesions of varicella, the relatively frequent ophthalmic zoster is often accompanied by keratouveitis that varies in severity according to the immune status of the patient. Thus, although children with zoster keratouveitis usually have benign disease, the aged have severe and sometimes blinding disease. Corneal complications in ophthalmic zoster can be anticipated if there is a skin eruption along the branches of the nasociliary nerve.

Unlike recurrent HSV keratitis that affects only the epithelium, VZV keratitis affects the stroma and anterior uvea at onset. The epithelial lesions are blotchy and amorphous except for an occasional linear pseudodendrite that only vaguely resembles the true dentrites of HSV keratitis. Stromal opacities are prominent, characteristically nummular in shape, and largely but not exclusively subepithelial. A disciform keratitis sometimes develops and resembles HSV disciform keratitis. Loss of corneal sensation is always a prominent feature and often persists for months after the corneal lesion appears to have healed. The associated uveitis tends to persist for weeks or months, but unless corticosteroid preparations have been used it eventually heals.

There is no specific treatment for VZV keratitis. Corticosteroid preparations, although giving temporary relief, have prolonged the course of the disease and worsened its prognosis. Opportunistic superinfection, which did not occur prior to 1952, is now a common complication. Of the various complications, postherpetic neuralgia, which is particularly severe in elderly patients, is the most troublesome. Fortunately it is self-limited, and reassurance can be helpful as a supplement to analgesics.

Although the future of specific antiviral treatment looks bleak, the future of immunotherapy is promising. Since zoster is a disease of immunosuppression, the restoration of immunocompetence by such immunopotentiators as human interferon is logical and can be looked upon as the hope of the future. The early results of the study of a number of immunopotentiating procedures are definitely encouraging.

Variola Virus Keratitis

Variola virus corneal ulcers were once a common cause of corneal scarring and blindness in developing countries. The lesions usually involved the pupillary area, and perforations with resultant adherent leukomas were common. This is one ocular disease that will be seen no more, however, for according to the World Health Organization, smallpox is now extinct.

Vaccinial Keratitis

On rare occasions vaccinial keratitis used to occur as a complication of vaccination for the prevention of smallpox. It was either a blotchy epithelial keratitis or a true corneal ulcer and was usually associated with lesions on the lid margin. Atypically, disciform keratitis sometimes occurred. Topical rifampin was apparently sometimes beneficial. Of academic interest (since vaccinial keratitis, like variolar keratitis, is no longer a problem) is the fact that intramuscular vaccinia immune globulin sometimes increased the severity of the disciform lesion.

Adenovirus Keratitis

Keratitis usually accompanies all types of adenoviral conjunctivitis, reaching its peak 5–7 days after onset of the conjunctivitis. It is a fine epithelial keratitis best seen with the slit lamp after instillation of fluorescein. The minute lesions may group together to make up larger ones.

The epithelial keratitis is often followed by subepithelial opacities. In epidemic keratoconjunctivitis (EKC), which is due to adenovirus types 8 and 19, the subepithelial lesions are round and grossly visible. They appear 8–15 days after onset of the conjunctivitis and may persist for months or even (rarely) for several years. Similar lesions occur very exceptionally in other adenoviral infections, eg, those caused by types 3, 4, and 7, but tend to be transitory and mild, lasting a few weeks at most.

Although the corneal opacities of adenoviral keratoconjunctivitis tend to fade temporarily with the use of topical corticosteroids, and although the patient is often made temporarily more comfortable thereby, corticosteroid therapy prolongs the disease and is therefore not recommended. No medication is needed.

Other Viral Keratitides

A fine epithelial keratitis may be seen in other viral infections such as measles (in which the central cornea is affected predominantly), rubella, mumps, infectious mononucleosis, acute hemorrhagic conjunctivitis, Newcastle disease conjunctivitis, and verruca of the lid margin. A superior epithelial keratitis and pannus often accompany molluscum contagiosum nodules on the lid margin. Rare cases of orf virus keratitis have been seen in sheepherders in California and Nevada. The corneal lesions resembled those of the now extinct vaccinial keratitis.

CHLAMYDIAL KERATITIS

All 5 principal types of chlamydial conjunctivitis (trachoma, inclusion conjunctivitis, primary ocular lymphogranuloma venereum, parakeet or psittacosis conjunctivitis, and feline pneumonitis conjunctivitis) are accompanied by corneal lesions. Only in trachoma and lymphogranuloma venereum, however, have they been blinding or visually damaging. The corneal lesions of trachoma have been the most studied and are of great diagnostic importance. In order of appearance they consist of (1) epithelial microerosions affecting the upper third of the cornea; (2) micropannus; (3) subepithelial round opacities, commonly called trachoma pustules; (4) limbal follicles and their cicatricial remains, known as Herbert's peripheral pits; (5) gross pannus; and (6) extensive, diffuse, subepithelial cicatrization. Mild cases of trachoma may show only epithelial keratitis and micropannus and may heal without impairing vision.

The rare cases of lymphogranuloma venereum have shown fewer characteristic changes but are known to have caused blindness by diffuse corneal scarring and total pannus. The remaining types of chlamydial infection cause only micropannus, epithelial keratitis, and rare subepithelial opacities not visually significant.

Chlamydial keratoconjunctivitis responds to treatment with the sulfonamides (except for the rare *C psittaci* infections, which are sulfonamide-resistant), and to tetracyclines and erythromycin.

DRUG-INDUCED EPITHELIAL KERATITIS

An epithelial keratitis is not uncommonly seen in patients using antiviral medications (idoxuridine and vidarabine) and the broad-spectrum and medium-spectrum antibiotics. It is usually a blotchy keratitis affecting predominantly the lower half of the cornea and interpalpebral fissure.

KERATOCONJUNCTIVITIS SICCA
(Sjögren's Syndrome)

Epithelial filaments in the lower quadrants of the cornea are the cardinal signs of this autoimmune disease in which secretion of the lacrimal and accessory lacrimal glands is diminished or eliminated. There is also a blotchy epithelial keratitis that affects mainly the lower quadrants. Severe cases show mucous pseudofilaments that stick to the dry corneal epithelium.

This keratitis of Sjögren's syndrome must be distinguished from the keratitis sicca of such cicatrizing diseases as trachoma and pemphigoid, in which the goblet cells of the conjunctiva have been destroyed. Such cases sometimes still produce tears, but without mucus the corneal epithelium sheds the tears and continues to be dry.

Treatment of keratoconjunctivitis sicca calls for the frequent use of tear substitutes, of which there are many commercial preparations. When goblet cells have been destroyed, as in the cicatricial conjunctivitides, mucus substitutes must be used in addition to artificial tears.

PERIPHERAL CORNEAL ULCERS

Marginal Infiltrates & Ulcers

The majority of marginal corneal ulcers are benign but extremely painful. They are secondary to acute or chronic bacterial conjunctivitis, particularly staphylococcal blepharoconjunctivitis and less often Koch-Weeks (*Haemophilus aegyptius*) conjunctivitis. They are not an infectious process, however, and scrapings do not contain the causal bacteria. They are the result of sensitization to bacterial products, antibody from the limbus vessels reacting with antigen that has diffused through the corneal epithelium.

Marginal infiltrates and ulcers (Fig 8–7) start as oval or linear infiltrates, separated from the limbus by a lucid interval, and only later may ulcerate and vascularize. They are self-limited, usually lasting from 7–10 days, but those associated with staphylococcal blepharoconjunctivitis usually recur. Topical corticosteroid preparations shorten their course and relieve symptoms, which are often severe, but treatment of the underlying conjunctivitis is essential if recurrences are to be prevented. Before starting corticosteroid therapy, great care must be taken to distinguish this entity, formerly known as "catarrhal corneal ulceration,"

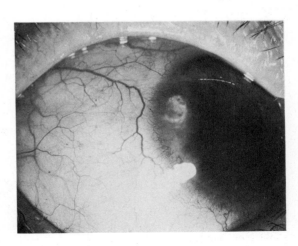

Figure 8–7. Marginal ulcer of temporal cornea, right eye. (Courtesy of P Thygeson.)

from marginal herpetic keratitis. Since marginal herpetic keratitis is usually almost symptomless because of corneal anesthesia, differentiating it from the painful, hypersensitivity-type marginal ulcer is not difficult.

Ring Ulcers (Fig 8–8)

Ring ulcers are rare but more destructive than marginal ulcers. They occasionally result from the confluence of multiple marginal ulcers secondary to conjunctivitis but are more often associated with systemic disease. They have been seen in the convalescent period of such infectious diseases as influenza and bacillary dysentery but can also be a complication of autoimmune disease. A few ring ulcers have been seen in ocular diphtheria, in severe beta-hemolytic streptococcal conjunctival infection, and (more often) in gonococcal conjunctivitis. They may also occur as a secondary manifestation of infectious endophthalmitis; in this event, the ulceration is preceded by a massive infiltration of neutrophils.

Treatment—often unsatisfactory—depends on identification of the underlying cause. Infectious ring ulcer may respond to appropriate systemic and topical antibiotics and the hypersensitivity types to topical corticosteroid therapy.

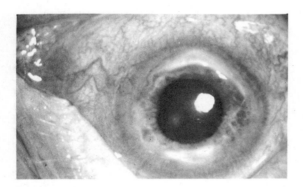

Figure 8–8. Ring ulcer of the cornea. (Courtesy of M Hogan.)

Mooren's Ulcer (Fig 8–9)

The cause of Mooren's ulcer is still unknown, but an autoimmune origin is suspected. It is a marginal ulcer, unilateral in 60–80% of cases and characterized by painful, progressive excavation of the limbus and peripheral cornea that often leads to loss of the eye. It occurs most commonly in old age but does not seem to be related to any of the systemic diseases that most often afflict the aged. It is unresponsive to both antibiotics and corticosteroids. Surgical excision of the limbal conjunctiva in an effort to remove sensitizing substances has recently been advocated. Past generations of ophthalmologists used repeated paracentesis with some success.

Phlyctenular Keratoconjunctivitis

This hypersensitivity disease (due to delayed hypersensitivity to bacterial products, mainly of the human tubercle bacillus) was formerly a major cause of visual loss in the USA, particularly among the Eskimos and Native Americans. Phlyctenules are localized accumulations of lymphocytes, monocytes, macrophages, and finally neutrophils. They appear first at the limbus, but in recurrent attacks they may involve the bulbar conjunctiva and cornea. Corneal phlyctenules, usually bilateral, cicatrize and vascularize, but conjunctival phlyctenules leave no trace.

Most cases of phlyctenular keratoconjunctivitis in the USA today are caused by delayed hypersensitivity to *S aureus*. The antigen is released locally from staphylococci that proliferate on the lid margin in staphylococcal blepharitis. Rare phlyctenules have occurred in San Joaquin Valley fever, a result of hypersensitivity to a primary infection with *Coccidioides immitis*. In this disease they are not visually important, however.

In the tuberculous type, the attack may be triggered by an acute bacterial conjunctivitis but is associated typically with a transient increase in the activity of a childhood tuberculosis. Untreated phlyctenules run a course to healing in 10–14 days, but topical therapy with corticosteroid preparations dramatically shortens the course to a day or two. The corticosteroid response in the staphylococcal type is poor, however, and treatment consists essentially of eliminating the causal bacterial infection. In resistant staphylococcal cases, desensitization with *Staphylococcus* toxoid or Staphage Lysate has been useful.

Marginal Keratitis in Autoimmune Disease

The corneal periphery receives its nourishment from the aqueous humor, the limbal capillaries, and the tear film. It is contiguous with the subconjunctival lymphoid tissue and the lymphatic arcades at the limbus. The perilimbal conjunctiva appears to play an important role in the pathogenesis of corneal lesions that arise both from local ocular disease and from

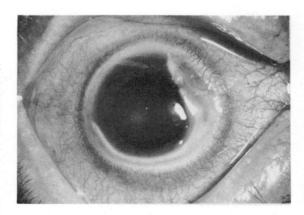

Figure 8–9. Mooren's ulcer. (Courtesy of M Hogan.)

systemic disorders, particularly those of autoimmune origin. There is a striking similarity between the limbal capillary network and the renal glomerular capillary network: On the endothelial basement membranes of the capillaries of both networks, immune complexes are deposited and immunologic disease results. Thus, the peripheral cornea often participates in such autoimmune diseases as rheumatoid arthritis, polyarteritis nodosa, systemic lupus erythematosus, scleroderma, midline lethal and Wegener's granulomatosis, ulcerative colitis, Crohn's disease, psoriasis, relapsing polychondritis, and Reiter's syndrome. These diseases are characteristically associated with infiltration, ulceration, thinning, and (rarely) perforation of the peripheral cornea. The corneal lesions range in severity from benign and even self-limited changes to perforation and loss of the eye. Treatment is directed toward control of the underlying disease but is for the most part unsatisfactory.

CORNEAL ULCER
DUE TO VITAMIN A DEFICIENCY

The typical corneal ulcer associated with avitaminosis A is centrally located and bilateral, gray and indolent, with a definite lack of corneal luster in the surrounding area (Fig 8–10). The cornea becomes soft and necrotic (hence the term, "keratomalacia"), and perforation is common. The epithelium of the conjunctiva is keratinized, as evidenced by the presence of a Bitot spot. This is a foamy, wedge-shaped area in the conjunctiva, usually on the temporal side, with the base of the wedge at the limbus and the apex extending toward the lateral canthus. Within the triangle the conjunctiva is furrowed concentrically with the limbus, and dry flaky material can be seen falling from the area into the inferior cul-de-sac. A stained conjunctival

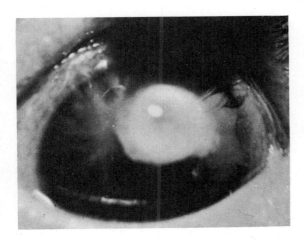

Figure 8–10. Keratomalacia with ulceration associated with xerophthalmia (dietary) in an infant. (Photo by Diane Beeston.)

scraping from a Bitot spot will show many saprophytic xerosis bacilli (*Corynebacterium xerosis*; small curved rods) and keratinized epithelial cells.

Avitaminosis A corneal ulceration results from dietary lack of vitamin A or impaired absorption from the gastrointestinal tract and impaired utilization by the body. It may develop in an infant who has a feeding problem; in an adult who is on a restricted or generally inadequate diet; or in any person with a biliary obstruction since bile in the gastrointestinal tract is necessary for the absorption of vitamin A. Lack of vitamin A causes a generalized keratinization of the epithelium throughout the body. The conjunctival and corneal changes together are known as **xerophthalmia.** Since the epithelium of the air passages is affected, many patients, if not treated, will die of pneumonia. Avitaminosis A also causes a generalized retardation of osseous growth. This is extremely important in infants; for example, if the skull bones do not grow and the brain continues to grow, increased intracranial pressure and papilledema can result.

Vitamin A should be administered in a dosage of at least 20,000 IU/d intramuscularly. Sulfonamide or antibiotic ointment can be used locally in the eye to prevent secondary bacterial infection. The average daily requirement of vitamin A is 1500–5000 IU for children, according to age, and 5000 IU for adults.

NEUROTROPHIC CORNEAL ULCERS

If the trigeminal nerve, which supplies the cornea, is interrupted by trauma, surgery, tumor, inflammation, or in any other way, the cornea loses its sensitivity and one of its best defenses against degeneration, ulceration, and infection. In the early stages of a typical neurotrophic ulcer, fluorescein solution will produce punctate staining of the superficial epithelium. As this process progresses, patchy areas of denudation appear. Occasionally the epithelium may be absent from a large area of the cornea.

The progress of the condition depends on the treatment. Without treatment, the denuded areas become infected. The integrity of the cornea can be maintained as long as the corneal surface is kept moist by wearing a Buller shield,* by suturing the lids together, by using a conjunctival flap, or by using a therapeutic soft contact lens. Artificial tears may be of benefit. Under the best conditions, however, the prognosis is poor, and repeated epithelial breakdown often occurs.

EXPOSURE KERATITIS

Exposure keratitis may develop in any situation in which the cornea is not properly moistened and covered by the eyelids. Examples include exophthalmos

---

*The Buller shield is a water-tight cone of exposed x-ray film secured to the surrounding skin with adhesive tape.

from any cause, ectropion, the absence of part of an eyelid as a result of trauma, and inability to close the lids properly, as in Bell's palsy. The 2 factors at work are the drying of the cornea and its exposure to minor trauma. The uncovered cornea is particularly subject to drying during sleeping hours. If an ulcer develops it usually follows minor trauma and occurs in the inferior third of the cornea.

This type of keratitis will be sterile unless it is secondarily infected, and the therapeutic objective is to provide protection and moisture for the entire corneal surface. The method depends upon the underlying condition: a plastic procedure on the eyelids, a Buller shield,* soft lens, or surgical relief of exophthalmos.

DEGENERATIVE CORNEAL CONDITIONS

KERATOCONUS

Keratoconus is an uncommon degenerative bilateral disease that is inherited as an autosomal recessive trait. Unilateral cases of unknown cause occur rarely. Symptoms appear in the second decade of life. The disease affects all races. Keratoconus has been associated with a number of diseases, including Down's syndrome, atopic dermatitis, retinitis pigmentosa, aniridia, vernal catarrh, Marfan's syndrome, Apert's syndrome, and Ehlers-Danlos syndrome. Pathologically, there are generalized thinning and anterior protrusion of the central cornea, ruptures in Descemet's membrane, and irregular, superficial linear scars at the apex of the cone that is formed.

Acute hydrops of the cornea may occur, in which there is sudden diminution of vision associated with central corneal edema. This usually arises as a conse-

*The Buller shield is a water-tight cone of exposed x-ray film secured to the surrounding skin with adhesive tape.

quence of rupture of Descemet's membrane and may be triggered by the patient rubbing the eye. Acute hydrops usually clears gradually without treatment.

Blurred vision is the only symptom. Signs include cone-shaped cornea (Fig 8–11), indentation of the lower lid by the cornea when the patient looks down (Munson's sign), an irregular shadow on retinoscopy, and a distorted corneal reflection with Placido's disk or the keratoscope. The fundi cannot be clearly seen because of corneal distortion.

Corneal perforation may occur in advanced cases. When this happens, the eye should be bandaged and the dressing changed daily until a corneal scar seals the wound. Corneal transplantation may be necessary. Keratoconus is one of the most common indications for keratoplasty.

Contact lenses improve visual acuity in the early stages. A corneal transplant is indicated when the corrected visual acuity decreases to the point where it interferes with the patient's normal activities.

Keratoconus is often slowly progressive between the ages of 20 and 60, although an arrest in progression of the keratoconus may occur at any time. If a corneal transplant is done before extreme corneal thinning occurs, the prognosis is excellent; about 80–95% obtain reading vision.

CORNEAL DEGENERATION

The corneal dystrophies are a rare group of slowly progressive, bilateral, degenerative disorders that usually appear in the second or third decades of life. Some are hereditary. Other cases follow ocular inflammatory disease, and some are of unknown cause.

Fatty or Lipoid Degeneration
This disorder may begin in infancy or adulthood. The cause is not known. There is a generalized deposition of lipid material within the corneal stroma, replacement of Bowman's membrane by macrophages, and thickening of the epithelium with some infiltration

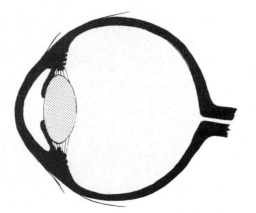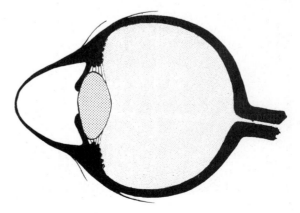

Figure 8–11. *Left:* Side view of normal cornea. *Right:* Keratoconus.

of lipid material. Clinical findings include blurred vision and haziness and thickening of the cornea, particularly in the central zone.

Symptoms and signs are slowly progressive until useful vision is lost. Corneal transplant improves vision significantly in most cases.

Marginal Degeneration of the Cornea (Terrien's Disease)

This is a rare bilateral symmetric degeneration characterized by marginal thinning of the upper nasal quadrants of the cornea. Males are more commonly affected than females, and the condition occurs more frequently in the third and fourth decades. There are no symptoms except for mild irritation, and the condition is slowly progressive. The clinical picture consists of marginal thinning, arcuate opacity distal to the thinned area simulating arcus senilis, and vascularization. Perforation is a known complication of this condition and may lead to iris prolapse. Histopathologic studies of affected corneas have revealed vascularized connective tissue with fibrillary degeneration and fatty infiltration of collagen fibers.

Because the course of progression is slow and the central cornea is spared, the prognosis is good.

Calcific Band Keratopathy (Fig 8–12)

This disorder is characterized by the deposition of calcium salts in the anterior layers of the cornea. The keratopathy is usually limited to the interpalpebral area and appears as a band. The calcium deposits are noted in the basement membrane, Bowman's membrane, and anterior stromal lamellas. A clear margin separates the calcific band from the limbus, and clear holes may be seen in the band, giving the swiss cheese appearance. Symptoms include irritation, injection, and blurring of vision.

Calcific band keratopathy has been described in a number of inflammatory, metabolic, and degenerative conditions. It is characteristically associated with juvenile rheumatoid arthritis. It has been described in long-standing inflammatory conditions of the eye, glaucoma, and chronic cyclitis. Band keratopathy may also be associated with hyperparathyroidism, vitamin D intoxication, sarcoidosis, and leprosy. Treatment consists of ablation of the corneal epithelium by curettement under topical anesthesia followed by irrigation of the cornea with a sterile 0.01 M solution of ethylenediaminetetraacetic acid (EDTA) or application of EDTA with a cotton applicator.

Climatic Droplet Keratopathy (Pearl Diver's Keratopathy, Bietti's Keratopathy, Labrador Keratopathy, Spheroid Degeneration of the Cornea) (Fig 8–13)

This is a relatively new clinical entity—an acquired keratopathy affecting mainly male adults who spend most of their working hours out of doors. The corneal degeneration is thought to be caused by exposure to ultraviolet light and is characterized in the early stages by fine subepithelial yellow droplets in the peripheral cornea. As the disease advances, the droplets become central, with subsequent corneal clouding causing blurred vision. Treatment in advanced cases is by corneal transplantation.

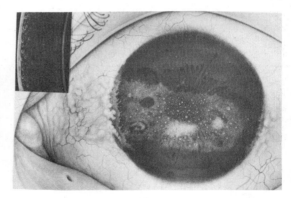

Figure 8–13. Climatic droplet keratopathy. Inset shows slit lamp view. (Courtesy of A Ahmad.)

Salzmann's Nodular Degeneration

This disorder is always preceded by corneal inflammation, particularly phlyctenular keratoconjunctivitis or trachoma. There is vascularization and degeneration of the superficial cornea that involves the stroma, Bowman's membrane, and epithelium. Symptoms include redness, irritation, and blurring of vision. There is a superficial vascularization, with whitish

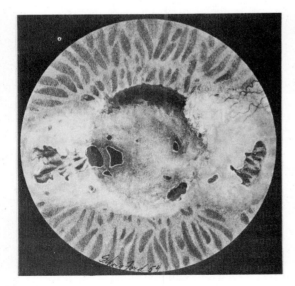

Figure 8–12. Calcific band keratopathy. (Courtesy of M Hogan.)

elevated nodules sometimes occurring in chains interspersed among the blood vessels.

Corneal transplantation will significantly improve the visual acuity in most cases.

HEREDITARY CORNEAL DYSTROPHIES

This is a group of rare hereditary disorders of the cornea of unknown cause characterized by bilateral abnormal deposition of substances and associated with alteration in the normal corneal architecture that may or may not interfere with vision. These corneal dystrophies usually manifest themselves during the first or second decade but sometimes later. They may be stationary or slowly progressive throughout life. Corneal transplantation improves vision in most patients with hereditary corneal dystrophy.

Anatomically, corneal dystrophies may be classified as anterior limiting membrane, stromal, and posterior limiting membrane dystrophies.

Anterior Limiting Membrane Corneal Dystrophies

A. Meesman's Dystrophy: This slowly progressive disorder is characterized by microcystic areas in the epithelium. The onset is in early childhood (first 1–2 years of life). The main symptom is slight irritation, and vision is slightly affected. The inheritance is autosomal dominant.

B. Cogan's Dystrophy: This condition is characterized by discrete comma-shaped or rounded, gray-white intraepithelial opacities located in the pupillary area. Fingerprint or maplike fine opacities may be seen at the level of the basement membrane. The disease is more common in females. Patients may develop recurrent erosion. Visual acuity is affected very slightly.

C. Fingerprint Dystrophy: This entity refers to fine wavy concentric lines located anterior to Bowman's membrane that can be seen best by retroillumination with the slit lamp. These lines may be associated with a map- or dotlike pattern. The condition is asymptomatic but may be associated with recurrent erosion. The findings are noted during routine examination.

D. Recurrent Corneal Erosion: See p 102.

E. Others: Reis-Bücklers dystrophy is a dominantly inherited dystrophy affecting primarily Bowman's membrane. The disease begins within the first decade of life with symptoms of recurrent erosion. Opacification of Bowman's membrane gradually occurs and the epithelium is irregular. No vascularization is usually noted. Vision may be markedly reduced.

Vortex dystrophy, or cornea verticillata, is characterized by pigmented lines occurring in Bowman's membrane or the underlying stroma and spreading over the entire corneal surface. Visual acuity is not markedly affected. Such a pattern of radiating pigmented lines may also be seen in patients suffering from chlorpromazine, chloroquine, or indomethacin toxicity as well as Fabry's disease.

Stromal Corneal Dystrophies

There are 3 types of stromal corneal dystrophies:

A. Granular Dystrophy: This usually asymptomatic, slowly progressive corneal dystrophy most often begins in early childhood. The lesions consist of central, fine, whitish "granular" lesions in the stroma of the cornea. The epithelium and Bowman's membrane may be affected late in the disease. Visual acuity is slightly reduced. Histologically, the cornea shows uniform deposition of hyaline material. Corneal transplant is not needed except in very severe and late cases. The inheritance is autosomal dominant.

B. Macular Dystrophy: This type of stromal corneal dystrophy is manifested by a dense gray central opacity that starts in Bowman's membrane. The opacity tends to spread toward the periphery and later involves the deeper stromal layers. Recurrent corneal erosion may occur, and vision is severely impaired. Histologic examination shows deposition of acid mucopolysaccharide in the stroma and degeneration of Bowman's membrane.

The inheritance is autosomal recessive.

C. Lattice Dystrophy: Lattice dystrophy starts as fine, branching linear opacities in Bowman's membrane in the central area and spreads to the periphery. The deep stroma may become involved, but the process does not reach Descemet's membrane. Recurrent erosion may occur. Histologic examination reveals amyloid deposits in the collagen fibers.

Posterior Limiting Membrane Corneal Dystrophies

A. Fuchs's Dystrophy: This disorder begins in the third or fourth decade and is slowly progressive throughout life. Women are more commonly affected than men. There are central wartlike deposits on Descemet's membrane, thickening of Descemet's membrane, and defects in the endothelium. Decompensation of the endothelium occurs and leads to edema of the corneal stroma and epithelium, causing blurring of vision. The cornea becomes progressively more opaque. Glaucoma or iris atrophy may be associated with this disorder. Histologic examination of the cornea reveals the wartlike excrescences over Descemet's membrane that are secreted by the endothelial cells. Thinning and pigmentation of the endothelium and thickening of Descemet's membrane are characteristic.

B. Posterior Polymorphous Dystrophy: This is a common disorder with onset in early childhood. Polymorphous plaques of calcium crystals are observed in the deep stromal layers. Vesicular lesions may be seen in the endothelium. Edema occurs in the deep stroma. The condition is asymptomatic in most cases, but in severe cases epithelial and total stromal edema may occur. The inheritance is autosomal dominant.

ARCUS SENILIS
(Corneal Annulus, Anterior Embryotoxon)

Arcus senilis is an extremely common, bilateral, benign peripheral corneal degeneration that may occur at any age but is far more common in elderly people as part of the aging process. When arcus senilis is present prior to age 50, hypercholesterolemia is usually associated with it.

Pathologically, lipid droplets involve the entire corneal thickness but are more concentrated in the superficial and deep layers, being relatively sparse in the corneal stroma.

There are no symptoms. Clinically, arcus senilis appears as a peripheral, annular, hazy gray ring about 2 mm in width and with a clear space between it and the limbus (Fig 8–14). No treatment is necessary, and there are no complications. Since arcus senilis causes no visual defect, it is not always classified with the corneal dystrophies.

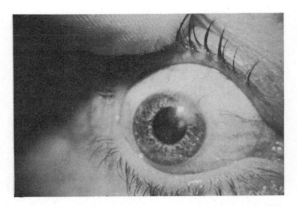

Figure 8–15. Sclerokeratitis. Note fibrovascular scar in upper nasal quadrant of cornea.

No specific treatment is available. The pupil should be kept dilated with atropine, 2%, 2 drops once daily. Warm compresses and local corticosteroid drops are used to relieve the discomfort. Although the process starts as a small area of infiltration, it may progress to total corneal opacification. It may, however, subside after months or years.

SUPERFICIAL PUNCTATE KERATITIS

Superficial punctate keratitis is an uncommon chronic and recurrent bilateral disorder without regard to sex or age. It is characterized by discrete and elevated oval epithelial opacities that show punctate staining with fluorescein, mainly in the pupillary area. The opacities are not visible grossly but can be easily seen with the slit lamp or loupe. Subepithelial opacities underlying the epithelial lesions (ghosts) are often observed in patients who have been misdiagnosed as having herpes simplex keratitis and treated with topical idoxuridine.

No causative organism has been identified, but a virus is suspected. A varicella-zoster virus has been isolated from the corneal scrapings of one case.

Mild irritation, slight blurring of vision, and photophobia are the only symptoms. The conjunctiva is not involved.

Epithelial keratitis secondary to staphylococcal blepharoconjunctivitis is differentiated from superficial punctate keratitis by its involvement of the lower third of the cornea. Epithelial keratitis in trachoma is ruled out by its location in the upper third of the cornea and the presence of pannus. Many other forms of keratitis involving the superficial cornea are unilateral or are eliminated by their histories.

Short-term instillation of corticosteroid drops will often cause disappearance of the opacities and subjective improvement, but recurrences are the rule. The ultimate prognosis is good since there is no scarring or vascularization of the cornea. Untreated, the disease runs a protracted course of 1–3 years. Long-term

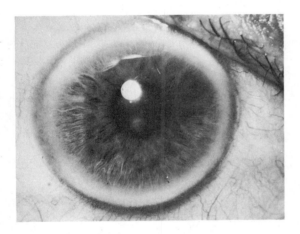

Figure 8–14. Arcus senilis. (Photo by Diane Beeston.)

MISCELLANEOUS CORNEAL DISORDERS

SCLEROKERATITIS
(Sclerosing Keratitis)

Sclerokeratitis is an uncommon, unilateral, localized inflammation of the sclera and cornea. The cause is not known, but tuberculosis was formerly implicated. However, antituberculosis therapy is not effective. Pathologically, there are many chronic inflammatory cells (small round cells) in the involved portion of both structures. Fibrosis occurs in the later stages (Fig 8–15). The patient complains of pain, photophobia, and irritation, but there is no discharge. A moderately severe iritis (anterior nongranulomatous uveitis) is usually associated.

treatment with topical corticosteroids may prolong the course of the disease for many years and lead to steroid-induced cataract and glaucoma.

RECURRENT CORNEAL EROSION

This is a fairly common and serious mechanical corneal disorder that presents some classic signs and symptoms but may be easily missed if the physician does not look for it specifically. The patient is usually awakened during the early morning hours by a pain in the affected eye. The pain is continuous, and the eye becomes red, irritated, and photophobic. When the patient attempts to open the eyes in the morning, the lid pulls off the loose epithelium, resulting in pain and redness.

Three types of recurrent corneal erosions can be recognized:

(1) Acquired recurrent erosion (traumatic): The patient usually gives a history of previous corneal injury. It is unilateral, occurs with equal frequency in males and females, and the family history is negative. The recurrent erosion occurs most frequently in the center below the pupil no matter where the site of the previous corneal injury was.

(2) Familial recurrent erosion: This condition is bilateral and occurs more frequently in women. Patients give a family history of similar cases. There is usually no history of trauma.

(3) Recurrent erosion associated with corneal dystrophies: (See above.) Recurrent erosions of the cornea may be observed in patients with Cogan's microcystic corneal dystrophy, fingerprint dystrophy, and Reis-Bücklers corneal dystrophy.

Recurrent corneal erosion is due to a defect in the basement membrane of the corneal epithelium. The hemidesmosomes of the basal layer of the corneal epithelium fail to adhere to the basement membrane and the corneal epithelium remains loose over the basement membrane with very slight subepithelial edema. The loose epithelial layers are vulnerable to separation and erosion.

Instillation of a local anesthetic relieves the symptoms immediately, and fluorescein staining will show the eroded area. This is typically a small area in the lower central cornea.

Treatment consists of a pressure bandage on the eye to promote healing. Mechanical denuding of the corneal epithelium may be necessary. The other eye should be kept closed most of the time to minimize movement of the lid over the affected eye. Bed rest is desirable for 24 hours. The cornea usually heals in 2–3 days. To prevent recurrence and to promote continued healing, it is important for these patients to use a bland ointment (eg, boric acid or other ocular lubricant) at bedtime for several months. In more severe cases, artificial tears are instilled during the day. The use of hypertonic ointment (glucose 40%) or 5% saline drops (Adsorbonac 5%) is often of value.

Rare instances of bilateral atraumatic dystrophic recurrent corneal erosion with a poor prognosis have also been reported.

INTERSTITIAL KERATITIS DUE TO CONGENITAL SYPHILIS

This self-limited inflammatory disease of the cornea is a late manifestation of congenital syphilis. There has been a sharp decrease in the incidence of the disease in recent years—almost to the point of extinction in some parts of the USA. It occasionally starts unilaterally but almost always becomes bilateral weeks to months later. It affects all races and is more common in females than males. Symptoms appear between the ages of 5 and 20. Pathologic findings include edema, lymphocytic infiltration, and vascularization of the corneal stroma.

Interstitial keratitis may be allergic in nature since *Treponema pallidum* is not found in the cornea during the acute phase. It has been postulated that these organisms enter the cornea at birth and that later in life there is a violent allergic reaction in the cornea to the organisms circulating in the bloodstream.

Clinical Findings

A. Symptoms and Signs: Other signs of congenital syphilis may be present, such as saddle nose and Hutchinson's triad (interstitial keratitis, deafness, and notched upper central incisors). The patient complains of pain, photophobia, and blurring of vision. Physical signs include conjunctival injection, corneal edema, vascularization of the deeper corneal layers, and miosis. There is an associated severe anterior granulomatous uveitis and blepharospasm due to photophobia. The grayish-pink appearance of the cornea (due to edema and vascularization) that occurs in the acute phase is sometimes referred to as a "salmon patch."

B. Laboratory Findings: Serologic tests for syphilis are positive.

Complications & Sequelae

Corneal scarring occurs if the process has been particularly severe and prolonged. Secondary glaucoma may result from the uveitis.

Treatment

There are no specific measures. Treatment is aimed at preventing the development of posterior synechiae, which will occur if the pupil is not dilated.

Both eyes should be dilated with frequent instillation of 2% atropine solution. Corticosteroid drops often relieve the symptoms dramatically but must be continued for long periods to prevent recurrence of symptoms. Dark glasses and a darkened room may be necessary if photophobia is severe. Treatment should be given for systemic syphilis, even though this usually has little effect on the ocular condition.

Corneal scarring may necessitate corneal transplant, and glaucoma, if present, may be difficult to control.

Course & Prognosis

The corneal disease process itself is not affected by treatment, which is aimed at prevention of complications. The inflammatory phase lasts 3 or 4 weeks. The corneas then gradually clear, leaving ghost vessels and scars in the corneal stroma.

INTERSTITIAL KERATITIS DUE TO OTHER CAUSES

Although congenital syphilis is no longer a common cause of interstitial keratitis, the disease still occurs as a complication of other granulomatous diseases, eg, tuberculosis and leprosy. Treatment is usually symptomatic, but it is important to establish the cause.

Cogan's syndrome is a rare disorder generally believed to be a vascular hypersensitivity reaction of unknown origin. It is a disease of young adults and is characterized by nonsyphilitic interstitial keratitis and a vestibuloauditory difficulty. Corticosteroids are reputed to be of value, but some degree of visual impairment and complete nerve deafness, with unresponsive labyrinths, usually supervenes.

CORNEAL PIGMENTATION

Pigmentation of the cornea may occur with or without ocular or systemic disease. There are several distinct varieties.

Krukenberg's Spindle

In this disorder, brown uveal pigment is deposited bilaterally upon the central endothelial surface in a vertical spindle-shaped fashion. It occurs in a small percentage of people over age 20, usually in myopic women. It can be seen grossly but is best observed with the loupe or slit lamp. The visual acuity is only slightly affected, and the progression is extremely slow. Pigmentary glaucoma should be ruled out.

Blood Staining

This disorder occurs occasionally as a complication of traumatic hyphema and is due to hemosiderin in the corneal stroma. The cornea is golden brown, and vision is blurred. In most cases the cornea gradually clears in 1–2 years.

Kayser-Fleischer Ring

This is a pigmented ring whose color varies widely from ruby red to bright green, blue, yellow, or brown. The ring is 1–3 mm in diameter and located just inside the limbus posteriorly. In exceptional cases there is a second ring. The pigment is composed of fine granules immediately below the endothelium. It involves Descemet's membrane, rarely the stroma. Electron microscopic studies suggest that the pigment is a copper compound. The intensity of the pigmentation can be reduced markedly by the use of chelating agents.

These rings, which were long considered to be pathognomonic of hepatolenticular degeneration (Wilson's disease), have recently been described in 3 non-wilsonian patients with chronic hepatobiliary disease and in one patient with chronic cholestatic jaundice. Recognition of the Kayser-Fleischer rings, however, remains important, since they call attention to the possibility that the patient has Wilson's disease. Specific medical treatment with the copper chelating agent penicillamine may dramatically improve a disease that would otherwise inevitably be fatal.

Stähli's Line

Stähli's line (Hudson's brown line, Hudson-Stähli line) is an uncommon phenomenon that occurs only in elderly persons. It is seen with the slit lamp as a horizontal brown line in the inferior third of the cornea. It does not extend to the limbus on either side. The line probably represents iron deposits in Bowman's membrane. It causes no visual disturbance.

Fleischer's Ring

Fleischer's ring is a brownish or greenish line around the base of the cone of the cornea that occurs almost regularly in keratoconus. It is probably due to deposits of iron (hemosiderin). Like Stähli's line, it probably represents tears in Bowman's membrane.

CORNEAL TRANSPLANTATION OPERATION

Corneal transplantation (keratoplasty) is indicated for a number of serious corneal conditions, eg, scarring, edema, thinning, and distortion. The term penetrating keratoplasty denotes full-thickness corneal replacement; lamellar keratoplasty denotes a partial-thickness procedure.

Young donors are preferred for penetrating keratoplasties; there is a direct relationship between age and the health of the endothelial cells. Because of the rapid endothelial cell death rate, the eyes should be enucleated soon after death and should be used within 48 hours, preferably within 24 hours.

For lamellar keratoplasty, corneas can be frozen, dehydrated, or refrigerated for several weeks; the endothelial cells are not important in this partial-thickness procedure.

Technique

The recipient eye is prepared by a partial-thickness cutting of a circle of diseased cornea with a

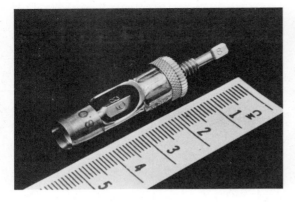

Figure 8–16. Eight-mm Castroviejo disposable trephine. (Courtesy of R Biswell and T King.)

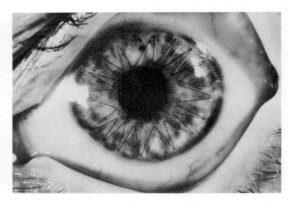

Figure 8–17. Penetrating keratoplasty with 10-0 nylon running suture, 3 months after operation. (Courtesy of R Biswell and T King.)

trephine (cookie cutter action) (Fig 8–16) and full-thickness removal with scissors or partial-thickness removal with dissection.

The donor eye is prepared in 2 ways. For penetrating keratoplasty, the entire cornea is placed endothelium up on a Teflon block; the trephine is pressed down into the cornea, and a full-thickness button is punched out. In lamellar keratoplasty, a partial-thickness trephine incision is made in the cornea and

the lamellar button is dissected free. Certain refinements in technique, such as free hand grafts, may be necessary.

In recent years, refined sutures (Fig 8–17) and instruments and sophisticated operating microscopes and illuminating systems have significantly improved the prognosis in all patients requiring corneal transplants.

● ● ●

References

Ahmad A et al: Climatic droplet keratopathy in a 16-year-old boy. *Arch Ophthalmol* 1977;**95**:149.

Angell LK et al: Visual prognosis in patients with ruptures in Descemet's membrane due to forceps injuries. *Arch Ophthalmol* 1981;**99**:2137.

Boger WP III et al: Keratoconus and acute hydrops. *Am J Ophthalmol* 1981;**91**:231.

Brown N, Bron A: Recurrent erosion of the cornea. *Br J Ophthalmol* 1976;**60**:84.

Brown SI: Mooren's ulcer treatment by conjunctival excision. *Br J Ophthalmol* 1975;**59**:675.

Brown SI, Bloomfield SE, Pearce DB: Alkali-burned cornea. *Am J Ophthalmol* 1974;**77**:538.

Burns RP, Potter MH: Epidemic keratoconjunctivitis due to adenovirus type 19. *Am J Ophthalmol* 1976;**81**:27.

Cogan DG: Applied anatomy and physiology of the cornea. *Trans Am Acad Ophthalmol* 1951;**55**:329.

Collum LMT et al: Randomised double-blind trial of acyclovir and idoxuridine in dendritic corneal ulceration. *Br J Ophthalmol* 1980;**64**:766.

Dawson CR et al: Adenovirus type 8 keratoconjunctivitis in the United States. *Am J Ophthalmol* 1970;**69**:473.

Dingle J et al: Ophthalmoscopic changes in a patient with Wilson's disease during long-term penicillamine therapy. *Ann Ophthalmol* 1978;**10**:1227.

Forrest WM, Kaufman HE: Zosteriform herpes simplex. *Am J Ophthalmol* 1976;**81**:86.

Forster RK, Rebell G: The diagnosis and management of keratomycoses. *Arch Ophthalmol* 1975;**93**:975.

Fraunfelder FT: Spheroidal degeneration. *Am J Ophthalmol* 1973;**76**:41.

Frommer D et al: Kayser-Fleischer-like rings in patients without Wilson's disease. *Gastroenterology* 1977;**72**:1331.

Gasset AR, Kaufman HE: Hydrophilic lens therapy of superficial sterile corneal ulcers. *Ann Ophthalmol* 1973;**5**:139.

Hutton WL, Sexton RR: Atypical pseudomonas corneal ulcers in semicomatose patients. *Am J Ophthalmol* 1972;**73**:37.

Jones BR: Principles in the management of oculomycosis: The 31st Edward Jackson memorial lecture. *Am J Ophthalmol* 1975;**79**:719.

Kenyon KR, Maumenee AE: Further studies of congenital hereditary endothelial dystrophy of the cornea. *Am J Ophthalmol* 1973;**76**:419.

Kim HB, Ostler HB: Marginal corneal ulcer due to β-streptococcus. *Arch Ophthalmol* 1977;**95**:454.

Klintworth GK et al: Recurrence of lattice corneal dystrophy type 1 in the corneal grafts of two siblings. *Am J Ophthalmol* 1982;**94**:540.

Laing RA et al: The human corneal endothelium in keratoconus. *Arch Ophthalmol* 1979;**97**:1867.

Lemp MA: Cornea and sclera: Annual review. *Arch Ophthalmol* 1976;**94**:473.

Lemp MA et al: Ocular surface defense mechanisms. *Ann Ophthalmol* 1981;**13**:61.

Malbran ES: Corneal dystrophies: A clinical, pathological, and surgical approach: The 28th Edward Jackson memorial lecture. *Am J Ophthalmol* 1972;**74**:771.

McGill J: Comparative trial of acyclovir and adenine arabinoside in the treatment of herpes simplex corneal ulcers. *Br J Ophthalmol* 1981;**65**:610.

Naumann G, Green WR, Zimmerman LE: Mycotic keratitis: A histopathologic study of 73 cases. *Am J Ophthalmol* 1967;**64**:668.

O'Connor GR: Calcific band keratopathy. *Trans Am Acad Ophthalmol Otolaryngol* 1972;**70**:58.

Olson RJ et al: Visual results after penetrating keratoplasty for aphakic bullous keratopathy and Fuchs's dystrophy. *Am J Ophthalmol* 1979;**88**:1000.

Ostler HB, Okumoto M, Wilkey C: The changing pattern of the etiology of central bacterial corneal (hypopyon) ulcer. *Trans Pac Coast Otoophthalmol Soc* 1976;**57**:235.

Ostler HB, Thygeson P, Okumoto M: Infectious diseases of the eye. 3. Infections of the cornea. *J Cont Educ Ophthalmol* (Sept) 1978;**40**:13.

Pavan-Langston D et al: Ganglionic herpes simplex and systemic acyclovir. *Arch Ophthalmol* 1981;**99**:1417.

Pettit TH, Holland GN: Chronic keratoconjunctivitis associated with ocular adenovirus infection. *Am J Ophthalmol* 1979;**88**:748.

Rabb MF, Blodi F, Boniuk M: Unilateral lattice dystrophy of the cornea. *Trans Am Acad Ophthalmol Otolaryngol* 1974;**78**:440.

Ruben M, Colebrook E, Guillon M: Keratoconus, keratoplasty thickness, and endothelial morphology. *Br J Ophthalmol* 1979;**63**:790.

Sanders N: Repair of corneal lacerations. *Ann Ophthalmol* 1975;**7**:1515.

Sanford-Smith JH, Whittle HC: Corneal ulceration following measles in Nigerian children. *Br J Ophthalmol* 1979;**63**:720.

Sen DK: Surgery of pterygium. *Br J Ophthalmol* 1970;**54**:606.

Shimeld C: Isolation of herpes simplex virus from the cornea in chronic stromal keratitis. *Br J Ophthalmol* 1982;**66**:643.

Slansky HH, Dohlman CH: Collagenase and the cornea. *Surv Ophthalmol* 1970;**14**:402.

Smolin G: Report of a case of rubella keratitis. *Am J Ophthalmol* 1972;**74**:436.

Smolin G, Okumoto M: Herpes simplex keratitis. *Arch Ophthalmol* 1970;**83**:746.

Sommer A et al: Corneal xerophthalmia and keratomalacia. *Arch Ophthalmol* 1982;**100**:404.

Sommer A et al: Nutritional factors in corneal xerophthalmia and keratomalacia. *Arch Ophthalmol* 1982;**100**:399.

Süveges MD, Levai G, Alberth B: Pathology of Terrien's disease. *Am J Ophthalmol* 1972;**74**:1191.

Tabbara KF, Shammas HF: Bilateral corneal perforations in Stevens-Johnson syndrome. *Can J Ophthalmol* 1975;**10**:514.

Thygeson P: Clinical and laboratory observations on superficial punctate keratitis. *Am J Ophthalmol* 1960;**61**:1344.

Thygeson P, Okumoto M: Keratomycosis: A preventable disease. *Trans Am Acad Ophthalmol Otolaryngol* 1974;**78**:433.

Tripathi RC, Bron AJ: Ultrastructural study of nontraumatic recurrent corneal erosion. *Ophthalmol Digest* 1973;**35**:38.

Valenton MJ: Deep stromal involvement in Dimmers' nummular keratitis. *Am J Ophthalmol* 1974;**78**:897.

Valenton MJ: Secondary ocular bacterial infection in hypovitaminosis A xerophthalmia. *Am J Ophthalmol* 1975;**80**:673.

Vannas A, Hogan MJ, Wood I: Salzmann's nodular degeneration of the cornea. *Am J Ophthalmol* 1975;**79**:211.

Waring GO, Baum JL, Jones DB (editors): Viewpoints: Initial therapy of suspected microbial corneal ulcers. (2 parts.) *Br J Ophthalmol* 1979;**24**:2, 97.

Werb A: Keratoconus. *Br J Ophthalmol* 1972;**56**:565.

Whitcher JP et al: Herpes simplex keratitis in a developing country. *Arch Ophthalmol* 1976;**94**:587.

Wilson FM II, Grayson M, Ellis FD: Treatment of peripheral corneal ulcers by limbal conjunctivectomy. *Br J Ophthalmol* 1976;**60**:713.

Wilson LA et al: Corneal ulcers and soft contact lenses. *Am J Ophthalmol* 1981;**92**:546.

9 | Sclera

ANATOMY & FUNCTION

The sclera is the fibrous outer protective coating of the eye. It is dense and white and continuous with the cornea anteriorly and with the dural sheath of the optic nerve posteriorly. At the insertion of the rectus muscles, it is about 0.3 mm thick; elsewhere, about 1 mm thick. A few strands of scleral tissue pass over the optic disk. This sievelike structure is known as the lamina cribrosa. Around the optic nerve, the sclera is penetrated by the long and short posterior ciliary arteries and the long and short ciliary nerves. Slightly posterior to the equator, the 4 vortex veins exit through the sclera, usually one in each quadrant. About 4 mm posterior to the limbus, the 4 anterior ciliary arteries and veins penetrate the sclera. Each set penetrates slightly anterior to the insertion of a rectus muscle.

The outer surface of the sclera is covered by a thin layer of fine elastic tissue, the episclera, containing numerous blood vessels that nourish the sclera. The brown pigment layer on the inner surface is the lamina fusca, which is continuous with the sclera and the choroid. On the inner surface at 180 degrees (in a horizontal plane through 9 and 3 o'clock), there is a shallow groove from the optic nerve to the ciliary body in which are embedded the long posterior ciliary artery and the long ciliary nerve. The nerve supply to the sclera is from the ciliary nerves.

Histologically, the sclera consists of many dense bands of parallel and interlacing fibrous tissue bundles each of which is 10–16 μm thick and 100–140 μm wide. The histologic structure of the sclera is remarkably similar to that of the cornea, which raises the question why the cornea is transparent and the sclera opaque. The apparent physiologic reason is the relative deturgescence of the cornea and the less uniform structure of the sclera. The cornea has the ability to absorb a great deal of water, whereupon it becomes opaque; the sclera is almost completely hydrated in its normal state.

DISEASES & DISORDERS OF THE SCLERA

BLUE SCLERAS

The normal sclera is white and opaque, so that the underlying uveal structures are not visible. Structural changes of the scleral collagen fibers and thinning of the sclera may allow the underlying uveal pigment to be seen, giving the sclera a bluish discoloration. Blue sclera occurs in several disorders that lead to disturbances in the connective tissues, particularly the collagen fibers. Blue scleras are part of the clinical picture in osteogenesis imperfecta, Ehlers-Danlos syndrome, pseudoxanthoma elasticum, Marfan's syndrome, and pseudohypoparathyroidism and may occur with prolonged use of corticosteroids. Blue scleras are sometimes noted in normal newborn infants, in keratoconus, and in keratoglobus.

SCLERAL ECTASIA

Prolonged elevation of intraocular pressure early in infancy, such as occurs in cases of congenital glaucoma, may lead to stretching and ectasia of the sclera. Scleral ectasia may occur as a congenital anomaly surrounding the disk or occasionally in the macular area. It may also follow inflammation or injury of the sclera.

STAPHYLOMA

Staphyloma results from bulging of the uvea into a thinned and stretched sclera. Staphylomas can be characterized as ectatic dark blue, bulging areas involving a localized segment of the eyeball. The staphyloma may be anterior, equatorial, or posterior. Anterior staphylomas are generally located over the ciliary body (ciliary staphyloma) (Fig 9–1) or between the ciliary body and the limbus (intercalary staphyloma). Equatorial staphylomas are located at the equator and posterior staphylomas posterior to the equator. Posterior staphylomas are most commonly seen at the optic nerve head. They affect the lamina

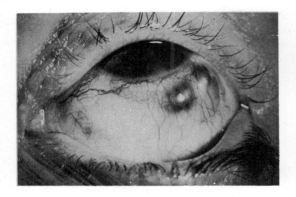

Figure 9–1. Ciliary staphyloma. (Courtesy of P Thygeson.)

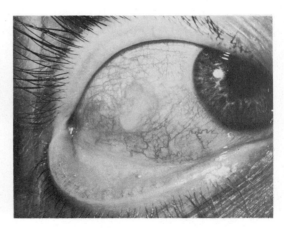

Figure 9–2. Nodular episcleritis, right eye. (Photo by Diane Beeston.)

cribrosa and may follow extreme myopia. Large congenital posterior staphylomas associated with poor vision have been observed. Patients having such conditions are generally extremely myopic. Cases of congenital peripapillary staphylomas in patients with normal or nearly normal vision have been reported. Posterior staphyloma is usually associated with areas of pronounced choroidal atrophy.

Staphyloma must be differentiated from extreme myopia and scleral ectasia in a coloboma of the optic nerve head.

INTRASCLERAL NERVE LOOPS OF AXENFELD

The intrascleral nerve loops are sites of branches of the long ciliary nerves. They enter the sclera close to the ciliary body and about 3.5 mm from the limbus. They are more commonly seen nasally. They may be pigmented and are usually accompanied by the small anterior ciliary artery in its inward course.

INFLAMMATION OF THE SCLERA & EPISCLERA

Inflammation involving the episclera, the thin layer of vascular elastic tissue overlying the sclera, is referred to as **episcleritis.** **Scleritis** is inflammation of the sclera itself, with or without inflammation of the episclera. The 2 diseases are considered distinct clinical entities and will be considered separately.

Episcleritis

This is a relatively common localized inflammation of the episclera. It is unilateral in about two-thirds of cases, and the sex incidence is equal. It may recur at the same or adjacent sites in the palpebral fissure.

The cause is not known, but hypersensitivity reactions may play a role. Certain systemic diseases such as rheumatoid arthritis, Sjögren's syndrome, coccidioidomycosis, syphilis, herpes zoster, and tuberculosis have been associated with episcleritis.

Symptoms of episcleritis include redness, pain, photophobia, tenderness, and lacrimation. Ocular examination reveals localized hyperemia that gives the eyeball a pink or purple color. There is also infiltration, congestion, and edema of the episclera, the overlying conjunctiva, and the underlying Tenon capsule. Two types of episcleritis are recognized: simple and nodular (Fig 9–2). The sclera itself is not involved. About 15% of patients with episcleritis develop mild iritis.

Conjunctivitis is ruled out by the localized nature of episcleritis and the lack of palpebral conjunctival involvement.

The condition is benign, and the course is generally self-limited in 1–2 weeks. However, recurrences may torment the patient for years. Topical therapy with corticosteroids (dexamethasone, 0.1%) resolves the inflammatory changes in 3 or 4 days. Corticosteroids are more effective in simple episcleritis than in nodular episcleritis.

Scleritis

Inflammation of the sclera is less common than episcleritis (Fig 9–3). Scleritis is a relatively rare chronic inflammation of the sclera that is frequently associated with systemic diseases. The causes of scleritis are listed in Table 9–1. The disease may be unilateral or bilateral, and women are more commonly affected than men.

Scleritis is classified according to its clinical and pathologic features. Two types are recognized: anterior and posterior. Anterior scleritis may be subdivided into diffuse, nodular, or necrotizing scleritis with or without adjacent inflammation.

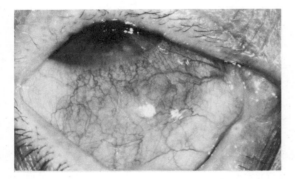

Figure 9–3. Nodular scleritis, left eye, associated with rheumatoid arthritis. (Courtesy of GR O'Connor.)

The symptoms of scleritis include pain, redness, photophobia, tenderness, and lacrimation. Pain is usually more severe than in episcleritis.

Examination reveals an intense violaceous, purple-bluish discoloration that may be diffuse. Episcleral and conjunctival tissues are also involved, and the vessels are characteristically dilated. A practical aid in diagnosis is the topical application of 1 drop of epinephrine, 1:1000, which constricts the superficial vessels but not the deeper scleral vessels. Areas of avascularity may suggest occlusive vasculitis and imply a grave prognosis. Elevated nodules are noted in nodular scleritis. These are often encountered in rheumatoid arthritis as well.

A. Necrotizing Scleritis: The most severe form of scleritis is necrotizing scleritis with adjacent inflammation, otherwise known as **brawny scleritis.** This disorder is characterized by an acute, painful, tender area of localized congestion and necrosis that leads to thinning and destruction of the scleral collagen fibers. There may be an avascular area in the overlying

Table 9–1. Causes of scleritis.

Collagen diseases:
    Ankylosing spondylitis
    Rheumatoid arthritis
    Polyarteritis nodosa
    Relapsing polychondritis
    Wegener's granulomatosis
    Systemic lupus erythematosus
Granulomatous diseases:
    Tuberculosis
    Syphilis
    Sarcoidosis
    Leprosy
Metabolic disorders: Gout, thyrotoxicosis, active rheumatic
    heart disease, psoriatic arthritis
Infections: Onchocerciasis, herpes zoster, herpes simplex
Others:
    Physical (irradiation, thermal burns)
    Chemical (alkali and acid burns)
    Mechanical (penetrating injuries)
Unknown

episcleral tissue. The disease may remain localized or may progress to involve the entire anterior sclera, allowing visualization of the underlying uvea. Elevation of the intraocular pressure may exacerbate scleral ectasia. Corticosteroids may exacerbate both scleral thinning and destruction of collagen fibers.

B. Necrotizing Scleromalacia (Scleromalacia Perforans): This is a rare scleral disease characterized by thinning and melting of the scleral tissue, leading to areas of dehiscence without any history or clinical evidence of inflammation of the sclera. This form of "scleral melting" is usually associated with severe forms of rheumatoid arthritis. As is true also of necrotizing scleritis, uveal pigment may be visualized through the areas of scleral thinning. Such thinning may lead to bulging. Rupture of the globe secondary to minor trauma may occur, but this is rare. The prognosis depends on the area of the globe affected but is in general poor. Corticosteroids are contraindicated. In cases of perforation or impending perforation, treatment may consist of repair of the dehiscence with a segment of homologous preserved sclera.

C. Posterior Scleritis: This is an uncommon disorder and is difficult to diagnose because of the absence of signs in the anterior segment. The disease should be suspected in patients with pain, proptosis, papilledema, and exudative retinal detachment. The disease is unilateral and is associated with severe pain, a decrease in visual acuity, diplopia, and limitation in ocular movements. Posterior scleritis is usually associated with severe rheumatoid arthritis. Recurrences may lead to extreme thinning of the sclera, giving rise to posterior staphyloma or perforation, especially when intraocular pressure is elevated. Ocular complications other than perforation include keratitis, uveitis, cataract, and glaucoma.

Scleritis is generally resistant to treatment. Topical corticosteroids should be used only with extreme caution because of their potential thinning effects on the scleral tissue and because of the possibility of increasing the intraocular pressure in certain patients. Systemic nonsteroidal anti-inflammatory agents such as salicylates, indomethacin, or ibuprofen appear to be effective in some patients. Systemic immunosuppressive agents are rarely indicated for the treatment of severe resistant forms of scleritis.

INJURIES OF THE SCLERA

The most frequently encountered injuries of the sclera are trauma (penetrating and blunt), physical damage (irradiation, thermal burns), and chemical injuries (alkali and acid burns).

Scleral wounds (lacerations) may result either from blunt trauma or from penetrating trauma caused by sharp instruments or flying objects. Scleral lacerations may be associated with intraocular hemorrhage and injury to other ocular structures. The management of scleral lacerations includes microbiologic control (surface antisepsis and the preparation of a sterile field), suturing of the wound, and excision of any prolapsed uveal tissue. Lacerations of the conjunctiva and Tenon's capsule must be approximated over the scleral wound.

HYALINE DEGENERATION

Hyaline degeneration is a fairly frequent finding in the scleras of persons over age 60. It is manifested by small, round, translucent gray areas that are usually about 2–3 mm in diameter and are located anterior to the insertion of the rectus muscles. They cause no symptoms or complications.

•   •   •

References

Bernardino ME et al: Scleral thickening: CT sign of orbital pseudotumor. *Am J Roentgenol* 1977;**129:**703.

Brown SI, Rosen J: Scleral perforation. *Arch Ophthalmol* 1975;**93:**1047.

Caldwell J, Sears M, Gilman M: Bilateral peripapillary staphyloma with normal vision. *Am J Ophthalmol* 1971;**71:**423.

Friedman AH, Henkind P: Unusual causes of episcleritis. *Trans Am Acad Ophthalmol Otolaryngol* 1974;**78:**890.

Goldberg M, Ryan S: Intercalary staphyloma in Marfan's syndrome. *Am J Ophthalmol* 1969;**67:**329.

Gregoratos N, Bartsocas C, Pappas K: Blue sclerae with keratoglobus and brittle cornea. *Br J Ophthalmol* 1971;**55:**424.

Hazleman BL: Rheumatoid arthritis and scleritis. *Trans Ophthalmol Soc UK* 1974;**94:**62.

Kielar RA: Exudative retinal detachment and scleritis in polyarteritis. *Am J Ophthalmol* 1976;**82:**694.

Lemp MA: Cornea and sclera: Annual review. *Arch Ophthalmol* 1974;**92:**158.

McGavin DDM et al: Episcleritis and scleritis: A study of their clinical manifestations and association with rheumatoid arthritis. *Br J Ophthalmol* 1976;**60:**192.

O'Connor GR: The uvea: Annual review. *Am J Ophthalmol* 1975;**93:**675.

Peyman GA, Sanders DR, Fishman GA: Sclerochorioretinal biopsy: Approach to tissue diagnosis and study of choroidal and retinal disease. *Trans Ophthalmol Soc NZ* 1977;**29:**101.

Pinnell SR: Osteogenesis imperfecta. Page 1380 in: *The Metabolic Basis of Inherited Disease.* Stanbury JB, Wyngaarden JB, Fredrickson DS (editors). McGraw-Hill, 1978.

Roper-Hall MJ: A retrospective study of eye injuries. *Ophthalmologica* 1969;**158:**12.

Ruedemann A: Osteogenesis imperfecta congenita and blue sclerotics. *Arch Ophthalmol* 1953;**49:**6.

Watson PG, Hazleman BL: *The Sclera and Systemic Disorders.* Saunders, 1976.

Wilhemus KR et al: Scleritis and glaucoma. *Am J Ophthalmol* 1981;**91:**697.

10 | Uveal Tract

The uveal tract is composed of 3 parts: the iris, the ciliary body, and the choroid. It is the middle, vascular layer of the eye, protected externally by the cornea and sclera. It contributes to the blood supply of the retina.

Anatomy of the Iris

The iris is the anterior extension of the ciliary body. It presents a relatively flat surface with a round aperture in the middle called the pupil. It forms the posterior wall of the anterior chamber and the anterior wall of the posterior chamber. The pupil varies in size and has the same form and function as the aperture of a camera lens. The iris is in contact with the lens and the aqueous posteriorly and with the aqueous anteriorly. It has 2 zones on its anterior surface, the ciliary and pupillary zones. The sphincter and dilator muscles, which serve to constrict and dilate the pupil, are in the iris stroma.

Because of the presence of a thick collagenous adventitia, normal iris vessels have the histologic appearance of being quite sclerotic. The iris capillaries have an unfenestrated endothelium and hence do not normally leak intravenously injected fluorescein. The 2 layers of epithelium on the posterior surface are heavily pigmented and represent the anterior extension of the pigmented epithelium of the retina as well as the retina proper. The blood supply is from the major circle of the iris (Fig 1–9). The nerve supply is described in Chapter 17.

When the iris is cut, as in doing a small peripheral iridectomy for acute angle-closure glaucoma, it seldom bleeds, and the wound remains permanently with no tendency to heal. Pain fibers are present, as is shown by the pain caused by traction on the iris during surgery.

Anatomy of the Ciliary Body

The ciliary body, roughly triangular in cross section, extends forward from the anterior termination of the choroid to the root of the iris, a distance of about 6 mm. Grossly it consists of 2 zones: the corona ciliaris, the corrugated anterior 2 mm; and the pars plana, the smoother and flatter posterior 4 mm. The surface of the corona ciliaris consists of many elevations and depressions.

There are 2 layers of ciliary epithelium, the external pigmented and the internal nonpigmented, both of which continue as pigmented layers over the posterior surface of the iris. The pigment epithelium represents the forward extension of the pigment epithelium of the retina.

The ciliary muscle consists of longitudinal, radial, and circular portions. Its function is to contract and relax the zonular fibers. This results in altered tension on the capsule of the lens, which gives the lens variable focus for both near and more distant objects in the field of vision. The ciliary processes themselves are composed mainly of capillaries and veins that drain through vortex veins. The capillaries are large and fenestrated and hence leak intravenously injected fluorescein.

The pars plana consists of a thin layer of ciliary muscle and vessels covered by ciliary epithelium. The zonular fibers, which hold the lens in place, originate in the valleys between the ciliary processes (Fig 10–1). The blood vessels to the ciliary body come from the

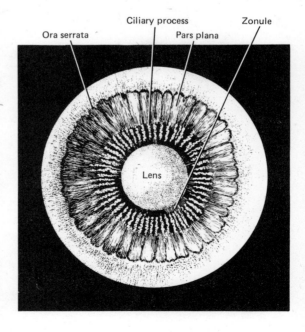

Figure 10–1. Posterior view of ciliary body, zonule, lens, and ora serrata. (Redrawn and reproduced, with permission, from Wolff E: *Anatomy of the Eye and Orbit,* 4th ed. Blakiston-McGraw, 1954.)

major circle of the iris (Fig 1–9). The sensory nerve supply is through the ciliary nerves.

Anatomy of the Choroid (Fig 10–2)

The choroid (the posterior portion of the uveal tract and the middle coat of the eye) lies between the retina and the sclera. It is largely composed of blood vessels. The choroidal vessels are bounded by Bruch's membrane internally and the suprachoroid externally. The avascular suprachoroid is composed of lamellas of collagenous and elastic tissue. Bruch's membrane can be divided into 3 portions: an outer elastic sheath, a middle collagenous sheath, and an inner cuticular sheath. (The latter is actually the basement membrane of the retinal pigment epithelium.)

The lumens of the blood vessels increase the deeper they are located in the choroid. There are 3 layers of blood vessels: large, medium, and small. The innermost layer of small blood vessels is known as the choriocapillaris and consists of large capillaries that nourish the outer portion of the retina. The endothelium of these capillaries is fenestrated and hence leaks intravenously injected fluorescein. Most of the large vessels consist of veins. These coalesce and leave the eye as the 4 vortex veins, one in each of the 4 posterior quadrants. The vessel layers of the choroid also contain some elastic fibers and chromatophores.

The choroid is firmly attached to the margin of the optic nerve posteriorly and extends to the ora serrata anteriorly, where it joins the ciliary body.

Functions of Uveal Structures

The function of the iris is to control the amount of light that enters the eye. This occurs by reflex constriction of the pupil under the stimulus of light and dilatation of the pupil in darkness. The ciliary body forms the root of the iris and serves, through the zonular fibers, to govern the size of the lens in accommodation. Aqueous humor is secreted by the ciliary processes into the posterior chamber. The choroid consists of abundant blood vessels; its function is to nourish the outer portion of the underlying retina.

Physiology of Symptoms

Symptoms of uveal tract disorders depend upon the site of the disease process. For example, since there are pain fibers in the iris, the patient with iritis will complain of moderate pain and photophobia. Inflammation of the iris itself does not cause blurring of vision unless the process is severe or advanced enough to cause clouding of the aqueous, cornea, or lens. Choroidal disease itself does not cause pain or blurred vision. Because of the close contact of the choroid with the retina, choroidal disease almost always affects the retina (eg, chorioretinitis). If the macular area of the retina is involved, central vision will be impaired.

The vitreous may also become cloudy as a result of posterior uveitis. The impairment of vision is in proportion to the density of vitreous opacity and is reversible as the inflammation subsides and the vitreous haze clears.

The physician examines for disease of the anterior uveal tract with the flashlight and loupe or slit lamp, and disease of the posterior uveal tract with the ophthalmoscope.

UVEITIS*

Inflammation of the uveal tract has many causes and may involve one or all 3 portions simultaneously. The most frequent form of uveitis is acute anterior

*"Uveitis" is a general term for inflammatory disorders of the uveal tract. "Anterior uveitis" is the preferred general term for iritis and iridocyclitis. "Posterior uveitis" is the preferred term for choroiditis and chorioretinitis. The term "iritis," used above, means acute anterior nongranulomatous uveitis.

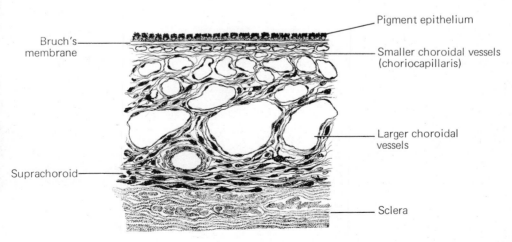

Figure 10–2. Cross section of choroid. (Redrawn and reproduced, with permission, from Wolff E: *Anatomy of the Eye and Orbit,* 4th ed. Blakiston-McGraw, 1954.)

Table 10–1. Differentiation of granulomatous and nongranulomatous uveitis.

	Nongranulomatous	Granulomatous
Onset	Acute	Insidious
Pain	Marked	None or minimal
Photophobia	Marked	Slight
Blurred vision	Moderate	Marked
Circumcorneal flush	Marked	Slight
Keratic precipitates	Fine white	Large gray ("mutton fat")
Pupil	Small and irregular	Small and irregular (variable)
Posterior synechiae	Sometimes	Sometimes
Anterior chamber	Flare predominates	Cells predominate
Iris nodules	Sometimes	Sometimes
Vitreous haze	Absent	Sometimes
Site	Anterior tract	Posterior tract (variable)
Course	Acute	Chronic
Prognosis	Good	Fair to poor
Recurrence	Common	Sometimes

uveitis (iritis), usually unilateral and characterized by a history of pain, photophobia, and blurring of vision; a red eye (circumcorneal flush) without purulent discharge; and a small pupil. It is important to make the diagnosis early and to dilate the pupil to prevent the formation of permanent posterior synechiae.

Inflammatory disorders of the uveal tract, usually unilateral, are common principally in the young and middle age groups. In most cases the cause is not known. In posterior uveitis the retina is almost always secondarily affected. This is known as chorioretinitis.

Two major types of uveitis may be distinguished upon clinical as well as pathologic grounds: nongranulomatous (more common) and granulomatous (Table 10–1).* Because pathogenic organisms have not been found in the nongranulomatous type and because it responds to corticosteroid therapy, it is thought to be a hypersensitivity phenomenon. Granulomatous uveitis usually follows active microbial invasion of the tissues by the causative organism (eg, *Mycobacterium tuberculosis* or *Toxoplasma gondii*). However, these pathogens are rarely recovered, and a definite etiologic diagnosis is seldom possible. The possibilities can often be narrowed down by clinical and laboratory examination.

Nongranulomatous uveitis occurs mainly in the anterior portion of the tract, ie, the iris and ciliary body. There is an inflammatory reaction, as evidenced by the cellular infiltration of lymphocytes and plasma cells in significant numbers and an occasional mononuclear cell. In severe cases, a large fibrin clot or a hypopyon may form in the anterior chamber.

Granulomatous uveitis may involve any portion

*The clinical differentiation of the 2 types is not always clear. In some clinics, this classification has been discarded in favor of an anatomic differentiation into 3 types: anterior, posterior, and diffuse.

of the uveal tract but has a predilection for the posterior uvea. Nodular collections of epithelioid cells and giant cells surrounded by lymphocytes are present in the affected areas. Inflammatory deposits on the posterior surface of the cornea are composed mainly of macrophages and epithelioid cells. It is possible to make a specific etiologic diagnosis histologically in an enucleated eye by identifying the cysts of *Toxoplasma,* the acid-fast bacillus of tuberculosis, the spirochete of syphilis, the distinctive granulomatous appearance of sarcoidosis and sympathetic ophthalmia, and a few other rare specific causes.

Clinical Findings

A. Symptoms and Signs: In the nongranulomatous form, the onset is characteristically acute, with pain, injection, photophobia, and blurred vision. There is a circumcorneal flush caused by dilated limbal blood vessels. Fine white deposits (keratic precipitates, "KPs") on the posterior surface of the cornea can be seen with the slit lamp or with a loupe. The pupil is small, and there may be a collection of fibrin with cells in the anterior chamber. If posterior synechiae are present, the pupil will be irregular in shape (Figs 10–3 to 10–6). Posterior uveitis is generally classified as granulomatous.

The patient should be asked about previous episodes of arthritis and possible exposure to toxoplasmosis, histoplasmosis, tuberculosis, and syphilis. The remote possibility of a focus of infection elsewhere in the body should also be investigated.

In granulomatous uveitis (which may cause anterior uveitis, posterior uveitis, or both), the onset is usually insidious. Vision gradually becomes blurred, and the affected eye becomes diffusely red with circumcorneal flush. Pain is minimal, and photophobia is less marked than in the nongranulomatous form. The pupil is often constricted and becomes irregular as posterior synechiae form. Large "mutton fat" KPs on the posterior surface of the cornea may be seen with the slit lamp. Flare and cells are seen in the anterior chamber, and nodules consisting of clusters of white cells are seen on the pupillary margin of the iris (Koeppe nodules). These nodules are the equivalent of the mutton fat KPs.

Fresh active lesions of the choroid and retina appear as yellowish-white patches seen hazily with the ophthalmoscope through the cloudy vitreous. Such posterior cases are generally classified as granulomatous disease. Because of the intimate relationship of the choroid and retina, the retina is nearly always involved (chorioretinitis). As healing progresses, the vitreous haze lessens, and pigmentation occurs gradually at the edges of the yellowish-white spots. In the healed stage, there is usually considerable pigment deposition. If the macula has not been involved, recovery of central vision is complete. The patient is usually not aware of the scotoma in the peripheral field corresponding to the scarred area.

B. Laboratory Findings: Extensive laboratory investigation is usually not indicated in anterior

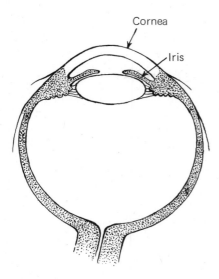

Figure 10–3. Normal anterior chamber.

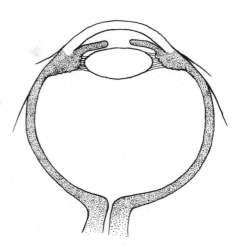

Figure 10–4. Anterior synechiae (adhesions). The peripheral iris adheres to the cornea.

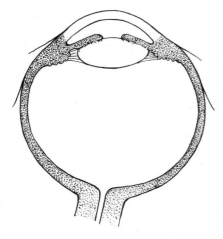

Figure 10–5. Posterior synechiae. The iris adheres to the lens.

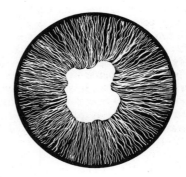

Figure 10–6. Posterior synechiae (anterior view). The iris is adherent to the lens in several places as a result of previous inflammation, causing an irregular fixed pupil.

uveitis, particularly if it is nongranulomatous or is readily responsive to nonspecific treatment. In persistent nonresponsive anterior or posterior uveitis, an attempt should be made to arrive at an etiologic diagnosis. Skin tests for tuberculosis and histoplasmosis may be helpful, as well as complement fixation tests and methylene blue dye tests (toxoplasmosis). On the basis of these tests and the clinical appearance, it is often possible to make an etiologic diagnosis.

Differential Diagnosis

In conjunctivitis, vision is not blurred, pupillary responses are normal, a discharge is present, and there is usually no pain, photophobia, or ciliary injection.

In keratitis or keratoconjunctivitis, vision may be blurred and pain and photophobia may be present. Some causes of keratitis such as herpes simplex and herpes zoster may be associated with a true anterior uveitis.

In acute glaucoma the pupil is dilated, there are no posterior synechiae, and the cornea is steamy.

After repeated attacks, nongranulomatous uveitis may acquire the characteristics of granulomatous uveitis. In recent years there has been less emphasis on this differentiation, and some authorities are disregarding it completely. Nevertheless, the differentiation is still of value as a guide to treatment and prognosis.

Complications & Sequelae

Anterior uveitis may produce peripheral anterior

Table 10–2. Treatment of granulomatous uveitis.

	Anti-infective Chemotherapy	Use of Corticosteroids
Toxoplasmosis	If central vision is threatened, give pyrimethamine (Daraprim), 75 mg orally as a loading dose for 2 days followed by 25 mg once daily for 4 weeks, in combination with trisulfapyrimidines (sulfadiazine, sulfamerazine, and sulfamethazine, 0.167 g of each per tablet), 4 g orally as loading dose followed by 1 g 4 times daily for 4 weeks. If a fall in the white or platelet count occurs during therapy, give folinic acid (leucovorin), 1 mL IM twice weekly or 3 mg orally 3 times a week.	If the response is not favorable after 2 weeks, continue anti-infective therapy and give systemic corticosteroids, eg, prednisolone, 20–25 mg 4 times a day for 1 week, followed by 60–120 mg every other day thereafter,* to protect the macula. Corticosteroids may activate the organisms of toxoplasmosis and tuberculosis but are given as a calculated risk to control the inflammatory response when it threatens vision.
Tuberculosis	Isoniazid, 100 mg 3 times daily, and aminosalicylic acid (PAS), 4 g 3 times daily after meals. If PAS is not tolerated, give streptomycin, 1 g IM twice weekly. Continue treatment for 4–6 months.	If a favorable response does not occur in 6 weeks, continue antimycobacterial therapy and give systemic corticosteroids, eg, prednisolone, 40–80 mg every other day for 2 months.*
Sarcoidosis	Treat with local corticosteroids and mydriatics and, during active stages, with systemic corticosteroids such as prednisolone, 40–80 mg every other day.* Give supplemental potassium chloride, 2 g 3 times daily. The usual contraindications to systemic corticosteroid therapy apply.	
Sympathetic ophthalmia	Treat with local corticosteroids and mydriatics and systemic corticosteroids in high doses, eg, prednisolone, 40–120 mg every other day.* The usual contraindications to systemic corticosteroid therapy apply, and the drugs may be needed in higher doses and for a longer time. Therefore, management of the side-effects is often more difficult. In severe cases that fail to respond to corticosteroids, treatment with antimetabolites and alkylating agents has met with some success. *Caution:* White blood counts and platelets must be monitored very carefully in these patients, and these drugs should not be used without careful consideration.	

*Administration every other day has been advocated to minimize the effects of stress and make drug withdrawal easier and safer.

synechiae (Fig 10–4), which impede aqueous outflow at the anterior chamber angle and cause glaucoma. Posterior synechiae can cause glaucoma by impeding the flow of aqueous from the posterior to the anterior chamber. Early and constant pupillary dilatation lessens the likelihood of posterior synechiae. Interference with lens metabolism may cause cataract. Retinal detachment occasionally occurs as a result of traction on the retina by vitreous strands. Cystoid macular edema and degeneration can result from long-standing anterior uveitis.

Treatment

A. Nongranulomatous Uveitis: Symptomatic measures include warm compresses for 10 minutes 3–4 times a day, systemic analgesics as necessary for pain, and dark glasses for photophobia. The pupil must be kept dilated with atropine, 1%, 1 drop at least twice daily. Local steroid drops are usually quite effective for their anti-inflammatory action. In severe and unresponsive cases, systemic steroids are given also.

B. Granulomatous Uveitis: If the process includes the anterior segment, pupillary dilatation with atropine, 2%, is indicated. Since it is often possible to make a tentative or likely diagnosis of the cause, an attempt at specific therapy is indicated as outlined in Table 10–2.

C. Treatment of Complications: Glaucoma is a common complication. Treatment of the uveitis is of primary importance, particularly dilating the pupil with atropine (not constricting the pupil, as with all forms of primary glaucoma). Carbonic anhydrase inhibitors often effectively reduce intraocular tension by depressing aqueous production. Epinephrine also lowers intraocular pressure by reducing ciliary body secretion of aqueous.

Cataract frequently develops in chronic uveitis. The eye tolerates removal of such cataracts very poorly; but if vision is poor enough, cataract surgery may be essential. Retinal detachment is also very difficult to treat successfully surgically when it occurs in association with uveitis.

Course & Prognosis

With treatment, an attack of nongranulomatous uveitis usually lasts a few days to weeks. Recurrences are common.

Granulomatous uveitis lasts months to years, sometimes with remissions and exacerbations, and may cause permanent damage with marked visual loss despite the best available treatment. The prognosis for a focal peripheral chorioretinal lesion is considerably better, often healing well with no significant visual loss.

SPECIFIC TYPES OF UVEITIS
(Uveitis Syndromes)

UVEITIS ASSOCIATED WITH JOINT DISEASE

About 20% of children with **rheumatoid arthritis (Still's disease)** develop a chronic bilateral nongranulomatous iridocyclitis. Females are far more commonly affected than males (4:1). The average age

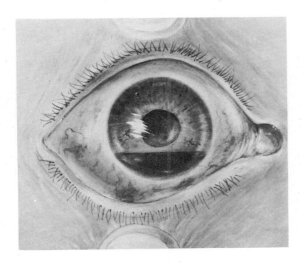

Figure 10–7. Blood in the anterior chamber (hyphema) associated with rheumatoid iridocyclitis. (Courtesy of M Hogan.)

at which the uveitis is detected is 5½ years. In most cases the onset is insidious, the disease being discovered only when the child is noted to have a difference in the color of the 2 eyes, a difference in the size or shape of the pupil, or the onset of strabismus. There is no correlation between the onset of the arthritis and of the uveitis. The uveitis may precede the arthritis by 3–10 years. The knee is the most common joint involved. The cardinal signs of the disease are calcific band keratopathy, cells and flare in the anterior chamber, small to medium-sized white keratic precipitates with or without flecks of fibrin on the endothelium, posterior synechiae, often progressing to seclusion of the pupil, complicated cataract, variable secondary glaucoma, and macular edema.

Corticosteroids and mydriatics are of value, especially in acute exacerbations, but their long-term effect seems merely to delay the inevitable, ie, severe visual impairment or phthisis bulbi. The prognosis is very poor because of the relentless and progressive character of the disease, which leads to serious complications. These patients tend to do poorly after surgery.

Iridocyclitis occurring in association with adult peripheral rheumatoid arthritis is strictly coincidental. The adult group is more likely to develop scleritis and sclero-uveitis. It is unfortunate that the associated cells and flare in the aqueous humor that accompany the scleritis have been misinterpreted as "iridocyclitis."

About 10–60% of patients with **Marie-Strümpell ankylosing spondylitis** develop an anterior uveitis. There is a marked preponderance in males. The uveitis presents as a mild to fairly severe nongranulomatous type of iridocyclitis with moderate to severe ciliary injection, pain, blurred vision, and photophobia. It is usually recurrent and eventually may lead to permanent damage if not adequately treated. Histocompatibility antigen HLA-B27 is present in approximately 90% of patients with ankylosing spondylitis.

Ocular examination shows ciliary injection, moderate cells and flare in the anterior chamber, and fine white keratic precipitates located mostly on the inferior cornea. Posterior synechiae, peripheral anterior synechiae, cataracts, and glaucoma are common complications after hyperacute attacks of inflammation. Macular edema occurs in 1% of cases with severe anterior iridocyclitis, which, if persistent, leads to cystoid degeneration and loss of central vision.

Confirmation of the diagnosis is by x-rays of the lumbosacral spine. In about 50% of patients, clinical signs and symptoms may all be absent so that the diagnosis may be made only by the radiologist.

The erythrocyte sedimentation rate, although nonspecific and sometimes normal in mild cases, is elevated in most patients, indicating active disease. The rheumatoid factor (F II) test, however, is negative in all but 5% of patients with this disease.

HETEROCHROMIC UVEITIS
(Fuchs's Heterochromic Iridocyclitis)

This disease of unknown cause accounts for about 3% of all cases of uveitis. It is essentially a quiet cyclitis associated with depigmentation of the iris in the affected eye. Pathologically, the iris and ciliary body show moderate atrophy, patchy depigmentation of the pigment layer, and diffuse infiltration of lymphocytes and plasma cells. Involvement is typically unilateral but may be bilateral, and the eyes are of different colors. Early in the course of the disease, the difference in color may not be readily apparent and is best noted in daylight.

The onset is insidious in the third or fourth decade, with no redness, pain, or photophobia; the patient is often unaware of the disorder until cataract formation results in blurred vision.

With the slit lamp (or loupe) one sees fine white deposits on the posterior corneal surface, flare and cells in the anterior chamber, and a slightly atrophic iris. Anterior vitreous floaters may be evident with the ophthalmoscope or slit lamp.

Cataract develops within a few years in about 15% of cases. Glaucoma occurs in 10–15% of cases. It is usually not necessary to dilate the pupil, as this is one type of uveitis in which posterior synechiae rarely form. The disease does not subside spontaneously, but the visual prognosis is good since the cataract can usually be removed safely despite the low-grade active uveitis.

CHRONIC CYCLITIS
(Pars Planitis)

The usual patient with chronic pars planitis is a young adult presenting with "floating spots" in the field of vision as the chief complaint. In the majority of cases, both eyes are affected. The sex distribution is equal. Pain, redness, and photophobia do not occur. The patient may be unaware of any ocular problem, but the physician detects vitreous opacities with the ophthalmoscope.

There are few, if any, signs of anterior uveitis. A few cells may occasionally be seen in the anterior chamber; rarely, anterior or posterior synechiae occur. Inflammatory cells are more likely to be seen in the retrolental space or in the anterior vitreous on slit lamp examination. Posterior subcapsular cataract occurs frequently.

Indirect ophthalmoscopy often reveals soft, round, white opacities over the peripheral retina. These cellular exudates may be confluent, often overlying the pars plana. Some of these patients may also have vasculitis, as shown by perivascular sheathing of retinal vessels.

In most patients, the disease remains stationary or gradually improves over a 5- to 10-year period. Some patients develop cystoid macular edema and permanent scarring as well as posterior subcapsular cataracts. In severe cases, cyclitic membranes and retinal detachments may occur. Secondary glaucoma is a rare complication.

The cause is unknown. Corticosteroids constitute the only helpful treatment and should only be used in more severe cases, especially when there is decreased vision secondary to macular edema. Topical corticosteroids are used first; if they fail, sub-Tenon or retrobulbar injections of corticosteroids may be effective. Such treatment increases the risk of cataract development. Fortunately, these patients do well following cataract surgery.

LENS-INDUCED UVEITIS

There are no data at present to substantiate the implication that lens material per se is toxic, so that the term phacotoxic uveitis should no longer be used to describe lens-induced uveitis. The terms phacogenic or lens-induced uveitis are more appropriate when referring to an autoimmune disease secondary to lens antigen. The classic case of lens-induced uveitis occurs when the lens develops a hypermature cataract. The lens capsule leaks and lens material passes into the anterior chamber, causing an inflammatory reaction characterized by the accumulation of plasma cells, mononuclear phagocytes, and a few polymorphonuclear cells. The eye becomes red and moderately painful; the pupil is small; and vision is markedly reduced (at times to light perception only). Lens-induced uveitis may also occur following traumatic cataracts.

Endophthalmitis phaco-anaphylactica, the term used for the more severe form of lens-induced uveitis, occurs following an extracapsular lens extraction when the same operation has already been performed on the fellow eye and the patient has been sensitized to his or her own lens material. Many polymorphonuclear leukocytes and mononuclear phagocytes appear in the anterior chamber. The eye becomes red and painful, and vision is blurred. Since most of the lens material has already been removed, treatment is conservative, consisting of corticosteroids locally and systemically plus atropine drops to keep the pupil dilated. If this is ineffective, the cataract incision must be opened and the anterior chamber irrigated.

Glaucoma (phacolytic glaucoma) is a common complication of lens-induced uveitis. Treatment consists of lens extraction after intraocular pressure has been brought under control. If this is done, both the uveitis and the glaucoma are cured, and the visual prognosis is good if the process has not been present for more than 1–2 weeks.

SYMPATHETIC OPHTHALMIA
(Sympathetic Uveitis)

Sympathetic ophthalmia is a rare but devastating granulomatous bilateral uveitis that comes on 10 days to many years following a perforating eye injury in the region of the ciliary body, or following retained foreign body. The cause is not known, but the disease is probably related to hypersensitivity to uveal pigment. It very rarely occurs following uncomplicated intraocular surgery for cataract or glaucoma.

The injured (exciting) eye becomes inflamed first and the fellow (sympathizing) eye second. Pathologically, there is a diffuse granulomatous uveitis. The epithelioid cells, together with giant cells and lymphocytes (Fig 10–8), form noncaseating tubercles. From the uveal tract the inflammatory process spreads to the optic nerve and to the pia and arachnoid surrounding the optic nerve.

The patient complains of photophobia, redness, and blurring of vision. If a history of trauma is obtained, look for a scar representing the wound of entry in the exciting eye. With the slit lamp or loupe one sees

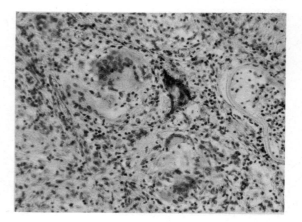

Figure 10–8. Microscopic section of giant cells and lymphocytes in sympathetic ophthalmia involving the choroid. (Courtesy of R Carriker.)

KPs and a flare in the anterior chamber of both eyes. Iris nodules may be present.

Sympathetic ophthalmia may be differentiated from other granulomatous uveitides by the history of trauma or ocular surgery and by the fact that it is bilateral, diffuse, and (usually) acute rather than unilateral, localized, and chronic.

The recommended treatment of a severely injured sightless eye (eg, a penetrating injury through the sclera, ciliary body, and lens, with loss of vitreous) is immediate enucleation to prevent sympathetic ophthalmia, and every effort must be made to secure the patient's informed consent to the operation. If enucleation can be performed within 10 days after injury, there is almost no chance that sympathetic ophthalmia will develop. However, when the inflammation in the sympathizing eye is advanced, it is wise not to enucleate the injured eye, since it may eventually prove to be the better of 2 very bad eyes.

If inflammation appears in the sympathizing eye, treat at once with local corticosteroids and atropine. Systemic corticosteroids may be required.

Without treatment, the disease progresses slowly but relentlessly over a period of months or years to complete bilateral blindness.

TUBERCULOUS UVEITIS

Tuberculosis causes a granulomatous type of uveitis. Tuberculous uveitis is diagnosed clinically far more often than the disease can be proved by positive identification of tubercle bacilli in the tissues. Although the infection is said to be transmitted from a primary focus elsewhere in the body, uveal tuberculosis is rare in patients with active pulmonary tuberculosis.

Tuberculous uveitis may be diffuse but is characteristically localized in the form of a severe caseating granulomatous chorioretinitis. The tubercle itself consists of giant cells and epithelioid cells. Caseation necrosis commonly occurs.

The patient complains of blurred vision, and the eye is moderately injected. If the anterior segment is involved, iris nodules and "mutton fat" KPs are visible on slit lamp examination. If the choroid and retina are primarily affected, one can see a localized yellowish mass partially obscured by a hazy vitreous.

The nodules and the localized nature of tuberculous uveitis help to make a clinical differentiation from sympathetic ophthalmia, and the caseation necrosis differentiates it pathologically from sympathetic ophthalmia and Boeck's sarcoid.

The pupil should be kept dilated with atropine, 1%, 1 drop 2–3 times daily. Antituberculosis drugs should be prescribed systemically if a reasonably certain clinical diagnosis can be made. (See Table 10–2.)

After a prolonged course of several months, the disease usually resolves, leaving permanently damaged tissue and blurred vision because of scarring of the retina.

SARCOIDOSIS
(Boeck's Sarcoid)

Sarcoidosis is a chronic granulomatous disease of unknown cause characterized by multiple cutaneous and subcutaneous nodules with similar invasions in the viscera and bones and periodic exacerbations and remissions. The onset is usually in the third decade. The tissue reaction is much less severe than in tuberculous uveitis, and caseation does not occur. The tuberculin skin test is usually negative or only faintly positive. When the parotid glands are involved, the disease is called uveoparotid fever (Heerfordt's disease); when the lacrimal glands are involved, it is called Mikulicz's syndrome.

Thirty percent of cases are complicated by chronic bilateral anterior uveitis, whereas posterior uveitis is far less common. Anterior uveitis is nodular, and in prolonged cases it may lead to severe visual impairment due to cataract and secondary glaucoma. Posterior uveitis is characterized by multiple whitish-yellow retinal exudates and perivasculitis.

Diagnosis is best aided by positive biopsy of the cutaneous nodules. In a small number of cases, typical nodules were also found on the tarsal or bulbar conjunctiva.

Corticosteroid therapy (Table 10–2) given early in the disease may be effective, but recurrences are common and the long-term visual prognosis is poor.

TOXOPLASMIC UVEITIS

Toxoplasmosis is primarily an inflammation of the central nervous system caused by *T gondii*, a protozoan parasite. In congenital toxoplasmosis, chorioretinitis is almost invariably present. Toxoplasmosis acquired in later life does not usually involve the eye in the acute stage, but chorioretinitis may occur in the chronic form.

The disease is more common in tropical countries.* Pathologically, there is a granulomatous retinochoroiditis. The retina is characteristically necrotic, and *Toxoplasma* organisms are found in the retinal tissues. The clinical picture is variable, but typically there is a chorioretinal lesion or lesions, usually in the macular area, which in the early stages appear as elevated white masses partially obscured by a hazy vitreous. In the later stages, a punched-out pigmented chorioretinal lesion develops through which the sclera may be clearly visible. The methylene blue dye test on the patient's serum is positive, ie, antibodies in the

---

*The cat is the definitive host of *T gondii*. The parasite is a coccidian undergoing typical schizogonic cycles and gametogony in the intestinal epithelial cells of the cat. Intermediate hosts such as rodents, birds, or humans become infected by ingestion of the oocysts passed in cat feces. Additional means of transmission among intermediate hosts include carnivorousness with ingestion of trophozoites or cysts present mainly in brain and muscle tissue. The ingestion of raw meat is an established source of the disease.

serum prevent the dye from staining *Toxoplasma* organisms.

Although the pathology of the retinochoroiditis is essentially the same, there are 2 distinct clinical types of ocular toxoplasmosis: congenital and acquired. The congenital type is due to intrauterine infection. As in the acquired (adult) type, the chorioretinitis is usually confined to the macular area. The inflammatory process is more severe in congenital than in acquired toxoplasmosis and is frequently bilateral. Cerebral involvement, with radiopaque calcification and mental deficiency, is present in 10% of cases of the congenital type.

Acquired ocular toxoplasmosis is usually milder than congenital toxoplasmosis. It may appear at any age, is often unilateral, and frequently occurs in the absence of central nervous system involvement. The patient complains of blurred vision if the macula is involved.

For treatment, see Table 10–2.

Clindamycin, a chlorinated lincomycin derivative, appears to hold great promise for the treatment of ocular toxoplasmosis. A combination of subconjunctival and intramuscular injections of clindamycin phosphate has brought about rapid healing of the ocular lesions in rabbits and has made it impossible to recover *Toxoplasma* organisms from the minced tissues of experimentally infected eyes. It appears also that clindamycin may be able to penetrate *Toxoplasma* cysts (Fig 10–9).

Although the search for new, more efficacious drugs for the treatment of ocular toxoplasmosis will continue, many investigators believe that the ultimate cure of the disease must come from destruction of the organism by macrophages. Research on ways to promote or augment the effects of activated macrophages on *Toxoplasma* continues.

The chorioretinitis progresses to a healed stage, leaving a scarred retina and choroid. If the macula has been involved, loss of central vision is permanent.

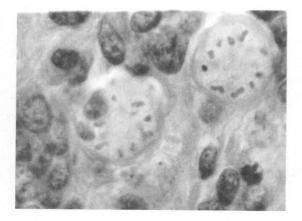

Figure 10–9. *Toxoplasma* cysts in the retina. (Courtesy of K Tabbara.)

HISTOPLASMOSIS

In some areas of the USA where histoplasmosis is endemic (eg, Cincinnati, Baltimore), the diagnosis of choroiditis presumably due to histoplasmosis is being made with increasing frequency. The patient usually has a positive skin test to histoplasmin and demonstrates "punched-out" spots in the peripheral fundus. These spots are small, irregularly round or oval, depigmented areas, sometimes with a fine pigmented border. They are smaller and have less pigment than the usual healed chorioretinal lesion. Peripapillary atrophy and hyperpigmentation are usually present. Macular lesions that begin as small edematous areas and may progress to hemorrhagic detachments are the most visually threatening feature of the disease. Vitreous haze does not occur.

It has been postulated that in areas where histoplasmosis is endemic, many persons develop a benign form of asymptomatic peripheral chorioretinitis. These lesions soon heal, leaving "histo" spots. This exposure sensitizes the choroid. A later antigenic insult to the choroid results in the observed macular changes. However, this hypothesis has not been verified.

Many types of treatment have been advocated, including systemic corticosteroids, amphotericin B (Fungizone), antihistamines, intradermal desensitization with histoplasmin, and photocoagulation of areas of perimacular leakage. The results have been questionable in all cases, and treatment with amphotericin B is now contraindicated.

Xenon and laser photocoagulation can be effective treatment for those paramacular lesions that cause leaks demonstrable by fluorescein angiography. This form of treatment has limited application since most lesions involve the macula directly and are thus not suitable for coagulation.

TOXOCARIASIS

Toxocara canis and *Toxocara cati* are common dog and cat ascarids that can cause uveitis, usually in children, and nearly always unilaterally. The ova are excreted in the feces of affected animals and contaminate dirt. They are then ingested, usually by children who have handled the contaminated soil. The ova hatch in the intestine and burrow into the intestinal wall to reach the bloodstream, which can carry the organism to any part of the body, including the eye.

The ocular involvement most often takes the form of a localized choroidal granuloma, but a chronic endophthalmitis can occur. Such extensive involvement can closely resemble retinoblastoma, Coats's disease, bacterial or fungal endophthalmitis, or exudative retinitis, thus making differential diagnosis most important.

There is no effective treatment.

• • •

References

Aaberg TM, Cesarz TJ, Flickinger RR: Treatment of peripheral uveoretinitis by cryotherapy. *Am J Ophthalmol* 1973;**75**:685.

Abrams J, Schlaegel TF Jr: The role of the isoniazid therapeutic test in tuberculous uveitis. *Am J Ophthalmol* 1982;**94**:511.

Allen JC: Sympathetic uveitis and phacoanaphylaxis. *Am J Ophthalmol* 1967;**63**:280.

Asbury T: The status of presumed ocular histoplasmosis, including a report of a survey. *Trans Am Ophthalmol Soc* 1966;**64**:371.

Barr CC et al: Uveal melanoma in children and adolescents. *Arch Ophthalmol* 1981;**99**:2133.

Bell R, Font RL: Granulomatous anterior uveitis caused by *Coccidioides immitis. Am J Ophthalmol* 1972;**74**:93.

Biglan AW, Glickman LT, Lobes LA: Serum and vitreous *Toxocara* antibody in nematode endophthalmitis. *Am J Ophthalmol* 1979;**88**:898.

Campinchi R et al: *Uveitis: Immunologic and Allergic Phenomena.* Thomas, 1973.

Chamberlain MA: Behçet's syndrome in 32 patients in Yorkshire. *Ann Rheum Dis* 1977;**36**:491.

Coles RS: Uveitis associated with systemic disease. (2 parts.) *Surv Ophthalmol* 1963;**8**:377, 479.

Duane TD (editor): *Clinical Ophthalmology,* Vol 4. Harper & Row, 1981.

Dunlap EA (editor): *Gordon's Medical Management of Ocular Disease,* 2nd ed. Harper & Row, 1976.

Elliott JH et al: Mycotic endophthalmitis in drug abusers. *Am J Ophthalmol* 1979;**88**:66.

Fraunfelder FT: *Drug-Induced Ocular Side-Effects and Drug Interactions.* Lea & Febiger, 1976.

Gass JD: Observation of suspected choroidal and ciliary body melanomas for evidence of growth prior to enucleation. *Ophthalmology* 1980;**87**:523.

Gibson JD et al: Re-examination of histocompatibility antigens found in patients with juvenile rheumatoid arthritis. *N Engl J Med* 1975;**293**:636.

Havener WH: *Ocular Pharmacology,* 4th ed. Mosby, 1978.

Hunter PFL, Fowler PD, Wilkinson P: Treatment of anterior uveitis. *Br J Ophthalmol* 1973;**57**:892.

Irvine SR, Irvine AR Jr: Lens induced uveitis and glaucoma. (4 parts.) *Am J Ophthalmol* 1952;**35**:177, 370, 375, 498.

Kazdan JJ, McCulloch JC, Crawford JS: Uveitis in children. *Can Med Assoc J* 1967;**96**:385.

Kimura SJ, Caygill WM (editors): *Differential Diagnostic Problems of Posterior Uveitis.* Lea & Febiger, 1966.

Kimura SJ, Hogan MJ: Chronic cyclitis. *Arch Ophthalmol* 1964;**71**:193.

Makley TA, Azar A: Sympathetic ophthalmia. *Arch Ophthalmol* 1978;**96**:257.

Mapstone R, Woodrow JC: HL-A 27 and acute anterior uveitis. *Br J Ophthalmol* 1975;**59**:270.

Maumenee AE: Uveitis in relation to connective tissue disease. *Trans Ophthalmol Soc UK* 1974;**94**:807.

Morse PH, Duke JR: Sympathetic ophthalmitis. *Am J Ophthalmol* 1969;**68**:508.

Newman PE et al: The role of hypersensitivity to *Toxoplasma* antigens in experimental ocular toxoplasmosis in non-human primates. *Am J Ophthalmol* 1982;**94**:159.

Obenauf CD et al: Sarcoidosis and its ocular manifestations. *Am J Ophthalmol* 1973;**75**:82.

O'Connor GR: Current concepts in ophthalmology: Uveitis and the immunologically compromised host. *N Engl J Med* 1978;**299**:130.

Ohno S et al: Vogt-Koyanagi-Harada syndrome. *Am J Ophthalmol* 1977;**83**:735.

Rollins DF et al: Minocycline in experimental ocular toxoplasmosis in the rabbit. *Am J Ophthalmol* 1982;**93**:361.

Roth AM: *Histoplasma capsulatum* in the presumed ocular histoplasmosis syndrome. *Am J Ophthalmol* 1977;**84**:293.

Sawelson H et al: Presumed ocular histoplasmosis syndrome. *Arch Ophthalmol* 1976;**94**:221.

Schlaegel TF Jr: Histoplasmic choroiditis. *Ann Ophthalmol* 1974;**6**:123.

Shields JA et al: The differential diagnosis of posterior uveal melanoma. *Ophthalmology* 1980;**87**:518.

Smith RE, O'Connor GR: Cataract extraction in Fuchs syndrome. *Arch Ophthalmol* 1974;**91**:39.

Smith RE, Godfrey WA, Kimura SJ: Chronic cyclitis. 1. Course and visual prognosis. *Trans Am Acad Ophthalmol Otolaryngol* 1973;**77**:OP760.

Stephens RF, Shields JA: Diagnosis and management of cancer metastatic to the uvea: A study of 70 cases. *Ophthalmology* 1979;**86**:1336.

Sugar HS: Heterochromia iridis with special consideration of its relation to cyclitic disease. *Am J Ophthalmol* 1965;**60**:1.

Tabbara KF, O'Connor GR: Treatment of ocular toxoplasmosis with clindamycin and sulfadiazine. *Ophthalmology* 1980;**87**:129.

Van Metre TE Jr, Knox DL, Maumenee AE: Specific ocular uveal lesions in patients with evidence of histoplasmosis and toxoplasmosis. *South Med J* 1965;**58**:479.

Weinreb RN, Kimura SJ: Uveitis associated with sarcoidosis and angiotensin converting enzyme. *Am J Ophthalmol* 1980;**89**:180.

Witmer R: Etiology of uveitis. *Ann Ophthalmol* 1972;**4**:615.

11 | Lens

ANATOMY & FUNCTION

The lens is a biconvex, avascular, colorless and almost completely transparent structure, about 4 mm thick and 9 mm in diameter. It is suspended behind the iris by the zonule, which connects it with the ciliary body. Anterior to the lens is the aqueous; posterior to it, the vitreous. The lens capsule (see below) is a semipermeable membrane (slightly more permeable than a capillary wall) that will admit water and electrolytes.

A subcapsular epithelium is present anteriorly (Fig 11–1). The lens nucleus is harder than the cortex. With age, subepithelial lamellar fibers are continu-ously produced, so that the lens gradually becomes larger and less elastic throughout life. The nucleus and cortex are made up of long concentric lamellas. The suture lines formed by the end-to-end joining of these lamellar fibers are Y-shaped when viewed with the slit lamp (Fig 11–2). The Y is erect anteriorly and inverted posteriorly.

Each lamellar fiber contains a flattened nucleus. These nuclei are evident microscopically in the peripheral portion of the lens near the equator and are continuous with the subcapsular epithelium.

The lens is held in place by a suspensory ligament known as the zonule (zonule of Zinn). This is composed of numerous fibrils that arise from the surface of

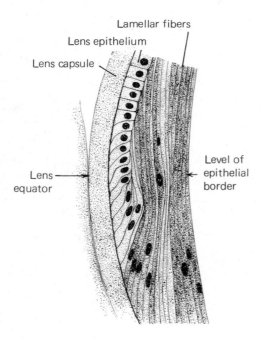

Figure 11–1. Magnified view of lens showing termination of subcapsular epithelium (vertical section).

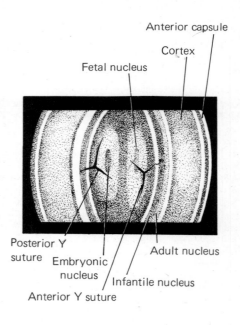

Figure 11–2. Zones of lens showing Y sutures.

[Figs 11–1 and 11–2 are redrawn from Duke-Elder WS: *Textbook of Ophthalmology.* Vol 1. Mosby, 1942. Drawings first appeared in Salzmann M: *Anatomy and Histology of the Human Eyeball in the Normal State.* Univ of Chicago Press, 1912.]

the ciliary body and insert into the lens equator.

The sole function of the lens is to focus light rays upon the retina. In order to focus light from a distant object, the ciliary muscle relaxes, tautening the zonular fibers and reducing the anteroposterior diameter of the lens to its minimal dimension; in this position the refractive power of the lens is minimized, and parallel rays are thus focused upon the retina. In order to focus light from a near object, the ciliary muscle contracts, pulling the choroid forward and releasing the tension on the zonules. The elastic lens capsule then molds the lens into a more spherical body with correspondingly greater refractive power. The physiologic interplay of the ciliary body, zonule, and lens that results in focusing near objects upon the retina is known as **accommodation.** As the lens ages, its accommodative power is gradually reduced.

Composition

The lens consists of about 65% water, about 35% protein (the highest protein content of any tissue of the body), and a trace of minerals common to other body tissues. Potassium is more concentrated in the lens than in most tissues. Ascorbic acid and glutathione are present in both the oxidized and reduced forms.

There are no pain fibers, blood vessels, or nerves in the lens.

Physiology of Symptoms

The only disorders of the lens are opacification and dislocation. Consequently, the patient with an opacity or dislocation of the lens will complain of blurred vision without pain. The physician examines for diseases of the lens by testing the visual acuity and by viewing the lens with an ophthalmoscope, a hand flashlight, or a slit lamp or loupe, preferably through a dilated pupil.

CATARACT

A cataract is a lens opacity. Cataracts vary markedly in degree of density and may be due to a variety of causes but are usually associated with aging. Some degree of cataract formation is to be expected in persons over age 70. Most are bilateral, although the rate of progression in each eye is seldom equal. Traumatic cataract, congenital cataract, and other types are less common.

Cataractous lenses are characterized by lens edema, protein alteration, necrosis, and disruption of the normal continuity of the lens fibers. In general, lens edema varies directly with the stage of cataract development. The immature (incipient) cataract is only slightly opaque. A completely opaque mature (moderately advanced) cataractous lens is somewhat edematous. If the water content is maximal and the lens capsule is stretched, the cataract is called intumescent (swollen). In the hypermature (far-advanced) cataract, water has escaped from the lens, leaving a relatively dehydrated, very opaque lens and a wrinkled capsule.

Most cataracts are not visible to the casual observer until they become dense enough (mature or hypermature) to cause blindness. However, a cataract in its earliest stages of development can be observed through a well-dilated pupil with an ophthalmoscope, loupe, or slit lamp.

The ocular fundus becomes increasingly more difficult to visualize as the lens opacity becomes denser, until the fundus reflection is completely absent. At this stage the cataract is usually mature and the pupil may be white.

The clinical degree of cataract formation, assuming that no other eye disease is present, is judged primarily by the visual acuity. Generally speaking, the decrease in visual acuity is directly proportionate to the density of the cataract. However, some individuals who have clinically significant cataracts when examined with the opthalmoscope or slit lamp see well enough to carry on with their normal activities. Others have a decrease in visual acuity out of proportion to the degree of lens opacification. This is due to distortion of the image by the partially opaque lens.

Cataract formation is characterized chemically by a reduction in oxygen uptake and an initial increase in water content followed by dehydration. Sodium and calcium content is increased; potassium, ascorbic acid, and protein content is decreased. Glutathione is not present in cataractous lenses. Attempts to accelerate or retard these chemical changes by medical treatment have not been successful, and their causes and implications are not known.

During the past few years, there has been increasing evidence implicating ultraviolet radiation as a significant factor in the occurrence of senile cataracts. Epidemiologic investigations have shown that for persons age 65 years or older there is an increased incidence of cataracts in geographic areas where there are long periods of strong sunlight. Further investigation of the effects of ultraviolet light on the lens is warranted.

SENILE CATARACT

Senile cataract (Figs 11–3, 11–4, 11–5) is by far the most common type. Progressively blurred vision is the only symptom. Paradoxically, although distant vision is blurred in the incipient cataract stage, near vision may be somewhat improved. Consequently, these patients read better without glasses (''second sight''). The artificial myopia is due to the greater convexity of the lens in the incipient stage of cataract formation. Glaucoma and lens-induced uveitis are uncommon complications. There is no medical treatment for cataract. Lens extraction (see p 126) is indicated when visual impairment interferes with the patient's normal activities. If glaucoma secondary to lens swelling (intumescent lens) occurs, surgical extraction of

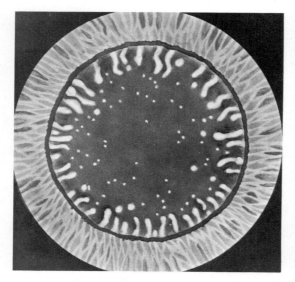

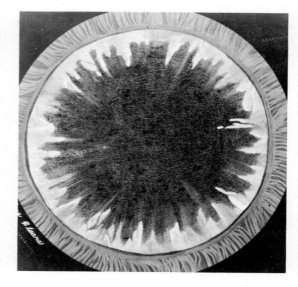

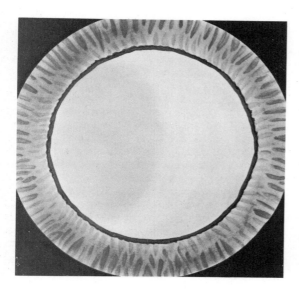

Figure 11–3. Cataract types. *Above, left:* Senile cataract, "coronary" type: club-shaped peripheral opacities with clear central lens; slowly progressive. *Above, right:* Senile cataract, "cuneiform" type: peripheral spicules and central clear lens; slowly progressive. *Left:* Senile cataract, "morgagnian" type (hypermature lens); the entire lens is opaque, and the lens nucleus has fallen inferiorly. (Reproduced, with permission, from Cordes FC: *Cataract Types,* 3rd ed. American Academy of Ophthalmology and Otolaryngology, 1954.)

the lens is indicated. Lens-induced uveitis requires surgical extraction of the lens to remove the source of the offending lens products.

Senile cataract is usually slowly progressive over a period of years, and the patient frequently dies before surgery becomes necessary. If surgery is indicated, lens extraction definitely improves the visual acuity in well over 90% of cases. The remainder either have preexisting retinal damage or develop serious postsurgical complications such as glaucoma, retinal detachment, vitreous hemorrhage, infection, or epithelial downgrowth into the anterior chamber that prevents significant visual improvement.

Corneal contact lenses have made it possible for the patient who has been operated on for cataract to adjust to a new world of sight much more easily, since the corneal lens allows almost normal vision without the distortion, magnification, and diminished peripheral vision caused by the thick cataract glasses. Corneal lenses are of particular value for the patient who has undergone surgery for unilateral cataract since these patients were unable to obtain binocular visual function until the development of contact lenses.

Implantation of **intraocular lenses** at the time of cataract removal has become increasingly popular within the past few years. The original intraocular lenses developed in London by Ridley in 1949 proved to be disastrous. However, greatly improved lens design has made the concept more attractive to patients, despite the increased risk as compared with the standard intracapsular operation. There are a number of preexisting ocular diseases, including diabetes and uveitis, which cause intraocular lenses to be poorly tolerated.

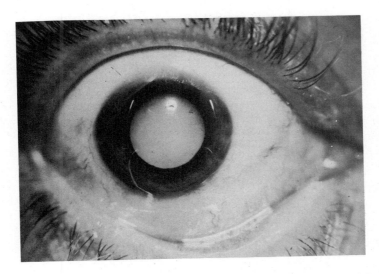

Figure 11–4. Mature senile cataract viewed through a dilated pupil. (Courtesy of A Rosenberg.)

An alternative to the intraocular lens is the continuous wear soft contact lens that can be worn day and night for weeks to months at a time. Considerable improvement in this device has also occurred within recent years.

Intraocular lenses are being inserted by an increasing number of cataract surgeons throughout the world. However, because the complication rate is higher than with the standard procedure, most conservative cataract surgeons favor the standard intracapsular operation.

CONGENITAL CATARACT
(Figs 11–6, 11–7)

Congenital cataracts are common but usually do not cause significant visual loss. Most are bilateral and are probably genetically determined. They occasionally occur as a consequence of maternal rubella during the first trimester of pregnancy. Only those congenital cataracts that cause a marked loss of vision are discussed here.

The parent notices that the child does not see well during the first few months or years of life. The pupil may be white. The opacities vary greatly in density.

If the cataracts are bilateral and dense enough so that the retinas are not clearly visible, lens extraction through a small limbal incision (2–6 mm) by aspiration, irrigation, ultrasonic fragmentation, or with a motor-driven lens and vitreous cutter should be done in one eye by the age of 2 months to permit normal development of vision and to prevent nystagmus. If surgery on the first eye has been successful, surgery on the second eye can be performed soon after. Otherwise, surgery on the second eye should be delayed 1–2

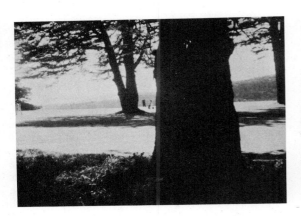

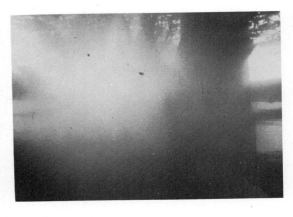

Figure 11–5. Senile cataract. In the photo at right the scene shown at left is reproduced as if seen by a person with a moderately advanced senile cataract (opacity denser centrally). (Courtesy of E Goodner.)

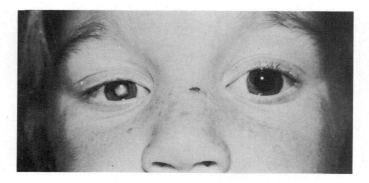

Figure 11–6. Congenital cataract.

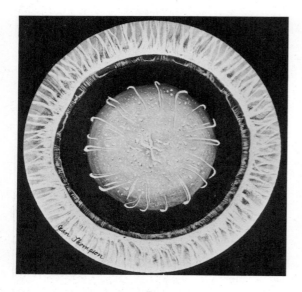

Figure 11–7. Congenital cataract, zonular type. One zone of lens involved. The cortex is relatively clear. (From Cordes FC: See next page.)

years until the eye is larger and there is less risk of operative complications.

Months or years following surgery, vitreous strands may develop that upon contraction produce retinal detachment. Retinal detachment may be successfully treated by surgery in the majority of such cases. Recent improved techniques of aspiration and irrigation have materially reduced the incidence of vitreous loss and therefore the late complication of retinal detachment.

Most congenital cataracts are not dense enough to blur the vision significantly and are not progressive. Others progress slowly and may not require surgery until the child is 10–15 years of age.

The visual prognosis for congenital cataract patients requiring surgery is not as good as that for patients with senile cataract. The complications of the operation, associated amblyopia, and occasional as-

sociated anomalies of the optic nerve or retina lower the degree of useful vision obtainable in this group of patients. The prognosis for improvement of visual acuity is worst following surgery for unilateral congenital cataracts and best for incomplete bilateral congenital cataracts that are slowly progressive.

TRAUMATIC CATARACT

Traumatic cataract (Figs 11–8, 11–9, 11–10) is most commonly due to a foreign body injury to the lens or blunt trauma to the eyeball. BB shot is a frequent cause; less frequent causes include arrows, rocks, contusions, overexposure to heat (''glassblower's cataract''), x-rays, and radioactive materials. Most traumatic cataracts are preventable. In industry, the best safety measure is a good pair of safety goggles.

The lens becomes white soon after the entry of the foreign body since the interruption of the lens capsule allows aqueous and sometimes vitreous to penetrate into the lens structure. The patient is often an industrial worker who gives a history of striking steel upon steel. A minute fragment of a steel hammer, for example, may pass through the cornea and lens at a tremendous rate of speed and lodge in the vitreous, where it can usually be seen with the ophthalmoscope.

The patient complains immediately of blurred vision. The eye becomes red, the lens opaque, and there may be an intraocular hemorrhage. If aqueous or vitreous escapes from the eye, the eye becomes extremely soft. Complications include infection, uveitis, retinal detachment, and glaucoma.

A magnetic intraocular foreign body should be removed without delay.

Antibiotics and corticosteroids should be given systemically and locally over a period of several days to minimize the chance of infection and uveitis. Atropine sulfate, 1%, 1 drop 3 times daily, is recommended to keep the pupil dilated and to prevent the formation of posterior synechiae.

The cataract can be removed at the same time the foreign body is removed or after the inflammation subsides. If glaucoma occurs during the waiting

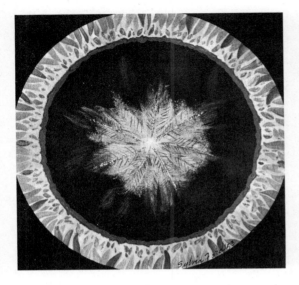

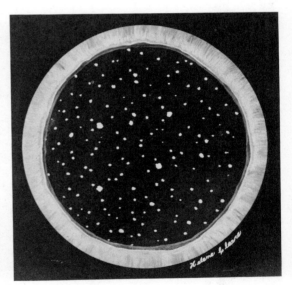

Figure 11—8. Traumatic "star-shaped" cataract in the posterior lens. This is usually due to ocular contusion and is only detectable through a well-dilated pupil.

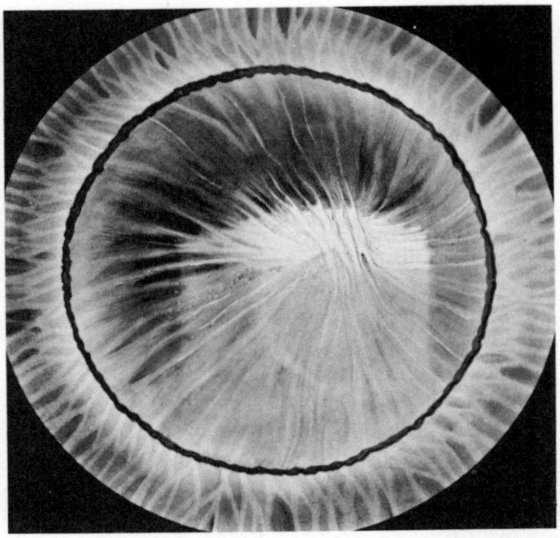

Figure 11—9. Traumatic cataract with wrinkled anterior capsule.

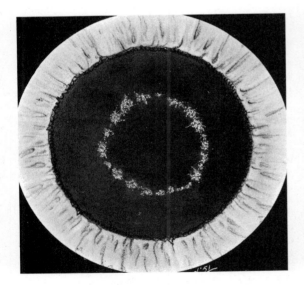

Figure 11—10. "Vossius' ring." Traumatic cataract caused by the imprint of the iris pigment on the anterior surface of the lens. The remainder of the lens is clear, and vision is not impaired.

Figure 11—11. Punctate dot cataract. This type of cataract is sometimes seen as an ocular complication of diabetes mellitus. It may also be congenital.

[Figs 11—7 to 11—12 are reproduced, with permission, from Cordes FC: *Cataract Types,* 3rd ed. American Academy of Ophthalmology and Otolaryngology, 1954.]

period, cataract surgery should not be delayed even though inflammation is still present. Some time after cataract surgery, a thin opaque membrane may occur, in which case discission (needling) may be necessary to improve vision. The same techniques utilized for removal of congenital cataracts are generally used for the removal of traumatic cataracts, especially in patients under 30 years of age.

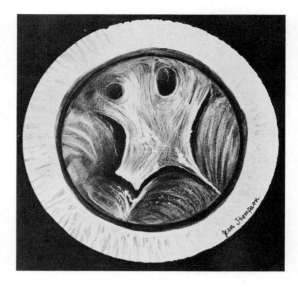

Figure 11–12. "After-cataract."

CATARACT SECONDARY TO INTRAOCULAR DISEASE ("Complicated Cataract")

Cataract may develop as a direct effect of intraocular disease upon the physiology of the lens (eg, severe recurrent uveitis). The cataract usually begins in the posterior subcapsular area and eventually involves the entire lens structure. Intraocular diseases commonly associated with the development of cataracts are chronic or recurrent uveitis, glaucoma, retinitis pigmentosa, and retinal detachment.

These cataracts are usually unilateral. The visual prognosis is not as good as in ordinary senile cataract.

CATARACT ASSOCIATED WITH SYSTEMIC DISEASE

Bilateral cataracts may occur in association with the following systemic disorders: diabetes mellitus (Fig 11–11), hypoparathyroidism, myotonic dystrophy, atopic dermatitis, galactosemia, and Lowe's, Werner's, and Down's syndromes.

TOXIC CATARACT

Toxic cataract is uncommon. Many cases appeared in the 1930s as a result of ingestion of dinitrophenol, a drug taken to suppress appetite. Other offenders are triparanol (MER/29) and corticosteroids administered over a long period of time. It has been suggested that echothiophate iodide, a strong miotic used in the treatment of glaucoma, may cause cataracts.

AFTER-CATARACT

After-cataract (Fig 11–12) is the term applied to the portion of the lens remaining after an extracapsular cataract extraction or a partially absorbed traumatic cataract. The opacity usually consists of capsular and cortical material.

If vision is reduced, discission of the membrane is the treatment of choice. Since discission is a simple, safe, and usually successful procedure, it may be performed when visual loss is relatively minor (VA 6/15 [20/50] to 6/18 [20/60]) if this loss is a definite handicap to the patient. If the after-cataract is thick and fibrous, removal is more difficult and may require the use of one of the vitrectomy devices that aspirate and cut small pieces of the membrane away until the pupillary axis is clear.

CATARACT SURGERY

In a cataract operation, the lens is removed from the eye (lens extraction). There are 2 principal types of lens extraction for cataracts in older patients—intracapsular and extracapsular. The former consists of removing the lens in toto, ie, within its capsule through a 140- to 160-degree superior limbal incision. In extracapsular operation, a superior limbal incision is also made, the anterior portion of the capsule is ruptured and removed, the nucleus is extracted, and the lens cortex is either irrigated or aspirated from the eye, leaving the posterior capsule behind. Some patients develop a secondary opacity of the posterior capsule that requires discission. However, in some older patients the extracapsular operation is preferred in an effort to reduce long-term postoperative vitreous and retinal complications. Examples would be patients with high myopia and retinal degeneration, previous retinal detachment in the same eye, or vitreous loss and retinal detachment in the fellow eye after intracapsular operation.

The intracapsular operation is still the procedure of choice for most standard senile cataracts. Extracapsular extraction (ultrasonic or aspiration irrigation) through a small limbal incision is the procedure of choice for congenital and traumatic cataracts.

Enzymatic zonulolysis is an important technique in intracapsular cataract surgery. It involves the injection of chymotrypsin, a fibrinolytic and proteolytic enzyme, in strengths not greater than 1:5000, into the anterior chamber of the eye. The material is left in the chamber for 1–3 minutes and the lens is then extracted.

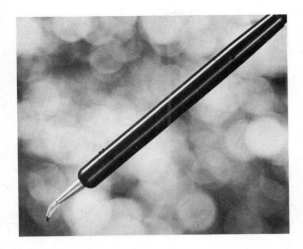

Figure 11–13. Amoils curved cataract cryopencil. (Courtesy of Keeler Optical Products, Inc.)

This substance has a specific lytic action on the zonules and so makes possible much easier removal of the cataractous lens. Chymotrypsin can cause temporary postoperative glaucoma associated with poor wound healing and iris prolapse. This unique secondary glaucoma can be prevented by giving acetazolamide (Diamox) postoperatively. Zonulolysis is used primarily in the younger age group (20–50), in whom the toughness of the zonules creates operative difficulties. The method is contraindicated in patients under 20 (congenital cataract) because up to this approximate age the lens is attached to the vitreous, and intracapsular extraction will surely lead to considerable loss of vitreous.

Cataract surgery can be performed successfully in many ways. The variables relate mainly to the size of the wound and the actual method of lens delivery. In performing the intracapsular procedure in senile cataracts, the time-honored method has been to make a large limbal incision superiorly, grasp the lens with a metal capsule forceps, and remove the lens intracapsularly. In recent years, the cryoprobe (Fig 11–13) has become popular as a replacement for the capsule forceps. The cryoprobe affords a firmer attachment to the lens and tends to result in fewer ruptures of the lens capsule.

Phacoemulsification and aspiration and phacofragmentation and irrigation, using ultrasonic vibrations and a small limbal incision, are relatively new extracapsular techniques that are frequently used in removing congenital, juvenile, and presenile cataracts.

Postoperative Care (Senile Cataract)*
The patient may be ambulatory on the day of surgery but is advised to move cautiously and to avoid

---

*If an ultrasonic technique is used (younger age group), the postoperative phase is greatly shortened.

straining of any type for about a month. The eye is usually kept bandaged for a few days, but if the eye is comfortable the bandage can be removed and the eye protected by spectacles or by a shield during the day. Protection at night by a metal shield is required for several weeks.

The patient may be given a pair of temporary thick, convex cataract glasses that can be worn a few days after surgery. These should be worn at first only when sitting down, since there is considerable visual distortion for the patient to adjust to. The patient gradually learns to adjust to a new world where everything is 30% larger by the time permanent glasses are ordered (approximately 2 months postoperatively). If the patient can tolerate contact lenses, visual distortion is eliminated.

DISLOCATED LENS
(Ectopia Lentis)
(Figs 11–14, 11–15)

Partial or complete lens dislocation may be hereditary or may result from trauma.

Hereditary Lens Dislocation
Hereditary lens dislocation is usually bilateral and may be associated with coloboma of the lens, homocystinuria, Marfan's syndrome, and Marchesani's syndrome. The vision is blurred, particularly if the lens is dislocated out of the line of vision. If dislocation is partial, the edge of the lens and the zonular fibers holding it in place can be seen in the pupil. If the lens is completely dislocated into the vitreous, it can be seen with the ophthalmoscope.

A partially dislocated lens is often complicated by

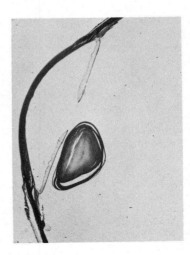

Figure 11–14. Dislocated lens. (Courtesy of R Carriker.)

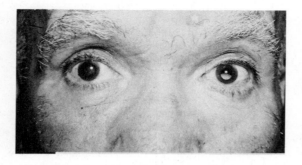

Figure 11–15. Dislocated lens.

cataract formation. If so, the cataract may have to be removed, but this should be delayed as long as possible because vitreous loss, predisposing to subsequent retinal detachment, is prone to occur during surgery. If the lens is free in the vitreous, it may lead in later life to the development of glaucoma of a type that responds poorly to treatment.

If dislocation is partial and the lens is clear, the visual prognosis is good.

Traumatic Lens Dislocation

Partial or complete traumatic lens dislocation may occur following a contusion injury such as a blow to the eye with a fist. If the dislocation is partial, there may be no symptoms; but if the lens is floating in the vitreous, the patient has blurred vision and usually a red eye. **Iridodonesis,** a quivering of the iris when the patient moves the eye, is a common sign of lens dislocation and is due to the lack of lens support. This is present both in partially and completely dislocated lenses but is more marked in the latter.

Iritis and glaucoma are common complications of dislocated lens, particularly if dislocation is complete.

If there are no complications, dislocated lenses are best left untreated. If uncontrollable glaucoma occurs, lens extraction must be done despite the poor results of this operation. The technique of choice is pars plana lensectomy using a motor-driven lens and vitreous cutter.

•   •   •

References

Allen HF, Mangiaracine AB: Bacterial endophthalmitis after cataract extraction. *Arch Ophthalmol* 1974;**91**:3.

Becker B: The side effects of corticosteroids. *Invest Ophthalmol* 1964;**3**:492.

Cataract surgery. *Ophthalmic Surg* 1979;**10**:1. [Entire issue.]

Chandler AC, Wadsworth JAC: Cataract surgery: Review of 500 consecutive cases. *Ann Ophthalmol* 1975;**7**:1597.

DeVoe AG: Critical evaluation of current concepts in cataract surgery: The George K. Smelser lecture. *Am J Ophthalmol* 1976;**81**:715.

Emery JM (editor): *Current Concepts in Cataract Surgery.* Mosby, 1978.

Frayer WC: What's new in surgery? Ophthalmic surgery. *Bull Am Coll Surg* 1982;**67**:32.

Heller R, Giacometti L, Yuen K: Sunlight and cataract: An epidemiologic investigation. *Am J Epidemiol* 1977;**105**:450.

Irvine AR: Extracapsular cataract extraction and pseudophakos implantation in primates: A clinico-pathologic study. *Ophthalmic Surg* 1981;**12**:27.

Jaffe NS, Clayman HM, Jaffe MS: Cystoid macular edema after intracapsular and extracapsular cataract extraction with and without an intraocular lens. *Ophthalmology* 1982;**89**:25.

Kirsch RE: The lens: Annual review. *Arch Ophthalmol* 1975; **93**:284.

Lerman S: Human ultraviolet radiation cataracts. *Ophthalmol Res* 1980;**12**:303.

Lerman S: Ultraviolet radiation and human cataractogenesis. *Invest Ophthalmol Vis Sci* 1979;**18(Suppl)**:128.

Lerman S: Ultraviolet radiation photodamage to the ocular lens: Diagnosis and treatment. *Ann Ophthalmol* 1982;**14**:411.

McDonald PR: Evolution of cataract surgery since the deSchweinitz era. *Ophthalmic Surg* 1979;**10**:44.

Nordan LT, Pettit TH: Hazards of bilateral intraocular lens implantation. *Am J Ophthalmol* 1979;**87**:322.

Rice NSC: Congenital cataract: A cause of preventable blindness in children. *Br Med J* 1982;**285**:581.

Shoch D: Management of unilateral senile cataract: Questions and answers. *JAMA* 1979;**242**:1082.

Shock JP: Phacofragmentation and irrigation. *Ann Ophthalmol* 1976;**8**:591.

Sommer A: Cataracts as an epidemiologic problem. *Am J Ophthalmol* 1977;**83**:334.

Stark WJ et al: Extended-wear contact lenses and intraocular lenses for aphakic correction. *Am J Ophthalmol* 1979;**88**:535.

Stern AL et al: Pseudophakic cystoid maculopathy. *Ophthalmology* 1981;**88**:942.

Varma SD, Mizuno A, Kinoshita JH: Diabetic cataracts and flavonoids. *Science* 1977;**195**:205.

Weinstein GW et al: Cataract surgery. *Ophthalmic Surg* 1979;**10**:19. [Entire issue.]

Vitreous | 12

COMPOSITION & ANATOMY

The vitreous is about 99% water. The remaining 1% includes 2 components, collagen and hyaluronic acid, which give it its specific physical character.

The vitreous owes its gel-like form and consistency to a loose syncytium of long-chain collagen molecules capable of binding about 200 times their own weight in water.

The hyaluronic acid molecules are very large, loose skeins capable of binding about 60 times their weight in water. Combined with the collagen element, they account for the physical characteristics of normal vitreous.

The vitreous is a clear, avascular, gelatinous body that comprises two-thirds of the volume and weight of the eye. It fills the space bounded by the lens, retina, and optic disk (Fig 12–1). Since it is quite inelastic and impervious to cells and debris, it plays an important role in maintaining the transparency and form of the eye. If the vitreous were removed, the eye would collapse. When the vitreous is replaced by saline, as in certain forms of vitreous surgery, cellular matter and particulate debris are free to migrate into the optical pathway.

The outer surface of the vitreous—the hyaloid membrane—is normally in contact with the following structures: the posterior lens capsule, the zonular fibers, the pars plana epithelium, the retina, and the optic nerve head. The base of the vitreous maintains a firm attachment throughout life to the pars plana epithelium and the retina immediately behind the ora serrata. The attachment to the lens capsule and the optic nerve head is firm in early life but soon disappears. This is the principal reason that intracapsular cataract extraction without vitreous prolapse or "loss" is possible in adults and not in children. In addition, the vitreous is prone to vitreoretinal adhesions at the site of lattice degeneration of the retina, congenital retinal rosettes, meridional retinal folds, vitreoretinal scars, and new retinal blood vessels, as in diabetes and central retinal vein occlusion.

The hyaloid canal (Cloquet's canal), which in the fetus contains the hyaloid artery, passes anteroposteriorly from the lens to the optic nerve head. The hyaloid artery usually disappears soon after birth, but the hyaloid canal remains throughout life. It is not visible ophthalmoscopically. A rudimentary portion of the hyaloid artery occasionally remains and can be seen floating in the vitreous with its anterior portion attached to the posterior surface of the lens. This point of attachment can be seen as a black dot (Mittendorf's dot) with the ophthalmoscope.

EXAMINATION OF THE VITREOUS

Normal vitreous is not visible by either direct or indirect ophthalmoscopy. The numerous ophthalmoscopically visible features are anomalies attributable either to structural changes such as the "floaters" of syneresis and the ringlike form associated with posterior vitreous detachment (Fig 12–2) or to invasive elements such as blood, white cell masses, or fibrovascular proliferations from adjacent tissues. Normal vitreous in situ and a variety of very important anomalies such as the retraction, condensation, and shrinkage characteristic of diabetes, injury, etc can be viewed only with a slit lamp. Although slit lamp examination of the vitreous is quite easy to learn and plays an important role in the management of vitreous disease, too few ophthalmologists are at present making optimal use of this instrument.

Slit lamps are microscopes with specialized illuminating systems that make transparent and near-

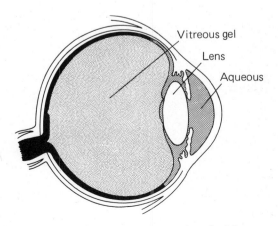

Figure 12–1. Schematic cross section of adult eye.

Vitreous gel

Lens

Aqueous

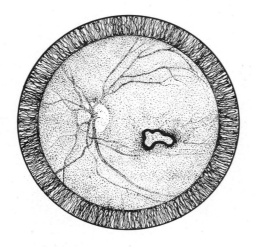

Figure 12–2. Vitreous detachment as seen with the +8 lens of the ophthalmoscope.

transparent ocular fluids and tissues visible. The anterior central vitreous (the anterior vitreous) can be seen by slit lamp alone; the posterior vitreous can be seen only with the additional aid of a contact lens; and the peripheral vitreous requires a specialized contact lens equipped with mirrors for off-axis illumination (Chapter 3.)

B-scan ultrasonography is an important diagnostic and prognostic tool in the management of many posterior segment problems associated with gross vitreous opacification (Figs 12–3, 12–4, and 12–5). Where x-ray techniques are useless and light-dependent ophthalmoscopes and slit lamps are of limited value, the skillful use of B-scan ultrasonography can extract much pertinent information about the state of the vitreous and adjacent structures. For example, it is possible in this way to identify and locate vitreous membranes (Fig 12–8), vitreoretinal relationships and retinal detachments greater than 1 mm in depth (Figs 12–5, 12–6, 12–7, and 12–8), scleral ruptures, and intraocular foreign bodies—even nonlucent plastic and glass.

AGING OF THE VITREOUS

Like all types of gel, the vitreous, with the passage of time, becomes increasingly prone to a degenerative process known as syneresis. Syneresis usually starts in and most severely affects the anterior central area, sparing the base or anterior peripheral sector. It is a multifocal process associated with breakdown of the gel and formation of fluid-filled cavities, and a large variety of collagen forms. It affects at least 65% of persons over 60 years of age. Myopes are especially susceptible, even in childhood.

The enlarging fluid-filled cavities coalesce and may discharge abruptly into the potential space anterior to the posterior retina (Fig 12–9). The patient may be aware of the collapse and detachment of the vitreous as an acute condition. The most common complaint is of "vitreous floaters," often with "flashing lights," and the patient may be eager to relate it to trauma but should be assured that it is a spontaneous occurrence. The mobility of the collapsed vitreous on eye movement and consequent potential for stress on

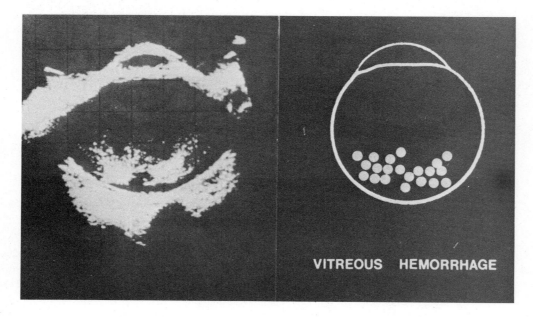

VITREOUS HEMORRHAGE

Figure 12–3. Vitreous hemorrhage limited to posterior vitreous region in aphakic eye. (Reproduced, with permission, from Coleman DJ: Ultrasound in vitreous surgery. *Trans Am Acad Ophthalmol Otolaryngol* 1972;**76**:469.)

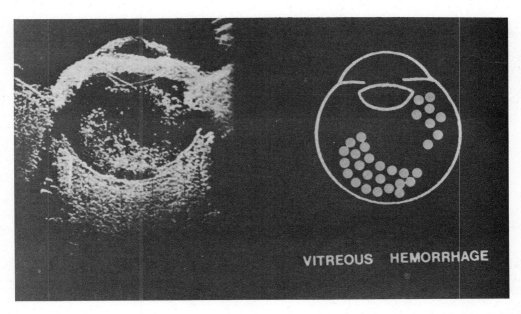

Figure 12–4. Diffuse vitreous hemorrhage scattered throughout entire vitreous body. Lens and retina are in normal position. (Reproduced, with permission, from Coleman DJ: Ultrasound in vitreous surgery. *Trans Am Acad Ophthalmol Otolaryngol* 1972;**76**:469.)

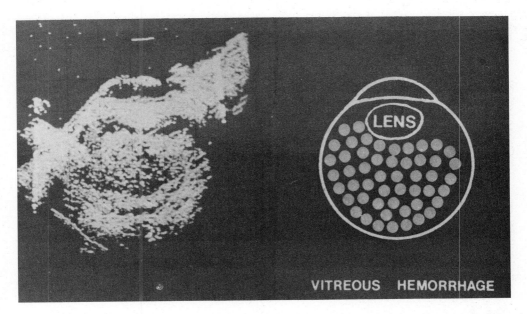

Figure 12–5. Dense vitreous hemorrhage filling entire vitreous compartment. Lens and retina are in place. (Reproduced, with permission, from Coleman DJ: Ultrasound in vitreous surgery. *Trans Am Acad Ophthalmol Otolaryngol* 1972;**76**:470.)

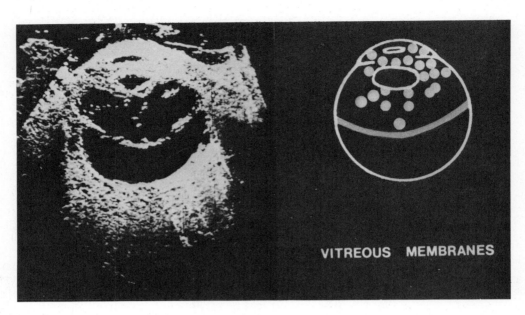

Figure 12–6. Vitreous membrane extending along posterior limiting membrane of vitreous from ora to ora. Retina is in place. (Reproduced, with permission, from Coleman DJ: Ultrasound in vitreous surgery. *Trans Am Acad Ophthalmol Otolaryngol* 1972;**76**:473.)

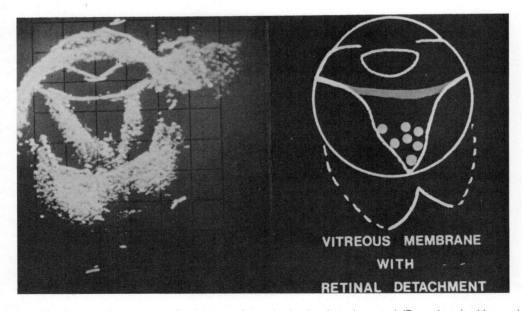

Figure 12–7. Vitreous membrane connecting 2 leaves of detached retina. Lens is normal. (Reproduced, with permission, from Coleman DJ: Ultrasound in vitreous surgery. *Trans Am Acad Ophthalmol Otolaryngol* 1972;**76**:474.)

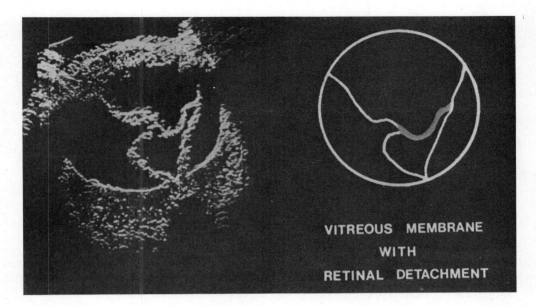

Figure 12–8. Total retinal detachment viewed horizontally below iris plane. A vitreous membrane connecting 2 leaves of retina is clearly demonstrated. (Reproduced, with permission, from Coleman DJ: Ultrasound in vitreous surgery. *Trans Am Acad Ophthalmol Otolaryngol* 1972;**76**:474.)

hitherto subclinical vitreoretinal adhesions may also cause vitreous hemorrhage, retinal tears, and retinal detachment.

"FLASHING LIGHTS"

"Flashing lights" are a common symptom. The patient is aware of a localized "light," "glow," "streak of light," or "flashing" (as of a neon tube) in the field of vision for which there is no reasonable explanation. The patient can usually point to the disturbance and often describes an arc-shaped flicker in the periphery of one or 2 quadrants. The light seldom persists for more than a fraction of a second. It frequently recurs at short intervals for a few minutes and then disappears for hours, days, or even weeks. It is most readily identified on moving the eye and when illumination is dim or absent.

Although this phenomenon is unilateral, a similar episode commonly occurs in the other visual field. The 2 episodes may occur simultaneously but more commonly are separated by an interval of days to many years.

The light represents a cerebral awareness of a new abnormal vitreous stimulation of the retina. It is most commonly associated with recent collapse and detachment of the vitreous due to syneresis with focal vitreous traction on vitreoretinal lesions such as lattice degeneration, meridional folds, congenital rosettes, and other visually subclinical vitreoretinal adhesions. A careful history will readily distinguish it from the scintillating scotoma of migraine, which is characterized by a symmetric quivering scotoma in both eyes, predictable configuration and progression, and variable nausea or headache.

Flashing lights require no treatment. The patient may be reassured that the symptom will pass. However, as the causative mechanism may also induce retinal tears, retinal detachment (Fig 12–10), or vitreous hemorrhage, every new case requires a survey of the vitreoretinal relationship, especially in the periphery.

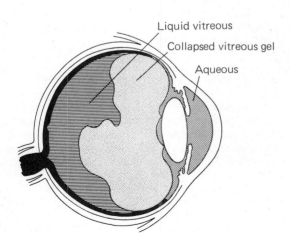

Liquid vitreous

Collapsed vitreous gel

Aqueous

Figure 12–9. Schematic drawing of collapse and detachment of the vitreous.

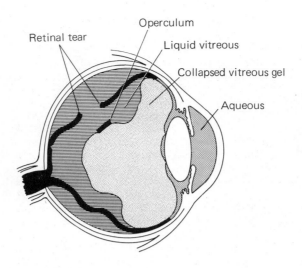

Retinal tear
Operculum
Liquid vitreous
Collapsed vitreous gel
Aqueous

Figure 12–10. Schematic representation of vitreous collapse causing the retina to tear and detach.

"VITREOUS FLOATERS"

A vitreous floater is a fine vitreous opacity that can stimulate the retina by casting a shadow upon it. The mind projects the corresponding dark form onto the appropriate area of the visual field.

The term vitreous floaters embraces a common and potentially serious symptom that was formerly called muscae volitantes—Latin for flies that flit, flutter, or fly to and fro.

The onset may be either insidious or acute and unilateral or bilateral. The patient is aware of one or more (or even many) fine, dark forms in the field of vision. Their configuration is usually so pronounced that the patient spontaneously classifies them as "spots," "soot," "particles," "spiders," "cobwebs," "threads," "worms," "dark streaks," "a ring," etc. Various combinations are often reported. The objects continue to migrate after the eye comes to rest—hence the name floaters.

Central, relatively immobile floaters are visually annoying and may even be disabling. Peripheral ones are readily overlooked as they are intermittent and require large eye motion or special positions merely to see them. Unlike "flashing lights," they are most readily seen against bright lights or a uniform light background. They are extremely common in myopes and people with syneresis.

Red cells not uncommonly cause the symptoms as a result of small hemorrhages into the vitreous due to retinal tears or hemorrhagic diseases such as diabetic retinopathy, hypertension, leukemia, old branch occlusion of the retinal vein, Eales's disease, Coats's disease, and subacute bacterial endocarditis.

White cell invasion of the vitreous gel associated with pars planitis may also cause "spots before the eyes."

Vitreous floaters due to pigment are usually a consequence of long-standing tear-induced detachment of the retina that has not yet reached the macula.

Vitreous floaters should never be dismissed as harmless or imaginary. A careful survey of the vitreous and retina is always indicated in order to identify their nature and origin and to decide on management. Failure to make such an examination not infrequently leads to missed diagnosis. In the absence of a serious causative pathologic process, the patient may be reassured that the condition is harmless.

ASTEROID HYALOSIS

Asteroid hyalosis is an uncommon condition that occurs in otherwise healthy eyes in elderly people. It is unilateral 3 times more often than bilateral. Hundreds of small yellow spheres consisting of calcium soaps are seen in the vitreous. These move when the eyes move but always return to their original positions because they are attached to interlacing fibers. There are no related ocular or systemic diseases. The opacities have little or no effect upon vision and are of no clinical significance.

SYNCHYSIS SCINTILLANS

Synchysis scintillans is an uncommon, usually bilateral condition in which the examiner sees numerous glistening white cholesterol crystals that tend to settle in the lowest part of very fluid vitreous when the eyes are motionless. When the eyes are moved, the crystals spring up in great showers and fly around the vitreous cavity until movement of the eyes stops.

Synchysis scintillans usually has its onset before age 40. There is usually no predisposing cause, but it may follow chronic uveitis. No relationship has been established with elevated blood cholesterol levels or any other systemic abnormality.

There is no blurring of vision, and the patient is unaware of this condition. The visual prognosis is excellent, as the condition does not progress.

MASSIVE VITREOUS RETRACTION

Massive vitreous retraction is a grave vitreous disease of unknown cause. The central area becomes a large fluid-filled cavity whose walls are condensed, shrunken, and rubbery. The residual posterior vitreous is invaded at several points by scar-forming elements from the retina.

The consequent traction distorts, detaches, and may tear the retina, causing gross visual impairment.

Tear-induced detachments complicated by this condition respond poorly to surgical repair since the tears are less favorable for closure and the residual retinal distortion and detachment compromise vision postoperatively.

INJURY TO THE VITREOUS

Contusion

Because the vitreous is inelastic compared with the adjacent tissues, contusions that abruptly though briefly alter the shape of the eye are apt to cause injuries where the vitreous is adherent.

Disinsertion of the vitreous base is not uncommon. It is frequently associated with tearing of the pars plana or retina, vitreous hemorrhage, or detachment of the retina—as long as 20 years later.

Less commonly, "flashing lights," "vitreous floaters," and even vitreous hemorrhage or detachment of the retina may result from stress behind the vitreous base. The affected sites may be hitherto subclinical anomalous vitreoretinal adhesions (eg, lattice degeneration) or areas of frank vitreoretinal disease such as diabetic retinopathy.

Rupture of the Globe

Rupture of the globe is always a serious injury that may result in early or late blindness or even loss of the eyeball. Prolapse of the vitreous through the wound is a severe complication often associated with acute secondary tearing or detachment of the retina. A seemingly uncomplicated prolapse may be followed by late retinal detachment with or without tears due to fibrous ingrowth from the orbit and subsequent contraction. The latter may be visible as membranes or bands in the vitreous. Various forms of vitreous surgery are used to prevent or treat such complications.

Penetration of the Globe

An almost endless variety of material may accidentally penetrate the globe. Common examples are needles, BB shot, and small particles of metal, stone, or plastic that fly into the eye at high velocity.

Prolapse of the vitreous may occur at the site of entry or exit or both. The part traversed by the foreign body is permanently damaged and is often marked by visible condensation, shrinkage, or fibrous elements. Vitreous surgery is increasingly used to prevent or treat complications such as retinal detachment with or without tears.

Vitreous Loss

Vitreous loss is an iatrogenic complication. The vitreous gel prolapses through a surgical wound, usually at (but not limited to) the corneal limbus during the course of operating on the lens, iris, or cornea.

Fibrous tissue invasion and contraction are frequent sequels that are prone to cause traction complications involving the retina. Corneal edema and iris displacement (eg, "updrawn pupil") may also occur. An acute prolapse can be effectively excised. An old prolapse may require surgery for release of vitreous traction.

VITREOUS INFLAMMATION

Vitreous inflammation includes a wide spectrum of disorders ranging from a few scattered white cells to abscess formation. Most commonly, one or more focal inflammatory lesions in the choroid or retina—as in chorioretinitis or retinitis—are responsible for a secondary cellular invasion of the liquid vitreous or relatively resistant gel. There may be a mild localized blurring of the fundus landmarks and lesions that provoke little or no visual complaint except for a possible "vitreous floater" effect. With greater infiltration, vision is decreased and the fundus is invisible or almost so. The condition may be so marked that the red reflection is lost and the vitreous appears opaque and white. Since these conditions spare the anterior segment, there is no pain and the external eye appears normal. The prognosis and treatment depend upon the underlying condition. The vitreous usually clears when the primary defect is quiescent. Vitreous surgery is used to remove gross residual opacities that show no sign of clearing spontaneously.

Vitreous abscess (or endophthalmitis*) is a rare, painful condition associated with photophobia as well as redness and edema of the conjunctiva and lids. It is a unilateral infection usually caused by *Bacillus subtilis,* a common barnyard contaminant. In most reported cases, the organism has been introduced by a penetrating injury. The vitreous is an excellent culture medium for this organism, and the abscess characteristically progresses rapidly to destroy the eye despite injections of antibiotics into the vitreous. In rare instances, vitreous abscess is the result of blood-borne infection.

The treatment of hospital-acquired endophthalmitis following surgery for cataract or glaucoma is summarized on p 377.

VITREOUS HEMORRHAGE

Vitreous hemorrhage may vary from minimal bleeding recognizable to the patient merely as "vitreous floaters" to a dense mass of blood, loss of the red reflection, and a sudden reduction of vision to as low as "light perception only." With moderate bleeding, the initial hemorrhage is often graphically described as one or more dense "black streaks" that subsequently "broke up into numerous minute black dots."

Fresh blood is readily identified by slit lamp examination. Ophthalmoscopically, there is a variable loss of fundus detail and floating debris, which is often recognizably red. With time, there is a marked tendency to syneresis, loss of color, and clearing of the optical pathway. Blood staining that persists for 6 or more months is apt to be permanent and to cause retinal atrophy (hemosiderosis) and cataract formation.

---

*If all 3 coats of the eye as well as the vitreous are involved by an inflammatory process, the condition is known as panophthalmitis. The line of demarcation between endophthalmitis and panophthalmitis is usually obscure.

Many conditions may cause the bleeding. Traumatic breakdown of adjacent vascularized tissues by contusion, concussion, penetration, or rupture may occur. Systemic diseases that are apt to affect the retinal vessels—especially diabetes, but hypertension and leukemia also—are common causes. Hemorrhage is often due to vitreous traction on the new vessels that appear at the edge of prior branch occlusions of the retinal vein. Acute collapse of the vitreous, which is extremely common, will sometimes tear the retina and cause a vitreous hemorrhage and even subsequent retinal detachment (Fig 12–3).

No patient with a vitreous hemorrhage should be dismissed until a pertinent history has been taken and a thorough examination performed—especially of the retina.

The outlook and management will depend upon the primary condition. A persistent substantial opacity may be removed surgically, often with dramatic improvement in vision.

● ● ●

VITREOUS SURGERY

As recently as 1970, eighty percent of the interior of the eye from the lens to the disk and macula was inaccessible to direct intraocular surgical manipulation.

A host of dread vitreous and retinal disorders were virtually incurable until Machemer pioneered the basic microsurgical equipment and techniques that now make it possible to dissect and remove preretinal membranes and large amounts of abnormal vitreous and to replace them with a fortified Ringer's solution.

Definitive vitrectomy is performed with one of a number of fine instruments for engaging, cutting, and removing a train of minute fragments of vitreous and debris. The instrument is easily inserted through the pars plana, and the vitreous and retina are viewed through a special corneal contact lens with the aid of a fiberoptic light attached to the vitrectomy instrument. Persons with poor vision resulting from vitreous opacities and vitreous shrinkage have benefited most from this procedure.

The opacity may be blood—as in diabetes, branch vein occlusion, Eales's disease, trauma, or hyphema with extension into the vitreous shortly after lens removal—persistent inflammatory debris following uveitis, or an amyloid deposit.

Other indications for vitreous surgery include distortion of the macula or traction detachment of the retina due to "vitreous loss" at the time of anterior segment surgery, fibrous invasion following rupture or penetration of the globe, and advanced vasoproliferative disease such as diabetes or Eales's disease. Complicated detachments associated with retinal breaks may also benefit. In addition, a variety of dense proliferative and vasoproliferative vitreous strands and membranes may be divided readily, without bleeding, by electrodissection. This procedure is called electrovitreotomy. It is distinct from endodiathermy, which is also performed with an electrode inserted through the pars plana. Endodiathermy causes only coagulation as opposed to cutting with coagulation.

A recent advance in vitreous surgery, the O'Malley collapsing technique, now allows full view of the retina to and including the ciliary body. An extensive vitrectomy is performed. The lens, if present, must be removed. Liquid equal to 20–30% of the ocular volume is removed from the vitreous cavity. The sclera is depressed toward the pupil with a cotton applicator until the desired area of retina and ciliary body is clearly visible behind the pupil. A corneal contact lens is not used. This simple, well tolerated maneuver makes any part of the anterior retina and ciliary body readily accessible for definitive surgery.

● ● ●

References

Boyd BF (editor): Chaps 1–4, pp 46–214 in: *Highlights of Ophthalmology*. 2 vols. Highlights of Ophthalmology Press, 1981.

Lincoff H, Kreissig I: The conservative management of vitreous hemorrhage. *Trans Am Acad Ophthalmol Otolaryngol* 1975;**79**:858.

Machemer R: *Vitrectomy: A Pars Plana Approach*. Grune & Stratton, 1975.

Morse PH: *Vitreoretinal Disease*. Year Book, 1979.

Peyman GA, Sanders DR: *Advances in Uveal Surgery, Vitreous Surgery, and the Treatment of Endophthalmitis*. Appleton-Century-Crofts, 1975.

Peyman G et al: Four hundred consecutive pars plana vitrectomies with vitrophage. *Arch Ophthalmol* 1978;**96**:45.

Treister G, Machemer R: Pars plana surgical approach for various anterior segment problems. *Arch Ophthalmol* 1979;**97**:909.

The retina covers the inner aspect of the posterior two-thirds of the wall of the globe. A fundus photo of the posterior pole of a normal retina is shown in Fig 13–1. The principal landmarks of the retina are illustrated and labeled in Fig 3–3.

The retina is a multilayered sheet of neural tissue closely applied to a single layer of pigmented epithelial cells, which in turn is attached to Bruch's membrane (Fig 13–2). The anterior extremity of the retina is firmly bound to the pigment epithelium. Posteriorly, the optic nerve fixes the retina to the wall of the globe. Elsewhere, the retina and the pigment epithelium are easily separated. In adults, the ora serrata—the partly serrated anterior end of the retina—is about 6.5 mm behind Schwalbe's line on the temporal side of the eye and 5.7 mm behind it nasally.

The retina is 0.1 mm thick at the ora serrata and 0.23 mm thick at the posterior pole. It is thinnest at the fovea centralis, the center of the macula. The retina is normally transparent, and some of the incident light is reflected at the vitreoretinal interface. The resulting sheen is especially noticeable when young, heavily

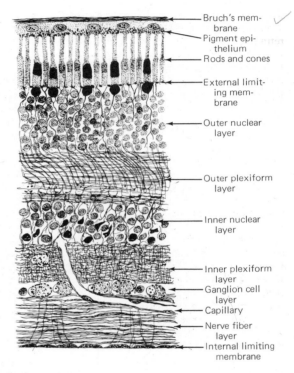

Figure 13–2. Layers of the retina. (Redrawn and reproduced, with permission, from Wolff E: *Anatomy of the Eye and Orbit,* 4th ed. Blakiston-McGraw, 1954.)

pigmented patients are examined with an indirect ophthalmoscope. On examination with the direct ophthalmoscope, the concave foveal surface produces a clearly visible inverted image of the lamp. Absence of this foveal reflection may indicate disease, but the reflection may be absent in blond or elderly patients even though the retina is normal.

The fovea centralis, which lies about 3.5 mm lateral to the optic disk, is specialized for fine visual discrimination. In the fovea, the receptors are all cones; the outer nuclear layer is thinned; the other parenchymal layers are displaced centrifugally; and the internal limiting membrane is thin. Throughout most of the retina, the axons of the receptor cells pass directly to the inner side of the outer plexiform layer

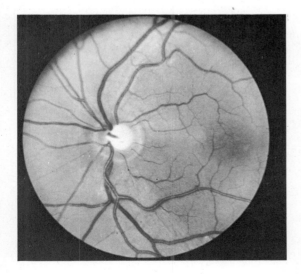

Figure 13–1. Ophthalmoscopic view of a normal retina. Note deep physiologic cup. (Courtesy of S Mettier, Jr.)

where they connect with dendrites of horizontal and bipolar cells, which extend outward from the inner nuclear layer. In the macula, however, the receptor cell axons follow an oblique course and are called the Henle fiber layer. The normally empty extracellular space of the retina is potentially greatest at the macula, and diseases that lead to accumulation of extracellular material cause considerable thickening of this area.

The axons of the bipolar cells are connected with amacrine and ganglion cells in the densely woven inner plexiform layer. The long axons of the ganglion cells pass in the nerve fiber layer to the optic nerve.

The retina receives its blood supply from 2 sources. The choriocapillaris is a single layer of closely spaced capillaries intimately attached to the outer surface of Bruch's membrane. The choriocapillaris supplies the outer third of the retina, including the outer plexiform and outer nuclear layers, the photoreceptors, and the pigment epithelium. The inner two-thirds of the retina receive branches of the central retinal artery. As the choriocapillaris is the only blood supply to the fovea centralis, this, the most important part of the retina, is susceptible to irreparable damage when the retina is detached.

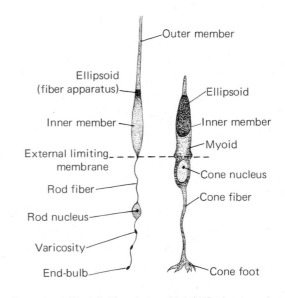

Figure 13–3. Rod *(left)* and cone *(right)*. (Redrawn and reproduced, with permission, from Wolff E: *Anatomy of the Eye and Orbit,* 4th ed. Blakiston-McGraw, 1954.)

PHYSIOLOGY

The optical system of the eye focuses a miniature image of the world upon the outer segments of the rods and cones, where the light starts a complex chain of chemical reactions beginning with a light-sensitive pigment composed of a small molecule, retinal (vitamin A aldehyde), bound to a large protein, opsin. The retinal is the same in both rods and cones, but the opsin differs. Light isomerizes the retinal from the 11-cis to an all-trans shape, so that it no longer remains adherent to the opsin. The liberated all-trans retinal may be metabolized to the 11-cis form and reattached to opsin, or it may be stored as vitamin A to be used later as the need arises.

The chemical sequence following the isomerization of retinal produces a transient excitation of the receptor that is propagated along its axon. A complex system of interconnections between the receptor axon and the cell processes of the horizontal and bipolar cells begins the process of analyzing the raw data from the receptors. The bipolar cells transmit this refined information to the inner plexiform layer, where it is once more modified through connections between amacrine, bipolar, and ganglion cells. The ganglion cells pass this reanalyzed information to the brain.

The cones are used for detailed vision (eg, reading) and color perception. They predominate at the macula, the center of visual attention; and they alone are present at the fovea, the site of best visual acuity. The rods, which predominate elsewhere, function best in reduced illumination. The principal roles of the extramacular retina are night vision and visual orientation. Examples of the latter are the ability to walk

without tripping over objects or to fix one's gaze on a moving object.

Physiology of Symptoms

The function of the retina is to receive visual images, to partly analyze them, and to dispatch this modified information to the brain. In the absence of refractive errors or opacities of the media, the images are seen in sharp focus. If the macular area of the retina is diseased, the patient's central visual acuity is affected, causing difficulty in reading and in discerning small objects in the distance (eg, street signs). If the peripheral portion of the retina is diseased, side vision is impaired but the patient continues to read well. With extreme contraction of peripheral visual field, the patient can read the finest print but bumps into large objects such as chairs and desks.

The retina has no pain nerve fibers, so that diseases of the retina are painless. In addition, they do not cause the eye to become red. The clinical evaluation of patients with retinal disease includes history, visual acuity, refraction, biomicroscopy, ophthalmoscopy, visual fields, color vision tests, and fluorescein angioscopy. Other helpful diagnostic tests in the study of retinal disorders include fluorescein angiography (see p 28), electroretinography (ERG), electro-oculography (EOG), dark adaptation, and echo-ophthalmography. (See Chapter 3.)

DISEASES OF THE RETINA

RETINAL ARTERY OCCLUSION

Blockage of the central retinal artery or one of its branches is an uncommon unilateral disorder of older patients. The obstruction may be due to an embolus or may be caused by intimal atherosclerosis. When the central retinal artery is affected, the result is sudden complete or almost complete loss of vision. Ophthalmoscopic examination within 2 hours of the occlusion shows segmentation of the blood column. Later, the vessel may appear normal, but emboli are often visible at its bifurcations. The posterior retina is pale and opaque because of changes in the axons of the nerve fiber layer (Fig 13–4). Lacking the inner retinal layers, the fovea remains transparent with the choroid showing through as a cherry-red spot. The direct pupillary response is absent. The consensual light reaction is normal.

As the retina has a dual blood supply, allowing it to survive longer than might be expected in the presence of central retinal artery occlusion, one should attempt to restore the blood flow if the patient is seen within 2 hours of the onset of symptoms. The suggested treatment is massaging the globe and anterior chamber paracentesis. The globe is massaged by pressing firmly through the closed lids for several seconds and then abruptly releasing the pressure. This maneuver is repeated several times.

Anterior chamber paracentesis is performed after anesthesia is achieved by instillation of drops and by local infiltration of the conjunctiva. The conjunctiva is held with a forceps, and a short 30-gauge needle, which is not attached to a syringe, is passed obliquely

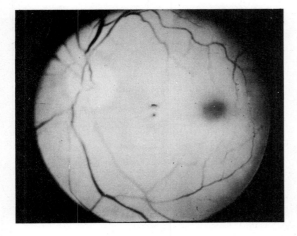

Figure 13–4. Twenty-four hours after left central retinal artery occlusion. Ischemic changes have made the nerve fiber layer pale and opaque. Because the fovea lacks this layer, the choroid can be seen as a cherry-red spot.

through the limbus at 4:30 or 7:30 o'clock. The needle is aimed at the 6 o'clock chamber angle so as to avoid the lens. One or two drops of aqueous are expressed through the needle by pressing on the globe, and the needle is removed. The rationale of the procedure is that the sudden lowering of the intraocular pressure might allow the blood in the central retinal artery to dislodge the embolus to a more peripheral branch of the vessel.

There is experimental evidence that 100% oxygen at atmospheric pressure may prolong retinal survival. However, if complete loss of vision persists for more than 2 hours, the value of therapy is questionable.

RETINAL VEIN OCCLUSION

1. CENTRAL VEIN OCCLUSION

Central retinal vein occlusion is an uncommon, usually monocular condition in which the retina and disk are swollen, the retinal veins are dilated and tortuous, and there are many retinal hemorrhages with a variable number of cotton wool patches. These findings, which are due to blockage of the central retinal vein at the level of the lamina cribrosa or behind it, are most prominent in the posterior pole and are less intense in the peripheral retina. The choriocapillaris protects the retina from ischemic death.

The patient generally presents with a slow, painless loss of vision. Predisposing systemic diseases are hypertension, diabetes, and conditions that slow venous blood flow. Many patients have elevated intraocular tension in both eyes.

One may divide the patients into 2 fairly distinct subgroups. In the less severely affected group, the retinal bleeding is mild and there are few, if any, cotton wool patches. The visual acuity is generally no worse than 6/24 (20/80) and the peripheral visual field is relatively normal. A few of the patients in this group may get worse, so that they will be included in the more severely affected group, but most dry out spontaneously when, in the course of weeks or months, the shunt vessels enlarge. Many regain normal vision, although some, in whom the fovea is permanently damaged by the edema, have a persistent central scotoma.

The usually older patients in the more severely affected subgroup are felt to have a deficient retinal arterial supply compounding the venous obstruction. In these patients, whose condition is sometimes labeled hemorrhagic retinopathy—as opposed to the name, venous stasis retinopathy, applied to the less severely affected group—the congestion and bleeding of the disk and retina are more pronounced and there may be many cotton wool exudates. These hemorrhagic retinopathy patients have a reduced peripheral visual field. Their visual acuity is 6/60 (20/200) or worse. Fluorescein demonstrates absence of blood flow through the greater part of the retinal capillary bed, and histologically there is no viable retinal vascu-

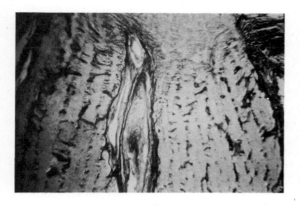

Figure 13–5. Microscopic section showing thrombus in the central retinal vein. (Courtesy of M Hogan and L Garron.)

lar endothelium. The protracted course of hemorrhagic retinopathy leads to the following states: cystoid degeneration and irreversible loss of foveal function; alterations of all parts of the retinal parenchyma; degeneration of the pigment epithelium; and liquefaction of the vitreous. When the vitreous is severely liquefied and thus no longer serves as a diffusion barrier to angiogenesis stimuli coming from the retina, new vessels often develop on the surface of the iris and the anterior chamber angle, causing peripheral anterior synechiae and intractable glaucoma.

Treatment

Many of the patients with venous stasis retinopathy recover spontaneously and require no treatment.

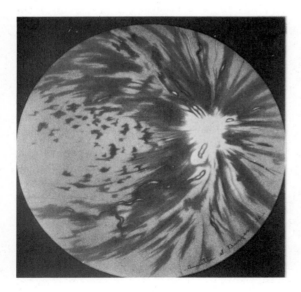

Figure 13–6. Thrombosis of the central retinal vein (drawing). (Reproduced, with permission, from Wilmer L: *Atlas Fundus Oculi.* Macmillan, 1934.)

Failing this, steroids may be considered.

Some practitioners advocate photocoagulation for those with hemorrhagic retinopathy. Anticoagulants, if they do anything, make matters worse.

In the hope of preventing neovascular glaucoma, the iris surface should be periodically checked for new vessels. Fluorescein angiography helps visualize these vessels, which first appear at the pupillary margin. If they occur, panretinal photocoagulation—a polka-dot distribution of coagulations covering areas of the retina other than the macula—usually arrests the process. If the media are too opaque for photocoagulation, the equivalent—transscleral cryotherapy—may help.

The possibilities of systemic vascular occlusive disease or blood sludging problems should be considered.

2. RETINAL BRANCH VEIN OCCLUSION

Retinal branch vein occlusion is more common than central retinal vein occlusion. The obstruction occurs at the site of an arteriovenous crossing. Distal to the obstruction, the vein is engorged and tortuous, the retina is edematous, and there are hemorrhages, microaneurysms, and sometimes cotton wool exudates. Fluorescein angioscopy emphasizes the venous dilation and demonstrates segmental dilation and leakiness of the retinal capillary bed.

The superior temporal vein is most often affected. When the macular area is involved, the vision is reduced. If one-quarter or less of the macula is edematous, the prognosis for spontaneous recovery is good. If more, the prognosis is poor.

A significant number of patients with occlusion of a branch of the retinal vein will subsequently develop new vessels. These proliferate from the surrounding, relatively normal retinal or disk vessels. If the vitreous still is against the retina, they fan out on its back surface and may bleed both behind the vitreous and into its substance, when eventually the vitreous detaches. Rarely, traction by the vitreous may tear the retina at the site of origin of the neovascular frond.

In the presence of preexisting vitreous detachment, the new vessels present as minute protrusions at the inner retinal surface. Such vessels also may bleed, apparently because the mobile vitreous brushes against them.

Three-fourths of patients with branch vein occlusion have high blood pressure. Diabetes, sickle cell disease, polycythemia vera, lymphoma, leukemia, macroglobulinemia, and multiple myeloma are less common causes.

Treatment

There is no known treatment for vision lost because of the macular edema associated with branch vein occlusion.

Photocoagulation of the involved retinal sector causes regression of the more common, fanlike, new vessel proliferations. Focal photocoagulation takes care of the new vessels that have not become adherent to the back of the vitreous. Scleral buckling may be necessary for retinal detachment and vitrectomy for extensive blood staining of the vitreous.

A medical work-up is recommended for patients with retinal branch vein occlusion.

DIABETIC RETINOPATHY

Both juvenile onset and maturity onset diabetics are prone to develop diabetic retinopathy, a disease of the retinal blood vessels that has become a leading cause of blindness in the western world. The incidence and severity of diabetic retinopathy increase with the duration of the diabetes, and the retinopathy is worse if the diabetes is poorly controlled in the early years after onset.

It is useful, though somewhat artificial, to divide diabetic retinopathy into background (nonproliferative) retinopathy and proliferative retinopathy. Background retinal abnormalities are confined to the retina. New vessels on the back of the vitreous are the hallmark of proliferative retinopathy. The former may exist without the latter, but the reverse is not true.

1. BACKGROUND RETINOPATHY

Pathologic Features & Clinical Findings
(Fig 13–7)

The earliest histologic change is loss of mural cells and thickening of the retinal capillary walls. This results clinically in leakage of fluid with focal or diffuse thickening and opacification of the retina. Yel-

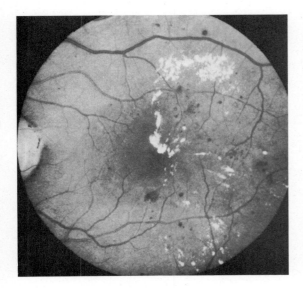

Figure 13–7. Background diabetic retinopathy. (Courtesy of P O'Malley.)

lowish deposits (hard exudates) collect where the fluid is being resorbed. Blood ceases to flow through some capillaries, and others are irregularly dilated (intraretinal microangiopathy; IRMA). There is abortive intraretinal budding of new capillaries (microaneurysms). Ruptured capillaries cause small intraretinal hemorrhages. Microinfarcts of the nerve fiber layer look like tufts of cotton (cotton wool exudates). The retinal veins may be engorged, irregularly dilated, or reduplicated, with shunts bypassing focal obstructions. Initially, the arteries may look normal. Later, they may progressively occlude from the periphery inward.

With the exception of capillary leakage, which is always present, each of the above features may be present or absent and may vary in severity with time.

A sensation of glare (due to scattering of light by the edematous retina) is a common complaint. Surprisingly, the lack of blood perfusion through large areas of the extramacular retina may be asymptomatic. However, if the macula is deprived of its blood supply or if edema or hard exudates encroach on the macula, visual acuity is decreased.

Treatment

If diabetes is well controlled in its early years, the onset of retinopathy is delayed and its severity is reduced. Once retinopathy is established, it is little affected by the day-to-day control of the diabetes. High blood pressure, if present, should be vigorously treated.

Photocoagulation may help, at least for a few years, when vision is affected by a focal area of retinal edema (circinate retinopathy), the edge of which is encroaching on the fovea. The edema clears and the usual surrounding ring of yellow exudates slowly resorbs, presumably because the leaking capillaries atrophy once the outer retinal layers, pigment epithelium, and choriocapillaris have been coagulated.

There is evidence (but no proof) that photocoagulation of background retinopathy delays the onset of proliferative retinopathy.

Prognosis

A patient can enjoy many years of useful vision after background retinopathy is first detected, and it is difficult to predict what the course will be.

2. PROLIFERATIVE RETINOPATHY

Pathology

In certain patients with background retinopathy, apparently in response to a chemical stimulus from the hypoxic retina, fragile new vessels with delicate supportive tissue grow from the retina or optic nerve head. When this happens, the vitreous is still attached to the retina and the neovascular tissue adheres to its posterior surface.

In time, this contractile vascular membrane on the back of the vitreous contracts, pulling the vitreous away from the retina. The resulting traction on the new

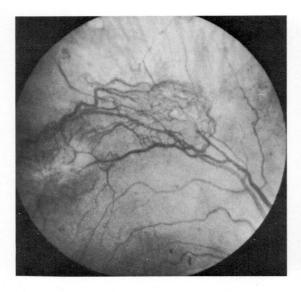

Figure 13–8. Proliferative retinopathy. New vessels at the vitreoretinal interface. (Courtesy of P O'Malley.)

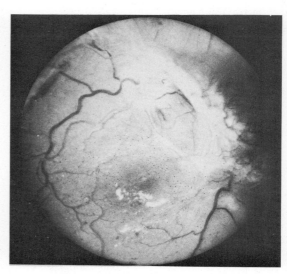

Figure 13–9. Proliferative diabetic retinopathy with extensive fibrosis. (Courtesy of L Sorenson.)

vessels may cause bleeding into the retrohyaloid space or into the vitreous body, or it may cause retinoschisis, tractional retinal detachment, or rhegmatogenous retinal detachment, or it may simply distort the retina by tangential traction. The fibrous tissue on the vitreous may in itself constitute a significant opacity.

Clinical Findings

The patient with proliferative retinopathy is relatively asymptomatic until the axial vitreous transparency is lost as a result of blood staining, with symptoms ranging from a few inconspicuous floaters to total loss of vision; or formation of scar tissue, which causes a permanent blur. Symptoms due to traction are dependent upon the site and degree of the retinal damage.

The pathologic changes of proliferative retinopathy as well as all of the findings observed in patients with background retinopathy (with the single exception of capillary nonperfusion, which can only be seen by fluorescein angioscopy) are visible to the examiner, especially if ophthalmoscopy or slit lamp examination is done with red-free light. When ophthalmoscopy isimpossible because of opacity of the media, B-scan ultrasonography is indicated.

Treatment

If little fibrous tissue is present and if the neovascular tissue is still in contact with the retina or disk, photocoagulation, by mechanisms that are not clearly understood, helps prevent the late catastrophic complications of proliferative retinopathy, although it does not necessarily preserve macular function. A xenon arc or laser is used as the light source with which the choriocapillaris, pigment epithelium, and outer retinal layers are destroyed by heat, which is generated primarily at the level of the pigment epithelium. A

carpet of contiguous retinal coagulations is placed beneath and surrounding the areas of new vessels (Fig 13–10), no attempt being made to actually coagulate the vessels. Elsewhere, coagulations are spotted at random in the postequatorial retina, sparing the perimacular zone (panretinal photocoagulation).

As the natural history of proliferative retinopathy is variable, it is difficult to say precisely when to photocoagulate. Thus, one or 2 small foci of new vessels flat on the retinal surface away from the disk may be observed and treatment withheld. If vitreous bleeding has begun, if there is extensive neovasculari-

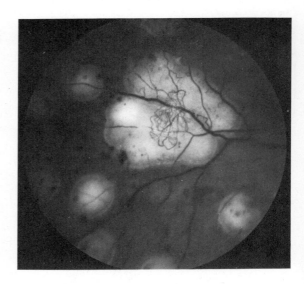

Figure 13–10. Photocoagulation for proliferative diabetic retinopathy. (Courtesy of P O'Malley.)

zation away from the disk area, or if there are any new vessels on the disk or in its vicinity, start therapy promptly.

Trans-pars plana vitrectomy with miniaturized endosurgical instruments helps about 75% of patients with diabetic retinopathy who have sustained severe loss of vision due to blood staining of the vitreous or formation of scar tissue along the visual axis. Similar therapy is often helpful for tractional retinal detachment and preretinal membranes. Rhegmatogenous retinal detachment is treated by scleral buckling.

Prognosis

Although proliferative retinopathy will sometimes regress spontaneously, it is usually progressive. Serious complications may be expected if the neovascular tissue is extensive; if new vessels are in the vicinity of the disk; if there is vitreous bleeding; or if the new vessels are pulled away from the retina.

EDEMA OF THE RETINA

Between the retinal cells there is a potential space that fills with fluid when the retinal capillaries leak. The accumulation is greatest in the outer part of the outer plexiform layer, less in the outer and inner nuclear layers, and negligible in the remaining tightly woven layers. Because of the oblique course of the receptor cell axons in the Henle fiber layer, the macula swells more than the rest of the retina and the fluid is often visibly loculated in varicose tunnels radiating from the fovea, which itself becomes a single cystlike cavity.

Chronic edema is often accompanied by minute yellow deposits, mainly in the outer plexiform layer or beneath the retina. In the Henle fiber layer, the aggregates have a striking stellate distribution. Elsewhere, a nidus of edema is surrounded by a circular belt of these deposits. If the circinate figure is close to the macula, it spreads along the spaces of the Henle fiber layer, forming one arm of a star figure. Beneath the retina, the fatty material is irregularly clumped like the aggregates sometimes seen when new vessels grow through Bruch's membrane.

The causes of retinal edema include diabetes, retinal vein obstruction, hypertension, retinal angiomas or telangiectases, traction by the vitreous or preretinal membranes, macroaneurysms, and inflammations involving the vitreous or retina. A special case of retinal edema is the **Irvine-Gass syndrome,** which consists of rapid, usually temporary loss of visual acuity in aphakic patients. It occurs more commonly after intracapsular extraction, which allows the vitreous to adhere to the iris. It is probably due to chemicals in the anterior segment having free access to the retina through the liquefied vitreous core.

Clinical Findings

Blurred vision occurs only when the macula is edematous. Visual acuity may be only slightly affected or may be as low as finger counting. The elevation and ground glass appearance of the macular area can be quite striking, and one may discern a cystoid accumulation of fluid. When retinal edema is widespread, with relative sparing of the macula—as can be the case in diabetic patients—the ophthalmoscopic diagnosis is difficult. The only clues are retinal pallor and difficulty in distinguishing details of the pigment epithelium and choroid.

Intravenous fluorescein confirms the diagnosis of retinal edema, because the dye leaks from the normally impermeable vessels and stains the extracellular fluid and because cystoid collections at the macula (which cannot be discerned with the ophthalmoscope) will become easily visible. Later, if there is frank cystoid degeneration, the cavity contents no longer stain. Fluorescein does not stain the waxy yellow deposits observed in chronic edema.

Treatment

If macular edema is due to inflammation, corticosteroids may help when given systemically or by parabulbar injection.

Most patients with the Irvine-Gass syndrome need only explanation and encouragement, since they will improve without treatment. Prophylactic therapy with indomethacin reduces the incidence of this complication. If the vitreous is detached from the retina and is extensively adherent to the iris and the cataract incision, the macular edema often persists until the fovea is irreversibly damaged. Patients with these developments are sometimes helped by vitrectomy.

Focal edema due to vasculopathies—including diabetic retinopathy—responds to photocoagulation.

Prognosis

Persistent macular edema may eventually become transformed into cystoid generation, with irreversible loss of central vision. In some cases, this is compounded by development of an atrophic hole at the fovea.

RETINAL MACROANEURYSMS

Sometimes, patients with hypertension or other systemic vascular diseases develop focal aneurysmal dilation of a retinal arteriole.

The aneurysm may bleed, but this usually clears spontaneously.

Surrounding the aneurysm is a ring of retinal edema. If this is away from the macula, nothing need be done, for it will clear on its own. If the exudate encroaches on the macula, however, it reduces the visual acuity and usually causes irreversible cystoid degeneration before resorbing. Photocoagulation helps if done before the macula is irreparably damaged.

RETROLENTAL FIBROPLASIA

Retrolental fibroplasia is a bilateral retinal disease of premature infants. It was first reported in 1942 and caused total blindness in a large number of patients until 1954, when the usual cause was found to be excessive oxygen given during the first few weeks of life.

A high oxygen concentration causes spasm of the retinal blood vessels. The spasm is followed by edema of the immature peripheral retina with later vascular dilatation and fibrovascular proliferation into the vitreous. Total retinal detachment often follows.

Retrolental fibroplasia usually has its onset in the first few days of life and may progress rapidly to blindness over a period of weeks. Once blindness occurs, there is no hope for restoration of sight. In many early cases, there is partial or complete regression in both eyes. Less commonly, the disease process regresses in one eye, allowing it to develop normal vision. Myopia and strabismus are common among those who retain useful vision, and in later life there is a tendency to rhegmatogenous retinal detachment (see p 149).

In advanced cases, one sees in both eyes a white retrolental membrane containing blood vessels. The anterior chamber is shallow, and the pupillary light reflex is absent. The lens is clear, and transillumination is normal. The contracting retrolental tissue draws the ciliary processes inward so that they can be seen at the periphery of the dilated pupil.

Differentiation from persistent hyperplastic vitreous usually is not difficult, since the latter condition is unilateral. Retinoblastoma has a later onset, may not transilluminate, and has an anterior chamber of normal depth. If bilateral, the tumor is usually more advanced in one eye.

Glaucoma, uveitis, cataract, or phthisis bulbi frequently occurs months or years after the onset of retrolental fibroplasia.

Infants of low birth weight and infants who require supplemental oxygen should have their pupils widely dilated for examination by indirect ophthalmoscopy and scleral depression in order to detect the earlier stages of retrolental fibroplasia. At first there is avascularity of the (usually temporal) peripheral retina. Later, a discrete intraretinal band appears at the junction of the vascular and avascular retina, with dilated retinal vessels and arteriovenous shunts behind this junction. Subsequently, new vessels grow into the vitreous at this site. It is the contraction of this fibrovascular tissue that causes the serious complications to the vitreous and retina. If the condition is aborted in the earlier stages, spontaneous regression may be quite complete. Regression is signaled by vessels growing into the previously avascular peripheral retina.

RETINITIS PIGMENTOSA

Retinitis pigmentosa is a group of hereditary dystrophies of the retinal receptors transmitted as autosomal recessive, autosomal dominant, or X-linked traits. The rods are slowly destroyed, with secondary atrophy of the remainder of the retina and the pigment epithelium. Cells filled with epithelial pigment aggregate along the retinal vessels to give the typical bone corpuscular appearance (Fig 13–11). These changes begin in the mid periphery, sparing the macular and

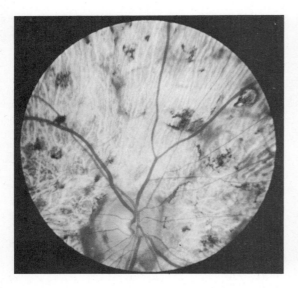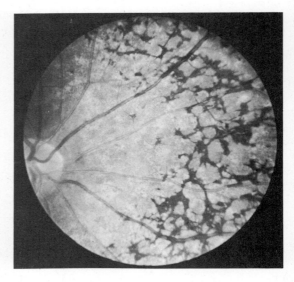

Figure 13–11. Retinitis pigmentosa. *Left:* Typical "bone spicule" arrangement of pigmentary changes. *Right:* Clumped, scattered pigment, attenuated arteries, and choroidal sclerosis. (Photos by L Arlinghaus.)

peripheral regions until later. The retinal problems are often associated with deafness, mental retardation, and other systemic findings, making several distinct syndromes. The most common of these is Laurence-Moon-Biedl syndrome, which combines retinitis pigmentosa, obesity, mental retardation, polydactyly, and hypogenitalism.

Night blindness—the first symptom of retinitis pigmentosa—usually occurs in early youth. Thereafter, the visual fields gradually constrict ("gun barrel vision") to become disabling in the fifth or sixth decade, at which time macular vision may also be lost. The fundi may appear normal at first. Later, most patients have the typical scattered black pigmentary disturbance. The retinal arterioles become attenuated, and the disk becomes pale and waxy. In rare instances, the disease may affect only one eye or just one sector of an eye.

The electroretinogram is reduced or absent, and the electro-oculogram gives a flat curve (see Chapter 3). Commonly associated eye findings are myopia, posterior polar cataract, and glaucoma.

In rare instances where retinitis pigmentosa is due to abetalipoproteinemia (Bassen-Kornzweig syndrome: steatorrhea, ataxia, and retinitis pigmentosa), its progress may be arrested in the early stages by massive doses of vitamin A. There is no specific therapy for the other causes of retinitis pigmentosa. Genetic counseling should be offered in an attempt to prevent propagation of the disease.

PERIPHERAL CYSTOID DEGENERATION
(Fig 13–12)

Cystoid degeneration of the retina consists of the permanent accumulation between the neural elements of a clear material that compresses the glial tissue into columns separating cystlike spaces. Some degree of cystoid degeneration is present in the peripheral retina of many infants and of everybody over age 8. It invariably begins at the ora serrata and progresses backward as a maze of contiguous varicose tunnels. It can extend behind the equator in later life, but not to the point

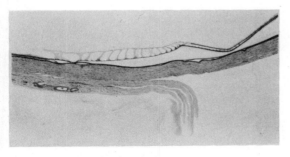

Figure 13–12. Peripheral cystoid degeneration of the retina. (Reproduced, with permission, from Arruga H: *Detachment of the Retina.* Salvat, 1936.)

where it causes symptoms or encroaches significantly on the peripheral field of vision.

Close to the ora serrata, the cystoid cavities are large and often cause the retina to have a moth-eaten appearance. Otherwise, the low magnification of the indirect ophthalmoscope does not normally allow the examiner to see this essentially innocuous condition.

SENILE RETINOSCHISIS

Peripheral cystoid degeneration may lead to splitting of the retina into 2 layers. Such "senile" retinoschisis occurs in about 3% of the population, increasing in frequency from the second decade onward.

The bulging internal wall of the cavity is thin and immobile and often has a "beaten metal" appearance. The thick external wall is hard to see in its usual position against the pigment epithelium, but there are often defects in it—in contrast to the inner layer, which usually is intact. Further diagnostic features include a band of prominent cystoid degeneration separating the cavity from the ora serrata and the presence of other areas of retinoschisis in the temporal half of the same eye or of the fellow eye.

If the contents of the cavity leak through a hole in the outer wall, a self-limited, usually harmless retinal detachment results. Rhegmatogenous detachment may develop when there is a hole in both walls. This rare complication is the only serious consequence of senile retinoschisis.

The bulging internal wall must not be mistaken for a retinal detachment and treated as such. Only when rhegmatogenous detachment has occurred or is imminent is it warranted to intervene with light coagulation, cryothermy, diathermy, or scleral buckling. In extremely rare instances, the retinal splitting threatens the macula and should be treated.

PAVING STONE DEGENERATION OF THE RETINA
(Fig 13–13)

Paving stone degeneration is a striking but harmless condition of the peripheral retina in which the pigment epithelium and outer retinal layers are damaged or absent. The intact inner retina is adherent to the exposed Bruch's membrane and also to the pigment epithelium at the edge of the lesion. The vitreous and the outer choroidal structures are normal.

The sharply outlined, rounded lesions are pale yellow, often with a partial rim of increased pigmentation. They range in size up to 1 disk diameter and may occur singly or in clusters. Several lesions may coalesce to form a circumferential band with a scalloped margin.

The process occurs mainly in the lower quadrants, though it is found in any part of the peripheral fundus. It is fairly common in young adults, and its incidence and the frequency of bilateral occurrence

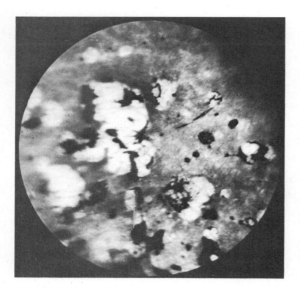

Figure 13–13. Paving stone degeneration. (Reproduced, with permission, from O'Malley C, O'Malley P: *The Peripheral Fundus of the Eye.* Medcom, 1973.)

increase with age. It is quite innocuous, and the patient is unaware of its presence.

LATTICE DEGENERATION

Lattice degeneration (Fig 13–14) of the retina is characterized by elongated, excavated troughs in the peripheral retina. The lesions are surrounded by a distinct narrow rim, which projects above the level of the normal adjacent retina. The vitreous is firmly adherent to the rim and forms a canopy, which envelops a pocket of fluid lying in the trough. Close to their insertion, the vitreous fibrils are condensed and may be visible as a white frill.

Glistening white spots are common on the retinal surface, giving a snail-track appearance to some lattice areas. Although the pigment epithelium beneath the lesions may appear normal, it is often disturbed and may vary from subtle disarray to gross disorganization. The walls of the retinal vessels are thickened where they cross the abnormal retina in over 10% of lesions. These sclerosed vessels form a white latticework that inspired the name.

The above features are often not visible on routine inspection, and areas of lattice might be missed were it not for the edge-on view afforded by scleral depression. With this aid to examination, the sharp rim and roughened, depressed surface of the trough are readily seen.

The individual lesions are about one-third disk diameter in width and one-half disk diameter to 1 quadrant long. They generally lie parallel to the ora serrata, are confined to the equatorial and oral zones, and are concentrated toward the vertical meridian. There may be as many as 20 lesions in one eye forming 2 or more parallel rows. Both eyes are affected in about a third of cases.

About 8% of the population have lattice degeneration, and the incidence is constant in each age group after 10. Surprisingly, teenagers may have heavily pigmented lesions with extreme thinning of the retina,

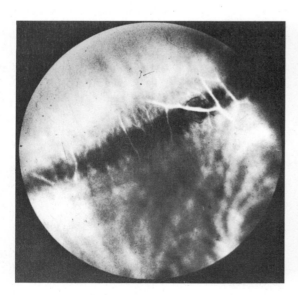

Figure 13–14. Lattice degeneration. (Reproduced, with permission, from O'Malley C, O'Malley P: *The Peripheral Fundus of the Eye.* Medcom, 1973.)

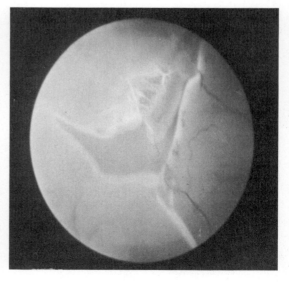

Figure 13–15. Retinal tear at an area of lattice degeneration. Operculum still attached to retina. (Reproduced, with permission, from O'Malley C, O'Malley P: *The Peripheral Fundus of the Eye.* Medcom, 1973.)

whereas septuagenarians will often have rather superficial nonpigmented lesions. Atrophic round holes are common in all age groups.

Lattice degeneration is an etiologic factor in about one-third of all cases of rhegmatogenous retinal detachment. One of 2 distinct mechanisms is responsible for the detachment. In one group of patients, the leakage is through an atrophic hole. This may result in tiny localized areas of detachment that rarely spread and require no treatment other than periodic observation. In younger patients, such a detachment sometimes spreads slowly, with multiple demarcation lines, and surgery is required.

The more common mechanism by which lattice degeneration leads to retinal detachment derives from the fact that, owing to their posterior location, about two-thirds of the lesions have established a firm vitreoretinal adhesion behind the vitreous base. If the vitreous detaches posteriorly, the stress at the ends and the posterior border of the lattice may be enough to produce a tear. The break is in the relatively normal retina beneath the rim and not through the thinned retina. Small lesions far back may be completely avulsed. Much more often, the tear is J-shaped and located at one end of the lattice. As the vitreous continues to tug on the retina, these tears usually cause extensive retinal detachment.

The threat of retinal detachment has given lattice degeneration notoriety in excess of what it deserves. Most people with this condition enjoy a normal asymptomatic existence. They should, however, be checked periodically, and they must be seen immediately if they report symptoms suggestive of vitreous detachment. If it is obvious that retinal detachment is likely—because of retinal detachment in the fellow eye, a family history of retinal detachment, or local findings—then one should perform prophylactic cryothermy or photocoagulation.

RETINAL HOLES

Retinal holes are either tears, which have an operculum (lid) of retinal tissue, or atrophic holes, which do not. The fovea and the peripheral retina are the sites of predilection for retinal holes. In both places, the internal limiting membrane and retinal parenchyma are thin. Extramacular tears and holes are described here. (For foveal holes, see p 154.)

1. RETINAL TEARS
(Fig 13–16)

The retina is torn by mechanical force, usually vitreous traction. The distinctive feature of a retinal tear is an operculum of avulsed tissue. The size of the tear may vary tremendously.

When the retina is torn, metaplastic pigment epithelial cells may enter the vitreous. If these tobacco-dustlike cells are found, a retinal tear is almost

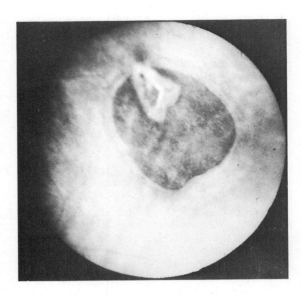

Figure 13–16. Retinal tear. Completely avulsed operculum. (Reproduced, with permission, from O'Malley C, O'Malley P: *The Peripheral Fundus of the Eye.* Medcom, 1973.)

certainly present and must be sought.

Retinal tears may be due to constant or intermittent vitreous traction.

Tears due to constant vitreous traction. Proliferative diabetic retinopathy, penetrating injuries, and a variety of other disorders cause scarring of the vitreous. Contraction of the scarred vitreous may tear the retina at its point of attachment. Only a small percentage of retinal tears occurs by this mechanism, but it is important to recognize and treat them promptly for they may lead to extensive retinal detachment.

Tears due to intermittent vitreous traction. When the vitreous is partly liquefied and detached from the retina, acceleration or deceleration of the globe—either as a result of normal eye movements or trauma—will cause whiplike motions of the gel that may exert sufficient stress to tear the retina at normal and abnormal points of vitreoretinal attachments. The latter may be due to a number of anatomic anomalies and pathologic processes that may not be recognizable before the tear appears.

The greater the space inside the eye, the greater the force that can be exerted to tear the retina. This may explain why aphakia, the large globe commonly associated with myopia, forward displacement of the lens by miotics, and localized scleral ectasia predispose to retinal tears.

The operculum of most tears retains a partial attachment at the anterior margin of the break, so that the vitreous continues to tug on the retina. Even so, such retinal tears should be watched and not treated unless (1) the vitreous cavity is unduly large; (2) the holes are multiple, large, or far behind the ora serrata; (3) there is a history of retinal detachment in the fellow eye or a family history of retinal detachment; or (4) there are recent symptoms of vitreous detachment. In these situations, even though treatment is not always successful, the danger of retinal detachment outweighs the risk of complications of prophylactic therapy.

Retinal tissue may be torn completely free if the area of vitreoretinal adhesion is small. Such tears are generally round or oval and rarely exceed the diameter of the disk. They are much less likely to lead to retinal detachment than if the operculum is still adherent to the retina.

Relationship of Blood Vessels to Retinal Tears

At the time the retina is torn, capillaries are often ruptured and the patient reports a shower of black spots that represent shadows on the macula caused by red blood cells in the retrovitreal space. If a larger vessel is broken, the subvitreal bleeding may be so severe that the retina is obscured. A few hours of bed rest with bilateral eye patches and elevation of the head will generally allow the blood to settle enough to permit visualization of the retina.

As a rule, the larger vessels do not break, so that the retina either continues to tear beyond the vessel and a segment of the vessel is elevated off the retina or the vessel arrests the shearing force.

In younger patients, the acquired posterior extension of the vitreous base is narrow, so that tears may occur close to the ora serrata. Since the mechanical reinforcement of the retinal vessels is lacking here, the rip can extend a considerable distance around the circumference of the globe.

Causes of Retinal Tears

Vitreous traction, either intermittent or constant, accounts for the vast majority of retinal tears. This usually happens spontaneously, but indirect trauma occasionally precipitates a retinal tear in a predisposed individual.

Direct trauma deforms the globe transiently and can cause conventional tears, giant tears at the posterior margin of the vitreous base, or tears in the nonpigmented epithelium of the pars plana at the anterior margin of the vitreous base (see p 155).

Anomalous zonular attachments to the retina are also believed to cause tears. The detaching retina (for whatever reason) may also tear at the site of chorioretinal adhesions resulting from previous therapy, paving stone degeneration, or chorioretinitis, but this is rare. In these latter cases, the torn fragment remains adherent to the external structure—not in its usual location at or central to the detached retina.

2. ATROPHIC RETINAL HOLES

In addition to the atrophic holes associated with lattice degeneration and retinoschisis, about 1% of people have small, round, nonoperculated holes of unknown cause in the peripheral retina. These are usually close to the ora serrata and rarely cause significant retinal detachment, though a tiny self-limiting detachment is often present.

Most atrophic retinal holes are asymptomatic. Some are accompanied by symptoms of vitreous detachment (see Chapter 12).

Treatment of Retinal Holes

The greatest problem in treating retinal holes is deciding whether or not treatment is necessary. Unfortunately, the decision must be made with an inadequate knowledge of the natural history of most types of holes and almost total ignorance of the qualitative and quantitative parameters of vitreous traction. However, careful observation does give some clues, for with the passage of time the lips of a retinal hole become white and rounded because of gliosis; opercula slowly shrink; the subjacent pigment epithelium is often altered; and a ring of pigment epithelial reaction may appear at the edge of the narrow halo of retinal detachment, which often accompanies even innocuous holes. In the absence of frank retinal detachment, these findings tell the examiner that the potentially dangerous lesion has been present for some time without causing trouble; thus, a conservative attitude toward prophylactic therapy is required.

The objective of prophylactic treatment is to establish a firm chorioretinal bond around the retinal break. The scar should be broader on the side nearest the ora serrata, since this is usually the site of greatest vitreous pull. Indeed, it is often safest to treat forward to the vitreous base to forestall future vitreous traction.

There are 3 ways to seal a retinal hole: freezing, burning by light, or burning by electricity. The mechanism in each case is to cause an inflammatory response of the retina and choroid that subsequently binds them together.

A. Cryothermy: A supercooled metal probe is placed on the conjunctiva in an area corresponding to the borders of the retinal hole. The instrument must have an adequate heat sink to propagate a dome of ice through the wall of the eye. The surgeon ophthalmoscopically controls the freezing, which selectively destroys cells but leaves the fibrous structures intact.

B. Photocoagulation: A bright light focused on the pigment epithelium will coagulate it and the overlying retina. One may use a xenon arc or argon laser as the light source. This form of therapy is excellent for posterior lesions but is awkward to administer anterior to the equator.

C. Diathermy: The energy of a high-frequency current, when applied to the sclera, is transformed to heat, which coagulates choroid and retina.

RETINAL DETACHMENT

Because the retina is only loosely adherent to the pigment epithelium, the 2 may separate, allowing fluid to accumulate between them. The fluid usually comes from the vitreous, having passed through a hole in the retina. Less often, it leaks from blood vessels, as happens with central serous retinopathy, choroidal tumors, some inflammatory conditions, malignant hypertension, or when vitreous traction creates a subretinal space without perforating the retina.

Mechanism of Rhegmatogenous Retinal Detachment

Rhegmatogenous (tear-induced) retinal detachment is dependent upon 3 factors: (1) a retinal hole, (2) liquid in the vitreous compartment with free access to the hole, and (3) a force sufficient to break the bond between the retina and the pigment epithelium and transfer fluid from in front of to behind the retina. The vitreous supplies this force in essentially the same way as it causes retinal tears (see p 148).

Until one or more of these factors is nullified, the detachment will continue to spread. Most of the retina may become detached in a few hours, or it may take years for this to happen.

Clinical Findings

The common sequence is for the symptoms of vitreous detachment (see Chapter 12) to be followed minutes to years later by a "shadow" or "curtain" spreading across the field of vision. When the detachment spreads very slowly, the patient may be unaware of any problem until the macula is affected.

On ophthalmoscopic examination, the detached retina bulges inward and is gently rippled or thrown into folds (Figs 13–18, 13–19, and 13–20). It is translucent, obscuring the details of the pigment epithelium and choroid, and trembles with each movement of the eye. A careful search will almost always reveal one or more holes. If the detachment is of long standing, the retina will usually be more transparent and a characteristic demarcation line of pigment epithelial disturbance separates detached from normal retina.

The other eye must be examined, since it often has retinal holes or vitreoretinal adhesions that might lead to tears. These should be mapped carefully and treated prophylactically.

Differential Diagnosis

One must consider senile retinoschisis, choroidal detachment, and malignant melanoma of the choroid. The retinoschisis cavity has a thin, immobile inner wall. The honeycomb appearance and large breaks of the outer wall are pathognomonic but are not always present. There may be other areas of retinoschisis on the temporal side of the same or fellow eye.

A detached choroid is not limited by the ora serrata but is prevented from spreading where the vortex vessels enter the sclera. The pigment epithelium is still visible, but the choroidal structures are not.

In malignant melanoma of the choroid, the subretinal fluid shifts on changing the patient's position. The tumor usually does not transilluminate, and its position disregards both ora serrata and vortex vessels.

Treatment

Surgical repair is mandatory in the treatment of rhegmatogenous retinal detachment, since spontaneous reattachment is extremely rare. The first step is ophthalmoscopic examination of the entire retina and construction of a detailed map showing each hole and each area of vitreoretinal traction. The goal is to seal the holes and prevent further holes from developing. By reducing the volume of the vitreous compartment and distorting it in various ways, vitreous traction is relieved. The retina is thus placed in contact with choroid, and the tissues are stimulated by diathermy, cryothermy, or photocoagulation to establish a permanent chorioretinal bond around the hole.

Course & Prognosis

With care, 90% of retinal detachments can be repaired by one operation. Subsequent procedures salvage another 6%. If the retina is still in place after 6 months, it is unlikely to become detached again.

The fovea may suffer irreparable damage in a brief period of separation from its only blood supply, the choriocapillaris. By contrast, on reattaching the retina, extrafoveal function may recover to a remarkable degree even after several months of detachment.

PRERETINAL MEMBRANES

These thin sheets of contractile tissue on the inner retinal surface are produced by glia or by pigment epithelium that has undergone metaplasia. They arise in association with a variety of conditions, including spontaneous vitreous detachment, retinal tears with or without retinal detachment, diabetic retinopathy, occlusion of retinal veins, and penetrating injuries. The associated condition apparently provides a vitreous-free retinal surface in combination with a break in the inner limiting lamina, or a full-thickness retinal hole through which the offending cells migrate.

In the beginning, the membrane, which covers part or all of the retina behind the vitreous base, is composed of elongated cells and delicate supportive tissue; later it contracts, exerting traction through scattered focal retinal attachments. This causes retinal folds if the retina is detached and mobile or if it causes the lips of a retinal tear to roll inward. If a large area of detached retina is involved, the condition is called **massive preretinal retraction.** In contrast, there is very little puckering when the retina is attached— whence the name **surface wrinkling retinopathy.**

Clinical Findings

Vision is rapidly lost when a contracting preretinal membrane in the presence of a retinal hole causes retinal detachment. At the opposite end of the spectrum, if the retina is attached and a membrane is some distance from the macula, the patient is asymptomatic. If the macula is wrinkled, however, visual acuity may be reduced to less than 6/60 (20/200).

It is usually impossible to detect an early preretinal membrane with the ophthalmoscope, since it is virtually transparent. When the membrane contracts, it

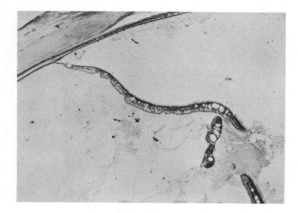

Figs 13–17 to 13–21 are reproduced, with permission, from Arruga H: *Detachment of the Retina.* Salvat, 1936.

Figure 13–17. Tear in retina causing retinal detachment (microscopic section). Also shows cystoid degeneration of retina.

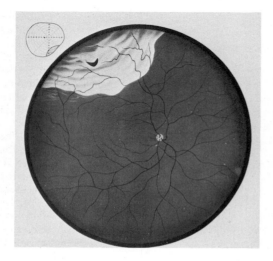

Figure 13–18. Retinal detachment 3 days after onset with crescent-shaped retinal tear.

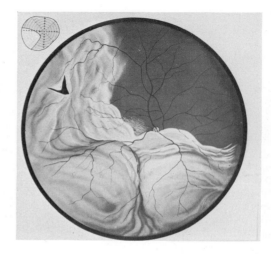

Figure 13–20. Appearance of retinal detachment 40 days after onset.

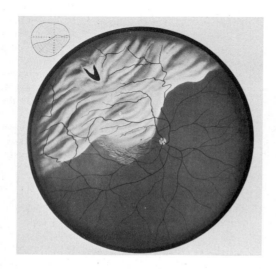

Figure 13–19. Retinal detachment and retinal tear 6 days after onset.

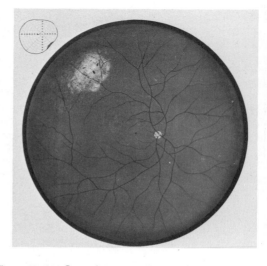

Figure 13–21. Operative cure of retinal detachment. Appearance of retina 2 months after surgical repair.

may become visible, especially with the aid of red-free light. The membrane is slightly opaque, with an irregular, ill-defined outline. It bridges the apexes of the retinal folds when the retina is detached and is at the focus of the retinal wrinkles and has a shiny surface when the retina is attached.

Treatment

Treatment is usually not necessary for surface wrinkling retinopathy. However, if severe visual loss occurs, one must attempt the hazardous task of surgically cutting the membrane on the surface of the retina. If retinal detachment is present, scleral buckling and sometimes vitrectomy are indicated.

THE MACULA

CENTRAL SEROUS DETACHMENT OF THE RETINA
(Fig 13–22)

This disorder occurs at any age past the early teens and affects males more often than females. Although it is usually monocular, both eyes may be affected either concurrently or sequentially. One or more small defects appear in the pigment epithelial layer of an otherwise normal-appearing fundus, and fluid leaks from the choriocapillaris to the subretinal space. This transudate is either clear or partly opaque. The resulting smooth retinal detachment may extend up to 6 disk diameters in circumference.

The main symptom is blurred vision, and—as with most macular problems—exposure to bright light makes this worse. Visual acuity is reduced to a variable degree, and there is a slight shift toward hyperopia. Ophthalmoscopic and slit lamp examinations reveal a shallow retinal detachment with loss of the foveal reflection. Intravenous fluorescein demonstrates the site of leakage. Because the fresh fluorescein-stained fluid is warm, it rises by convection in the cooler preexisting fluid. The new fluid eventually becomes mixed with the old, and detectable fluorescence persists for about 30 minutes.

In most cases the leak closes spontaneously, and the subretinal fluid is resorbed within 3 months of the onset of the disease. Most of these patients recover good vision. Sometimes the detachment persists longer, increasing the likelihood of secondary cystoid degeneration of the macula. Permanent damage to the retina is also more likely if there are repeated episodes of central serous detachment.

If the pigment epithelial leakage persists longer than 3 months and if it is not directly beneath the fovea, photocoagulation is indicated. This seals the leakage site and the subretinal fluid is resorbed, with improvement in vision.

Although central serous retinopathy appears to be a distinct entity, it must be stressed that any condition damaging Bruch's membrane and the pigment epithelium may cause leakage of serous fluid beneath the central retina. The differential diagnosis thus includes senile degeneration of Bruch's membrane, angioid streaks, tumors such as choroidal angioma, nevus, and malignant melanoma, familial drusen, high myopia, and trauma.

Very rarely, a pit of the optic nerve may be associated with detachment in the posterior polar retina. In these cases, there is no demonstrable leak in the pigment epithelium, and it is thought that the fluid may be cerebrospinal or from the vitreous.

DETACHMENT OF PIGMENT EPITHELIUM

Focal detachment of the pigment epithelium appears to be a manifestation of damage to Bruch's membrane. It may develop in a normal-looking fundus or may be associated with the conditions described above as sometimes causing central serous retinal detachment. Indeed, detachment of the pigment epithelium and central serous retinopathy are often concurrent, with one of them dominating the clinical picture.

When the lesion is away from the macula, the patient is usually asymptomatic. Even when the lesion is beneath the fovea, vision may be surprisingly good. As viewed with the ophthalmoscope, the lesion is a sharply outlined low elevation of the pigment epithelium that masks the choroidal details. The slit lamp readily confirms the blisterlike elevation, and retroillumination reveals the clarity of its contents together with the commonly present irregular opaque lines on its anterior wall.

Fluorescein promptly stains the cavity contents, which, though the pigment epithelium may be quite opaque, shine brightly in contrast with the rest of the fundus. This is probably explained by the fact that the layer of fluorescein-stained fluid is much thicker here than elsewhere. If there is an associated serous detachment of the retina, the fluorescein may show a discrete leak in the pigment epithelium.

Pigment epithelial detachments either regress spontaneously, spread, result in atrophy of the pigment epithelium, or lead to neovascularization beneath the pigment epithelium.

Photocoagulation is of value if the pigment epithelial detachment has not developed new vessels and if the surrounding pigment epithelium is healthy.

NEW VESSELS BENEATH THE PIGMENT EPITHELIUM & DISCIFORM DEGENERATION OF THE MACULA

New blood vessels may grow into the potential space between the mesodermal portion of Bruch's membrane and the basement membrane of the pigment epithelium. This happens mainly at the posterior pole, and there usually is some recognizable predisposing abnormality of Bruch's membrane, such as senile or hereditary degeneration, detachment of the pigment epithelium, presumed histoplasmic choroidal scars, angioid streaks, traumatic rupture, high myopia, or congenital rubella retinopathy. The new vessels arise from the choroid and pass through defects in Bruch's membrane or around its edge at the disk. They can be rendered visible by fluorescein perfusion.

These vessels may cause serous or hemorrhagic detachment of the pigment epithelium. The subsequent scar tissue usually breaks into the subretinal space, becoming irregularly pigmented and continuing for years to bleed and leak serous fluid, often with accumulation of yellow deposits. Blood usually leaks beneath the retina, and on rare occasions it may rupture through the retina into the vitreous, especially in the case of patients taking aspirin or other anticoagulants. Overlying these roughly circular (disciform) lesions, the retina suffers irreparable damage, and if the macula is involved, central vision is lost. However, these patients are not incapacitated because peripheral func-

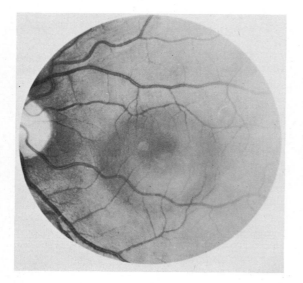
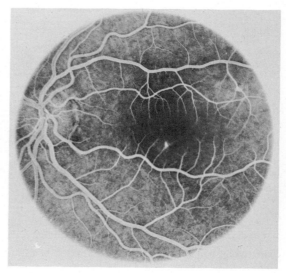
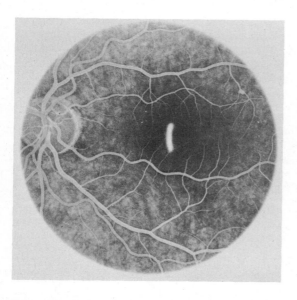
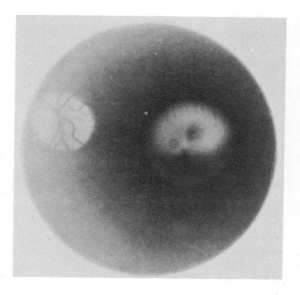

Figure 13–22. Central serous retinal detachment. *Top left:* Fundus photo of a 34-year-old man with serous detachment of the central retina. *Top right:* The arteriovenous phase of the fluorescein angiogram reveals a tiny defect in the pigment epithelium. *Bottom left:* The warm dye-stained serum leaks into the subretinal cavity and rises in the preexisting cooler fluid. *Bottom right:* In the course of time, the dye mixes through the fluid in the dome of the detachment. (Reproduced, with permission, from Gass J: *Stereoscopic Atlas of Macular Diseases.* Mosby, 1970.)

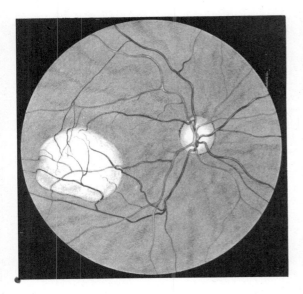

Figure 13-23. Quiescent disciform macular degeneration (drawing). (Courtesy of F Cordes.)

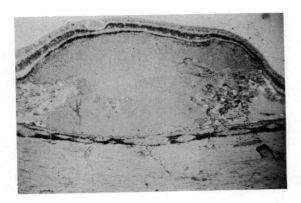

Figure 13-24. Microscopic section, disciform macular degeneration. (Courtesy of M Hogan.)

treat neovascularizations even closer to the center of the fovea.) Subretinal neovascularization as a complication of senile degeneration of Bruch's membrane progresses so rapidly that photocoagulation should be undertaken promptly. Where subretinal new vessels develop because of some other process, the eventual deterioration of the fovea is not so rapid nor is it inevitable; yet clinical experience indicates that photocoagulation should be performed.

SENILE DEGENERATION OF BRUCH'S MEMBRANE

Irregular thickening of Bruch's membrane and associated sclerosis of the choriocapillaris are frequent findings in elderly patients. The overlying pigment epithelium is disturbed, especially in the macula and at the disk margin. Drusen—tiny discrete deposits beneath the basement membrane of the pigment epithelium—may be present as further evidence of damage to Bruch's membrane.

These changes get worse with time. In some cases, areas of the pigment epithelium may atrophy completely; in others, serous detachment of the pigment epithelium may develop; and in still others new vessels may develop with subsequent bleeding. In the early stages—and, indeed, for many years—the symptoms are minimal, with only a small drop in visual acuity. However, the later complications cause severe loss of central vision.

Although serous detachment of the pigment epithelium, which may occur as a complication of

tion usually remains intact. They lose the ability to read but can ambulate easily, especially in familiar surroundings.

Malignant melanoma may be difficult to differentiate from disciform degeneration. Indeed, eyes with disciform degeneration have often been enucleated in error. It is sometimes necessary to follow the patient for months or years to see if the lesion is growing.

When the fovea is affected by serous or bloody leakage from subretinal new vessels, the patient usually presents with distorted, blurred vision. Visual acuity is reduced, and some abnormality is apparent with the Amsler grid. If fluorescein angiography shows the new vessel net to be no closer than 0.2 mm from the center of the fovea, treatment with the argon laser may be successful. (A krypton laser, producing red light, which is more appropriate than the blue-green light of the common argon lasers, allows one to

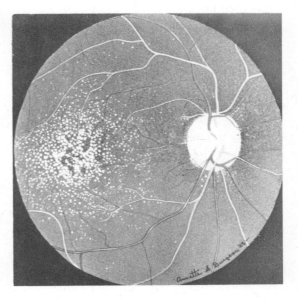

Figure 13-25. Drusen in the macula. (Reproduced, with permission, from Wilmer L: *Atlas Fundus Oculi.* Macmillan, 1934.)

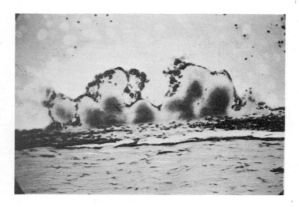

Figure 13–26. Microscopic section of drusen (excrescences of Bruch's membrane). Retina not shown. (Courtesy of M Hogan.)

senile degeneration, can sometimes be treated, there is no treatment for the primary changes in the capillaries and Bruch's membrane. Even so, with optical aids, many patients can be helped to continue reading.

Some younger patients with a family history of drusen may show similar changes in the macular area.

ANGIOID STREAKS
(Fig 13–27)

Linear breaks in the fibroelastic layer of Bruch's membrane look somewhat like blood vessels, for which reason they are called angioid streaks. They are brown, irregular bands radiating from the disk. As-

sociated findings are pseudoxanthoma elasticum (Groenblad-Strandberg syndrome), sickle cell disease, and Paget's disease (osteitis deformans). From a practical point of view, the lacquer breaks of high myopia and traumatic ruptures of Bruch's membrane can be grouped with angioid streaks. The pigment epithelium overlying all of these lesions slowly degenerates, and new vessels sometimes grow through the defect in Bruch's membrane to cause a disciform lesion.

In the absence of neovascularization, angioid streaks are usually asymptomatic. If new vessels are present, photocoagulation occasionally helps.

PRESUMED HISTOPLASMOSIS SYNDROME

A considerable number of patients from the eastern half of the USA have combinations of the following findings: positive skin test for histoplasmosis, miliary opacities of the lungs, tiny choroidal scars, peripapillary disruption of the choroid, and exudation or bleeding from subretinal neovascular lesions at or near the macula. Except for the macular complications, the condition is asymptomatic and benign. Once disciform changes commence, the prognosis is very poor. Photocoagulation usually arrests the course of active lesions that are eccentric to the fovea.

FOVEAL HOLE

As in the retinal periphery, the parenchyma and internal limiting membrane at the avascular fovea are thin and prone to hole formation (Fig 13–28). These

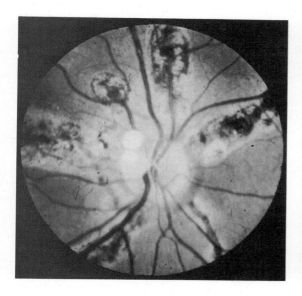

Figure 13–27. Retinal photograph showing angioid streaks in retina. (Courtesy of M Hogan and S Aiken.)

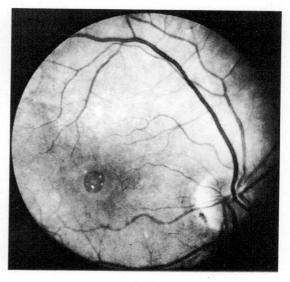

Figure 13–28. Atrophic macular hole. (Reproduced, with permission, from O'Malley C, O'Malley P: *The Peripheral Fundus of the Eye*. Medcom, 1973.)

atrophic macular holes are fairly common and can be caused by prolonged macular edema or traction by a preretinal membrane. In older patients, they may develop spontaneously.

The loss of vision is proportionate to the size of the hole and the associated findings. If the retina is flat, it is often difficult to tell if the macula is really perforated. However, one can be reasonably confident of the diagnosis if the view of the underlying pigment epithelium is sharp, the hole margin is rounded and more opaque than the contiguous retina, and the background choroidal fluorescence shows through clearly.

There is no effective treatment for macular atrophic holes. They very rarely lead to retinal detachment and should merely be watched.

HEREDITARY DISEASES OF THE MACULA

The hereditary diseases of the macula—all of which are untreatable—can be loosely divided into those that involve primarily the choriocapillaris and those that initially affect the pigment epithelium.

Central areolar choroidal sclerosis is an example of the former group. This autosomal dominant or recessive disease leads to slow loss of central vision in middle life. Abnormalities of the choriocapillaris and pigment epithelium are apparent early. By the time symptoms occur, there may be complete atrophy of the central pigment epithelium.

Stargardt-Behr disease and Best's disease are examples of macular diseases primarily affecting the pigment epithelium. Stargardt-Behr disease is usually transmitted in an autosomal recessive manner. Commencing at different ages, the macular pigment epithelium slowly degenerates. The intensity of the pigment epithelial changes and the degree of visual loss vary from family to family.

In Best's vitelliform macular degeneration, there is a diffuse abnormality of the pigment epithelium, but the visible changes are confined to the macula. Initially in this autosomal dominant disease—though the vision is good—there are deposits in the pigment epithelium, giving the appearance of a poached egg "sunny side up." Later, when the yolk of the egg appears scrambled, macular vision is seriously reduced.

TRAUMA

Though the eye as a whole must be considered when dealing with an injury (see Chapter 23), some details particular to the retina are described here.

BLUNT TRAUMA

A nonpenetrating injury to the globe may tear the retina or produce commotio retinae, or it may indirectly damage the retina as a result of fracturing Bruch's membrane.

Traumatic Retinal Tears

The severe, almost instantaneous distortion of the globe caused by blunt trauma can tear the retina, primarily because of the different rates at which the vitreous and the eye wall change shape. The nonuniform structure of the vitreous and the attachments of the vitreous to the retina dictate where the tears will occur. Thus, the vitreous base, the ribbon of very firm vitreoretinal adhesion extending 1–2 mm in front of and behind the ora, may be disinserted, or the tears may be confined to the retina at the posterior margin of the vitreous base or the nonpigmented epithelium of the pars plana at its anterior margin. Such tears can lead to retinal detachment and usually require treatment.

Trauma may prematurely cause a posterior vitreous detachment, such as normally happens as an aging phenomenon to most people. On detaching, the vitreous may tear the retina at focal vitreoretinal adhesions situated behind the vitreous base. These tears and the associated bleeding into the vitreous are handled the same way as those that occur spontaneously.

Commotio Retinae (Berlin's "Edema")

A blow to the front of the eye can sometimes avulse the outer segments of the retinal receptor cells in a discrete area at the back of the eye. In the following weeks, this debris is phagocytosed by the pigment epithelium. At first, the white subretinal material is easily visible. Eventually, little ophthalmoscopic evidence of it remains other than a localized mild disturbance of the underlying pigment epithelium. There is a permanent scotoma in the affected area. When it includes the macula, the symptoms are distressing. Otherwise, the loss of visual field may go unnoticed.

With involvement of the peripheral retina or the fovea, where the retina and its internal limiting membrane are thinnest, an atrophic retinal hole may later develop at the site of the contrecoup injury (Fig 23–1). Such holes rarely cause a significant retinal detachment.

Fracture of Bruch's Membrane (See Fig 23–2.)

Blunt trauma will sometimes cause one or more easily visible linear fractures of Bruch's membrane, which are usually accompanied by subretinal bleeding. The break may occur anywhere. Those in the posterior pole are curved and are concentric with the optic nerve head. In the course of time, the subretinal blood resorbs, but the pigment epithelium bordering the fracture atrophies over the areas of choriocapillaris supplied by the affected ciliary arterioles. Later still, new vessels may grow into the subretinal space through the breaks in Bruch's membrane (see Disciform Degeneration of the Macula, above).

If they are some distance from the macula, fractures of Bruch's membrane and possible complications are of little consequence to the patient. However, a fracture beneath the fovea usually causes permanent loss of function, though vision sometimes improves when the subretinal blood is resorbed. Late involvement of the macula by a disciform lesion usually causes permanent loss of macular vision. These disciform cases are occasionally helped by photocoagulation.

PENETRATING INJURY

At the time of a penetrating injury, the retina may be directly damaged by the penetrating object or indirectly damaged through traction on the vitreous. The findings are protean and are handled surgically according to the anatomic situation.

Quite often, an injury involving the vitreous will cause late traction on the retina owing either to contraction of fibrous tissue, which grows along the penetration tract, or to the delayed detachment of the vitreous, which was initiated by the injury. In either case, the retina may be distorted or detached and may require surgical intervention.

COLOR VISION & COLOR BLINDNESS

Light may be defined as that portion of the electromagnetic spectrum (400–700 nm) that readily stimulates human retinal receptors. To other species, "light" may encompass a different set of wavelengths.

The cones mediate color vision. In order to be stimulated, they require a greater intensity of light than the rods. Thus, one cannot detect color in moonlight. Each cone has one of 3 distinct spectral sensitivity patterns. These curves are overlapping, with maxima at red, green, or blue. A given light elicits different degrees of response in each type of cone. This generates data which the neural computer interprets as a specific color.

Color is dependent upon hue, saturation, and brightness. Objects appear to have a particular **hue** primarily because they reflect, irradiate, or transmit light of certain wavelengths. The addition of black to a given hue produces the various **shades.**

Saturation is an index of purity of a hue. For example, scarlet is more saturated than pink because pink is made up of red and white mixed together.

Brightness is that aspect of perception most closely related to light intensity.

Color blindness is a misleading term, since most color-blind people have normal visual acuity. According to Marriott, 8% of men and 0.4% of women interpret colors differently than the rest of mankind. They are classified as follows:

(1) Cone monochromats: These individuals have only one type of cone. The incidence is about 1:1,000,000.

(2) Dichromats: Persons having 2 rather than 3 types of cones. They are divided into 3 groups: Protanopes, or red-blind subjects, are insensitive to deep red light. Deuteranopes confuse shades of red, green, and yellow. Tritanopes are blue-blind subjects who confuse blue and green shades and, generally, orange and pink shades.

(3) Anomalous trichromats: This is by far the largest group. Protans have similar but milder defects than occur in protanopia; deutans have similar but milder defects than occur in deuteranopia; and tritans have similar but milder defects than occur in tritanopia.

(4) Rod monochromats: Rod monochromatism is a very rare disorder in which there is complete lack of cone function. It is always associated with photophobia, nystagmus, and poor visual acuity.

The common types of color blindness are inherited as X-linked characteristics. Acquired causes of color blindness include retinal disease and poisoning. In the acquired cases, the patient may be color-blind in only one area of the visual field.

The detection of color blindness is described in Chapter 3. Because of the relationship to choice of occupation, color vision testing should be done early in life (eg, age 8–12). However, the physician must be wary of attributing too much importance to a hereditary anomaly that in its more common milder forms is little more than an occasional social inconvenience.

Treatment is of no value.

•   •   •

References

Brown GC, Magargal LE: Central retinal artery obstruction and visual acuity. *J Am Acad Ophthalmol* 1982;**89**:14.

Byer NE: The natural history of senile retinoschisis. *Trans Am Acad Ophthalmol Otolaryngol* 1976;**81**:459.

Chawla HB: A review of techniques employed in 1100 cases of retinal detachment. *Br J Ophthalmol* 1982;**66**:636.

Cunha-Vas JG et al: A follow-up study by vitreous fluorophotometry of early retinal involvement in diabetics. *Am J Ophthalmol* 1978;**86**:467.

DeLuise VP et al: Syphilitic retinal detachment and uveal effusion. *Am J Ophthalmol* 1982;**94**:757.

Diabetic Retinopathy Study Research Group: Preliminary report on effects of photocoagulation therapy. *Am J Ophthalmol* 1976;**81**:383.

Duke-Elder S, Dobree GH: *System of Ophthalmology.* Vol 10: *Diseases of the Retina.* Mosby, 1967.

Foos RY: Vitreoretinal junction: Topographical variations. *Invest Ophthalmol* 1972;**11**:801.

François J et al: Neovascularization after argon laser photocoagulation of macular lesions. *Am J Ophthalmol* 1975;**79**:206.

Frank KE, Purnell EW: Subretinal neovascularization following rubella retinopathy. *Am J Ophthalmol* 1978;**86**:462.

Galainena MC: Solar retinopathy. *Ann Ophthalmol* 1976;**8**:304.

Gass JDM: *Stereoscopic Atlas of Macular Diseases,* 2nd ed. Mosby, 1977.

Gass JDM: Treatment of retinal vascular abnormalities. *Trans Am Acad Ophthalmol Otolaryngol* 1977;**83**:432.

Haimann MH, Burton TC, Brown MS: Epidemiology of retinal detachment. *Arch Ophthalmol* 1982;**100**:289.

Hamilton AM, Taylor W: Significance of pigment granules in the vitreous. *Br J Ophthalmol* 1972;**56**:700.

Hayreh SS: So-called "central retinal vein occlusion." 2. Venous stasis retinopathy. *Ophthalmologica* 1976;**172**:14.

Heller MD, Straatsma BR, Foos RY: Detachment of the posterior vitreous in phakic and aphakic eyes. *Mod Probl Ophthalmol* 1972;**10**:23.

Hogan MJ, Alvarado JA, Weddell JE: *Histology of the Human Eye.* Saunders, 1971.

Jackson RL et al: Retinopathy in adolescents and young adults with onset of insulin-dependent diabetes in childhood. *J Am Acad Ophthalmol* 1982;**89**:7.

Jaffe NS, Clayman HM, Jaffe MS: Cystoid macular edema after intracapsular and extracapsular cataract extraction with and without an intraocular lens. *J Am Acad Ophthalmol* 1982;**89**:25.

Kalina RE, Karr DJ: Retrolental fibroplasia: Experience over two decades in one institution. *J Am Acad Ophthalmol* 1982;**89**:91.

Kohner EM: Symposium on retinal vascular disease. 1. Morphological, circulatory and histopathologic response to retinal vein occlusion: Pathophysiology of retinal vein occlusion.

Trans Ophthalmol Soc UK 1976;**96**:189.

Kolker AE, Becker B: Epinephrine maculopathy. *Arch Ophthalmol* 1968;**79**:552.

Kreissig I, Lincoff H: Mechanism of retinal attachment after cryosurgery. *Trans Ophthalmol Soc UK* 1975;**95**:148.

Lincoff J, Gieser R: Finding the retinal hole. *Arch Ophthalmol* 1971;**85**:565.

Lyons DE: Conservative management of central serous retinopathy. *Trans Ophthalmol Soc UK* 1977;**97**:214.

Macular Photocoagulation Study Group: Argon laser photocoagulation for senile macular degeneration. *Arch Ophthalmol* 1982;**100**:912.

Mandelcorn MS, Blankenship G, Machemer R: Pars plana vitrectomy for the management of severe diabetic retinopathy. *Am J Ophthalmol* 1976;**81**:561.

Maumenee AE, Emery JM: An anatomic classification of diseases of the macula. *Am J Ophthalmol* 1972;**74**:594.

Merin S, Auerbach E: Review: Retinitis pigmentosa. *Surv Ophthalmol* 1976;**20**:303.

Miami Study Group: Cystoid macular edema in aphakic and pseudophakic eyes. *Am J Ophthalmol* 1979;**88**:45.

Moses RA: *Adler's Physiology of the Eye,* 7th ed. Mosby, 1981.

Norton EWD: The past 25 years of retinal detachment surgery. *Am J Ophthalmol* 1975;**80**:450.

O'Malley P et al: Paving-stone degeneration of the retina. *Arch Ophthalmol* 1965;**73**:169.

Palestine AG, Robertson DM, Goldstein BG: Macroaneurysms of the retinal arteries. *Am J Ophthalmol* 1982;**93**:164.

Patz A: Clinical and experimental studies on retinal neovascularization: The 29th Edward Jackson memorial lecture. *Am J Ophthalmol* 1982;**94**:715.

Patz A et al: Diseases of the macula: Diagnosis and management of choroidal neovascularization. *Trans Am Acad Ophthalmol Otolaryngol* 1977;**83**:468.

Schlagel TF Jr: The presumed ocular histoplasmosis syndrome. Pages 720–731 in: *Controversy in Ophthalmology.* Brockhurst RJ et al (editors). Saunders, 1977.

Sipperly JO, Quigley HA, Gass JD: Explanation of commotio retinae: Traumatic retinopathy in primates. *Arch Ophthalmol* 1978;**96**:2267.

Straatsma BR et al: Lattice degeneration of retina: The 30th Edward Jackson memorial lecture. *Trans Am Acad Ophthalmol Otolaryngol* 1974;**78**:87.

Tasman W: Retina and optic nerve: Annual review. *Arch Ophthalmol* 1976;**94**:1201.

Verdaguer J: Juvenile retinal detachment. *Am J Ophthalmol* 1982;**93**:145.

Virdi PS, Hayreh SS: Ocular neovascularization with retinal vascular occlusion. *Arch Ophthalmol* 1982;**100**:331.

Zinn KM, Marmor MF (editors): *The Retinal Pigment Epithelium.* Harvard Univ Press, 1979.

14 | Glaucoma

Glaucoma includes a complex of disease entities that have in common an increase in intraocular pressure sufficient to cause degeneration of the optic disk and defects in the visual field. An estimated 50,000 persons in the USA are blind as a result of glaucoma. The incidence of glaucoma in unselected persons over age 40 is about 1.5%.

The chief threat of chronic (open-angle) glaucoma is insidious visual impairment. The degree of interference with vision varies from slight blurring to complete blindness. The disease is bilateral and is genetically determined, probably by multifactorial or polygenic inheritance. Infantile glaucoma usually has an autosomal recessive mode of inheritance, whereas some specific glaucoma syndromes are transmitted as autosomal dominant diseases. Acute glaucoma (angle-closure glaucoma) comprises less than 5% of primary glaucoma cases.

In most cases, blindness can be prevented if treatment is instituted early. The objective of therapy is to facilitate the outflow of aqueous through existing drainage channels by the use of miotics and in some cases to inhibit the secretion of aqueous by the ciliary processes, using systemically and topically administered drugs. The most commonly used miotic is pilocarpine. The most commonly used secretory suppressants are epinephrine and timolol maleate, which are applied topically, and acetazolamide, which is given orally. Operative treatment is sometimes indicated in the later stages when medical management is no longer sufficient to control the intraocular pressure.

The management of glaucoma is best left to the ophthalmologist, but all physicians should participate in the diagnosis by making ophthalmoscopy and tonometry a part of the routine physical examination of all patients old enough to cooperate. This is especially important in patients with a family history of glaucoma. The physician should learn to recognize optic nerve changes associated with glaucoma as seen with the ophthalmoscope. Doubtful cases should be referred to an ophthalmologist for confirmation and management.

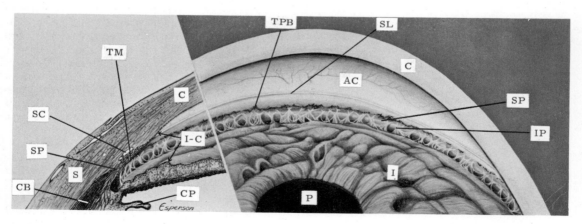

AC = anterior chamber	I = iris	S = sclera	TM = trabecular meshwork
C = cornea	I-C = iris-corneal angle	SC = Schlemm's canal	TPB = trabecular pigment band
CB = ciliary body	IP = iris processes	SL = Schwalbe's line	
CP = ciliary process	P = pupil	SP = scleral spur	

Figure 14–1. Composite illustration showing anatomic *(left)* and gonioscopic *(right)* view of normal anterior chamber angle. (Courtesy of R Shaffer.)

Classification

A generally accepted classification of glaucoma is as follows:

A. Primary Glaucoma:

1. **Open-angle glaucoma**–Also called simple glaucoma, chronic simple glaucoma. The most common form.
2. **Angle-closure glaucoma**–Also called narrow-angle glaucoma, closed-angle glaucoma.
   a. Acute.
   b. Subacute or chronic.
   c. Plateau iris.

B. Congenital Glaucoma:

1. **Primary congenital glaucoma, infantile glaucoma, trabeculodysgenesis.**
2. **Glaucoma associated with congenital anomalies**–
   a. Pigmentary glaucoma.
   b. Aniridia.
   c. Axenfeld's syndrome.
   d. Sturge-Weber syndrome.
   e. Infantile glaucoma developing late.
   f. Marfan's syndrome.
   g. Neurofibromatosis.
   h. Lowe's syndrome.
   i. Microcornea and megalocornea.

C. Secondary Glaucoma:

1. **Due to changes of the lens**–
   a. Dislocation.
   b. Intumescence.
   c. Phacolytic.
   d. Exfoliative syndrome (pseudoexfoliation of lens capsule, glaucoma capsulare).
2. **Due to changes of the uveal tract**–
   a. Peripheral anterior synechiae (PAS) (angle closure without pupillary block).
   b. Iridocyclitis.
   c. Tumor.
   d. Essential iris atrophy (iridocorneoendothelial [ICE] syndrome).
3. **Due to trauma**–
   a. Massive hemorrhage into the anterior chamber.
   b. Massive hemorrhage into the posterior chamber.
   c. Corneal or limbal laceration with iris prolapse into the wound.
   d. Retrodisplacement of iris root following contusion (angle recession).
4. **Following surgical procedures**–
   a. Epithelial ingrowth into the anterior chamber.
   b. Failure of prompt restoration of the anterior chamber following cataract extraction.
5. **Associated with rubeosis** (diabetes mellitus and central retinal vessel occlusion).
6. **Associated with pulsating exophthalmos.**
7. **Associated with topical corticosteroids.**
8. **Other rare causes** of secondary glaucoma.

D. Absolute Glaucoma: The end result of any uncontrolled glaucoma is a hard, sightless, and often painful eye.

PHYSIOLOGY OF GLAUCOMA

Aqueous Humor

The intraocular pressure is determined by the rate of aqueous production by the ciliary body epithelium and the resistance to outflow of aqueous from the eye. Some knowledge of the physiology of aqueous is necessary to an understanding of glaucoma.

A. Composition of Aqueous: The aqueous is a clear liquid that fills the anterior and posterior chambers of the eye. Its volume is about 125 μL. The osmotic pressure of aqueous is slightly higher than that of plasma. The total protein content is 0.02%. The albumin-globulin ratio is the same as that of blood serum (2:1). In general, the same electrolytes and other components are found in the aqueous as in plasma, although the concentrations differ.

Intraocular inflammation and surgical or traumatic emptying of the anterior chamber cause the formation of plasmoid aqueous, which closely resembles blood serum and has a much higher protein concentration than normal aqueous.

B. Formation and Flow of Aqueous: A great deal is known about the dynamics of aqueous humor, but the exact mechanism of production and elimination of aqueous is not completely understood. Water, electrolytes, and nonelectrolytes enter and leave the eye at varying rates. Water enters both by diffusion from the ciliary body and by secretion from the epithelium of the ciliary processes. From the posterior chamber the fluid passes through the pupil into the anterior chamber. The flow in the anterior chamber is peripheral, toward the filtering trabecular meshwork and into Schlemm's canal. Efferent channels from Schlemm's canal (about 30 collector channels and about 12 aqueous veins) conduct the fluid into the venous system. There is also a constant exchange of nonelectrolytes as well as a major exchange of water in and out of the iris stroma. A small amount of aqueous leaves the eye through the uveal vessels and the sclera.

Pressure Dynamics*

Intraocular pressure is such an important feature of glaucoma that a review of pressure dynamics is desirable.

A. Blood Flow: If blood were a newtonian fluid (like water), the rate of flow into the eye would be in direct proportion to the difference of blood pressure at the entrance of the eye and the intraocular pressure. When intraocular pressure equals blood pressure, there

---

*This section on pressure dynamics by Dr Orson White comprises important new information that should be carefully studied by all persons interested in the pathophysiology of glaucoma.

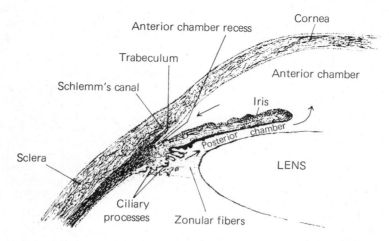

Figure 14–2. Anterior segment structures. Arrows indicate direction of flow of aqueous.

would be no flow. However, blood is not a newtonian fluid, probably because it contains corpuscles. Blood does not flow through capillaries until the pressure head is about 15 mm Hg, and at that level of pressure the flow should be linear with the difference of blood pressure and intraocular pressure. For example, if blood pressure at the entrance of the eye is 40 mm Hg, subtract 15 mm Hg for the "nonnewtonian factor" and 15 mm Hg for the intraocular pressure, leaving only a 10-mm Hg pressure head to supply the eye. It is thus easy to see that a small increase in intraocular pressure may cause a large decrease in blood flow.

B. Pressure-Tension-Strain Relationships: The terms "pressure," "tension," and "strain" are frequently used interchangeably and are defined as synonyms in some dictionaries. However, the precise distinctions between these related but different terms must be appreciated before pressure dynamics in glaucoma can be understood.

1. Pressure–Hydrostatic pressure is the force per unit area exerted by a fluid (gas or liquid). The force is exerted at a right angle (normal) to the surface subjected to the pressure. Compressing air in a blocked syringe is a good example of pressure. Hydrostatic pressure per se causes no damage. Using diving apparatus, one may rest on an ocean bottom 140 ft deep with no discomfort. At this depth, the total force being exerted on the body is about 9000 kg (10 tons).

The unit of pressure in the International System of Units (SI) is the pascal (Pa), which is 1 newton per square meter (N/m²). To convert mm Hg to kilopascals (kPa), divide mm Hg by 7.5. However, for calculation of pressure within the eye, it is helpful to convert mm Hg to g/cm². Multiply mm Hg by 1.36 to obtain g/cm².

2. Tension (tensile stress)–A jack supporting a car is subjected to *compressive stress*. A towline pulling a car is subjected to *tensile stress* or tension. Stresses are assigned a magnitude of force per unit area. In the case of the eye, the pressure force vector acts at a right angle to the scleral wall, whereas the tensile stress or tension force vector acts parallel to the

scleral wall (attempting to pull the sclera apart).

Trampolines and drumheads are examples of pure tension without pressure. The pressure is the same on either side of the tensed membrane. The tensions in the sclera, cornea, and lamina cribrosa are not the same but are related to the intraocular pressure, very nearly by the expression used for thin-walled spheres. The eye does not satisfy the criteria for definition of thin-walled spheres. A thin-walled sphere is one in which the tension in the wall is directly proportionate to the contained pressure multiplied by the radius of curvature and inversely proportionate to twice the thickness of the wall:

$$\text{Tension} = \frac{\text{Pressure} \times \text{Radius}}{2 \times \text{Thickness}}$$

An inflated surgical glove or balloon illustrates this relationship. The "palm" of the glove has relatively *high tension* and the tip of the "thumb" has relatively *low tension,* though the *pressure* within the glove is equal at all locations. The "thumb" has low tension, because the radius of curvature is small and the thickness is large relative to the same factors at the "palm." In the case of the eye, the tension is lower in the cornea or optic cup than in the sclera. Rupture of an eye resulting from high pressure occurs beneath the lateral rectus, as the relationship would suggest. The 140 ft used in the pressure example above was chosen because this is about the intraocular pressure which results, via tension and strain, in rupture of the eye.

3. Strain–Strain is stretch or displacement per unit length. A strain gauge measures displacement. Strain can result in damage, and in the body both pain and damage. Depending on the circumstances, one of 3 moduli of elasticity is used to determine strain or stretch in structures resulting from a given pressure or tension. Thomas Young (1773–1829), a physician, clarified these complex relationships. The modulus used for elasticity of cables, pressure vessels, submarines, etc *(and eyes)* is named in his honor. Young's modulus, *E,* is the tension required to stretch a material of unit cross section to double its length. Thus, the stretch of the sclera per unit length (strain) is given by the change in tension of the sclera divided by "Young's modulus of the sclera," *E*. (See discussion of tension regarding the relationship of intraocular pressure to tension.) Young's modulus is the proper one to use when considering elastic properties of the eye.

$$E = \frac{\Delta \text{ Tension}}{\Delta \text{ Length sclera per unit length}}$$

The second modulus is shear modulus, *G*, used for drive shafts, bolts, etc, and should not concern us in the discussion of elasticity of the eye. It is sometimes called the modulus of rigidity. The incorrect term "scleral rigidity" may have been derived from shear modulus (the wrong one).

The third modulus is bulk modulus, *K*, and should not concern us in elasticity of the eye except that it is wrongly used in most of the ophthalmologic literature at the present time. Bulk modulus is the hydrostatic force (compressive stress) required to compress (strain) a solid material to half its volume:

$$K = \frac{\text{Pressure}_2 - \text{Pressure}_1}{\Delta \text{ Volume per unit volume}}$$

The expression presently used in glaucoma literature for "scleral rigidity," *E* or *K*, was derived empirically and is

$$E = \frac{\text{Log pressure}_2 - \text{Log pressure}_1}{\Delta \text{ Volume}}$$

This "scleral rigidity" equation has some resemblance to the bulk modulus equation in that it depends on pressure change (as opposed to tension change in Young's modulus) and change in volume (as opposed to strain or stretch per unit length in Young's modulus). The difference of the "scleral rigidity" equation from the bulk modulus equation is the use of logarithm pressures and absolute volume change as opposed to volume change per unit volume. Bulk modulus would be valid only if the eye were solid sclera and were subjected to external hydrostatic pressure. The eye is nearly a spherical shell of sclera filled with a fluid under pressure and therefore qualifies, as do other pressure vessels, *only* for Young's modulus. It is apparent that the term "scleral rigidity" is not based on sound physical principles. Thus, one may appreciate that at present elasticity of the eye is one of the most confused areas of ophthalmology.

C. Local Exceptions to the Mathematical Theory of Elasticity: The tension and strain exerted on areas of discontinuity such as the optic disk are not easy to calculate. These relationships can be studied by various methods of photoelasticity on models or on actual eyes.

D. Biological Exceptions to the Mathematical Theory of Elasticity: Living tissue reacts like nonliv-

ing materials to brief changes in tensions and strains. However, long-term tensions and strains have a unique effect on living tissue, causing changes in growth, shape, and strength. This is the basis of the "orthodontic shift" of teeth and of the head, face, foot, and other deformations practiced at one time by some cultures. The cupping of the disk may be a similar response to long-term tension and strain. *Nerve damage in glaucoma is not directly due to intraocular pressure but may be due to deformation from long-term tension-strain effects.*

SPECIAL DIAGNOSTIC TECHNIQUES
(See also Chapter 3.)

A number of special diagnostic tests have been developed to help detect, classify, and follow the course of glaucoma.

Tonometry
This is an important test in establishing the diagnosis of glaucoma since it measures the intraocular pressure. A single normal reading either with the Schiotz or applanation tonometer does not rule out glaucoma, however, as the intraocular pressures may vary within wide limits. A single "high normal" reading (24–32 mm Hg) is suggestive of glaucoma but always requires repeated testing before a definite diagnosis can be made.

Gonioscopy
Visualization of the anterior chamber angle differentiates angle-closure from open-angle glaucoma, demonstrates the extent of peripheral anterior synechiae, and offers the only means of detecting an impending angle closure before there is any rise in intraocular pressure. It is an essential part of any glaucoma evaluation.

Ophthalmoscopy
Direct visualization of the optic disk is the single most important test in diagnosing glaucoma and evaluating the response to treatment. A patient with elevated intraocular pressure (eg, 32 mm Hg) and normal-appearing optic disks may not require active treatment but only periodic examinations.

Provocative Tests
A. Open-Angle Glaucoma: Provocative tests are not helpful in predicting what pressure level will damage the individual patient's optic nerve, which is the important consideration. Therefore, provocative tests are of little help in open-angle glaucoma.

B. Narrow-Angle Glaucoma:

1. Dark room test of Seidel–The patient sits in a dark room for 1 hour without going to sleep. A rise in intraocular pressure of more than 8 mm indicates that iris blockage is impeding outflow when the pupil is relatively dilated. Positive results must be confirmed

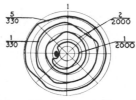

Baring of the blind spot. The earliest nerve fiber bundle defect.

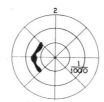

Incipient double nerve fiber bundle defect (Bjerrum scotoma).

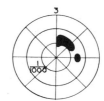

Bjerrum scotoma isolated from blind spot.

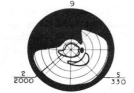

End stages in glaucoma field loss. Remnant of central field still shows nasal step.

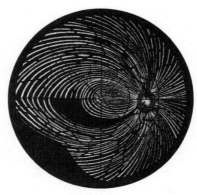

The basic visual field loss in glaucoma is the nerve fiber bundle defect with nasal step and peripheral nasal depression. It is here shown superimposed upon the nerve fiber layer of the retina and the retinal vascular tree. All perimetric changes in glaucoma are variations of these fundamental defects.

Fully developed nerve fiber bundle defect with nasal step (arcuate scotoma).

Peripheral depression with double nerve fiber bundle defect. Isolation of central field.

Double arcuate scotoma with peripheral breakthrough and nasal step.

Nasal depression connected with arcuate scotoma. Nasal step of Rönne.

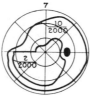

Peripheral breakthrough of large nerve fiber bundle defect with well developed nasal step.

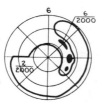

Seidel scotoma. Islands of greater visual loss within a nerve fiber bundle defect.

Figure 14–3. Visual field changes in glaucoma. (Reproduced, with permission, from Harrington DO: *The Visual Fields: A Textbook and Atlas of Clinical Perimetry,* 5th ed. Mosby, 1981.)

by gonioscopic evidence of angle closure. A negative result does not rule out a future attack of angle-closure glaucoma.

2. Prone position test–If a patient lies in a prone position and the intraocular pressure rises 8–10 mm Hg, this may indicate angle-closure glaucoma. As with test 1 (above), gonioscopy is necessary to confirm the angle closure if the pressure rises. This may be used in conjunction with the dark room test.

Visual Fields in Glaucoma

The visual field test is most important in detecting open-angle glaucoma and in following the course of visual deterioration caused by the disease. The tangent screen, the Goldmann perimeter, and various automated perimeters give important information. Small extensions of the blind spot or early nerve fiber bundle defects not necessarily connected to the blind spot are noted early in the disease. Ideally, the diagnosis is made before visual field loss occurs. Under these circumstances, medical control can usually prevent significant visual loss.

The nerve fibers are arranged in the retina as indicated in Fig 14–3. Increased intraocular pressure at the nerve head will gradually destroy the function of a bundle of these fibers, and the resulting visual field defect is spoken of as a "nerve fiber bundle defect." As the nerve fiber bundle defect enlarges, it takes an arcuate shape from the blind spot encircling the fixation area. It arches into either the superior or inferior field and ends at the horizontal meridian (Bjerrum scotoma). A double arcuate scotoma (one in the superior and one in the inferior field) forms a full-ring scotoma around the central fixation area.

Loss of peripheral field occurs later in the course of the disease. The nasal and superior fields are usually lost first. The last remnant of the visual field is usually a temporal island.

The field of vision may slowly contract in some cases down to 5 degrees from fixation, leaving the patient with good central vision but no peripheral vision. Central visual acuity, therefore, is not a reliable index of the progress of the disease. There is no substitute for careful periodic study of the visual field, applanation tonometry, and, most importantly, ophthalmoscopic visualization of the optic disks.

OPEN-ANGLE GLAUCOMA

At least 90% of cases of primary glaucoma are of the open-angle type. Open-angle glaucoma is bilateral, insidious in onset, and slowly progressive. There are no symptoms until visual impairment occurs, often too late to salvage useful vision. It is therefore the physician's responsibility to diagnose glaucoma before irreversible optic nerve damage has occurred. Early treatment prevents or delays visual deterioration.

Significant advances in the understanding of the course of open-angle glaucoma have been made in recent years, but unsolved problems remain and there

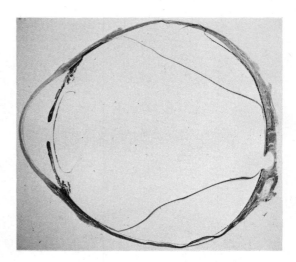

Figure 14–4. Cross section of an eye with open-angle glaucoma. Note open anterior chamber angle (peripheral iris is not in contact with the posterior corneal surface). Deep glaucomatous cupping ("bean-pot" appearance) shows the process to be well advanced. (Courtesy of R Carriker.)

are still differences of opinion among authorities on some issues. It now seems certain that increased intraocular pressure is caused by interference with aqueous outflow due to degenerative changes in the trabeculum, Schlemm's canal, and adjacent channels (see below). Increased pressure, whether caused by obstructed outflow or increased production of aqueous, affects primarily the retina and optic nerve, the functional elements of the eye.

Some authorities feel that in open-angle glaucoma there is also a primary degenerative disorder of the optic nerve due to vascular insufficiency. This view is supported by the observation that loss of function sometimes continues to progress even after the intraocular pressure has been normalized by miotic therapy or surgery. Also, patients with systemic disease (eg, diabetes, arteriosclerosis) are more likely than others to suffer optic nerve damage as a result of ocular hypertension.

There are few detectable histologic changes in the early stages. Nonspecific changes common to all forms of primary glaucoma occur in later stages. Studies of early open-angle glaucoma reveal primary degeneration in the trabecular meshwork, degeneration of the collagen and elastic fibers of the trabeculum, and endothelial proliferation and edema. The trabecular spaces tend to be obliterated. The collector channels also undergo degenerative changes.

If the pressure remains elevated, gross damage to the eye occurs. The optic nerve undergoes degeneration, often assuming a typical bean-pot cupping appearance (Fig 14–5). There is degeneration of ganglion cells and nerve fibers in the retina. The iris and ciliary body become atrophic, and the ciliary processes show hyaline degeneration.

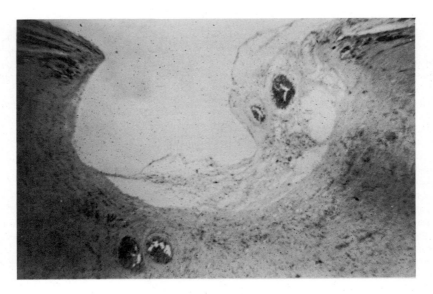

Figure 14–5. Glaucomatous ("bean-pot") cupping of the optic disk.

Genetic aspects. Open-angle glaucoma is a familial, genetically determined disorder, probably multifactorial or polygenic in origin. In any case, family history and routine systematic testing of relatives are most important in glaucoma detection.

Clinical Findings

Open-angle glaucoma causes no early symptoms. Subjective visual loss is nearly always a late finding. Although the disease is nearly always bilateral, one eye is frequently involved earlier and more severely than the other.

Optic disk changes are the most important early findings. The temporal disk margin thins (Fig 14–6)

and the cup gradually becomes wider and deeper. The large vessels become nasally displaced, and the affected area of the disk becomes atrophic (light gray or white rather than pink). The lamina cribrosa becomes more exposed.

The intraocular pressure is increased. The anterior chamber angle may be normal on gonioscopy. The loss of visual function from glaucoma can best be determined by repeated studies of the visual fields, preferably using a Goldmann type perimeter.

Treatment

A. Medical Treatment: Miotics facilitate aqueous outflow by increasing the efficiency of the outflow channels. The exact mechanism of their effect is not understood. The drug of choice is pilocarpine, 1–4%, instilled in each eye up to 5 times daily. Carbachol, 0.75–3%, may be effective when pilocarpine fails or in patients who are allergic to pilocarpine. These are cholinergic drugs.

Anticholinesterase drugs are the longest-acting miotics available. These include demecarium bromide (Humorsol), 0.06–0.25%, and echothiophate (Phospholine) iodide, 0.03–0.25%. These drugs are primarily useful in aphakic glaucoma. *Caution:* These drugs should not be used in the presence of a narrow anterior chamber angle or in chronic angle-closure glaucomas since the extreme miosis increases relative pupillary block and can lead to angle closure. They also have cataractogenic properties and therefore should be avoided, if possible, in the phakic eye. They may cause iritis, bleeding, and excessive conjunctival scarring if used before surgery. Also, systemic effects have been noted in children who receive succinylcholine during anesthesia. Because of their high complication rate, their use is generally reserved for patients with open-angle glaucoma who are not good surgical candi-

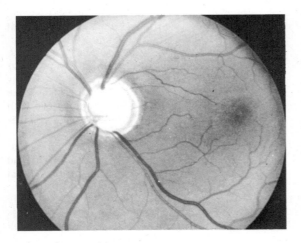

Figure 14–6. Typical glaucomatous cupping. Note the nasal displacement of the vessels and hollowed-out appearance of the optic disk except for a thin border. (Courtesy of S Mettier Jr.)

dates or who are aphakic.

Miotics frequently cause dimness of vision for 1–2 hours after instillation due to pupillary constriction, and younger glaucoma patients often have accommodative spasm with induced myopia.

Epinephrine, 0.5–2% instilled 1–2 times daily, decreases aqueous production and increases aqueous outflow. No miosis or myopia is induced, and it has a longer action than the miotics. For these reasons, epinephrine is often used as the primary drug in open-angle glaucoma (do not use in narrow angle eyes), with miotics and carbonic anhydrase inhibitors added later as necessary to lower the intraocular pressure.

Epinephrine instilled once or twice daily dramatically reduces the intraocular pressure in selected cases of aphakic glaucoma. Watch for macular edema as a complication.

Timolol maleate (Timoptic), a beta-adrenergic blocking agent with few side-effects, lowers intraocular pressure by decreasing aqueous production. It is available in 2 strengths, 0.25% and 0.5%, for use as eye drops instilled twice daily. Timolol can be used alone or in combination with other drugs. This drug has been used worldwide for over 5 years and continues to gain acceptance. It should be used with great caution in patients who have asthma or who are taking oral beta-adrenergic blocking agents.

Carbonic anhydrase inhibitors such as acetazolamide (Diamox), 125–250 mg 4 times daily, are used in open-angle glaucoma if strong antiglaucoma solutions do not adequately control intraocular pressure. Dichlorphenamide (Daranide), methazolamide (Neptazane), and ethoxzolamide (Cardrase, Ethamide) are similarly effective carbonic anhydrase inhibitors and, like acetazolamide, usually suppress aqueous production from 40 to 60%. Complications of long-term therapy with carbonic anhydrase inhibitors include renal calculi (see also p 374). Nevertheless, these drugs are indicated to avoid glaucoma surgery.

B. Laser Trabeculoplasty: Treatment of the trabecular meshwork by laser energy will reduce intraocular pressure by almost 25% in 80% of patients. It can be used as an adjunct to medical therapy before resorting to surgery. Its long-term effect has not yet been assessed.

C. Surgical Treatment: (See p 172.) Surgery for open-angle glaucoma may be performed if the intraocular pressure is not maintained within normal limits by medical therapy and there is progressive visual field loss associated with optic nerve damage. There is no operation that can be called uniformly successful in the treatment of open-angle glaucoma. Standard filtration procedures such as trephine, sclerectomy, and thermal sclerostomy all have their advocates. Trabeculectomy and other forms of filtering procedures beneath a scleral flap have recently become popular. This is not because they are more effective but because they have a lower complication rate, since the anterior chamber remains formed following the procedure. Cataract formation does not occur as rapidly or as frequently following these latter procedures as it did with standard filtering operations.

If a cataract is present that should be extracted, this alone will help control the glaucoma in a large percentage of cases. If the glaucoma is difficult to control or is uncontrolled prior to extraction, the cataract operation and glaucoma surgery may be done simultaneously. The success rate of glaucoma surgery in the aphakic patient is approximately 60%. If medical therapy fails, however, subscleral filtration procedures may be used. Some authorities still use cyclodialysis.

In patients under 40 years of age, filtration surgery of any type has a low success rate. Standard filtering techniques are somewhat mutilating to the eye. The external trabeculotomy is somewhat more successful in these patients and is less mutilating. In general, surgery is recommended in open-angle glaucoma only when maximum medical therapy has failed to halt the progression of visual field and optic nerve deterioration.

Course & Prognosis

Without treatment, open-angle glaucoma may be insidiously progressive to complete blindness. If antiglaucoma drops control the intraocular pressure in an eye that has not suffered extensive glaucomatous damage, the prognosis is good (although visual field loss sometimes continues to progress in spite of normalized intraocular pressure). When the process is detected early, most glaucoma patients can be successfully managed medically.

LOW PRESSURE GLAUCOMA

This term denotes a number of conditions in which there is evidence of intraocular glaucomatous damage (cupping of the optic disk, visual field defects, etc) with normal or low intraocular pressure. Most such cases can be classified in the following groups:

(1) Cases of open-angle glaucoma in which Schiotz tonometry shows falsely low intraocular pressure. The truly elevated intraocular pressure is determined by use of the applanation tonometer (see Chapter 3). These cases are being recognized with increasing frequency as applanation tonometry becomes more widely used in glaucoma evaluation.

(2) Cases in which some type of glaucoma, usually secondary, has caused permanent changes and then regressed spontaneously. Tonography may reveal a diminished facility of outflow.

(3) Diurnal variation: The pressure is usually normal when taken but is elevated at other times. This may be due to diurnal variation, so that if the pressure is measured at the same time of day it seems normal. Diurnal pressure curves disclose the real diagnosis.

(4) A variety of miscellaneous cases of damage to the optic nerve and retina due to vascular, congenital, degenerative, and other causes. Some of these are

apparently due to reduced blood pressure and blood flow to the optic nerve or perhaps to an easily distorted lamina cribrosa.

ANGLE-CLOSURE GLAUCOMA
(Acute Glaucoma)

Angle-closure glaucoma occurs when there is a sudden increase in the intraocular pressure due to a block of the anterior chamber angle by the root of the iris, which cuts off all aqueous outflow, causing severe pain and sudden visual loss.

An acute attack of angle-closure glaucoma can develop only in an eye in which the anterior chamber angle is anatomically narrow. The following factors may cause further encroachment upon the anterior chamber angle, setting the stage for angle-closure glaucoma.

(1) Physiologic pupillary block: When the anterior chamber angle is narrow, the iris has a relatively large arc of contact with the anterior surface of the lens. This may obstruct the free passage of aqueous from the posterior to the anterior chamber. As pressure builds up in the posterior chamber, the peripheral iris is pushed forward (iris bombé). If the iris is pushed forward far enough so that it lies against the trabeculum, aqueous humor drainage is impeded, resulting in acute angle-closure glaucoma.

(2) Increased size of the lens: Normally, the lens continues to enlarge slightly with age. During the act of accommodation there may be a further increase in the forward displacement of the lens, increasing the relative pupillary block.

Precipitating Factors

A sudden increase in the volume of the posterior chamber may push the iris forward against the trabeculum. This results from hemorrhage, conges-tion, or edema of the iris, ciliary body, or choroid.

Therapeutic or physiologic mydriasis in an eye with a narrow anterior chamber angle occasionally bunches the iris into the chamber angle sufficiently to precipitate an acute attack of angle-closure glaucoma. If the central anterior chamber of such an eye is of moderate depth, the diagnosis is **plateau iris. *Caution:*** Dilation of the pupil should be avoided if the anterior chamber is shallow. This is easily determined by oblique illumination of the anterior segment of the eye (Fig 14–7).

An eye that is predisposed to acute angle-closure glaucoma has a shallow anterior chamber. Otherwise the eye is normal, with complete permeability of the trabeculum, Schlemm's canal, and the aqueous veins. A rapid increase in intraocular pressure occurs when the peripheral iris is forced against the trabeculum, obstructing drainage into the outflow channels.

"Angle-closure kit." Patients with normal intraocular pressure and narrow anterior chamber angles and no history of symptoms referable to glaucoma should be warned about the symptoms of angle-closure glaucoma and what to do if they should suddenly occur. For some patients, it may be wise to provide a simple "angle-closure kit" consisting of pilocarpine, 2% solution, 15 mL; 30 tablets of 250 mg acetazolamide; glycerin (glycerol), 50% solution, 180 mL; and directions for use in case an attack of acute angle-closure glaucoma occurs when the patient is traveling, on vacation, or otherwise unable to secure the services of an ophthalmologist. Having the angle-closure kit available is doubly beneficial to these patients in that it relieves their anxiety and provides a source of immediate treatment when an attack occurs. A newer optional treatment for these patients is preventive laser iridectomy.

Pathology

The pathologic changes in acute glaucoma in-

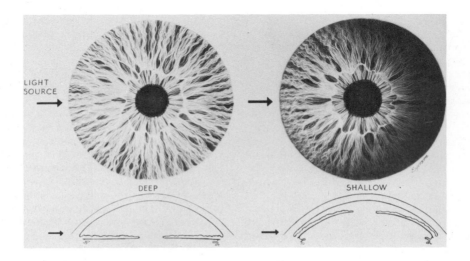

Figure 14–7. Estimation of depth of anterior chamber by oblique illumination (diagram). (Courtesy of R Shaffer.)

clude peripheral anterior synechiae and edema and congestion of the ciliary processes and iris. These are secondary to the vascular strangulation that results from the high pressure. Late changes are the result of interference with circulation and the continued high pressure. The iris and ciliary body become atrophic, and the ciliary processes show hyaline degeneration. Chronic edema of the cornea results in loosening of the corneal epithelium and the formation of epithelial bullae (bullous keratopathy). The most important pathologic change is damage to the nerve elements: degeneration of nerve fibers and a loss of substance of the optic cup associated with a backward bowing of the cribriform plate. The ganglion cell layer and the nerve fiber layer of the retina undergo degeneration. Eventually the lens may show cataractous change.

Clinical Findings

Angle-closure (acute) glaucoma is characterized by a sudden onset of blurred vision followed by excruciating pain, and a rainbow-colored halo is seen around lights. Nausea and vomiting are often present. The pain is usually localized in and around the eye. Other findings include markedly increased intraocular pressure, a shallow anterior chamber, an edematous cornea, decreased visual acuity (at times limited to light perception only), a fixed, moderately dilated pupil, and ciliary injection.

Differential Diagnosis

Acute iritis and conjunctivitis must be considered with acute angle-closure glaucoma in the differential diagnosis of any acutely inflamed eye. (1) Acute iritis causes more photophobia and less pain than acute glaucoma. Intraocular pressure may be normal, the pupil is constricted, and the cornea is not edematous. Marked flare and cells are present in the anterior chamber, and there is deep ciliary injection. (2) In acute conjunctivitis there is little or no pain and no visual loss. There is discharge from the eye and an intensely inflamed conjunctiva, but no ciliary injection. The pupillary responses are normal, the cornea is clear, and intraocular pressure is normal. (3) Iridocyclitis with secondary glaucoma occasionally presents a difficult problem of differentiation. Gonioscopy to define the type of angle is most helpful. If corneal or anterior chamber haze prevents good visibility, gonioscopy of the other eye will usually confirm the diagnosis.

Complications & Sequelae

A. Formation of Peripheral Anterior Synechiae: The peripheral iris adheres to the trabecular meshwork and blocks the outflow of aqueous.

B. Cataract Formation: The lens sometimes swells, and a cataract may develop. The enlarged lens pushes the iris even farther anteriorly; this increases the pupillary block, which in turn increases the degree of angle block.

C. Atrophy of the Retina and Optic Nerve: The nerve elements of the eye withstand increased in-

traocular pressure poorly. Glaucomatous cupping of the optic disk and retinal atrophy, particularly of the ganglion cell layer, occur.

D. Absolute Glaucoma: The end result of uncontrolled angle-closure glaucoma is absolute glaucoma. The eye is stony hard, sightless, and often quite painful, in which case enucleation or retrobulbar alcohol injection is necessary.

Prevention

Miotics may prevent attacks of acute glaucoma indefinitely in predisposed individuals.

Treatment

Angle-closure glaucoma is an ophthalmic surgical emergency.

A. Medical Treatment: Before surgery, every effort must be made to reduce the intraocular pressure by medical means. Osmotic agents, miotics, and acetazolamide are usually required. The immediate administration of oral glycerin (glycerol), 1 mL/kg of body weight in a cold 50% solution mixed with chilled lemon juice, nearly always interrupts the acute attack by making the blood hypertonic and drawing fluid from the eye. Pilocarpine, 4%, 2 drops every 15 minutes for several hours, will usually constrict the pupil and pull the iris away from the trabeculum, allowing aqueous outflow to be reestablished (unless permanent adhesions have formed).

If treatment with glycerin is not successful or if the patient is nauseated, intravenous hypertonic mannitol (20%) may be effective in total doses of 1.5–3 g/kg. Acetazolamide, 500 mg given intramuscularly if the patient is nauseated, will further reduce intraocular pressure by decreasing aqueous production.

Meperidine, 100 mg intramuscularly, or other systemic analgesic should be given as necessary to relieve pain.

B. Surgical Treatment: (See p 172.) In general, if the pressure has not begun to recede within 4–6 hours of medical treatment as outlined above, operation is mandatory. In recent years, surgical peripheral iridectomy has been replaced by laser iridectomy.

SUBACUTE OR CHRONIC ANGLE-CLOSURE GLAUCOMA

Chronic angle-closure glaucoma is caused by the same etiologic factors as acute angle-closure glaucoma. The difference is that there is no sudden complete block to aqueous outflow by the iris being pushed against the trabeculum. The iris extends its arc of contact with the trabeculum gradually until an adequate area of angle is no longer available for aqueous outflow. The pressure rises and glaucoma results that may be clinically similar to open-angle glaucoma.

Clinical Findings

Symptoms are minimal or absent. Occasional mild attacks of increased intraocular pressure cause transient blurring of vision, halos around lights, and possibly slight pain in or about the eyes. On examination, one finds a shallow anterior chamber, high intraocular pressure (25–50 mm Hg), and a partially closed chamber angle as seen on gonioscopic examination. The iris is in apposition to the trabeculum except in an area covering one-fifth or less of the chamber angle.

Complications & Sequelae
A. Acute Attack: If the last open segment of the chamber angle is suddenly blocked, a full-blown attack of glaucoma is the inevitable result. Untreated cases that escape an acute attack undergo slow degeneration much like that which occurs in open-angle glaucoma. The end result is absolute glaucoma: a sightless, stony hard, and often painful eye.

B. Ciliary Block Glaucoma (Malignant Glaucoma): Surgery upon an eye with markedly increased intraocular pressure and a closed angle can lead to ciliary block glaucoma. Immediately after surgery, the intraocular pressure increases markedly and the lens-iris diaphragm is pushed forward as a result of the collection of aqueous in and behind the vitreous body.

Treatment consists of cycloplegics, mydriatics, and hyperosmotic agents. Atropine, 2–4%, should be used topically every 2 hours for the first day and may need to be continued indefinitely on a daily basis therafter. Phenylephrine, 10%, is used 4 times a day. Hyperosmotic agents are used to shrink the vitreous body and let the lens-iris diaphragm fall posteriorly.

C. Other: These include cataract and atrophy of the optic nerve and retina as described for acute angle-closure glaucoma.

Treatment
A. Medical Treatment: Pilocarpine, 1–4%, or carbachol, 0.75–3%, 1 drop in the affected eye 5 times daily as necessary, may reduce the base pressure and prevent transient rises in intraocular pressure.

B. Surgical Treatment: Once the diagnosis of chronic angle-closure glaucoma has been made, an operation is indicated. Peripheral iridectomy (see p 172) may allow the iris to fall away from the posterior corneal surface if the iris is not permanently adherent to the trabeculum. This also relieves whatever physiologic pupillary block is present. Iridectomy may prove to be inadequate if too great an area of the filtration angle is blocked by permanent anterior synechiae. In these cases, a filtering operation is performed.

Course & Prognosis
Chronic angle-closure glaucoma causes transient episodes of intraocular pressure elevation. During these periods, insidious damage occurs to the nerve elements of the eye. Anterior peripheral synechiae slowly extend and further impede the aqueous outflow.

Permanent medical control of chronic angle-closure glaucoma is usually not possible. The sooner peripheral iridectomy is performed, the better the ultimate visual prognosis will be. If a significant cataract is present, lens extraction alone may permanently lower the intraocular pressure to normal.

PRIMARY CONGENITAL OR INFANTILE GLAUCOMA
(Trabeculodysgenesis)

Infantile glaucoma is a form of developmental glaucoma with onset in the first year of life. One-fourth of cases are present at birth. A few are diagnosed after the second year of life. The pathologic picture is produced by an arrest in development of the angle structures at about the seventh month of fetal life. The iris is hypoplastic and inserts onto the trabecular surface in front of a poorly developed scleral spur.

Clinical Findings
The earliest and most constant symptom is epiphora. Photophobia may be present. Increased intraocular pressure is the cardinal sign. Glaucomatous cupping of the optic disk is a relatively early and most important change. Later findings include increased corneal diameter (above 11.5 mm is considered significant), epithelial edema, tears of Descemet's membrane, and increased depth of the anterior chamber (associated with general enlargement of the anterior segment of the eye), as well as edema and opacity of the corneal stroma. The iris inserts anteriorly onto the trabeculum instead of into the ciliary body.

Differential Diagnosis
Megalocornea, secondary glaucoma, and traumatic corneal haze should be ruled out. Measurement of intraocular pressure, gonioscopy, and evaluation of the optic disk are important in making the differential diagnosis.

Treatment
Unlike open-angle glaucoma, in which the best treatment is often nonsurgical, infantile glaucoma

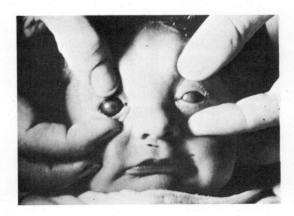

Figure 14–8. Infantile glaucoma (buphthalmos).

must be treated surgically to obtain lasting results. Medical treatment with miotics is at best a preoperative adjunctive measure.

Goniotomy is the treatment of choice. If repeated goniotomies fail or are not possible due to corneal haze, external trabeculotomy is often effective. Subscleral filtration (trabeculectomy) may be tried if these measures fail. The long-term visual prognosis is then much less favorable.

Course & Prognosis

In untreated cases, blindness occurs early. The eye undergoes marked stretching and may even rupture with minor trauma. Typical glaucomatous cupping occurs relatively soon, emphasizing the necessity of early effective treatment.

The earlier the disease becomes manifest, the less favorable the prognosis, since the early appearance of symptoms implies a more severe defect of aqueous drainage. Over 80% of cases are evident by age 3 months. Goniotomy controls the pressure permanently in 70–80% of cases. The long-term visual prognosis in such cases is good.

DEVELOPMENTAL GLAUCOMA ASSOCIATED WITH OTHER CONGENITAL ANOMALIES*

A number of syndromes characterized by increased intraocular pressure in persons under 40 have been grouped under this broad heading, which includes late-developing infantile glaucoma.

Pigmentary Glaucoma

This syndrome seems to be primarily a degeneration of the pigmented epithelium of the iris and ciliary body. The pigment granules flake off and are deposited on the posterior corneal surface (Krukenberg's spindle). The pigment becomes lodged in the trabecular meshwork and impedes the normal outflow of aqueous. The syndrome occurs most often in myopic males between the ages of 25 and 40 who have a deep anterior chamber with a wide anterior chamber angle.

A number of pedigrees of autosomal dominant inheritance of pigmentary glaucoma have been reported. The pigmentary changes may be present without glaucoma, but such persons must be considered "glaucoma suspects."

This type of glaucoma responds to timolol and to epinephrine. Miotics can seldom be used in these young patients because of induced myopia. The prognosis is not favorable if the process is severe enough to require a filtering operation. Laser trabeculoplasty may improve the prognosis.

Aniridia

The distinguishing feature of aniridia, as the name implies, is the vestigial iris. Often, little more

*Formerly classified as juvenile glaucoma.

than the root of the iris or a thin iris margin is present. Other deformities of the anterior segment of the eye may be present, most often congenital cataract and corneal dystrophy. Glaucoma frequently develops before adolescence and is usually refractory to medical or surgical management.

This rare syndrome is genetically determined. Numerous examples of both autosomal dominant and recessive inheritance have appeared in the literature.

If medical therapy is ineffective, goniotomy or trabeculotomy may occasionally normalize the intraocular pressure. Often, filtering operations are necessary, but the long-term visual prognosis is poor.

Iridocorneal Trabeculodysgenesis (Axenfeld's Syndrome, Rieger's Syndrome)

These rare diseases represent a spectrum of improper development of the mesodermal structures of the anterior segment. The result is an abnormally developed angle, iris, and cornea. Occasionally, lens changes are present. Usually there is some hypoplasia of the anterior stroma of the iris, with bridging filaments connecting the iris stroma to the cornea. If these bridging filaments occur peripherally and connect to a prominent, axially displaced Schwalbe's line (posterior embryotoxon), the disease is known as **Axenfeld's syndrome.** If adhesions are between the central iris and central posterior surface of the cornea, the disease is known as **Peters' anomaly** or **anterior chamber cleavage syndrome.** If there are broader iridocorneal adhesions associated with the disruption of the iris with polycoria and, in addition, skeletal and dental anomalies, the disorder is called **Rieger's syndrome.**

These diseases are usually dominantly inherited, although sporadic cases have been reported. Glaucoma occurs in approximately 50% of such eyes. Since no highly effective surgical procedure is available for these syndromes, they are treated as open-angle glaucomas. Filtering surgery or trabeculotomy may be used if medical therapy fails. The prognosis is poor for long-term retention of good visual function.

SECONDARY GLAUCOMA

Increased intraocular pressure occurring as one manifestation of intraocular disease is called secondary glaucoma. These diseases are difficult to classify satisfactorily.

In addition to treatment of the underlying disease, several drugs are of value in control of secondary glaucoma. With moderate elevation of intraocular pressure, reduction of aqueous production with epinephrine or timolol with or without acetazolamide is adequate management. With extreme elevations, osmotic agents are indicated. These ocular antihypertensive drugs may prevent permanent damage due to increased intraocular pressure until the underlying cause of secondary glaucoma can be controlled.

GLAUCOMA SECONDARY TO CHANGES IN THE LENS

Lens Dislocation (Traumatic)

The lens may dislocate anteriorly, pressing the iris against the posterior cornea and blocking aqueous outflow, or it may dislocate posteriorly. Secondary glaucoma is a frequent complication of posterior dislocation of the lens and is not easy to explain. Often it may be due to angle recession or trabecular damage that occurred at the time of the trauma. In other cases pupillary block occurs when a wedge of vitreous curls around the dislocated lens and plugs the pupillary opening. Surgery may be necessary if the intraocular pressure cannot be controlled medically.

Intumescence of the Lens

The lens may take up considerable fluid during cataractous change, increasing its size markedly. It may then encroach upon the anterior chamber, produce a pupillary block, or cause angle occlusion, resulting in angle-closure glaucoma. Treatment consists of lens extraction.

Phacolytic Glaucoma

As cataract formation proceeds, the lens cortex elements may undergo liquefaction and seep out through the lens capsule. Lens protein products may cause a phacoanaphylactic reaction within the eye. In this case, uveitis occurs, and the protein and cellular debris lodge in the outflow system to obstruct the free passage of aqueous. Edema of the trabeculum itself is probably associated, further decreasing the facility of aqueous outflow. Lens extraction is indicated.

Exfoliative Syndrome (Pseudoexfoliation of the Lens Capsule, Glaucoma Capsulare)

In exfoliative syndrome, deposits of unknown origin and composition are seen on the lens surface, ciliary processes, zonule, posterior iris surface, loose in the anterior chamber, and in the trabecular meshwork. The disease is usually found in patients over the age of 65. Glaucoma and sometimes cataract eventually develop. Lens extraction has no effect on the glaucoma. Miotics, timolol, and epinephrine are moderately effective, but laser trabeculoplasty or a filtering operation may be necessary.

GLAUCOMA SECONDARY TO CHANGES IN THE UVEAL TRACT

Uveitis

Often the intraocular pressure is below normal early in uveitis. This is because the inflamed ciliary body is functioning poorly and does not secrete the elements that produce the difference in osmotic pressure between aqueous and plasma. There is edema of the trabeculum as well as the ciliary body and iris, and this may result in a decreased facility of aqueous outflow. As long as there is no osmotic difference between blood and aqueous there will be no rise in pressure, but when the ciliary body begins secreting there will be an abrupt rise of pressure unless there has been a simultaneous improvement in the patency of the outflow channels. Long-standing or repeated attacks of iridocyclitis cause permanent anterior synechiae. In these cases, after the inflammatory reaction has subsided, miotics or even filtering procedures may be needed to control the intraocular pressure.

Tumor

Rapidly growing melanomas originating in the uveal tract can cause increased intraocular pressure by volume replacement, by encroachment on the filtration angle, or by blocking of a vortex vein. Enucleation is indicated.

Iridocorneoendothelial (ICE) Syndrome (Essential Iris Atrophy)

Slowly progressive atrophy of iris tissue is a rare disorder of unknown cause that is almost always associated with glaucoma. Anterior synechiae form and the degenerated iris elements block the trabecular meshwork, creating a glaucoma that is very difficult to control either medically or surgically. Endothelial degeneration occurs with edema of the cornea at relatively low intraocular pressures. The condition is nearly always unilateral.

GLAUCOMA SECONDARY TO TRAUMA

Massive Hemorrhage Into the Anterior Chamber

Contusion or penetrating injuries of the globe can cause tears in the iris or ciliary body and thus massive hemorrhage into the anterior chamber. The intraocular pressure is immediately elevated, and blood breakdown products or organized clots lodge in the outflow mechanism. One serious complication is blood staining of the cornea. Once well established, the staining may require several years to absorb. If the intraocular pressure cannot be controlled with systemic hypotensive drugs, the anterior chamber should be lavaged through a limbal incision.

Corneal or Limbal Laceration With Prolapse of Iris Into the Wound

Lacerations of the anterior eye or contusions causing anterior rupture of the eye are sealed spontaneously by prolapse of uveal tissue into the wound. This ordinarily causes loss of the anterior chamber and the rapid closure of the chamber angle by the adherence of the iris to the cornea. The primary objective of the treatment is the re-formation of the anterior chamber to prevent permanent anterior peripheral synechiae. Excision of prolapsed uvea, tight closure of the wound, and injection of saline into the anterior chamber are of paramount importance.

Contusion Causing Retrodisplacement of the Iris Root & Deepening of Anterior Chamber Angle (Angle Recession Glaucoma)

A number of clinicians have called attention to this type of trauma-induced unilateral secondary glaucoma. Following a contusion injury, the anterior chamber is observed to be significantly deeper than in the uninjured eye. Gonioscopically, one sees a recession of the angle and a torn ciliary body. Glaucoma occurs if there is sufficient associated damage to the trabecular meshwork to interfere with aqueous outflow. The condition often responds to standard open-angle glaucoma therapy, although occasionally a filtering operation is necessary.

GLAUCOMA FOLLOWING SURGERY

Epithelial Ingrowth Into the Anterior Chamber

Following cataract surgery with resultant poor healing of the wound edges, epithelium may grow into the anterior chamber and eventually line the anterior chamber angle structures, preventing normal outflow of aqueous. This is a difficult complication to treat once it is well established. An effort can be made to scrape the newly deposited epithelium off of the angle structures. Corneal transplant may be beneficial. The problem is primarily one of prevention.

Flat Anterior Chamber Following Cataract Surgery

Following cataract surgery, aqueous may escape through an imperfectly closed wound resulting in a flat (absent) anterior chamber. If the flat chamber persists more than a week, permanent anterior and posterior synechiae may form, with subsequent severe glaucoma.

GLAUCOMA SECONDARY TO RUBEOSIS IRIDIS

Rubeosis often follows central vessel occlusion and occurs frequently in advanced diabetes mellitus. Small vessels grow on the anterior surface of the iris and into the anterior chamber angle, interfering with normal aqueous outflow. Miotics are of little value. Cyclocryosurgery is the best therapeutic technique available, but results are poor. Early panretinal photocoagulation can arrest the blood vessel proliferation. Filtering surgery can then be successful in some cases.

GLAUCOMA SECONDARY TO ARTERIOVENOUS FISTULAS

Pulsating exophthalmos from arteriovenous fistula is usually accompanied by a slightly elevated intraocular pressure due to increased venous pressure. Treatment is directed at the underlying condition.

GLAUCOMA SECONDARY TO THE USE OF TOPICAL CORTICOSTEROIDS

Much interest has been aroused by the observation that topically administered corticosteroids may produce a type of glaucoma that simulates open-angle glaucoma. Most persons do not develop significant intraocular pressure elevations while on such treatment. In those that do, withdrawal of the medication eliminates the glaucoma; but permanent damage can occur if the condition goes unrecognized too long. If topical steroid therapy is absolutely necessary, miotics or other open-angle glaucoma therapy usually will control the glaucoma. It is imperative that patients receiving long-term topical steroid therapy should have periodic tonometry and ophthalmoscopy. It is equally important to beware of topical administration of corticosteroids in the eyes of patients known to have glaucoma or a family history of glaucoma. Less commonly, glaucoma can occur in patients being given long-term systemic corticosteroids over prolonged periods. Injections of corticosteroids under the conjunctiva and under Tenon's capsule may cause elevated intraocular pressure for several months. Surgical excision of the residual steroid deposit may allow the pressure to return to normal.

OCULAR HYPERTENSION

Ocular hypertension is the term coined to denote an elevated intraocular pressure (above the statistically normal level of 10–25 mm Hg) without evidence of anatomic or functional damage to the eye. Anatomic damage may be noted as enlargement of the optic disk cup, asymmetry of the disk cups (cup in one eye larger than the cup in the other), or increase of the size of the disk cup over a period of time. Obviously, functional loss represents visual field defects specific for glaucoma.

The patient with ocular hypertension should be considered a glaucoma suspect. Although no evidence of damage from the elevated intraocular pressure may be apparent, there is as yet no sure means of predicting which patient will subsequently develop damage. Frequent observation (1–3 times yearly) of the optic disk, tonometry, and visual field testing are indicated in order to make certain that proper treatment is initiated immediately if the optic nerve appears threatened.

SURGICAL PROCEDURES USED IN THE TREATMENT OF THE GLAUCOMAS

1. ANGLE-CLOSURE GLAUCOMA

PERIPHERAL IRIDECTOMY

In acute or chronic angle-closure glaucoma when extensive peripheral anterior synechiae have not formed, peripheral iridectomy is the operation of choice. It offers the one hope of a permanent cure by reestablishing ready communication between the posterior and anterior chambers. This relieves pupillary block and allows the iris root to drop away from the filtration angle, thus reestablishing the outflow of aqueous by normal channels.

In recent years, most peripheral iridectomies have been produced by laser iridectomy. The risk of intraocular surgery and the expense of hospitalization are avoided.

2. OPEN-ANGLE GLAUCOMA

LASER TRABECULOPLASTY

This procedure is gradually replacing standard cutting operations for open-angle glaucoma. The laser is applied to the trabecular meshwork through a special goniolens, and the procedure is safe and effective in 80–85% of cases. In the remaining 15–20%, the standard filtering procedures can still be performed.

Laser surgery of glaucoma is a remarkable advance. Robert Abraham of Los Angeles introduced laser iridectomy (1972) for angle-closure glaucoma; James Wise of Oklahoma City later pioneered laser trabeculoplasty for open-angle glaucoma.

CYCLOCRYOTHERMY

Cyclocryothermy has generally replaced cyclodiathermy in the treatment of aphakic glaucoma. It has the advantage of destroying the ciliary body without causing damage to either the conjunctiva or the sclera. No cutting is required. The highly vascular reaction in the ciliary body leads to fibrosis, decreased ciliary body function, and consequent decreased aqueous production.

Laser trabeculoplasty (see above) can also be tried in aphakic glaucoma, with an approximate success rate of 40%.

3. CONGENITAL GLAUCOMA

GONIOTOMY

Infantile glaucoma is best treated by goniotomy. This procedure was introduced for treatment of infantile glaucoma by Otto Barkan in 1938 and changed the prognosis of the disease from very bad to good (70–80% cure). The operation aims to establish normal aqueous outflow through physiologic channels.

● ● ●

References

Abraham RK, Miller GL: Argon laser iridectomy for angle-closure glaucoma. (Letter.) *Ann Ophthalmol* 1973;**5**:613.

Abraham RK, Miller GL: Argon laser iridectomy for angle-closure glaucoma: Preliminary report. Presented at the American Society for Contemporary Ophthalmology, Miami Beach, March 2, 1973.

Anderson DR: Pathology of the glaucomas. In: Cambridge Ophthalmological Symposium—Perrers Taylor Memorial (Sept 1971). *Br J Ophthalmol* 1972;**56**:146.

Armaly MF: Glaucoma: Annual review. *Arch Ophthalmol* 1975;**93**:146.

Becker B, Kolker AE: Glaucoma: A classic treatise. (7 parts.) *Eye Ear Nose Throat Mon* 1976;**54**:350, 379, 431, 460 and 1975;**55**:15, 58, 89.

Campbell DG: A comparison of diagnostic techniques in angle-closure glaucoma. *Am J Ophthalmol* 1979;**88**:197.

Carpel EF et al: Normal cup-disk ratio. *Am J Ophthalmol* 1981;**91**:588.

Chandler PA, Grant WM: *Lectures in Glaucoma.* Lea & Febiger, 1965.

Chandler PA, Simmons RJ, Grant WM: Malignant glaucoma: Medical and surgical treatment. *Am J Ophthalmol* 1968; **66**:495.

Chandler PA et al: *Glaucoma,* 2nd ed. Lea & Febiger, 1980.

Cristiansson J: Glaucoma simplex in diabetes mellitus. *Acta Ophthalmol (Kbh)* 1965;**43**:224.

David R et al: Genetic markers in glaucoma. *Br J Ophthalmol* 1980;**64**:227.

Drance SM: Chronic open-angle glaucoma: Present and future. (Second Spaeth Lecture.) *Can J Ophthalmol* 1977;**12**:251.

Drance SM: Some factors in the production of low tension glaucoma. In: Cambridge Opthalmological Symposium—Perrers Taylor Memorial (Sept 1971). *Br J Ophthalmol* 1972;**56**:229.

Drance SM et al: Multivariate analysis in glaucoma. *Arch Ophthalmol* 1981;**99**:1019.

Edwards RS: Behaviour of the fellow eye in acute angle-closure glaucoma. *Br J Ophthalmol* 1982;**66**:576.

François J: Corticosteroid glaucoma. *Metabol Ophthalmol* 1978;**2**:3.

Friedland BR, Malonee J, Anderson DR: Short-term dose-response of acetazolamide in man. *Arch Ophthalmol* 1977; **95**:1809.

Gaasterland DE, Jocson VL, Sears ML: Channels of aqueous outflow and related blood vessels. 3. Episcleral arteriovenous anastomoses in the rhesus monkey eye *(Macaca mulatta).* *Arch Ophthalmol* 1970;**84**:770.

Giles JT, Ellis PP: Glaucoma: Carbonic anhydrase inhibitors. Page 130 in: *Year Book of Ophthalmology, 1978*. Year Book, 1978.

Goldman H: An analysis of some concepts concerning chronic simple glaucoma. *Am J Ophthalmol* 1975;**80**:409.

Grant WM: Microsurgery of the outflow channels: Laboratory research. (Symposium.) *Trans Am Acad Ophthalmol Otolaryngol* 1972;**76**:398.

Harrington DO: *The Visual Fields: A Textbook and Atlas of Clinical Perimetry*, 5th ed. Mosby, 1981.

Hayreh SS: Pathogenesis of cupping of the optic disc. *Br J Ophthalmol* 1974;**58**:863.

Hetherington J: Treatment of juvenile glaucoma: Commentary. In: Cambridge Opthalmological Symposium—Perrers Taylor Memorial (Sept 1971). *Br J Ophthalmol* 1972;**56**:262.

Hoskins HD Jr: Evaluation techniques for the congenital glaucomas. *J Pediatr Ophthalmol* 1971;**8**:81.

Hoskins HD Jr: Neovascular glaucoma: Current concepts. *Trans Am Acad Ophthalmol Otolaryngol* 1974;**78**:330.

Hoskins HD Jr, Gelber EC: Optic disk topography and visual field defects in patients with increased intraocular pressure. *Am J Ophthalmol* 1975;**80**:284.

Hoyt WF: Ophthalmoscopy of the retinal nerve fibre layer in neuro-ophthalmologic diagnosis. *Aust J Ophthalmol* 1976;**4**:14.

Hoyt WF, Frisén L, Newman NM: Fundoscopy of nerve fiber layer defects in glaucoma. *Invest Ophthalmol* 1973;**12**:814.

Jocson VL, Sears ML: Channels of aqueous outflow and related blood vessels. 1. *Macaca mulatta* (rhesus). 2. *Cercopithecus ethiops*. *Arch Ophthalmol* 1968;**80**:104 and 1969;**81**:244.

Kitazawa Y, Horie T: Diurnal variation of intraocular pressure in primary open-angle glaucoma. *Am J Ophthalmol* 1975;**79**:557.

Kolker AE, Hetherington J: *Becker-Shaffer's Diagnosis and Therapy of the Glaucomas*, 5th ed. Mosby, 1982.

LeBlanc RP et al: Timolol: Canadian Multicenter Study. *Ophthalmology* 1981;**88**:244.

Miller SJH: Glaucoma simplex and the management of first-degree relatives. In: Cambridge Ophthalmological Symposium—Perrers Taylor Memorial (Sept 1971). *Br J Ophthalmol* 1972;**56**:284.

Pollack IP: Laser iridotomy in the treatment of angle-closure glaucoma. (Editorial.) *Ann Ophthalmol* 1981;**13**:549.

Quigley HA et al: Optic nerve damage in human glaucoma. *Arch Ophthalmol* 1982;**100**:135.

Radius RL, Maumenee AE: Visual field changes following acute elevation of intraocular pressure. *Trans Am Acad Ophthalmol Otolaryngol* 1977;**83**:61.

Schwartz B: Current concepts in ophthalmology: The glaucomas. *N Engl J Med* 1978;**299**:182.

Shaffer RN et al: The use of diagrams to record changes in glaucomatous discs. *Am J Ophthalmol* 1975;**80**:460.

Simmons RJ: Goniophotocoagulation for neovascular glaucoma. *Trans Am Acad Ophthalmol Otolaryngol* 1977;**83**:80.

Sommer A, Pollack I, Maumenee AE: Optic disc parameters and onset of glaucomatous field loss. 1. Methods and progressive changes in disc morphology. 2. Static screening criteria. *Arch Ophthalmol* 1979;**97**:1444, 1449.

Spencer WH: Microsurgery of the outflow channels: Histologic evaluation of microsurgical glaucoma techniques. (Symposium.) *Trans Am Acad Ophthalmol Otolaryngol* 1972;**76**:389.

Watson PG: Surgery of the glaucomas. In: Cambridge Ophthalmological Symposium—Perrers Taylor Memorial (Sept 1971). *Br J Ophthalmol* 1972;**56**:299.

Watson PG et al: The place of trabeculectomy in the treatment of glaucoma. *Ophthalmology* 1981;**88**:197.

Werblin TP, Pollack IP, Liss RA: Aplastic anemia and agranulocytosis in patients using methazolamide for glaucoma. *JAMA* 1979;**241**:2817.

Werner EB, Drance SM: Early visual field disturbances in glaucoma. *Arch Ophthalmol* 1977;**95**:1173.

Williams MT: Community screening for glaucoma and diabetes. *Sight Sav Rev* 1974;**44**:79.

Williams MT et al: Evolution of a prevention of blindness program in Santa Clara County. *JAMA* 1972;**219**:737.

Wise J: Long-term control of adult open-angle glaucoma by argon laser treatment. *Ophthalmology* 1981;**88**:197.

Zimmerman TJ (editor): Glaucoma symposium. (Special issue.) *Surv Ophthalmol* 1979;**23**:345.

Zimmerman TJ: Medication versus surgery: Are we doing it wrong? (Editorial.) *Ann Ophthalmol* 1981;**13**:783.

15 | Strabismus

Under normal conditions the image of the object of regard falls on the fovea of each eye. When the eyes are positioned so that the image falls upon the fovea of one eye but not the other, the second eye is deviating (squinting) and strabismus is present. The deviation may be inward, outward, up, or down. The amount of deviation is a measurement of the angle formed by the visual axes of the 2 eyes.

Strabismus is present in about 3% of children. Treatment should begin as soon as the diagnosis is definite in order to ensure the development of the best possible visual acuity and a good cosmetic result and increase the chance for normal binocular visual function. The idea that "the child may outgrow crossed eyes" should be discouraged.

ANATOMY

Muscles

Six extraocular muscles control the movement of each eye: 4 rectus and 2 oblique muscles.

A. Rectus Muscles: The 4 rectus muscles originate at a common ring tendon (annulus of Zinn) surrounding the optic nerve at the posterior apex of the orbit. They are named according to their insertion into the sclera on the medial, lateral, inferior, and superior surfaces of the eye. The muscles are about 40 mm long, becoming tendinous 4–6 mm from insertion, and are about 10 mm wide at the point of insertion. The approximate distances of insertion from the corneal limbus are as follows: medial rectus, 5 mm; inferior rectus, 6 mm; lateral rectus, 7 mm; and superior rectus, 8 mm (Fig 15–1).

B. Oblique Muscles: The 2 oblique muscles control primarily torsional movement and, to a lesser extent, upward and downward movement. The inferior

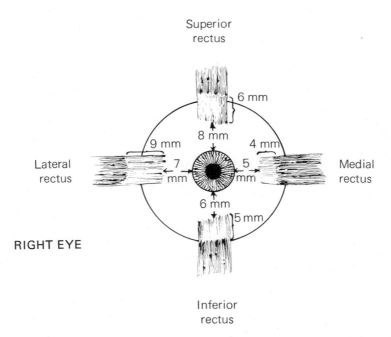

Figure 15–1. Approximate distances of the rectus muscles from the limbus, and the approximate lengths of tendons.

oblique muscle arises from the nasal orbital wall several millimeters behind the orbital rim; it passes under the inferior rectus and curves around the eyeball, making a large arc of scleral contact, and inserts in the posterior lateral quadrant of the eye just under the lateral rectus muscle. The main muscle body of the superior oblique muscle originates from the annulus of Zinn just above the origin of the superior rectus muscle and passes to the cartilaginous pulley (trochlea) attached to the nasal side of the superior orbital rim. At the pulley it is reflected downward, outward, and posteriorly, passing under the tendon of the superior rectus muscle to insert into the sclera. In the primary position, the muscle plane of the superior and inferior oblique muscles forms a 51-degree angle with the optical axis.

Innervation

The abducens nerve innervates the lateral rectus muscle; the trochlear nerve innervates the superior oblique muscle; and the oculomotor nerve innervates the other 3 rectus muscles and the inferior oblique muscle.

Fascia

The rectus and oblique muscles are ensheathed by fascia. Near the points of insertion of these muscles the fascia is continuous with Tenon's capsule, which is between the sclera and conjunctiva. Fascial condensations to adjacent orbital bony structures serve as check ligaments for the extraocular muscles and limit ocular rotation (Figs 15–2 and 15–3).

DEFINITIONS

Angle kappa: The angle between the visual axis and the central pupillary line. When fixing a light, if the corneal reflection is centered on the pupil, the visual axis and the central pupillary line coincide and the angle kappa is zero. Ordinarily, the light reflex is 2–4 degrees nasal to the pupillary center, giving the appearance of slight exotropia (positive angle kappa). A negative angle kappa gives the false impression of esotropia.

Ductions: Monocular rotations (other eye covered).
Adduction: Inward rotation.
Abduction: Outward rotation.
Infraduction: Downward movement.

Fusion: The cortical integration of the images received simultaneously by the 2 eyes.

Heterophoria (or phoria): A deviation of the eyes corrected by the fusion mechanism.
Esophoria: Tendency for one eye to turn inward.
Exophoria: Tendency for one eye to turn outward.
Hyperphoria: Tendency for one eye to deviate upward.
Hypophoria: Tendency for one eye to deviate downward.

Heterotropia (or tropia): Strabismus, or "squint"; deviation of the eyes not corrected by the fusion mechanism.

Esotropia: "Crossed eyes"; convergent strabismus.
Exotropia: "Wall eyes"; divergent strabismus.
Hypertropia: Deviation of one eye upward.
Hypotropia: Deviation of one eye downward. By common usage one usually refers to a vertical deviation in terms of hypertropia rather than hypotropia.

Orthophoria: The absence of any tendency of either eye to deviate when fusion is suspended. This state is rarely seen clinically. A small degree of phoria is "normal."

Primary deviation: The deviation measured with the normal eye fixing and the eye with the paretic muscle deviating.

Prism diopter (Δ): A unit to measure deviations. One Δ is that strength of prism which will deflect a ray of light 1 centimeter at a distance of 1 meter. The deflection is toward the base of the prism. Another commonly used unit, a degree (°), equals about 2 Δ. (For technique of measurement, see p 179.)

Secondary deviation: The deviation measured with the paretic eye fixing and the normal eye deviating.

Torsions: Wheel-like motion of the eye on its anteroposterior axis.
Intorsion (incycloduction): Torsion of superior limbus toward the nose.
Extorsion (excycloduction): Torsion of superior limbus away from the nose.

Vergences (disjunctive movements): Movement of the 2 eyes in opposite directions.
Convergence: The eyes turn inward.
Divergence: The eyes turn outward.

Versions: Binocular voluntary movement of the eyes in conjugate gaze.
Dextroversion (levoversion): Movement of the eyes to right (or left).
Supraversion (infraversion): Movement of the eyes up (or down).
Dextrocycloversion: Torsional movement of both eyes to the right (clockwise).
Levocycloversion: Torsional movement of both eyes to the left (counterclockwise).

PHYSIOLOGY: MOTOR ASPECTS

Individual Muscle Functions

The lateral rectus muscle has the lone function of abducting the eye; the medial rectus muscle, that of adducting the eye; the other muscles have both primary and secondary actions that vary according to the position of the eye.

The elevation-depression actions of the superior and inferior rectus muscles increase as the eye is abducted; the elevation-depression actions of the superior and inferior oblique muscles increase as the eye is adducted.

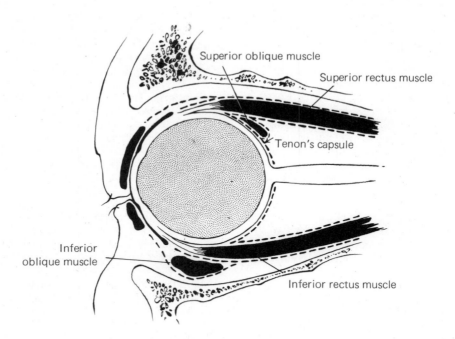

Figure 15–2. Fascia about muscles and eyeball (Tenon's capsule).

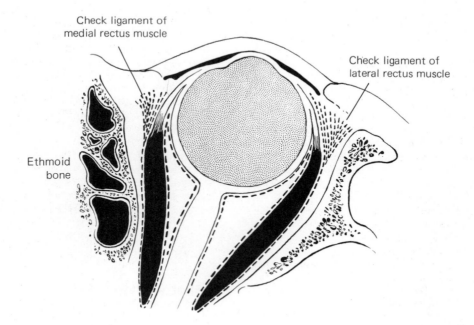

Figure 15–3. Check ligaments of medial and lateral rectus muscles, right eye (diagrammatic).

Table 15–1. Functions of the ocular muscles.

Muscle	Primary Action	Secondary Action
Lateral rectus	Abduction	None
Medial rectus	Adduction	None
Superior rectus	Elevation	Adduction, intorsion
Inferior rectus	Depression	Adduction, extorsion
Superior oblique	Depression	Intorsion, abduction
Inferior oblique	Elevation	Extorsion, abduction

Field of Action

The field of action of a muscle is that direction in which its primary action is greatest. Every movement of the eye involves the cooperation of all the muscles (each contracting or relaxing as its antagonist relaxes or contracts), but in each of the 6 cardinal directions of gaze there is always one muscle of each eye whose pull predominates.

Synergistic & Antagonistic Muscles (Sherrington's Law)

Two or 3 muscles of the same eye work together to produce a certain movement. In elevation, for example, the superior rectus and inferior oblique muscles are synergistic. Synergistic muscles for one function may be antagonists for another, eg, the superior rectus and inferior oblique are synergists for elevation but antagonists for torsional movement, since the superior rectus causes intorsion and the inferior oblique extorsion. When a muscle is stimulated, its antagonist is simultaneously and equally inhibited (Sherrington's law of reciprocal innervation). Thus, in dextroversion (eyes turning to the right), the right medial and left lateral rectus muscles receive inhibitory impulses that cause them to relax.

Yoke Muscles (Hering's Law)

In coordinated eye movements, a muscle of one eye is paired with a muscle of the opposite eye to produce movement in the 6 cardinal directions of gaze. (Eyes straight up and eyes down are not considered primary directions of gaze since no single pair of yoke muscles is primarily responsible for this action.) These paired primary movers are termed yoke muscles. In any conjugate movement, the yoke muscles receive equal innervation (Hering's law). Table 15–2 lists the yoke muscle combinations.

Table 15–2. Yoke muscle combinations.

Cardinal Direction of Gaze	Yoke Muscles
Eyes up, right	Right superior rectus and left inferior oblique
Eyes right	Right lateral rectus and left medial rectus
Eyes down, right	Right inferior rectus and left superior oblique
Eyes down, left	Right superior oblique and left inferior rectus
Eyes left	Right medial rectus and left lateral rectus
Eyes up, left	Right inferior oblique and left superior rectus

The Evolution of Binocular Movement

The movements of the eyes at birth are irregular and uncoordinated. By 4 weeks of age, the conjugate fixation reflexes are sufficiently developed so that the infant's eyes follow a slowly moving light. By 3 months of age the eyes will follow any moving object, but occasional deviations or "wandering" eye movements are seen until the age of 6 months. If a deviation is still present after 6 months, the child has strabismus and should be under the care of an ophthalmologist.

PHYSIOLOGY: SENSORY ASPECTS

Binocular Vision

In normal binocular vision, the image of the object of regard falls on the 2 foveas. The impulses travel along the optic pathways to the occipital cortex, where a single image is perceived. This is known as **fusion.** With normal use of the eye, the fovea looking at an object in space has a visual direction of "straight ahead." The foveas have a common visual direction and are the principal corresponding points. An extrafoveal point (or area) of one eye having the same visual direction as an extrafoveal point of the other eye is called a corresponding point. Fusion is a relative process regardless of the alignment of the eyes, and therefore it is classified into 3 grades or degrees (see p 182).

Sensory Changes in Strabismus

Up to the age of 6 or 7, the sensory pattern of the eyes is not entirely fixed and the eye is capable of adjusting to new mechanical alignments. If one eye deviates, the image of an object observed by the nondeviating eye falls on an extrafoveal retinal area of the deviating eye. If the sensory conditions are normal, **diplopia** will result. The fovea of the deviating eye will also be directed toward another object in space, and this second object will be perceived as if it were superimposed upon the object seen by the nondeviating eye. This causes confusion of images. Under these conditions of diplopia and visual confusion, suppression rapidly occurs. Suppression consists of the development of a scotoma that involves the macula as well as the point on which the image of regard falls (the image of the object being fixed by the dominant eye). Suppression exists only under binocular conditions and is a method of obtaining relief from the diplopia and confusion caused by the deviating eye. With the nondeviating eye covered, there is no discernible loss of vision or demonstrable scotoma. Under binocular conditions using suitable testing apparatus, a "suppression scotoma" can be elicited.

If monocular strabismus persists untreated, suppression will usually deepen into **amblyopia** of the deviating eye. In this case, the visual acuity may be reduced to finger counting only or perception of hand movement.

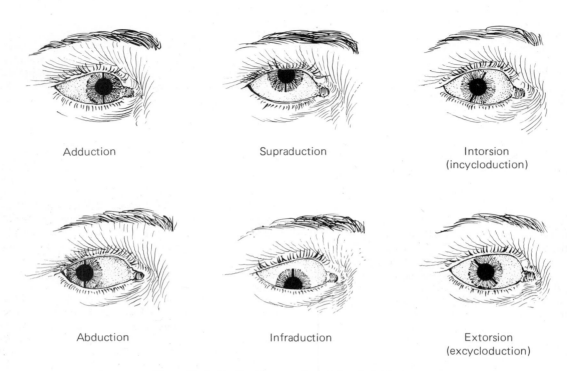

| Adduction | Supraduction | Intorsion (incycloduction) |
| Abduction | Infraduction | Extorsion (excycloduction) |

Figure 15–4. Ductions (monocular rotations), right eye.

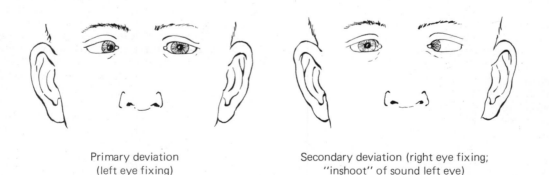

Primary deviation
(left eye fixing)

Secondary deviation (right eye fixing;
"inshoot" of sound left eye)

Figure 15–5. Paresis of horizontal muscle (right lateral rectus). Secondary deviation is greater than primary deviation because of Hering's law. With the left eye fixing, the right eye is deviated inward because of the paretic right lateral rectus. For the right eye to fix, the paretic right lateral rectus muscle must receive excessive stimulation. The yoke muscle, the left medial rectus, also receives the same excessive stimulation (Hering's law), which causes "inshoot" shown above.

Abnormal (Anomalous) Retinal Correspondence

An extrafoveal area of the deviating eye may adapt to give a new sense of "straight ahead." The fovea of the fixing eye and the extrafoveal area of the deviating eye will then experience a common visual direction. This is called anomalous retinal correspondence and represents a crude attempt at binocular vision in the presence of strabismus. In alternating strabismus the sensory pattern changes, depending upon which eye is fixing, so that when the right eye is being used for fixation the left eye is suppressed (and vice versa).

Eccentric Fixation

In eyes with amblyopia, an extrafoveal area is usually employed for fixation even when the dominant eye is covered (monocular conditions). This is termed eccentric fixation. It may be a retinal area near the fovea and detectable only with special pleoptic instruments (see p 185), or it may be an area distant from the fovea depending upon such variables as angle of deviation, duration of strabismus, age, and other poorly understood factors. Gross eccentric fixation can be readily identified clinically by occluding the dominant eye and directing the patient's attention to a light source held directly in front. An eye with gross eccentric fixation will not point toward the light source but will appear to be looking in a different direction.

**EXAMINATION:
STRABISMUS EVALUATION**

History

A careful history is of great aid in the diagnosis, prognosis, and treatment of strabismus.

A. Family History: Strabismus is frequently present; autosomal dominant inheritance is common.

B. Age at Onset: The single most important factor in prognosis. The earlier the onset, the worse the prognosis for fusion.

C. Type of Onset: May be gradual, sudden, intermittent, or associated with systemic disease.

D. Type of Deviation: Under what conditions does the patient notice strabismus? When viewing near objects? When tired? Is the amount of deviation constant? Does the patient shut one eye in the sunlight? It is most important to know if the eyes are straight at any time.

E. Fixation: Is it always the same eye that deviates? Alternating strabismus?

Visual Acuity

Visual acuity must be evaluated even if only a rough approximation or comparison of the 2 eyes is possible. The illiterate "E" chart can be used with children as young as 3½ years of age.

Determination of Refractive Error

It is important to determine the full cycloplegic refractive error by retinoscopy (see p 324). Up to 6 years of age, atropine, 0.5 or 1%, is used. Homatropine, 5%, or cyclopentolate (Cyclogyl), 1%, is adequate for older children.

Inspection

Inspection alone will show whether the strabismus is constant or intermittent, alternating or nonalternating, and variable or constant. Associated ptosis and abnormal position of the head may also be noted. The quality of fixation of each eye separately and both eyes together is important. Nystagmoid movements indicate poor fixation and reduced visual acuity.

Prominent epicanthal folds commonly confuse laymen as well as some physicians. The folds obscure a portion of the nasal sclera and may give the child the appearance of esotropia ("pseudoesotropia"). This pitfall can be avoided if the positions of the corneal reflections are noted. When the child is observing a light source, the corneal reflection of this light should be centered in the 2 pupillary areas. Prominent epicanthal folds usually disappear by 4 or 5 years of age.

Determination of Angle of Strabismus (Angle of Deviation)

A. Cover-Uncover Test (Fig 15–6): In addition to determining the presence of a heterophoria or heterotropia, its degree can be measured by placing the appropriate prism in front of one eye. For esodeviations, the prism is placed base-out in such strength that when the cover is moved from one eye to the other, the eye being uncovered no longer moves to obtain fixation upon the target light.

B. Maddox Rod Test (Fig 15–7): This test is an accurate method of measuring a deviation if normal retinal correspondence is present. It is particularly useful for measurement of heterophoria but can also be used in heterotropia. A Maddox rod consists of a series of thin red glass cylinders placed side by side, usually mounted in a circular holder that can be held before the eye. When a target light is seen through the Maddox rod, its image is a red focal line perpendicular to the axes of the cylinders. Thus, one eye sees the light directly, while the other views its image through the Maddox rod. In orthophoria the red line appears to run through the light. When the Maddox rod is held so that the cylinders are horizontal, a vertical red line is seen that in cases of horizontal deviation is displaced laterally. A prism can be held in front of one eye so that the red line appears to "run through the light." The strength of such a prism reflects the angle of deviation. By rotating the Maddox rod 90 degrees, a horizontal line is produced (cylinders of the rod are vertical). Its displacement can also be measured by prisms as described for horizontal deviations.

C. Objective Tests: If the patient is uncooperative or has eccentric fixation, some purely objective method of testing must be used to measure the deviation. Two methods are available. Results by both methods or any objective method must be modified by allowing for the angle kappa.

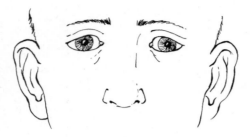

Eyes straight (maintained in position by fusion).

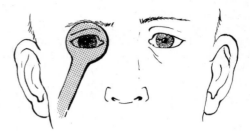

Position of eye under cover in orthophoria (fusion-free position). The right eye under cover has not moved.

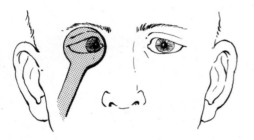

Position of eye under cover in esophoria (fusion-free position). Under cover, the right eye has deviated inward. Upon
removal of cover, the right eye will immediately resume its
straight-ahead position.

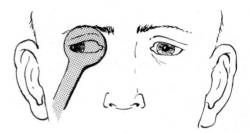

Position of eye under cover in exophoria (fusion-free position). Under cover, the right eye has deviated outward. Upon
removal of the cover, the right eye will immediately resume its
straight-ahead position.

Figure 15–6. Cover-uncover test. The patient is directed to look at a small light source at eye level 20 feet away. *Note:* In the
presence of heterotropia, the deviation will remain when the cover is removed.

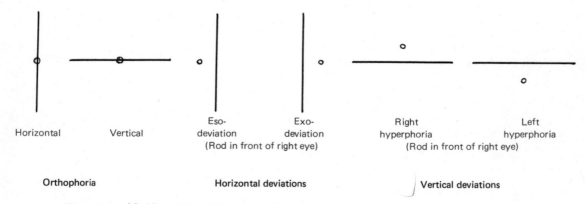

| Horizontal | Vertical | Eso-deviation (Rod in front of right eye) | Exo-deviation | Right hyperphoria (Rod in front of right eye) | Left hyperphoria |

Orthophoria   Horizontal deviations   Vertical deviations

Figure 15–7. Maddox rod test. Normal and abnormal responses. (Subjective view of the patient.)

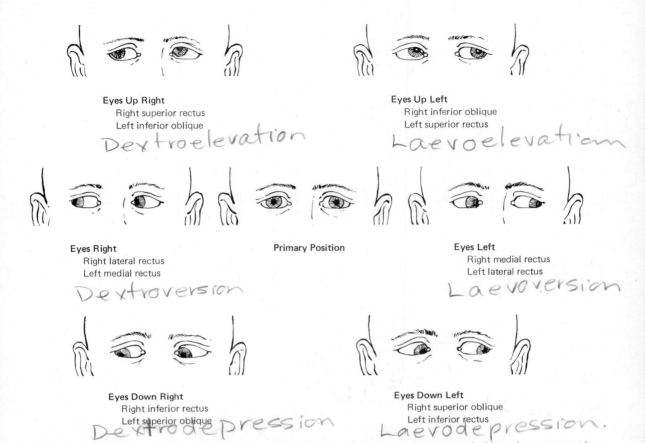

Eyes Up Right
  Right superior rectus
  Left inferior oblique

Dextroelevation

Eyes Up Left
  Right inferior oblique
  Left superior rectus

Laevoelevation

Eyes Right
  Right lateral rectus
  Left medial rectus

Dextroversion

Primary Position

Eyes Left
  Right medial rectus
  Left lateral rectus

Laevoversion

Eyes Down Right
  Right inferior rectus
  Left superior oblique

Dextrodepression

Eyes Down Left
  Right superior oblique
  Left inferior rectus

Laevodepression.

Figure 15–8. Normal version movement (binocular rotations). Yoke muscles primarily concerned with ocular movement in the cardinal directions are shown.

Eyes Up Right (Right Eye Fixing). Shows upshoot of left eye, indicating overaction of left inferior oblique. Excessive stimulation is needed to move right eye into position because of paretic right superior rectus muscle. The yoke muscle (left inferior oblique) receives the same excessive stimulation and "overacts." Secondary deviation; eye with paretic muscle is fixing.

Eyes Up Right (Left Eye Fixing). Shows underaction of right superior rectus. The left eye moves up and to the right with normal stimulation of the left inferior oblique muscle. The same normal impulse (Hering's law) to the right superior rectus muscle is insufficient to move the right eye up normally. Primary deviation; eye with nonparetic muscle is fixing.

Figure 15–9. Testing versions. Example of paretic right superior rectus muscle.

1. Hirschberg method—The patient fixes a light at a distance of about 33 cm (13 inches). The decentering of the light reflection is noted in the deviating eye. By allowing 15 diopters for each millimeter of decentration, an estimate of the angle of deviation can be made.

2. Prism reflex method (modified Krimsky test)—The patient fixes a light at any distance. The strength of a prism placed before the fixing eye required to center the corneal reflection of the deviating eye measures the angle of deviation.

Ductions (Monocular Rotations)

With one eye covered, the other eye follows a moving light in all directions of gaze so that any weakness of rotation can be noted. Such a weakness can be due to a muscle paralysis or to a mechanical anatomic anomaly.

Versions (Conjugate Ocular Movements)

According to Hering's law, yoke muscles receive equal stimulation during any conjugate ocular movement. The versions are tested by having the eyes follow a light at 33 cm in the cardinal directions of gaze and evaluating any "overaction" or "underaction" noted. First one eye and then the other is made to fix the light. "Overaction" of a muscle results when the eye with the paretic muscle is fixing the light placed in the cardinal directions of gaze controlled primarily by the set of yoke muscles in question (eg, eyes up and to the right for the right superior rectus and left inferior oblique muscles). The paretic muscle receives excessive innervation. Its yoke muscle receives the same excessive stimulation and therefore "overacts" (Figs 15–8 and 15–9).

The evaluation of versions is most important in diagnosing paretic muscles, particularly those acting vertically. They are more important than monocular rotations (ductions), which can appear normal in testing mildly paretic muscles.

Disjunctive Movements

A. Convergence (Fig 15–10): As the eyes follow an approaching object, they must turn inward in order to maintain alignment of the visual axes with the object of regard. The medial rectus muscles are contracting

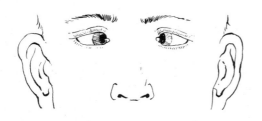

Figure 15–10. Convergence. The normal position of the eyes at the near point of convergence (NPC) is shown above. The break point is within 50 mm of the bridge of the nose.

and the lateral rectus muscles are relaxing under the influence of neural stimulation and inhibition. (Neural pathways of supranuclear control are discussed in Chapter 17.)

Convergence is an active process with a strong voluntary as well as involuntary component. An important consideration of extraocular movements in evaluating strabismus is the function of convergence.

To test convergence, a small object or light source is slowly brought toward the bridge of the nose. The patient's attention is directed to the object by saying, "Keep the light from going double as long as possible." Convergence can normally be maintained until the object is nearly to the bridge of the nose. An actual numerical value is placed on convergence by measuring the distance from the bridge of the nose (in millimeters) at which the eyes "break" (ie, when the nondominant eye swings laterally so that convergence is no longer maintained). This point is termed the near point of convergence (NPC), and a value of up to 50 mm is considered within normal limits.

B. Divergence: Electromyography has established that divergence is an active process, not merely a relaxation of convergence as previously believed by some authorities. Clinically, this function is seldom tested except in considering the amplitude of fusion (see below).

The Major Amblyoscope

(Grades of fusion, amplitude, suppression, retinal correspondence.)

This is an effective testing device for evaluation of the sensory status of the eyes. It consists essentially of 2 adjustable tubes that present an illuminated image to each eye separately, using a mirror system. The tubes can be moved horizontally or vertically, and they are calibrated. The light source illuminates the images separately, alternately, or together. Pairs of slides, one for each eye, are placed in the end of each tube. With appropriate slide pairs and a cooperative child (at least age 3), the sensory status can be evaluated. Orthoptic therapy can also be carried out with the aid of the amblyoscope.

A. Grades of Fusion: Grades of fusion as measured with the amblyoscope are as follows:

1. Grade I—(Simultaneous macular perception.) Dissimilar test targets (bird on one side, cage on the other side) are presented to the maculas. If the subject sees both objects (can see the bird in the cage), grade I fusion is present. If one object is not seen, the eye on the corresponding side is suppressing.

2. Grade II—(Fusion under stress with some amplitude.) Pairs of test targets are used which individually lack some detail but which when superimposed form a complete image. If these are perceived as a single image and this fusion is maintained as the tubes are moved from 5 to 10 diopters, grade II fusion exists.

3. Grade III—(Stereopsis.) The test targets are so devised that an impression of depth is given if the observer has normal binocular vision.

B. Amplitude of Fusion: If grade II or III fusion exists, it is important to evaluate the stability of fusion. This is done by measuring the amplitude of fusion. Starting at the zero point, the arms are gradually converged until diplopia occurs. Normally, this is at least 25 or 30 diopters. The same test is performed for divergence, with 5 diopters being a minimal normal value. Vertical dissociation is also tested, and a normal person should overcome at least 5 diopters.

C. Suppression: Although grade I targets may disclose suppression (as above), foveal suppression can only be tested by using targets with very small central check marks.

D. Retinal Correspondence: Normal retinal correspondence has been defined as being present when anatomically corresponding retinal areas have the same subjective visual direction in space. To test retinal correspondence, the amblyoscope is set at the patient's objective angle of strabismus (angle measured by cover test; see p 179). If the grade II test targets are superimposed, normal retinal correspondence exists. If the images are double, abnormal retinal correspondence exists. Conversely, as a check, the patient is asked to place the tubes so that the images are together or as close together as possible. If this coincides with the angle of strabismus, normal retinal correspondence exists.

After-Image Test

This is a good simple test for determining whether a constant deviation in one eye has caused an extrafoveal area to take on the rudimentary function of the fovea in binocular vision (abnormal retinal correspondence).

The room is darkened and the patient instructed to cover the right eye. The left eye is then exposed to a horizontal beam of light for 20 seconds. This procedure is then repeated, covering the left eye and exposing the right eye to a vertical beam of light for 10 seconds. The patient is then asked to describe what he or she "sees." If the after-images of the 2 lines cross at the center, the patient has normal retinal correspondence. If not, abnormal retinal correspondence is present.

ORTHOPTIC THERAPY
WITH THE AMBLYOSCOPE

Before or after strabismus surgery, orthoptic therapy may materially aid in the treatment of strabismus by improving the quality of fusion. An attempt can be made to eliminate suppression by stimulating the fovea of the suppressing eye, or to break down abnormal retinal correspondence by presenting the maculas simultaneously with grade II test targets (see p 182). If grade II fusion is present or is developed, the amplitude of fusion can be improved by using grade II targets and varying the angle while maintaining fusion. In association with glasses or, at times, as an aid in reducing the strength of glasses required or eliminating

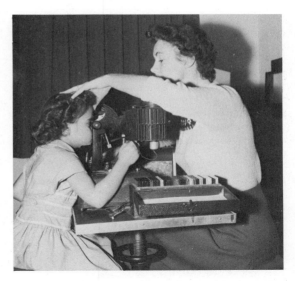

Figure 15–11. Giving eye exercises with the major amblyoscope.

them altogether, orthoptic exercises are useful in accommodative esotropia.

In special instances, heterophorias of significant degree in adults may be aided by various orthoptic exercises.

OBJECTIVES & PRINCIPLES OF
THERAPY OF STRABISMUS

There are 3 main objectives in the treatment of strabismus:

(1) Good visual acuity in each eye, achieved by occluding the good eye to force the child to use the deviating eye or, in some cases, by means of pleoptics (see p 185).

(2) A good cosmetic appearance. The eyes can be "straightened" by surgery or spectacles, or by a combination of both.

(3) Binocular vision (fusion, stereopsis). This also depends upon surgery, orthoptics, and refractive lenses, and often is an unobtainable goal.

Poor visual acuity and cosmetic defects are easier to correct if the child is seen early; the ideal age at which to begin therapy is 6 months. Normal fusion is difficult to obtain unless the child has already developed powers of binocular vision before the onset of strabismus; it is the ideal objective of therapy but is attained less than half the time. It is a satisfactory result in strabismus therapy to obtain 2 straight eyes with good vision but without good fusion. (Absence of fusion is not a serious handicap, affecting depth perception and estimation of distance to a limited degree.)

Occlusive therapy ("patching") may be required for variable periods depending upon the age at which strabismus is discovered and the presence of amblyopia. It is essential to secure (and maintain, if necessary by frequent urging) the complete cooperation of the child and the parents; they must understand that this simple procedure will prevent the loss of vision in one eye. Patching is effective up to age 7. In older children, pleoptics may be effective.

Surgical correction of muscle imbalance should not be undertaken until maximal visual acuity has been restored by means of patching or pleoptics. (It is important to emphasize that strabismus surgery does not correct the visual disturbance or the underlying cause of ocular deviation, but merely the cosmetic deformity.) Two or more operations may be required before the eyes are straightened, since there is no mathematically precise relationship between the number of millimeters the surgeon will recess or resect and the number of degrees of deviation corrected. However, the surgeon can usually make a good estimate of how many millimeters should be recessed or resected; these clinical estimates are based on the degree of deviation and the size of the muscle as observed at surgery.

In most cases it does not greatly matter whether surgery is performed on the straight eye or the deviating eye, but the deviating eye is usually chosen since this is easier to explain to parents.

Strabismus surgery is "trial and error" surgery, which creates an artificial defect in one or more extraocular muscles to compensate for an existing defect of unknown cause.

CLASSIFICATION OF STRABISMUS

A. Estropia:
   1. Nonparalytic (comitant)—The angle of deviation is constant in all directions of gaze.
      a. Nonaccommodative
      b. Accommodative
      c. Combined accommodative and nonaccommodative
   2. Paretic (noncomitant)—The angle of deviation varies in different directions of gaze.
B. Exotropia:
   1. Intermittent
   2. Constant
C. Hypertropia:
   1. Paralytic
   2. Nonparalytic

ESOTROPIA
(Convergent Strabismus, "Crossed Eyes")

Esotropia is by far the most common type of strabismus. It is divided into paralytic (due to paresis or paralysis of one or more extraocular muscles) and nonparalytic (comitant). Comitant esotropia is the most common type in infants and children; it may be accommodative, nonaccommodative, or a combination of both. Paralytic strabismus is uncommon in childhood but accounts for nearly all cases of adult onset of strabismus.

NONPARALYTIC ESOTROPIA

1. NONACCOMMODATIVE ESOTROPIA

Nearly half of all cases of esotropia fall into this group. In most cases the cause is obscure. Characteristically, the convergent deviation is manifest early in life, usually by the first year and often at birth. By definition, the deviation is comitant, ie, the angle of deviation is approximately the same in all directions of gaze and is not affected very much by accommodation. The cause, therefore, is not related to the refractive error or dependent upon a paretic extraocular muscle. It is probable that some cases are due to anomalous insertions of the horizontally acting muscles, abnormal check ligaments, or various other fascial abnormalities. It seems likely that most cases are due to faulty innervational control, most likely involving the supranuclear pathways for convergence and divergence and their neural connections to the medial longitudinal fasciculus.

There is also good evidence that "idiopathic" strabismus may occur on a genetically determined basis. Esophoria and esotropia are frequently passed on as an autosomal dominant trait. Siblings often have similar ocular deviations. At other times, when there is no apparent family history, the parents of an esotropic child may be found to have significant esophoria, and have passed on the defect in a more severe form. An accommodative element is often superimposed upon comitant esotropia, ie, a correction of the hyperopic refractive error corrects some but not all of the deviation.

Clinical Findings

Aside from the cosmetic defect and the personality problems it may create in older children, there are usually no symptoms due to strabismus.

The deviation may be monocular (ie, the same eye always deviates) or alternating (either eye may deviate). The refractive error in alternating esotropia is approximately the same in each eye; in monocular esotropia the refractive error is frequently more marked in one eye (anisometropia). Adduction is commonly increased and abduction decreased in one or both eyes. Convergence may be unaffected. Visual acuity is not affected in alternating esotropia, but it usually becomes reduced in the deviating eye in monocular esotropia. The deviation usually varies only slightly when the eyes are focused on near and distant objects, and correction of the refractive error does not appreciably affect the deviation.

If the strabismus has been present for several months, alternating esotropia will usually result in alternate suppression and often abnormal retinal correspondence (but not amblyopia). Monocular strabismus is most likely to cause amblyopia.

Treatment

A. Occlusive Therapy: The objective of occlusive therapy is to equalize the visual acuity in both eyes. Early diagnosis followed by patching the good eye is the best means of preventing amblyopia. However, even with patching and successful surgical correction, many patients (especially those who have strabismus at birth) do not develop normal fusion. In general, the earlier the deviation is discovered and the fixing eye patched, the sooner will the deviating eye develop useful visual acuity. Even a few days of patching may be sufficient prior to age 1, whereas several months may be necessary by age 5. After age 7, only pleoptics can help develop or restore visual function, and this is a very time-consuming procedure in which there is no assurance of success.

Occlusion has a favorable effect upon abnormal sensory patterns but rarely on the degree of deviation. When nothing further can be accomplished by occlusion, surgical realignment of the eyes is indicated.

Occlusive therapy may be combined with orthoptics (see p 183), utilizing the amblyoscope in an effort to develop better binocular function. The sensory abnormalities of suppression and abnormal retinal correspondence are also broken down, if possible, by orthoptic means.

B. Pleoptics: The value of pleoptics as a practical therapeutic tool has not lived up to early expectations. It is more widely used in Europe than in the USA. A wide variety of techniques have been utilized, all designed to disrupt eccentric fixation and establish foveal fixation. One frequently used technique is based on stimulating the dormant fovea while discouraging the eccentric fixation point by dazzling and blocking out appropriate retinal areas. The entire parafoveal area out to 30 degrees is dazzled with an ophthalmoscope light source that has a central dark shield to protect the macula from the dazzle. After the light is removed, the macula stands out as a positive after-image. Shortly thereafter, a negative after-image becomes apparent to the patient. The patient is then taught that the after-image is in the straight-ahead position, and in this way foveal vision can be gradually reoriented to the straight-ahead position. Many concentrated hours of pleoptic work are required to attain proper macular and foveal orientation so that improved visual acuity can occur. Some patients respond fairly quickly, but others require months or years of treatment. For ideal results, hospitalization is necessary—an almost prohibitive financial factor in the USA. The average visual improvement is from 6/60 (20/200) to 6/20 (20/70), but some exceptional cases have improved from hand movement visual acuity to 6/7.5 (20/25). Even many of these apparently successfully treated patients have reverted to previous visual levels shortly after cessation of treatment.

The best age group for treatment is from age 7 to 14, but a few remarkable results have been reported on amblyopic eyes of elderly patients who have lost the vision of the dominant eye from some organic cause.

C. Surgical Treatment: There are basically 2 surgical approaches to the correction of strabismus: strengthening a muscle or weakening a muscle. In the case of the horizontal muscles, the strengthening operation is usually resection and the weakening operation is usually recession. Other rarely used procedures include tucking and advancement for strengthening, and various types of tenotomy for weakening.

1. Recession of the medial rectus muscle—A conjunctival incision is made near the nasal limbus and carried down through Tenon's capsule. The muscle is isolated and exposed for a short distance away from its insertion. The immediate check ligaments are severed. The muscle is severed at the insertion and resutured to the sclera 4–5 mm behind this point, depending upon the amount of adjustment desired. The conjunctiva is then reapproximated.

The operation is usually done under general anesthesia, and the patient may be ambulatory within hours after surgery. The eye is often left unpatched or patched for only one day. Conjunctival injection is present immediately postoperatively but gradually disappears within 2–3 weeks.

2. Resection of the lateral rectus muscle—A limbal incision is made at the temporal limbus and carried through Tenon's capsule. The insertion of the lateral rectus is isolated and the muscle clamped and detached from the sclera. One or 2 sutures are then placed through the sclera at the original point of insertion. The sutures are then passed through the muscle 6–10 mm from its detached end and tied. The excess muscle tissue is dissected off, and the conjunctival incision reapproximated.

There is no precise rule for the amount of recession or resection needed to correct a given amount of deviation. There are many variables, including the technique of the surgeon, which determine how much correction will be achieved by a given amount of surgery. In general, the surgeon first decides how many muscles are to be operated on and then varies the amount of surgery within rather narrow limits. In the case of esotropia, deviations of less than 20 diopters can usually be corrected by surgery on one muscle (eg, 4- to 5-mm recession of one medial rectus muscle). For deviations of 20–35 diopters, it is usually necessary to operate on 2 muscles. Some surgeons prefer to operate upon 2 muscles of one eye, doing a recession of the medial rectus and a resection of the lateral rectus; others prefer so-called symmetric surgery, eg, bilateral recession of both medial rectus muscles.

To some extent the type of strabismus influences the type of surgery. In the case of monocular strabismus with an amblyopic eye, most surgeons prefer to operate upon the deviating eye. In the case of alternating esotropia, recession of both medial rectus muscles is preferable. In deviations above 45 diopters, it may be necessary to operate on 3 or even 4 muscles.

3. Adjustable sutures–In the past several years, a significant advance in strabismus surgery has been achieved by the use of adjustable sutures. In adults and in children old enough to cooperate (usually age 9 or older), sutures used in recession or resection are tied in bow knots. The day following surgery, adjustment can be made when necessary to obtain the best ocular alignment. The knots are then permanently secured,

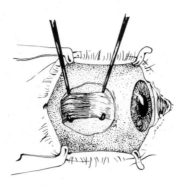

Exposure of lateral rectus

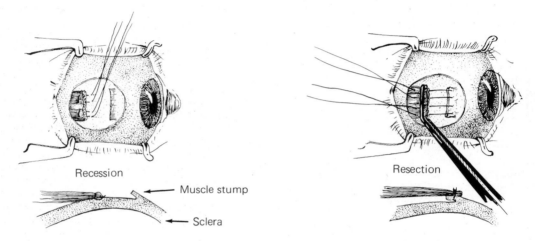

Recession

← Muscle stump

← Sclera

Resection

Figure 15–12. Surgical correction of strabismus (right eye).

and in this way the overall surgical results have been improved.

Prognosis

Strabismus surgery is empirical, and consistent results cannot be predicted. The family should be warned that 2 or more operations may be necessary before a good result is obtained. One of the best opportunities to improve fusion occurs just before and just after strabismus surgery, since the sensory status is made temporarily more flexible by strabismus surgery.

2. ACCOMMODATIVE ESOTROPIA

About one-third of cases of esotropia fall into this group; another 15–20% have some accommodative factor. These patients are hyperopic, usually 2 diopters or more. For this reason they must accommodate for clear distance vision. Accommodation is associated with a certain amount of convergence; if the amount of convergence is too great to be overcome by the available fusional amplitude, convergent strabismus results. Accommodative esotropia sometimes takes the

form of esophoria for distance and esotropia for near vision. In these cases there is an overresponse of convergence in association with accommodation.

Clinical Findings

The onset of this type of esotropia is characteristically between 18 months and 4 years of age (because the faculty of accommodation is not well developed until then). The deviation is most often monocular but may be alternating. The hyperopic refractive error is usually from +2 to +5 diopters. Sensory findings reveal that suppression develops rapidly in the deviating eye, but normal retinal correspondence is usually retained.

Treatment

Pure accommodative esotropia responds satisfactorily to correction of hyperopia with eyeglasses if treatment is instituted within a fairly short time, usually not more than 6 months after onset. If treatment is delayed beyond this time, the abnormal sensory pattern is apt to have become so well established that glasses alone will not correct the strabismus. In this event, treatment is generally as outlined above for nonaccommodative esotropia. If amblyopia has developed in one eye, occlusion is indicated, and this may so reverse the abnormal sensory pattern that nonsurgical cure is possible. More frequently, however, surgical treatment will be necessary in long-standing cases. In cases that have a partial accommodative factor, a prescription for hyperopic eyeglasses will reduce the amount of deviation, and the residual deviation must be corrected surgically. Bifocals may be prescribed if the deviation is much greater for near than for distance vision.

Long-acting miotics in weak strengths (echothiophate [Phospholine] iodide, 0.06 or 0.12% solution; or isoflurophate [Floropryl] ointment, 0.025%) applied once daily have been used with success in treating accommodative esotropia. In younger children (age 2–4), these drugs can be used instead of glasses if the hyperopia is less than 4 diopters and there is little astigmatism. Miotics are particularly useful in cases where hyperopic eyeglasses align the eyes for distance vision but esotropia remains at near vision. These drugs act by altering the accommodative convergence relationship in a favorable way so that fusion is maintained despite accommodation. In addition, the miotic effect allows a clear vision with less accommodation both for near and distance vision.

PARETIC (NONCOMITANT) ESOTROPIA
(Abducens Palsy)
(Fig 15–13)

In noncomitant strabismus there are always one or more paretic extraocular muscles. In the case of noncomitant esotropia, the paresis is always of one of the lateral rectus muscles, usually as a result of palsy of the abducens nerve. These cases are most often seen in adults who have had cerebrovascular accidents or diabetes, but abducens palsy may occasionally be the first sign of a tumor or of inflammatory disease involving the central nervous system. Head trauma is a frequent cause of abducens palsy.

Noncomitant esotropia is also seen in infants and children, but much less commonly than comitant esotropia. These cases result from birth injuries affecting the muscle directly, from injury to the nerve, or, less commonly, from a congenital anomaly of the lateral rectus muscle or its fascial attachments.

Clinical Findings

If the lateral rectus muscle is totally paralyzed, the eye will not move temporally beyond the midline. Paralysis of a right lateral rectus muscle causes a right esotropia, which becomes more marked as the eyes attempt to fix an object moving to the right of the midline. The deviation is absent upon conjugate movement of the eyes to the left.

In children age 6 or younger, suppression will develop under conditions of deviation but entirely normal binocular relationships may remain when the eyes are aligned in the field of gaze opposite the side of the paretic lateral rectus muscle. There may even be a change of retinal correspondence from normal to abnormal as one passes into the field of strabismus. In adults with a sudden onset of paralytic esotropia, the patient experiences diplopia whenever an eye deviates, since the sensory pattern is fixed and the object of regard falls on noncorresponding retinal areas.

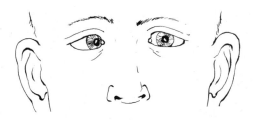

Primary position: right esotropia

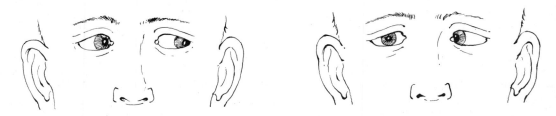

Left gaze: no deviation

Right gaze: left esotropia

Figure 15–13. Noncomitant strabismus (paralytic). Paralysis of right lateral rectus muscle, with left eye fixing.

Treatment

The treatment of persistent paralytic esotropia is exclusively surgical. In adults who have a sudden onset of strabismus, a period of at least 6 months is allowed to pass before surgery, since the condition may improve or even correct itself. During this period, occlusion of one eye is necessary to relieve diplopia.

In children, or in adults who have had no improvement after 6 months, surgical treatment is indicated. In paresis of the lateral rectus muscle, strengthening this muscle by resection combined with recession of the ipsilateral medial rectus is effective. In this operation the resection is carried out as described for nonparalytic esotropia. The type and amount of surgery will depend on the extent of the deviation. In the case of total paralysis of the lateral rectus muscle, strengthening by resection of the muscle will not attain the desired result. The best procedure, as advocated by Knapp, involves transplanting the entire superior and inferior rectus muscles to the insertion of the paralyzed lateral rectus. This not only greatly improves abduction but has the added advantage of not restricting upward or downward movement of the eye to any significant extent.

The surgical treatment of noncomitant (paralytic) esotropia is seldom completely successful, but some improvement can usually be achieved.

EXOTROPIA
(Divergent Strabismus)

Exotropia is less common than esotropia, particularly in infancy and childhood. Its incidence increases gradually with age. Not infrequently, a tendency to divergent strabismus beginning as exophoria progresses to intermittent exotropia and finally to constant exotropia if no treatment is given. Other cases begin as a constant or intermittent exotropia and remain stationary. As in esotropia, there is a strong hereditary element. Exophoria and exotropia (considered as a single entity of divergent deviation) are frequently passed on as autosomal dominant traits, so that one or both parents of an exotropic child may demonstrate exotropia or a high degree of exophoria.

INTERMITTENT EXOTROPIA

Intermittent exotropia (Fig 15–14) comprises well over half of cases of exotropia. The onset of the deviation may not be noted prior to age 2 or 3. The history reveals that the condition has become progressively worse. A characteristic sign is closing one eye in bright sunlight, as this avoids diplopia. There is usually a manifest exotropia for distance. The patient can fuse for near vision, overcoming a moderate to large angle exophoria. Convergence is frequently excellent. There is no correlation with a specific refractive error.

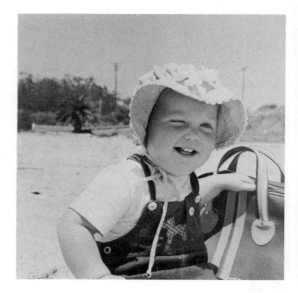

Figure 15–14. Child with intermittent exotropia squinting in sunlight.

Since the child fuses at least part of the time, there is usually no gross sensory abnormality. For distance, with one eye deviated, there is suppression but normal retinal correspondence and no amblyopia.

The definitive treatment is surgery of the extraocular muscles. The choice of surgical procedure is based on a number of considerations, the most important of which is the amount of deviation and a comparison of near and distance measurement. When the deviation is greater for distance than for near vision, recession of each lateral rectus muscle gives the best results. If the near deviation is approximately equal to the distance, many surgeons prefer a recession of one lateral rectus and a resection of the medial rectus of the same eye. As with other types of strabismus, one operation does not always accomplish the desired result and a second operation may be required.

CONSTANT EXOTROPIA

Constant exotropia is much less common than intermittent exotropia. It may be present at birth or may occur when intermittent exotropia progresses to constant exotropia. Some cases have their onset later in life, particularly following loss of vision in one eye.

As with esotropia, the cause of exotropia is usually not known. Congenital constant exotropia may be the result of anomalous insertions of the extraocular muscles, other defects of the muscles, or faulty innervation. It has been postulated that in infants and young children, a tendency toward excessive convergence may be present which is controlled by nuclear and infranuclear pathways and held in check by supranuclear influences which maintain the proper alignment

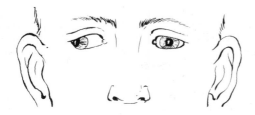

Figure 15–15. Right exotropia.

of the eyes. There probably also is a divergence center with similar supranuclear influences, and both esotropia and exotropia may well result from abnormalities of the supranuclear influences. Such common terms as "convergence excess and convergence insufficiency" and "divergence excess and divergence insufficiency" are merely descriptive. For example, "divergence excess" means an exodeviation, either phoria or tropia, which is greater for distance than for near vision; "convergence excess" means an esodeviation that is greater for near than for distance vision. It is true that the tendency toward divergence becomes greater as age increases. If there is no fusion, as in the case of one blind eye, the blind eye usually deviates inward in a person up to age 6 and usually deviates outward if the visual loss occurs after age 6. Many cases of exotropia develop as a result of loss of vision in one eye, with subsequent progressive exotropia.

The most important consideration is the psychic factor resulting from the cosmetic appearance. The loss of depth perception that occurs is seldom of much practical importance to the average person.

Constant exotropia is most often monocular (the same eye always deviating) but may be alternating. Abduction is frequently increased and adduction decreased in both eyes, with little or no convergence. Hypertropia of varying degree is often associated. The deviations vary from as little as 10 diopters to 80 diopters or more.

In children age 6 or under with alternating exotropia, alternate suppression characteristically develops. If the squint is monocular, amblyopia of the deviating eye results. Abnormal retinal correspondence is an infrequent sensory change. Eccentric fixation of the deviated eye almost never occurs. Exotropia very seldom has its onset in adulthood unless there is significant loss of visual acuity in the deviating eye, and diplopia is therefore not usually a troublesome symptom.

Surgery is the only treatment available. A practical goal is a good cosmetic appearance with maintenance of good vision in each eye. In general, slight overcorrection is attempted, since the resultant small angle esotropia is less likely to revert to exotropia. If surgery leaves a residual small angle exotropia, the eye is apt to deviate outward again.

Even in children with good vision in each eye, a good fusional result is seldom attained.

In monocular exotropia, it is usually necessary to operate upon at least the 2 horizontal muscles of the deviating eye, resecting the medial rectus and recessing the lateral rectus. (Technique is described under treatment of nonaccommodative esotropia, p 184.) In large deviations, 3 or all 4 horizontal muscles may have to be altered to straighten the eyes.

• • •

"A" & "V" SYNDROMES

Increasing importance has been attached to 2 types of horizontal strabismus in which the deviation is significantly different in upward and downward gaze. The terminology is intended to be descriptive of the position of the eyes where the deviation is greatest. In "A" esotropia, deviation is greater on eyes up than on eyes down; in "A" exotropia, deviation is greater on eyes down than on eyes up. Conversely, in "V" esotropia, deviation is greater on eyes down than on eyes up; and in "V" exotropia, deviation is greater on eyes up than on eyes down.

When these findings are present in significant degree, most ophthalmic surgeons alter their surgical approach.

HYPERTROPIA

Vertical deviations are designated according to the eye that is deviated upward. "Right hypertropia" means that the right eye deviates upward when the left eye is fixating (Fig 15–16). The same condition could be called a left hypotropia when the right eye is fixating, but this terminology is seldom used. Hypertropia is much less common than horizontal deviation and usually has its onset later in life.

There are many causes of hypertropia. Trauma may cause paralysis of a vertically acting muscle. Abnormal insertions, abnormal fascial attachments, and other congenital anomalies may also cause hypertropia.

Complications of systemic disease also account for a great number of cases, eg, myasthenia gravis, multiple sclerosis, thyrotoxicosis, orbital tumor, and brain stem disease. Many of the specific entities are

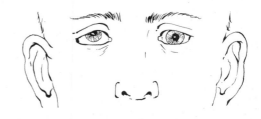

Figure 15–16. Right hypertropia.

considered in the chapter on neuro-ophthalmology. The discussion here will be limited to "idiopathic cases," ie, those due to paralysis of unknown cause involving one or more of the vertically acting muscles.

Clinical Findings (See also Figs 15–7 and 15–8.)

Hypertropia with onset after age 6 causes diplopia if both eyes have good visual acuity. There may be an associated head tilt or abnormal posture of the head.

The deviation may vary from slight (a few prism diopters) to marked. At onset and for a variable period thereafter, the deviation will be greater in one position or direction of gaze than in others. Subsequently, heterotropia tends to become comitant, since secondary contraction of the direct antagonist and the yoke muscle occurs. It is important to determine which muscle or muscles are at fault. This becomes more difficult if the disorder is of long duration. Many tests are available that are of aid in specific muscle diagnosis. In any one case all tests may not be consistent, but the bulk of evidence will point toward paresis of one or more specific muscles. Treatment is based upon these determinations.

The superior oblique is the most frequently involved, with the superior rectus the next most frequent. Isolated palsies of the inferior rectus and inferior oblique are uncommon.

A. Measurement of the Deviation: The deviation must be measured in the 6 cardinal directions of gaze both for near and for distance vision, and with each eye fixing. Secondary deviation is larger than primary deviation (see p 178); therefore, the deviation measured while the eye containing the paretic muscle

is fixing will be larger than that measured while the eye with the nonparetic muscle is fixing. In general, a deviation that is greater for near than for distance vision implicates an oblique muscle rather than a rectus muscle and vice versa, since in adduction (position of the eyes for near vision) the eyes depend more upon the oblique muscles than the rectus muscles for elevation and depression. With the eyes in the straight-ahead position (as for distance vision), the rectus muscles are more prominent as elevators and depressors than are the oblique muscles.

The deviation in the cardinal directions is measured with prisms. In general, if deviation is greater in one of the cardinal directions, this points toward a specific vertical muscle paralysis. For example, in right hypertropia, if the deviation is greater with the eyes up and to the right, this indicates underaction of the left inferior oblique muscle.

B. Head Tilt (Bielschowsky's) Test (Fig 15–17): A person with a paretic oblique muscle may tilt his or her head toward one shoulder. This is often useful in diagnosing paralysis of an oblique muscle. Normally, when tilting the head toward the right shoulder, the incycloductors of the right eye (superior oblique and superior rectus) and the excycloductors of the left eye (inferior oblique and inferior rectus) tend to cycloduct each eye to neutralize the tilted head position. The oblique muscle predominates in this torsion movement. For example, if the right superior oblique is paretic, the patient will have a right hypertropia and carry his or her head tilted to the left. This is because the intorsional movement of the right eye is in this instance produced by the right superior rectus; its

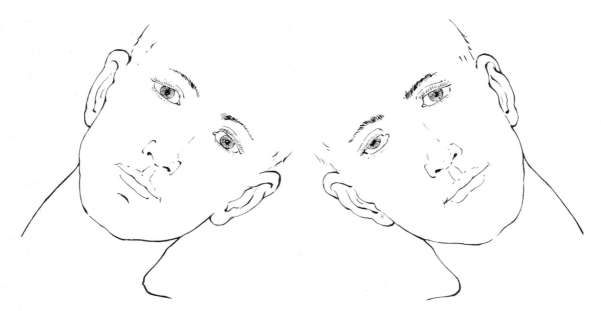

Figure 15–17. Head tilt test (Bielschowsky). *Left:* Paresis of right superior oblique muscle. Head is carried to shoulder on sound side (left), where fusion is obtained. This is a postural attitude called a "head tilt." *Right:* When the head is tilted to the shoulder on the paretic side, the right hypertropia becomes exaggerated. This is a positive forced head tilt test of Bielschowsky.

elevating action is unopposed, since its antagonist in vertical movement is the right superior oblique. With the head tilted to the left, the excycloduction (see p 178) required of the right eye is accomplished by the right inferior oblique and right inferior rectus. The vertical component is balanced, and no hypertropia is present. Thus, in order to avoid vertical diplopia, the patient will usually carry his or her head tilted to the left.

The head tilt test of Bielschowsky utilizes the above principle to aid in the diagnosis of paretic oblique muscles. The patient fixes a light at 6 meters (20 feet). The eye to be tested may be placed under cover (still visible to the examiner), but this is not necessary. The head is tilted first toward one shoulder and then the other. An increased hypertropia is diagnostic of oblique paralysis.

Example: The right eye is covered (may be left uncovered) and the head is tilted 45 degrees upon the right shoulder. The eye moves upward. This indicates paralysis of the right superior oblique muscle. This occurs upon tilting the head because the 2 incycloductors (right superior rectus and right superior oblique) receive impulses to contract (as above). In addition to their synergistic function of incycloduction, these muscles are antagonistic in the function of elevation and depression; the normal superior rectus (elevation) will not be balanced by the paretic superior oblique (depression), and the eye will elevate.

C. Sensory Changes in Hypertropia: As in other forms of strabismus, a sensory adaptation will take place if the strabismus has its onset before age 6. The sensory pattern may vary with the position of the eyes, so that suppression or even abnormal retinal correspondence may be present in the direction of gaze of strabismus and normal retinal correspondence without suppression in directions of gaze where strabismus is absent. If the onset is after age 6, there is no sensory adaptation and diplopia is constant.

Treatment

A. Conservative Treatment: In smaller deviations, usually under 10 diopters with relatively comitant strabismus, prisms may neutralize the hypertropia. In the case of a right hypertropia of 8 diopters, a 4-diopter prism base-down, right eye, and a 4-diopter prism base-up, left eye, may be incorporated into the eyeglasses and fusion reestablished. With larger deviations or in cases where the strabismus is noncomitant even though not of great magnitude, surgery is usually indicated. If there are medical contraindications, such as systemic disease, or if there is a good possibility that the strabismus may clear or improve subsequently, temporizing measures are necessary to relieve the diplopia. This frequently consists of patching one eye. When hypertropia is due to a complication of a systemic disease, treatment of the underlying disease will materially affect the hypertropia (eg, myasthenia gravis).

B. Surgical Treatment: Many approaches are used in the surgical treatment of hypertropia. The recent tendency has been to strengthen the weakened muscle. At times it may be necessary to weaken the direct antagonist or the yoke muscle, or both. The vertically acting rectus muscles can be recessed or resected in the same manner as the horizontally acting rectus muscles, although within somewhat smaller limits. The superior oblique muscle can be strengthened by tucking the tendon. This effectively shortens the superior oblique tendon by as much as 10 mm and therefore strengthens the muscle. The superior oblique muscle can also be weakened by intrasheath tenotomy in which the sheath of the superior oblique tendon is opened and a full tenotomy performed. The sheath is then resutured. This gives a fairly predictable amount of correction, usually about 15 diopters. The inferior oblique muscle can be effectively weakened by a recession of 8–10 mm, or by myotomy. A number of other operations that both strengthen and weaken the vertical muscles are available but are used less commonly.

HETEROPHORIA

Heterophoria is a deviation of the eyes that is held in check by the fusion mechanism. Almost all individuals have some degree of heterophoria, so that small amounts are considered normal. Larger degrees of heterophoria may be a cause of "eyestrain" (asthenopia), since a strain is placed upon the extraocular muscles to overcome the latent deviation. From a causative standpoint, heterophoria and heterotropia differ only in degree. The same causal concepts that have been discussed above apply to the 3 types of heterophoria. As with heterotropia, many of the causal factors are unknown. Heterophoria is clinically significant only if it causes symptoms. Symptoms will not always correlate well with the degree of heterophoria, since the personality and occupation of the individual are important in determining the nature of the complaints.

Asthenopia ("eyestrain") as a symptom of heterophoria takes a wide variety of forms. There may be a feeling of tiredness or discomfort of the eyes varying from a dull ache to deep pain located in or behind the eyes. Headaches of all types occur. Easy fatigability, blurring of vision, and diplopia, especially after prolonged, intense use of the eyes, also occur.

In general, the same diagnostic tests used in evaluating heterotropia are used for heterophoria. The most important test is the cover-uncover test, which allows one to differentiate a heterophoria from heterotropia.

The Maddox rod with prism measurement is especially useful in evaluating measurements in the cardinal directions of gaze when dealing with hyperphoria.

The sensory pattern as determined by the

amblyoscope is nearly always normal, including normal retinal correspondence and absence of suppression or amblyopia.

The **prism vergence test** determines whether an individual has the reserve fusional mechanism required to overcome any heterophoria that is present. The test is carried out by asking the patient to fixate on a small light at 6 meters (20 feet) with both eyes uncovered. Prisms of gradually increasing strength or the rotary prism of Risley in gradually increasing strengths are placed before one eye until diplopia occurs ("break point"). This is done with both base-in and base-out prism measurements for both near and distance vision. This measures the fusional convergence and divergence, respectively. Prisms are used base-up or base-down to measure the relative vertical divergence. (Positive vertical divergence if the right eye is directed upward; negative vertical divergence if the left eye is directed upward.) In calculating the numerical results of these tests, one must use the reading for distance heterophoria as a starting point. The normal values for prism vergence at 6 meters (20 feet) are as follows: prism divergence, 7 diopters; prism convergence, 20 diopters; vertical divergence, 5 diopters. At 33 cm (13 inches), the values are as follows: prism divergence, 20 diopters; prism convergence, 20 diopters; vertical divergence, 5 diopters.

DISCUSSION & TREATMENT OF HETEROPHORIA

Esophoria

Esophoria greater than 3 diopters for near or distance vision may cause asthenopic symptoms.

A. Significant Esophoria for Near and Distance Vision: If the patient has uncorrected hyperopia, the addition of plus sphere to the correction, or the prescription of eyeglasses if not previously worn, may relieve the symptoms. Less accommodation is thus required both for near and for distance vision, and so less convergence is induced. If full hyperopic correction still leaves a significant esophoria, base-out prism equally divided in the 2 spectacle lenses may be prescribed. One-half to one-third of the residual deviation is usually prescribed, although more than a total of 4 prism diopters is usually poorly tolerated. If symptoms persist and optical methods are unsatisfactory, surgery is indicated. It is usually necessary to operate on only one muscle, most often a recession of a medial rectus muscle.

B. Significant Esophoria for Near and Not for Distance Vision: In this instance, the complaint is "tired eyes" or other symptoms upon reading or using the eyes for close work. Treatment by optical methods is usually satisfactory. In the case of a hyperope who has been wearing full correction, the addition of more plus sphere for reading (up to 2 or 2.5 diopters) will often be helpful. This reduces necessary accommodation and accompanying convergence, so that it is pos-

sible to reduce or nullify the esophoria. In the case of a myopic individual, the same principle can be applied, giving less minus correction. If significant esophoria persists, base-out prism may be added to the prescription and adjusted until the symptoms disappear. In rare instances, if optical devices fail, a recession of one medial rectus muscle may be performed.

Exophoria

Larger amounts of exophoria are tolerated than of esophoria, particularly for near vision where it is not unusual to have a measurement of 7–10 diopters without symptoms. Exophoria above 3 diopters for distance vision is considered abnormal.

A. Significant Exophoria for Near and Distance Vision: With exophoria it is more difficult to overcome the phoria by manipulating the power of the eyeglasses. Undercorrection or no correction in the hyperope induces more accommodation and thus convergence, which helps to nullify exophoria. Similarly, overcorrection in myopes accomplishes the same result (stimulates accommodation). More commonly, base-in prism equally divided between the 2 eyes, correcting one-fourth to one-half of the deviation, is the treatment of choice. If the deviation is too large, usually above 15 diopters, or if spectacles with prisms do not relieve symptoms, recession of a lateral rectus muscle is indicated.

B. Significant Exophoria for Near and Not for Distance Vision: Base-in prisms are incorporated in spectacles used only for close work. One-fourth to one-half of the deviation is neutralized with prisms. If prisms fail, and particularly if poor convergence is also present, resection of one or both medial rectus muscles is indicated (depending on the degree of exophoria).

C. Significant Exophoria for Distance and Not for Near Vision: The same principle applies as above except that the prism correction must be placed in the distance glasses and a separate pair of eyeglasses used for near vision. Occasionally there will be a large exophoric deviation for distance and a relatively small one for near vision. If the deviation for distance is 15 diopters or more, surgery may be indicated, depending upon the severity of symptoms and the patient's occupation. The procedure of choice is recession of one or both lateral rectus muscles.

Hyperphoria

This is a frequent cause of asthenopia. Symptoms are often present if the deviation is 2–4 diopters or more. In very high degrees of hyperphoria, a paretic muscle may be diagnosed and surgery (as described for hypertropia) is indicated to strengthen the paretic muscle or weaken its antagonist or yoke muscle. Lesser degrees of deviation can be corrected with prisms. It is important to measure the hyperphoria in the cardinal directions of gaze for both near and distance vision. If the deviation proves to be comitant or nearly comitant, neutralizing vertical prisms, base-down in front of the higher eye and base-up in front of the lower eye, equally divided, are effective. It is usually necessary to neutralize one-third to one-half the deviation in this manner. If the deviation is noncomitant, treatment may be difficult. Symptoms will usually then be produced only under certain conditions. For example, in driving, if the deviation is greatest with the eyes straight ahead for distance, special prismatic driving glasses could be prescribed. In other cases the deviation is greatest for near vision in the reading position, in which case prisms could be incorporated into reading glasses or into the reading segment of bifocals.

Dissociated Vertical Divergence (Alternating Sursumduction, or Double Hyperphoria)

Dissociated vertical divergence is frequently associated with congenital esotropia, much less frequently with exotropia, sometimes with vertical muscle imbalances, and occasionally with otherwise normal muscle balance. The cause is not known. It is important to differentiate this condition from true hypertropia or hyperphoria to avoid inappropriate treatment. There are no symptoms, and no treatment is indicated except for cosmetic reasons (eg, one eye noticeably elevated much or all of the time).

The diagnosis is made by having the patient fixate a light at 6 meters (20 feet) while one eye is covered. The eye under cover is noted to deviate upward. When the cover is switched to the other eye, the opposite eye takes up fixation, while the one under cover now deviates upward. With the cover removed, the eyes usually return to straight ahead. As a rule, no true overaction of the inferior oblique muscles exists, and in most cases no A or V pattern is present. The deviation is often symmetric, but one eye sometimes goes up under cover much farther than the other eye.

Much interest has developed in the surgical treatment of cosmetically significant dissociated vertical divergence. Good results have been reported following large recessions (12–14 mm) of the superior rectus muscle and with the Faden operation, in which a small recession of the superior rectus is combined with a suture that anchors the muscle to the globe about 15 mm behind its insertion.

Cyclophoria

Cyclophoria is a rare disorder characterized by abnormal torsional movements held in check by fusion. There is some dispute about its importance, but it certainly may cause asthenopia. Treatment is quite difficult.

•   •   •

References

Apt L, Isenberg S: Eye position of strabismus patients under general anesthesia. *Am J Ophthalmol* 1977;**84**:574.

Burian HM: Strabismus: Past, present and future. *J Pediatr Ophthalmol* 1974;**11**:107.

Duke-Elder S: *System of Ophthalmology.* Vol 6. Mosby, 1973.

Dunlap EA: Inferior oblique weakening: Recession, myotomy, myectomy, or disinsertion? *Ann Ophthalmol* 1972;**4**:905.

Dyer JA: *Atlas of Extraocular Muscle Surgery.* Saunders, 1970.

Foster RS, Paul TO, Jampolsky A: Management of infantile esotropia. *Am J Ophthalmol* 1976;**82**:291.

Helveston EM: *Atlas of Strabismus Surgery,* 2nd ed. Mosby, 1977.

Hurtt J, Rasicovici A, Windsor CE: *Comprehensive Review of Orthoptics and Ocular Motility,* 2nd ed. Mosby, 1977.

Ingram RM: Refraction as a basis for screening children for squint and amblyopia. *Br J Ophthalmol* 1977;**61**:8.

Knapp P: Use of membrane prisms. *Trans Am Acad Ophthalmol Otolaryngol* 1975;**79**:718.

Moses RA (editor): *Adler's Physiology of the Eye: Clinical Application,* 7th ed. Mosby, 1981.

Magoon E, Cruciger M, Jampolsky A: Dissociated vertical deviation: An asymmetric condition treated with large superior rectus recession. *J Pediatr Ophthalmol Strabismus* 1982;**19**:152.

New Orleans Academy of Ophthalmology: *Symposium on Strabismus.* Mosby, 1977.

O'Malley ER, Helveston EM, Ellis FD: Duane's retraction syndrome-plus. *J Pediatr Ophthalmol Strabismus* 1982;**19**:161.

Parks MM: *Ocular Motility and Strabismus.* Harper & Row, 1975.

Parks MM: The weakening surgical procedures for eliminating overaction of the inferior oblique muscle. *Am J Ophthalmol* 1972;**73**:107.

Reinecke RD (editor): *Strabismus: Proceedings of the Third Meeting of the International Strabismological Association.* Grune & Stratton, 1979.

Romano PE, Robinson JA: General anesthesia morbidity and mortality in eye surgery at a children's hospital. *J Pediatr Ophthalmol Strabismus* 1981;**18**:17.

Rosenbaum AL, Jampolsky A, Scott AB: Bimedial recession in high AC/A esotropia. *Arch Ophthalmol* 1974;**91**:251.

Vasquez R, Calhoun JH, Harley RD: Development of monofixational syndrome in congenital esotropia. *J Pediatr Ophthalmol Strabismus* 1981;**18**:42.

Von Noorden GK: New clinical aspects of stimulus deprivation amblyopia. *Am J Ophthalmol* 1981;**92**:416.

Von Noorden GK: Nystagmus blockage syndrome. *Trans Am Ophthalmol Soc* 1976;**74**:220.

Von Noorden GK: *Von Noorden-Maumenee's Atlas of Strabismus,* 3rd ed. Mosby, 1977.

Watson PG (editor): Strabismus. (Symposium.) *Br J Ophthalmol* 1974;**58**:157.

16 | Orbit

ANATOMY

The orbital cavity is schematically represented as a pyramid of 4 walls that converge posteriorly. The medial walls of the right and left orbit are parallel and are separated by the nose. In each orbit the lateral and medial walls form an angle of 45 degrees, which results in a right angle between the 2 lateral walls. The orbit is compared to the shape of a pear, with the optic nerve representing its stem. The anterior circumference is somewhat smaller in diameter than the region just within the rim, which makes a sturdy protective margin.

The orbits are related to the frontal sinus above, the maxillary sinus below, and the ethmoid and sphenoid sinuses medially. The thin orbital floor is easily damaged by direct trauma to the globe, resulting in a "blowout" fracture with herniation of orbital contents into the maxillary antrum. Infection within

the sphenoid and ethmoid sinuses can erode the paper-thin medial wall (lamina papyracea) and involve the contents of the orbit. Erosion of the roof (eg, neurofibromatosis) may result in visible pulsations of the globe transmitted from the brain.

Orbital Walls

The roof of the orbit is composed principally of the orbital plate of the **frontal bone.** The lacrimal gland is located in the lacrimal fossa in the anterior lateral aspect of the roof. Posteriorly, the lesser wing of the **sphenoid bone** containing the optic canal completes the roof.

The lateral wall is separated from the roof by the superior orbital fissure, which divides the lesser from the greater wing of the **sphenoid bone.** The anterior portion of the lateral wall is formed by the orbital surface of the **zygomatic (malar) bone.** This is the strongest part of the bony orbit. Suspensory ligaments,

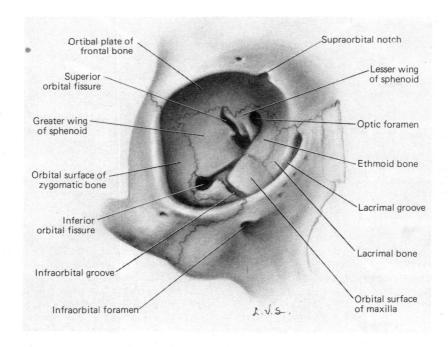

Figure 16–1. Anterior view of bones of right orbit.

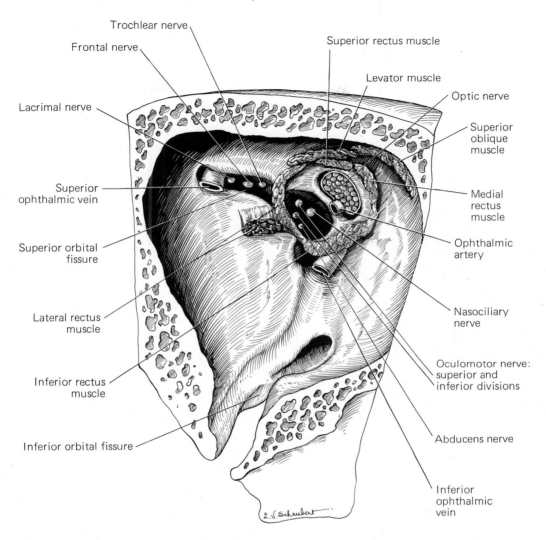

Figure 16–2. Anterior view of apex of right orbit.

the lateral palpebral tendon, and check ligaments have their connective tissue attachment to the lateral orbital tubercle.

The orbital floor is separated from the lateral wall by the inferior orbital fissure. The orbital plate of the **maxilla** forms the large central area of the floor and is the region where blowout fractures most frequently occur. The frontal process of the **maxilla** medially and the **zygomatic bone** laterally complete the inferior orbital rim. The orbital process of the **palatine bone** forms a small triangular area in the posterior floor.

The boundaries of the medial wall are less distinct. The **ethmoid** bone is paper-thin but thickens anteriorly as it meets the **lacrimal bone.** The body of the **sphenoid** forms the most posterior aspect of the medial wall, and the angular process of the **frontal bone** forms the upper part of the posterior lacrimal crest. The lower portion of the posterior lacrimal crest is made up of the **lacrimal bone.** The anterior lacrimal

crest is easily palpated through the lid and is composed of the frontal process of the **maxilla.** The lacrimal groove lies between the 2 crests and contains the lacrimal sac.

Contents of the Orbit

The volume of the adult orbit is approximately 30 mL, and the eyeball occupies only about one-fifth of the space. Fat and muscle account for the bulk of the remainder.

The anterior limit of the orbital cavity is the **orbital septum.** It is a thin sheet of fascia extending from the orbital rim to the tarsus in the lower lid and to a point slightly above the border of the tarsus in the upper lid. The orbital septum acts as a barrier between the eyelids and the orbit. The extraocular muscles are described and discussed in Chapter 15.

The principal arterial supply of the orbit and its structures derives from the **ophthalmic artery,** the

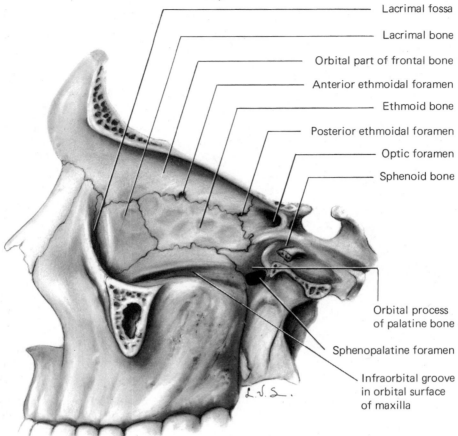

Lacrimal fossa

Lacrimal bone

Orbital part of frontal bone

Anterior ethmoidal foramen

Ethmoid bone

Posterior ethmoidal foramen

Optic foramen

Sphenoid bone

Orbital process
of palatine bone

Sphenopalatine foramen

Infraorbital groove
in orbital surface
of maxilla

Figure 16–3. Medial view of bony wall of left orbit.

first major branch of the intracranial portion of the internal carotid artery. This branch passes beneath the optic nerve and accompanies it through the optic canal into the orbit. The first intraorbital branch is the central retinal artery, which enters the optic nerve about 8–15 mm behind the globe. The ophthalmic artery also sends branches to the lacrimal gland as well as to the intraocular structures via the short, long, and anterior ciliary arteries. The most anterior branches contribute to the formation of the arterial arcades of the eyelids, which make an anastomosis with the external carotid circulation via the facial artery.

The venous drainage of the orbit is primarily through the superior and inferior orbital veins. The superior orbital vein is important because it drains the skin of the periorbital region directly to the cavernous sinus. This forms the basis of the potentially lethal septic cavernous sinus thrombosis resulting from a superficial infection in this region.

The apex of the orbit is the entry portal for all nerves and vessels to the eye and the site of origin of all extraocular muscles except the inferior oblique. Expanding lesions of the apex result in a predictable neurologic deficit known as the orbital apex syndrome. The nerves enter the orbit through the **superior orbital fissure.** In its pathway to the cavernous sinus, the

superior ophthalmic vein usually crosses at the highest point of the superior orbital fissure. Beneath the skin of the eyelid, this vein makes an anastomosis with the angular vein. The blood thus may drain posteriorly through the orbit or anteriorly to the facial vein.

The upper lateral aspect of the superior orbital fissure carries the **lacrimal nerve,** a branch of the first (ophthalmic) division of the trigeminal nerve. This small twig remains outside the area of origin of the rectus muscles (annulus of Zinn) and continues its lateral course in the orbit to terminate in the lacrimal gland, providing its sensory innervation. Slightly medial to the lacrimal nerve within the superior orbital fissure is the **frontal nerve,** which is the largest of the first division of branches of the trigeminal nerve. It also crosses over the annulus of Zinn and follows a course over the levator to the medial aspect of the orbit, where it divides into the supraorbital and supra-trochlear nerves. These provide sensation to the brow and forehead. The only other nerve to enter the orbit outside the annulus of Zinn is the **trochlear nerve.** Although the thinnest of the cranial nerves, the trochlear nerve has the longest intracranial course, and it is also the only nerve to originate on the dorsal surface of the brain stem. The fibers decussate before they emerge from the brain stem just before the inferior

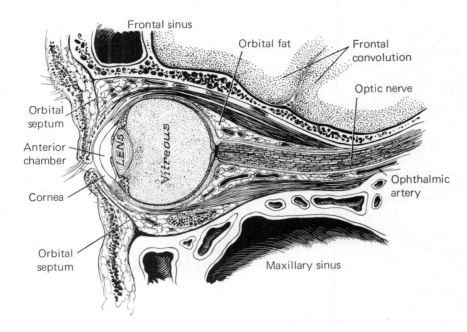

Figure 16—4. Orbital anatomy (right lateral view). (Redrawn and reproduced, with permission, from Wolff E: *Anatomy of the Eye and Orbit.* Blakiston-McGraw, 1954.)

colliculi, where they are subject to injury from the tentorium. The nerve pierces the dura behind the sella turcica and travels within the lateral wall of the cavernous sinus to enter the superior orbital fissure medial to the frontal nerve. From this point it travels within the periorbita of the roof over the levator muscle to the upper surface of the superior oblique muscle.

The rectus muscles originate from a fibrous ring (the annulus of Zinn), which surrounds the remainder of the superior orbital fissure as well as the optic canal. The superior division of the **oculomotor nerve** is adjacent to the trochlear nerve but lies within the annulus of Zinn at its highest point. The oculomotor nerve originates from between the cerebral peduncles and passes near the posterior communicating artery of the circle of Willis. Lateral to the pituitary gland, it is closely approximated to the optic tract, and here it pierces the dura to course in the lateral wall of the cavernous sinus. As the nerve leaves the cavernous sinus, it divides into superior and inferior divisions. The superior division enters high within the annulus of Zinn and passes over the optic nerve to innervate the levator and superior rectus muscles. The inferior division enters the annulus of Zinn low and passes below the optic nerve to supply the medial and inferior rectus muscles. A large branch from the inferior division extends forward to supply the inferior oblique. A small twig from the proximal end of the nerve to the inferior oblique carries parasympathetic fibers to the ciliary ganglion.

Between the superior and inferior divisions of the oculomotor nerve within the annulus of Zinn lie the last 2 orbital nerves. On the lateral aspect is the **abducens nerve,** and medially the **nasociliary nerve.** The abdu-

cens originates between the pons and medulla and pursues an extended course up the clivus to the posterior clinoid, penetrates the dura, and passes within the cavernous sinus. (All other nerves course through the lateral wall of the cavernous sinus.) After passing through the superior orbital fissure within the annulus of Zinn, the nerve continues laterally to innervate the lateral rectus muscle.

The nasociliary nerve is the third branch of the first (ophthalmic) division of the trigeminal nerve and is the sensory nerve of the eye. The trigeminal nerve originates from the pons, and its sensory roots form the trigeminal ganglion. The first of the 3 divisions passes through the lateral wall of the cavernous sinus and divides into the lacrimal, frontal, and nasociliary nerve. The nasociliary nerve, after entering through the annulus of Zinn, lies between the superior rectus and the optic nerve. It sends a branch to the ciliary ganglion and other branches to supply the cornea (the posterior ciliary nerves), eventually terminating near the tip of the nose. Thus, the skin on the tip of the nose may be affected with vesicular lesions prior to the onset of herpes zoster ophthalmicus.

The second (maxillary) division of the trigeminal nerve passes through the foramen rotundum and enters the orbit through the inferior orbital fissure. It passes through the infraorbital canal and exits via the infraorbital foramen, supplying sensation to the lower lid and adjacent cheek. It is frequently damaged in fractures of the orbital floor.

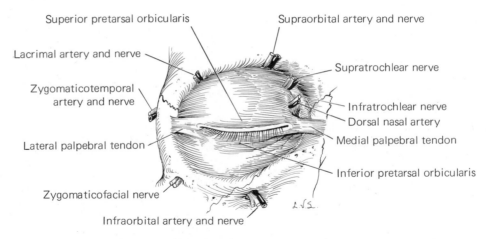

Superior pretarsal orbicularis

Lacrimal artery and nerve

Zygomaticotemporal artery and nerve

Lateral palpebral tendon

Zygomaticofacial nerve

Infraorbital artery and nerve

Supraorbital artery and nerve

Supratrochlear nerve

Infratrochlear nerve

Dorsal nasal artery

Medial palpebral tendon

Inferior pretarsal orbicularis

Figure 16–5. Vessels and nerves to extraocular structures.

PHYSIOLOGY OF SYMPTOMS

Owing to the rigid bony structure of the orbit, with only an anterior opening for expansion, any increase in the orbital contents taking place to the side of or behind the eyeball will displace that organ. Pressure behind the eyeball will push it forward (proptosis). Pressure on one side will displace the eyeball to the other side.

With the change in position of the eyeball, especially if it takes place rapidly, there may be enough interference with the movement of the eye to cause dissociation of ocular movements and diplopia (double vision). Pain is absent unless there is extreme swelling of the tissues or unless the eyelids are unable to protect the cornea adequately and there is irritation from exposure.

EXOPHTHALMOS
(Proptosis)

Etiology & Classification

Exophthalmos may be due to any of the following factors: (1) a space-occupying lesion in the rigid bony orbit, displacing the only moveable tissue, the eyeball; (2) swelling of the retrobulbar tissues through edema or hemorrhage, pushing the eyeball forward; (3) relaxation of the retracting effect of the extraocular muscles through paralysis or trauma; and (4) the apparent forward displacement (pseudoexophthalmos) seen with lid retraction (Graves's disease) and large eye (myopia, macrophthalmos).

A. Acute Exophthalmos:
1. Emphysema due to rupture of the medial orbital wall, allowing air from the sinus to enter the orbit.
2. Hemorrhage (traumatic or spontaneous).
3. Orbital cellulitis.

B. Pulsating Exophthalmos:
1. Carotid–cavernous sinus fistula.

2. Vascular tumors or aneurysms.
3. Cerebral pulsations due to a defect in the orbital roof.

C. Unilateral Exophthalmos:
1. Inflammatory—Cellulitis, pseudotumor of orbit, abscess, tenonitis, lacrimal gland inflammation, panophthalmitis, cavernous sinus thrombosis (may become bilateral).
2. Vascular—Hemorrhage, traumatic or spontaneous; varicosities, aneurysms.
3. Traumatic—Fracture, hemorrhage, rupture of the extraocular muscles, emphysema from sinuses, aneurysms.
4. Tumors—Primary, from the eye or orbital contents; spread from surrounding structures, metastatic.
5. Cysts—Congenital dermoid, parasitic, mucocele from surrounding sinuses.
6. Relaxation of retractors of eyeball, as with paralysis of the extraocular muscles.
7. General disease—Leukemia, lymphoma (frequently bilateral).

D. Bilateral Exophthalmos:
1. Endocrine—(Sometimes begins as unilateral exophthalmos.) Thyrotoxic (hyperthyroid, Graves's disease), thyrotropic (malignant, ophthalmoplegic).
2. Pseudoexophthalmos—Congenital macrophthalmos, high myopia, lid retraction (Graves's disease).

The most frequent primary orbital tumor in adults is cavernous hemangioma; the prognosis with surgery is good. The most common cause of proptosis—unilateral or bilateral—is Graves's disease. Mild exophthalmos and lid retraction associated with hyperthyroidism are usually completely reversible with appropriate medical therapy. Malignant exophthalmos (also called exophthalmic ophthalmoplegia and hyperophthalmic Graves's disease) is a progressive, more severe form. Eye signs may occur years before any detectable physical or biochemical abnormality. Tissue changes consist of lymphocytic infiltration and orbital edema. Massive hypertrophy of the extraocular muscles begins in the inferior oblique and inferior rectus. The resultant limitation of movement often becomes permanent when fibrosis ensues. Restricted upgaze with vertical diplopia is characteristic. In severe cases, there is intractable diplopia, corneal ulceration from inability to close the eyelids, and occasionally optic neuropathy from orbital compression. These changes are generally believed to originate in the pituitary gland, but as yet no laboratory correlation has been found. The diagnosis is made by demonstration of muscular hypertrophy on ultrasonography or CT scan.

Treatment of malignant exophthalmos is difficult. High doses of sytemic corticosteroids are sometimes effective. Orbital radiation has also been used with some success in selected cases. Lubrication of the cornea, particularly at night, may prevent serious damage. Optic neuropathy is an indication for surgical decompression of the orbit using the antral, temporal, or transcranial approach. Once the condition has stabilized, lid retraction can be corrected by retractor recession, scleral grafting, and tarsorraphy.

Sudden onset of unilateral proptosis in childhood is most frequently from malignant rhabdomyosarcoma. Bilateral proptosis in a child is usually a result of metastatic neuroblastoma. Optic nerve glioma also presents in children and is sometimes associated with café au lait spots.

Lymphomatous orbital tumors and most metastatic tumors occur after middle age and are usually suspected because of systemic involvement. Tumors originating from the lacrimal gland should be excised in toto rather than subjected to biopsy. Fifty percent of these tumors are malignant, and an incisional biopsy is associated with tumor seeding. When there is good evidence of a primary malignant lacrimal gland tumor, it is preferable to take a biopsy specimen through an incision of the eyelid to prevent seeding within the orbit. Exenteration plus x-ray therapy offers the only chance for survival of these highly malignant tumors.

A skilled clinician may suspect the diagnosis in a patient with proptosis but is greatly assisted by CT scan and ultrasonography. Venography is useful in the diagnosis of an orbital varix. Air or positive contrast orbitography is seldom indicated.

ENOPHTHALMOS

Retraction of the eye into the orbit is a normal change in elderly people that is due to senile atrophy of the orbital fat. Enophthalmos before age 25 occurs rarely as part of Horner's syndrome or because of atrophy of the orbital fat in hemifacial atrophy or following surgery.

The most common cause of enophthalmos is trauma. Fracture of the orbital floor results in herniation into the maxillary sinus. After severe contusion, orbital fat may absorb slowly for many months.

INFLAMMATORY ORBITAL DISEASES

ORBITAL CELLULITIS
(Fig 16–6)

Orbital cellulitis is usually caused by pneumococci, streptococci, or staphylococci, the same organisms that cause acute sinusitis. They enter the orbit by direct extension or through the vascular channels between the orbital contents and infected ethmoid, sphenoid, maxillary, or frontal sinuses.

Swelling and redness of the eyelids, chemosis, exophthalmos of varying degrees, and dull pain are usually present in mild cases. The onset is often sudden. More severe involvement may cause pain on rotation of the eyeball. Occasional intraocular hemorrhage and inflammatory signs are probably due to involvement of the vessels of the retina or choroid. Constitutional symptoms vary, according to the severity of the infection, from mild fever, malaise, and leukocytosis to high fever and marked debility. Infection may spread to the cavernous sinuses or meninges.

Orbital cellulitis must be differentiated from tenonitis, orbital periostitis, and cavernous sinus thrombosis. In children, rhabdomyosarcoma must be ruled out.

Almost all cases respond well to large doses of antibiotics. Hot compresses are useful to localize the inflammatory reaction. Unless the condition is growing steadily worse, surgical drainage should be delayed until absolutely necessary.

If antibiotics fail to bring the condition under control after a vigorous trial of 2–3 days, surgical drainage must be employed. The safest method is to make an incision into the area of greatest

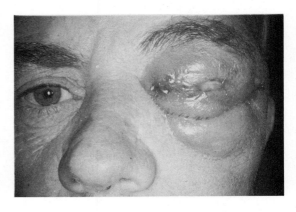

Figure 16–6. Orbital cellulitis. Abscess draining through upper eyelid.

fluctuation—avoiding, if possible, the areas of the trochlea of the superior oblique muscle and the lacrimal gland recess.

The response to antibiotics is generally good. If not, the infection may localize anteriorly and rupture or require drainage, or it may extend posteriorly, causing cavernous sinus thrombosis, meningitis, or brain abscess. Optic neuritis with secondary atrophy may follow severe inflammatory reactions. The visual prognosis is excellent in the absence of complications.

CAVERNOUS SINUS THROMBOSIS

Orbital signs and symptoms are usually associated with thrombosis of the cavernous sinus. Exophthalmos with edema of the orbit and eyelids, diminished or absent pupillary reflexes, impaired visual acuity, and papilledema are usually present. Since the third, fourth, and sixth cranial nerves and the ophthalmic division of the fifth cranial nerve traverse the cavernous sinus, involvement of these nerves leads to paresis of the respective muscles and limitations of ocular movement. Fever is of the septic type.

Thrombosis of the cavernous sinus is usually due to infection spreading along the venous channels that drain the orbit, central face, throat, and nasal cavities.

Differentiation from orbital cellulitis is sometimes necessary. Cavernous sinus thrombosis may be bilateral, whereas orbital cellulitis is almost always unilateral. In cellulitis the pupillary reflexes remain normal, there is no papilledema, and pain and tenderness are more severe.

Massive doses of systemic antibiotics are necessary. Prophylactic chemotherapy and avoidance of manipulation of pyogenic infections, which may drain into the cavernous sinus, are of the greatest importance.

Since the pyogenic bacteria are usually responsible, most patients can be saved with good visual recovery. Before the antibiotics became available, all patients died.

PSEUDOTUMOR OF ORBIT

Pseudotumor of the orbit is an uncommon inflammatory reaction, usually unilateral, that clinically resembles a neoplasm. The histopathologic features may vary from vasculitis to a generalized lymphocytic inflammation. Exophthalmos is a prominent clinical finding. Many bacteria, viruses, parasites, and other possible causes have been investigated, but the cause has not been determined.

Inflammatory pseudotumor is characterized by restriction of ocular movement, exophthalmos with occasional lateral displacement, swelling of the lids, and resistance to retrodisplacement of the eye with finger pressure. Pain and diplopia are present in about one-half of cases. The onset is usually gradual, and other signs of inflammation such as are seen with the more acute orbital cellulitis are not present.

The resemblance of pseudotumor to neoplasm may lead to exploratory orbital surgery; biopsy of the tissue reveals only signs of chronic inflammation or granuloma.

Treatment is often difficult. Anti-infective chemotherapeutic and antibiotic drugs and x-ray radiation have been tried without effect. Systemic steroids in high doses have proved to be effective in many cases. Therapy may have to be continued for weeks or months to prevent serious relapse. If the swollen, chronically inflamed tissues impinge upon the optic nerve, there may be permanent damage to the optic nerve. Corticosteroid therapy decreases the chances of optic atrophy.

A significant number of patients with orbital pseudotumor later manifest systemic neoplastic disease.

●   ●   ●

References

American Academy of Ophthalmology: Sec 9, pp 17–72, in: *Orbit Eyelids & Lacrimal System*. American Academy of Ophthalmology Manual, 1981.

Beard C, Quickert MH: *Anatomy of the Orbit*. Aesculapius, 1969.

Blodi FC: Pathology of orbital bones: The 32nd Edward Jackson memorial lecture. *Am J Ophthalmol* 1976;**81**:1.

Converse JM, Smith B: On the treatment of blowout fractures of the orbit. (Editorial.) *Plast Reconstr Surg* 1978;**62**:100.

Donaldson SS et al: Supervoltage orbital radiotherapy for Graves's ophthalmopathy. *J Clin Endocrinol Metab* 1973; **37**:276.

Garner A: Pathology of "pseudotumors" of the orbit: A review. *J Clin Pathol* 1973;**26**:639.

Grove AS: Evaluation of exophthalmos. *N Engl J Med* 1975;**292**:1005.

Grove AS et al: Symposium on orbital diseases. *Trans Am Acad Ophthalmol Otolaryngol* 1979;**86**:854.

Henderson JW: *Orbital Tumors,* 2nd ed. Saunders, 1980.

Jakobiec FA: *Ocular and Adnexal Tumors*. Aesculapius, 1978.

Jones IS, Jakobiec FA: *Diseases of the Orbit*. Harper & Row, 1979.

Koornneef L: Orbital septa: Anatomy and function. *Ophthalmology* 1979;**86**:876.

Londer L, Nelson DL: Orbital cellulitis due to *Haemophilus influenzae*. *Arch Ophthalmol* 1974;**91**:89.

Moseley I, Sanders M: *Computerized Tomography in Neuro-ophthalmology*. Saunders, 1982.

Ogura JH, Pratt LL: Transantral decompression for malignant exophthalmos. *Otolaryngol Clin North Am* 1971;**4**:193.

Trokel SL: The orbit: Annual review. *Arch Ophthalmol* 1974;**91**:223.

Trokel SL, Jakobiec FA: Correlation of CT scanning and pathologic features of ophthalmic Graves' disease. *Ophthalmology* 1981;**88**:553.

Unsöld R, Newton TH, De Groot J: CT-evaluation of extraocular muscles: Anatomic-CT-correlations. *Albrecht Von Graefes Arch Klin Exp Ophthalmol* 1980;**214**:155.

Von Noorden GK: Orbital cellulitis following extraocular muscle surgery. *Am J Ophthalmol* 1972;**74**:627.

Warwick R: *Eugene Wolff's Anatomy of the Eye and Orbit,* 7th ed. Saunders, 1976.

17 | Neuro-ophthalmology

The eyes are intimately related to the brain and frequently give important diagnostic clues to central nervous system disorders. Indeed, the optic nerve is a part of the central nervous system. Intracranial disease frequently causes visual disturbances because of destruction of or pressure upon some portion of the optic pathways. Cranial nerves III, IV, and VI, which control ocular movements, may be involved, and nerves V and VII are also intimately associated with ocular function.

THE SENSORY VISUAL PATHWAY

Topographic Overview (Fig 17–1)

The second cranial nerve subserves the special sense of vision. Light is detected by the rods and cones of the retina, which may be considered the special sensory end organ for vision. The cell bodies of these receptors extend processes that synapse with the bipolar cell, the second neuron in the visual pathway. The bipolar cells synapse, in turn, with the retinal ganglion cells. Ganglion cell axons comprise the nerve fiber layer of the retina and converge to form the optic nerve. The nerve emerges from the back of the globe and travels posteriorly within the muscle cone to enter the cranial cavity via the optic canal.

Intracranially, the 2 optic nerves join to form the optic chiasm. At the chiasm, more than half of the fibers (those from the nasal half of the retina) decussate and join the uncrossed temporal fibers of the opposite nerve to form the optic tracts. All of the fibers receiving impulses from the right half of the visual field thus make up the left optic tract and project to the left cerebral hemisphere. Similarly, the left half of the visual field projects to the right cerebral hemisphere. Each optic tract sweeps around the cerebral peduncle toward the lateral geniculate nucleus. Twenty percent of the fibers in the tract subserve pupillary function. These fibers leave the tract just anterior to the nucleus and pass via the brachium of the superior colliculus to the midbrain. The remaining fibers synapse in the lateral geniculate nucleus. The cell bodies of this structure give rise to the geniculocalcarine tract. This tract passes through the posterior limb of the internal capsule and then fans into the optic radiations that traverse parts of the temporal and parietal lobes en route to the occipital cortex.

Detection of Lesions in the Visual Pathways

The primary method of localizing lesions of the visual pathways is by central and peripheral visual field examination. The technique is discussed on p 19. Fig 17–2 shows the types of field defects caused by lesions in various locations of the pathway. Lesions anterior to the chiasm (of the retina or optic nerve) cause unilateral field defects; lesions anywhere in the visual pathway posterior to the chiasm cause contralateral homonymous defects. These may be congruent (ie, identical in size, shape, and location) or incongruent. Chiasmal lesions usually cause bitemporal defects.

Multiple isopters (field tests with several objects of different sizes) should be used in order to evaluate the defects thoroughly. A field defect shows evidence of actively spreading disease when there are areas of "relative scotoma" (ie, a larger field defect for a smaller test object). Such visual field defects are said to be "sloping." This is in contrast to vascular lesions with steep borders (ie, the defect is the same size no matter what size test object is used).

Another important generalization is that the more congruous the homonymous field defects (ie, the more similar the 2 fields), the farther posterior the lesion is in the visual pathway. A lesion in the occipital region causes identical defects in each field, whereas optic tract lesions cause incongruous (dissimilar) homonymous field defects. Also, the more posterior the lesion, the more likely that there will be macular sparing and, therefore, maintenance of good visual acuity.

THE OPTIC NERVE

Anatomy (Fig 17–3)

The optic nerve is a trunk consisting of about 1.1 million axons arising from the ganglion cells of the retina. The nerve emerges from the back of the globe through a short, circular opening (0.7 mm long, 1.5 mm in diameter) in the sclera situated 1 mm below and 3 mm nasal to the posterior pole of the eye. The orbital portion is 25–30 mm long and travels posteriorly within the muscle cone. The nerve then passes via the bony optic canal into the cranial cavity. This intracanalicular portion measures 4–9 mm. After a 10-mm intracranial course, the nerve joins the opposite optic nerve to form the optic chiasm.

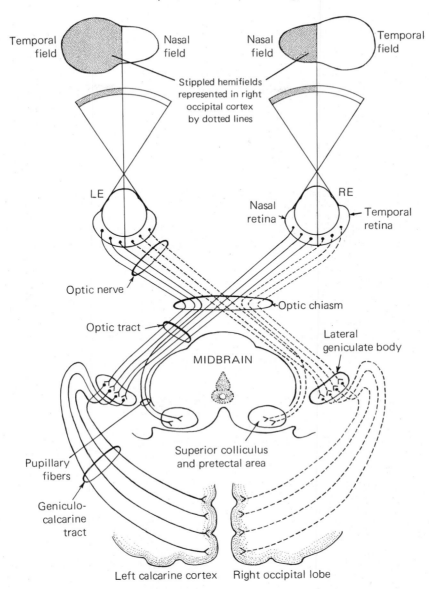

Figure 17–1. The optic pathway. The dotted lines represent nerve fibers from the retina to the occipital cortex that carry visual and pupillary afferent impulses from the left half of the visual field.

The nerve fibers become myelinated upon leaving the eye and are supported by neuroglia; this increases the diameter from 1.5 mm (within the sclera) to 3 mm (within the orbit). Eighty percent of the nerve is made up of visual fibers en route to synapse in the lateral geniculate nucleus. The twenty percent that are pupillary bypass the lateral geniculate nucleus en route to the pretectal area. Since the ganglion cells of the retina and their axons that make up the optic nerve are actually extensions of the central nervous system, they have no capacity to regenerate if severed.

Sheaths of the Optic Nerve (Fig 17–3)

The fibrous wrappings that ensheath the optic nerve are continuous with the meninges. The pia mater is loosely attached about the nerve near the chiasm and only for a short distance within the cranium, but it is closely attached around most of the intracanalicular and all of the intraorbital portions. The pia consists of some fibrous tissue with numerous small blood vessels. It divides the nerve fibers into bundles by sending numerous septa into the nerve substance. The pia continues to the sclera, with a few fibers running into the choroid and lamina cribrosa.

The arachnoid comes in contact with the optic nerve at the intracranial end of the optic canal and accompanies the nerve to the globe, where it ends in the sclera and overlying dura. This sheath is a diapha-

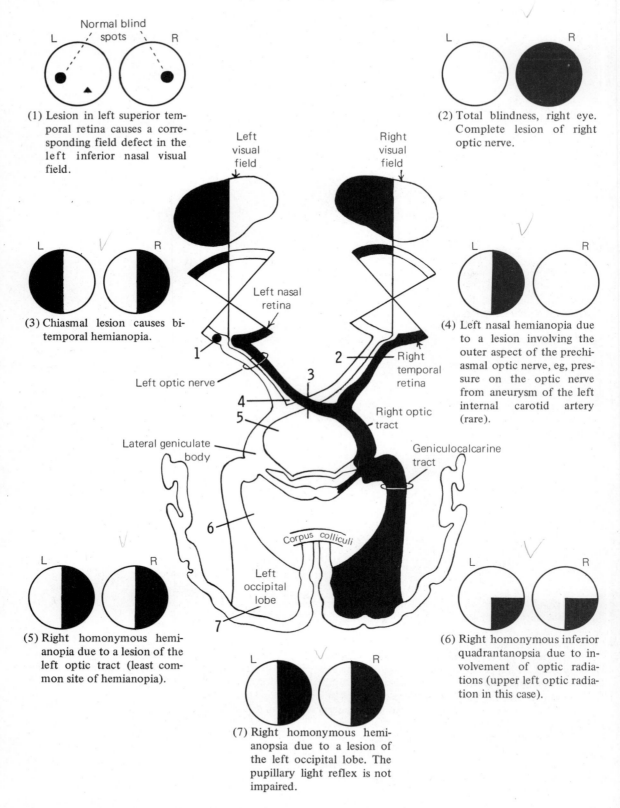

Normal blind spots

(1) Lesion in left superior temporal retina causes a corresponding field defect in the left inferior nasal visual field.

(2) Total blindness, right eye. Complete lesion of right optic nerve.

Left visual field

Right visual field

(3) Chiasmal lesion causes bitemporal hemianopia.

Left nasal retina

Left optic nerve

Right temporal retina

Right optic tract

Lateral geniculate body

Geniculocalcarine tract

Corpus colliculi

Left occipital lobe

(4) Left nasal hemianopia due to a lesion involving the outer aspect of the prechiasmal optic nerve, eg, pressure on the optic nerve from aneurysm of the left internal carotid artery (rare).

(5) Right homonymous hemianopia due to a lesion of the left optic tract (least common site of hemianopia).

(6) Right homonymous inferior quadrantanopsia due to involvement of optic radiations (upper left optic radiation in this case).

(7) Right homonymous hemianopsia due to a lesion of the left occipital lobe. The pupillary light reflex is not impaired.

Figure 17–2. The visual system; topographic diagnosis. (Modified and reproduced, with permission, from Chusid JG: *Correlative Neuroanatomy & Functional Neurology,* 18th ed. Lange, 1982.)

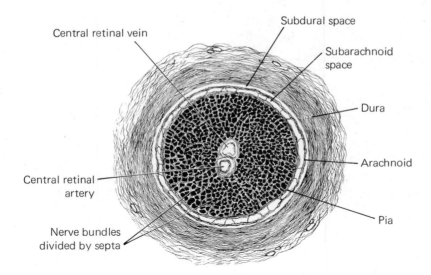

Figure 17–3. Cross section of the optic nerve. (Redrawn and reproduced, with permission, from Wolff E: *Anatomy of the Eye and Orbit,* 6th ed. Blakiston-McGraw, 1968.)

nous connective tissue membrane with many septate connections with the pia mater, which it closely resembles. It is more intimately associated with pia than with dura.

The dura mater lining the inner surface of the cranial vault comes in contact with the optic nerve as it leaves the optic canal. As the nerve enters the orbit from the optic canal, the dura splits, one layer (the periorbita) lining the orbital cavity and the other forming the outer dural covering of the optic nerve. The dura becomes continuous with the outer two-thirds of the sclera. The dura consists of tough, fibrous, relatively avascular tissue lined by endothelium on the inner surface.

The subdural space is between the dura and arachnoid; the subarachnoid space is between the pia

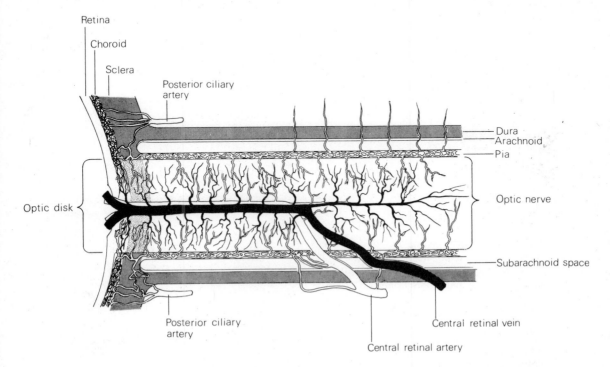

Figure 17–4. Blood supply of the optic nerve. (Redrawn and reproduced, with permission, from Hayreh SS: *Trans Am Acad Ophthalmol Otolaryngol* 1974;**78**:240.)

and the arachnoid. Both are more potential than actual spaces under normal conditions but are direct continuations of their corresponding intracranial spaces. Subarachnoid or subdural fluid under sufficient pressure will fill these potential spaces about the optic nerve. The meningeal layers are adherent to each other and to the optic nerve and the surrounding bone within the optic foramen, making the optic nerve resistant to traction from either end.

DISEASES OF THE OPTIC NERVE

Etiologic Classification
A. Idiopathic optic neuritis.
B. Demyelinating Diseases:
  1. Multiple sclerosis.
  2. Other rare demyelinating syndromes–
     a. Neuromyelitis optica (Devic's disease).
     b. Diffuse periaxial encephalitis (Schilder's disease).
C. Viral Infections:
  1. Postviral optic neuritis (measles, mumps, chickenpox, influenza).
  2. Postinfectious encephalomyelitis.
  3. Polyradiculoneuronitis (Guillain-Barré syndrome).
  4. Infectious mononucleosis.
  5. Herpes zoster.
D. Local Extension of Inflammatory Disease:
  1. Sinusitis.
  2. Intracranial–Meningitis, encephalitis.
  3. Orbital–Cellulitis, vasculitis.
  4. Intraocular–Chorioretinitis, endophthalmitis, iridocyclitis.
E. Systemic Infections and Inflammation:
  1. Syphilis.
  2. Tuberculosis.
  3. Cryptococcosis.
  4. Coccidioidomycosis.
  5. Infective endocarditis.
  6. Sarcoidosis.
F. Nutritional and Metabolic:
  1. Diabetes mellitus.
  2. Dysthyroidism.
  3. Vitamin deficiencies–Beriberi, pellagra.
G. Toxic:
  1. Tobacco-alcohol amblyopia.
  2. Heavy metal–Arsenic, lead, thallium.
  3. Drugs–Ethambutol, isoniazid, streptomycin, disulfiram, digitalis, chloramphenicol, chloroquine, chlorpropamide, halogenated hydroxyquinones (eg, iodochlorhydroxyquin).
  4. Methanol.
H. Hereditary Optic Atrophy:
  1. Leber's disease.
  2. Dominant (juvenile) optic atrophy.
  3. Recessive (infantile) optic atrophy.
  4. Behr's syndrome.
I. Vascular Disease:
  1. Cranial arteritis.
  2. Arteriosclerosis (anterior ischemic optic neuropathy).
  3. Polyarteritis nodosa.
  4. Takayasu's disease.
J. Neoplastic:
  1. Direct infiltration of optic nerve, leukemic or malignant.
  2. Compressive neuropathy.
  3. Paraneoplastic syndrome.
K. Trauma.
L. Radiation neuropathy.

OPTIC NEURITIS
(Figure 17–5)

Optic neuritis (papillitis) is a broad term denoting inflammation, degeneration, or demyelinization of the optic nerve. A wide variety of diseases can cause optic neuritis. Loss of vision is the cardinal symptom and serves to differentiate optic neuritis from papilledema, which it may resemble on ophthalmoscopic examination.

Retrobulbar neuritis is optic neuritis that occurs far enough behind the optic disk so that no early changes of the optic disk are visible by means of the ophthalmoscope. Visual acuity is markedly reduced. ("The patient sees nothing and the doctor sees nothing.")

The most frequent cause of retrobulbar neuritis is multiple sclerosis. A diagnosis of multiple sclerosis is eventually made in 25–50% of patients between 20 and 45 years of age who have an attack of retrobulbar neuritis. Other causes are late neurosyphilis, toxic amblyopias, other demyelinating diseases, Leber's optic atrophy, diabetes mellitus, and vitamin deficiency. If the process is sufficiently destructive, retrograde optic atrophy results. The disk loses its normal pink color and becomes pale. In very severe cases a chalky-white disk with sharp outlines in a blind eye results.

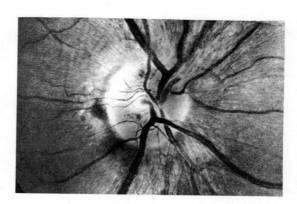

Figure 17–5. Optic neuritis. (Courtesy of WF Hoyt.)

Pathology

In the early stages of optic neuritis there is an outpouring of white blood cells, predominantly neutrophils, in the affected area. The nerve fibers are swollen and fragmented. Fat-bearing macrophages soon appear, carrying away degenerated myelin material. As the process becomes more chronic, lymphocytes and plasma cells predominate. In mild attacks of optic neuritis, the nerve fibers may be preserved with a minimum amount of scar tissue formation. When nerve tissue is permanently destroyed, fibrous gliosis replaces the nerve elements.

Clinical Findings

There is usually a temporary but severe loss of vision. There may be pain in the region of the eye, especially upon movement of the globe. Vision characteristically improves dramatically within 2–3 weeks.

Central scotomas are the most common visual field defect. They are usually circular, varying widely in size and density. Almost any unilateral field change is possible. The pupillary light reflex is sluggish.

Ophthalmoscopically, hyperemia of the optic disk and distention of large veins are early signs. Blurred disk margins and filling of the physiologic cup are common. The process may advance to marked edema of the nerve head, but elevations of more than 3 diopters (1 mm) are unusual. Extensive surrounding retinal edema may be present. Flame-shaped hemorrhages may occur in the nerve fiber layer near the optic disk.

Differential Diagnosis

Papilledema is the most common differential diagnostic problem. In papilledema there is often greater elevation of the optic nerve head, nearly normal visual acuity, normal pupillary response to light, associated increased intracranial pressure, and no visual field defect except an enlarged blind spot unless the visual pathway has been interrupted intracranially. Papilledema is usually bilateral, whereas papillitis is usually unilateral. Despite these obvious differences, differential diagnosis continues to be a problem because of the similarity of the ophthalmoscopic findings.

Treatment

Ideally, treatment is directed toward the underlying cause. If the cause cannot be effectively treated or is not known, treatment is often satisfactory. Systemic corticosteroids have not been proved to be helpful in persistent optic neuritis due to any cause. Since the tendency is in the direction of improvement, many drugs have been reported to be "successful" in the treatment of this disorder.

Course & Prognosis

Loss of vision occurs within the first few hours after onset and is maximal within several days. Visual acuity usually begins to improve 2–3 weeks after onset and sometimes returns to normal in a few days. Improvement may continue slowly over a period of several months. The appearance of optic atrophy indicates some permanent destruction of nerve fibers with permanent loss of function. Optic neuritis associated with systemic or local inflammatory disease or of unknown cause does not usually recur. Optic neuritis in demyelinating disease has a favorable prognosis without treatment for an individual attack, but over a period of years significant visual loss is the rule since permanent damage results from recurrent attacks.

DEMYELINATING DISEASES

MULTIPLE SCLEROSIS
(Fig 17–6)

Multiple sclerosis is a chronic, relapsing demyelinating disorder of the central nervous system of unknown cause. Onset is usually in young adult life; this disease rarely begins before 15 years or after 55 years of age. There is a tendency to involve the optic nerves and chiasm, brain stem, cerebellar peduncles, and spinal cord, although no part of the central nervous system is invulnerable. The peripheral nervous system is not often involved. Clinically, there are a variety of symptoms and signs that may vary in number and character from time to time. In addition to ocular disturbances, there may be muscle weakness, ataxia, urinary disturbances, paresthesis, dysarthria, intention tremors, sensory disturbances, and pyramidal signs.

Pathologically, multiple areas of demyelination are present in the white matter. Early, there is degeneration of the myelin sheaths and a relative sparing of the axons. Glial tissue overgrowth and complete nerve fiber destruction with some round cell infiltrations are seen later. The disease has a predilection for the optic nerve and chiasm.

Patients may first complain of blurring of vision, as if a mist or film covers the eye. This is due to optic neuritis (especially retrobulbar neuritis) and is characterized by acute unilateral loss of vision with a tendency toward recovery. Because of the transient nature of the visual defect and the absence of physical findings, the complaint is sometimes discussed as being of hysterical origin. The other eye is involved eventually. With each attack, there may be some residual permanent damage (eg, loss of visual acuity or defective color vision).

Because of the tendency toward selective involvement of the papillomacular bundle within the optic nerve, central scotoma is by far the most common visual field defect during the acute stage.

The pupil reacts sluggishly to light. If the optic neuritis is severe, there may be atrophy of the optic disk that is ophthalmoscopically visible as the so-called temporal pallor.

Diplopia is a frequent early symptom of extraocular muscle involvement, due most frequently to inter-

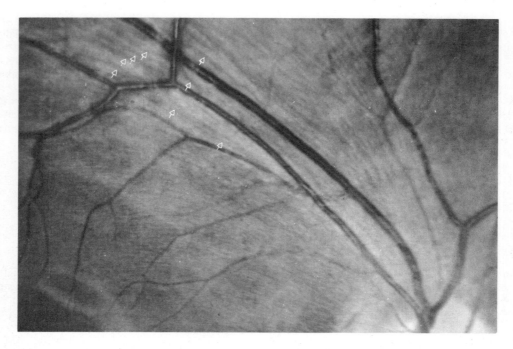

Figure 17–6. Retinal nerve fiber layer in demyelinative optic neuropathy of multiple sclerosis. The upper temporal nerve fiber bundles show multiple slitlike areas of thinning (arrows) representing retrograde axonal atrophy from subclinical disease in the optic nerve. Vision in the eye was 6/6 (20/20). (Courtesy of WF Hoyt.)

nuclear ophthalmoplegia. This condition, caused by a lesion of the medial longitudinal fasciculus, is characterized by paresis of one or both of the medial rectus muscles on conjugate lateral gaze to the opposite side and symptoms in the opposite (abducting) eye; medial rectus function is normal for convergence. Ptosis may also occur; less commonly, weakness of the lateral rectus or other muscles, singly or together, occurs.

Nystagmus is a common early sign, and—unlike most manifestations of the disease (which tend toward remission)—it is often permanent (70%).

Retinal vessel vasculitis and low-grade uveitis are occasionally associated with multiple sclerosis.

The cerebrospinal fluid gamma globulin concentration is frequently high, but some patients with multiple sclerosis have no spinal fluid abnormalities.

The visual evoked response (VER) may help confirm involvement of the visual pathway. The VER has been reported to be abnormal in 80% of definite, 43% of probable, and 22% of suspected cases of multiple sclerosis. A normal VER in suspected multiple sclerosis makes the diagnosis questionable.

There is no specific therapy for multiple sclerosis. Treatment is symptomatic and supportive. The course of the disease is unpredictable, and remissions and exacerbations may occur. The prognosis for vision in retrobulbar neuritis is fairly good, but with successive attacks there may be an increased permanent defect. Complete blindness may occur when there is severe optic atrophy. Death may occur within a decade, but survival for 25–30 years is not uncommon.

NEUROMYELITIS OPTICA
(Devic's Disease)

This rare demyelinating disease of the central nervous system (considered by many to be a form of multiple sclerosis) is characterized by bilateral optic neuritis and paraplegia. The cause is not known. There is usually a sudden onset of blindness in one eye, followed soon by blindness in the other eye and paraplegia. There is only a moderate tendency to recovery of both elements of the disease. The mortality rate is 50% in some series.

There is no treatment.

DIFFUSE PERIAXIAL ENCEPHALITIS
(Schilder's Disease)

This rare disease of young children is characterized pathologically by widespread demyelinization of the white matter in the brain. Clinically, there is an acute onset of rapidly developing cortical blindness,* mental deterioration, convulsions, bilateral spastic weakness, and paralysis progressing to coma and death.

*Cortical blindness is due to bilateral widespread destruction of the visual cortex. The pupils react normally to light. A striking feature of cortical blindness may be the patient's subjective unawareness of disability (Anton's syndrome). Despite being totally blind, the patient believes that he or she can see.

PAPILLEDEMA & OPTIC ATROPHY

PAPILLEDEMA
(Figs 17–7 to 17–10)

Papilledema (choked disk) is a noninflammatory congestion of the optic disk associated with increased intracranial pressure. Papilledema will occur in any condition causing persistent increased intracranial pressure; the most common causes are cerebral tumors, abscesses, subdural hematoma, hydrocephalus, and malignant hypertension. An important factor in the mechanism of papilledema is obstruction to the venous flow caused by pressure on the central retinal vein where it leaves the optic nerve and passes through the subarachnoid and subdural spaces.

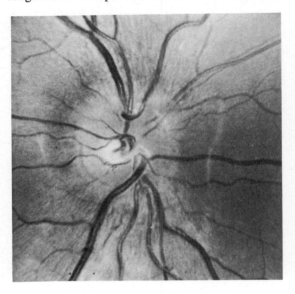

Figure 17–7. Early papilledema. The disk margins are blurred superiorly and inferiorly by the thickened layer of nerve fibers entering the disk. (Courtesy of WF Hoyt.)

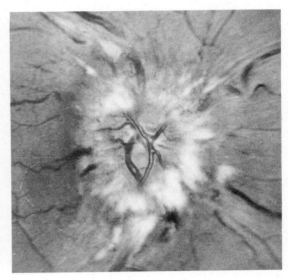

Figure 17–8. Papilledema with opaque (white) patches of swollen nerve fibers and hemorrhages. (Courtesy of WF Hoyt.)

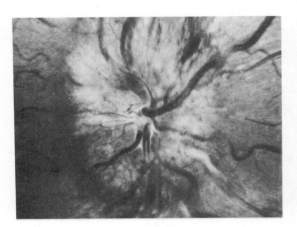

Figure 17–9. Fully developed papilledema. The disk tissue is swollen, elevated, and congested, and the retinal veins are markedly dilated. (Courtesy of WF Hoyt.)

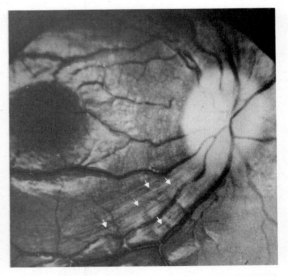

Figure 17–10. Chronic atrophic papilledema in a child with a cerebellar medulloblastoma. The disk is pale and slightly elevated and has blurred margins. The white areas surrounding the macula are reflected light from the vitreoretinal interface. The inferior temporal nerve fiber bundles are partially atrophic (arrows). (Courtesy of WF Hoyt.)

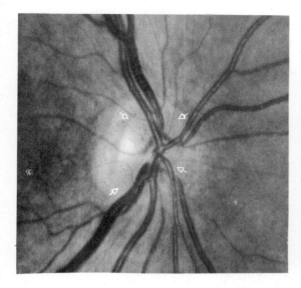

Figure 17–11. Optic nerve hypoplasia. The disk border (arrows) is small in circumference. Note the disproportion between the small disk and the normal-sized central retinal vessels. (Courtesy of WF Hoyt.)

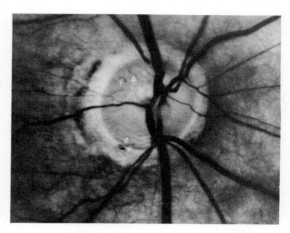

Figure 17–12. Chronic ischemic optic atrophy with loss of neuroglial tissue and exposure of the lamina cribrosa. The pale disk has a shallow cup without nasal displacement of the central retinal vessels. Multiple dark holes are present in the disk surface. The disk is ringed by a zone of choroidal atrophy. The retinal arterioles are narrowed irregularly. (Courtesy of WF Hoyt.)

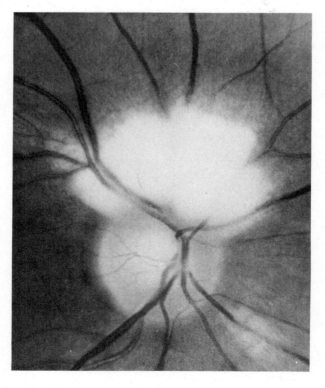

Figure 17–13. Large path of myelinated nerve fibers originating from superior edge of disk. Another smaller patch is present near inferior nasal border of disk. (Right eye.)

Edema of the optic nerve is the principal pathologic finding. Edema may also be present in the adjacent nerve fiber layer of the retina. Subhyaloid hemorrhages and hemorrhages in the nerve fiber layers are common. Inflammatory signs are minimal, and leukocytes are seen histologically only in the later stages. Degeneration of nerve fibers may eventually occur.

Clinical Findings

The blind spot is enlarged. Visual acuity and visual fields are otherwise normal. Early ophthalmoscopic findings include hyperemia of the disk, blurring of the disk margins, and distention of retinal veins. It is difficult to be sure about early papilledema. One helpful sign is the absence of pulsation of the central retinal vein or failure to produce a pulsation with light digital pressure on the globe. Frank (measurable) swelling of the disk, peripapillary retinal edema, and hemorrhages radially about the disk in the nerve fiber layers appear later. Papilledema may elevate the disk to 6 or 10 diopters, and hemorrhages in severe cases are subhyaloid, occasionally breaking into the vitreous and markedly affecting vision.

Differential Diagnosis

The common differential diagnostic problem of papilledema and optic neuritis is discussed above (p 206).

A condition known as pseudopapilledema is sometimes noted in normal optic disks, particularly in farsighted persons, that have a "blurred" disk margin which suggests papilledema. A normal blind spot and normal intracranial pressure rule out true papilledema.

Myelinated nerve fibers of the retina adjacent to the nerve head as well as drusen of the optic nerve may be confused with papilledema (Fig 17–13).

Complications

Papilledema may persist for a long time without permanently affecting vision, or secondary optic atrophy may occur as a complication. Following reduction of increased intracranial pressure, papilledema improves rapidly. Hemorrhages, exudates, and retinal edema usually clear promptly. If optic atrophy does follow, slight to total permanent loss of vision results.

Treatment

Treatment depends upon the underlying cause. Papilledema associated with hypertensive retinopathy is an indication for vigorous treatment with potent hypotensive drugs.

Caution: Although it is at times undertaken as a calculated risk with proper precautions, lumbar puncture is usually contraindicated in patients with papilledema because of the danger of herniation of the brain into the tentorial incisure or into the foramen magnum. Such herniation causes pressure particularly on the medulla and can cause sudden death. A CT scan should be obtained before lumbar puncture to rule out a supratentorial mass.

Course & Prognosis

In general, the more rapid the onset, the greater the danger of permanent visual loss. Papilledema of more than 5 diopters, extensive retinal hemorrhages and exudates, and macular stars imply a poor visual prognosis. Early pallor of the disk and attenuated arterioles, once the edema of the nerve head clears, indicates that some optic atrophy will follow. Gliosis of the disk is a particularly bad prognostic sign.

OPTIC NERVE ATROPHY
(Figs 17–11 to 17–13)

Etiologic Classification

A. Vascular: Occlusion of the central retinal vein or artery; arteriosclerotic changes within the optic nerve itself, disturbing its normal nutrition; or posthemorrhagic, due to sudden massive blood loss (eg, bleeding peptic ulcer, traumatic amputation).

B. Degenerative: Consecutive atrophy secondary to retinal disease, with destruction of ganglion cells (eg, retinitis); or as part of a systemic degenerative disease (eg, cerebromacular degeneration).

C. Secondary to Papilledema: See p 209.

D. Secondary to Optic Neuritis (Including Retrobulbar Neuritis): See p 206.

E. Pressure Against the Optic Nerve: Aneurysm of the anterior circle of Willis, bony pressure at the optic foramen (eg, osteitis deformans), intracanalicular or parasellar tumors.

F. Toxic: End result of toxic amblyopia (see pp 226–228).

G. Metabolic: Eg, diabetes mellitus, ganglioside disease.

H. Traumatic: Direct injury to a nerve (ie, severing, avulsion, or contusion).

I. Glaucomatous: See Chapter 14.

Clinical Findings

Loss of vision is the only symptom. Pallor of the optic disk and loss of pupillary reaction are usually proportionate to visual loss.

Treatment, Course, & Prognosis

It is rarely possible to treat the underlying cause effectively. Changes in visual function occur very slowly over weeks or months. It is difficult to assess prognosis on the basis of ophthalmoscopic findings alone. Atrophic cupping, attenuation and reduced number of vessels on the disk, and pallor with papilledema are unfavorable prognostic signs. Optic atrophy secondary to vascular, traumatic, degenerative, and some toxic causes usually has a very bad prognosis. Visual loss due to pressure on the optic nerve may be reversed, particularly if the cause is relieved early.

GENETICALLY DETERMINED OPTIC ATROPHY

Leber's Disease

This rare disease, characterized by sequential, rapidly progressive optic neuropathy, occurs in young men age 20–30 (very rarely in women). It has classically been considered to be due to an X-linked recessive gene, but its real mode of inheritance must still be considered to be in doubt. Vision is not totally lost. There is no known treatment. Other types of central nervous system involvement can be present and may cause confusion with multiple sclerosis.

Congenital or Infantile Hereditary Optic Atrophy

This occurs in a severe autosomal recessive form and a milder autosomal dominant form. The recessive form is present at birth or within 2 years and is accompanied by nystagmus. The more common dominant form has an insidious onset in childhood, with little progression thereafter. There is characteristically a centrocecal scotoma with variable loss of central visual acuity.

Behr's Hereditary Optic Atrophy

This rare autosomal recessive disease is characterized by (1) bilateral optic atrophy, rarely complete; and (2) associated neurologic findings such as mild ataxia, a positive Babinski sign, clubfoot, mental deficiency, nystagmus, and other findings, at times with generalized slow progression to a static condition by late adolescence. There is no known treatment.

DISEASES OF THE OPTIC CHIASM

Anatomy (Fig 17–14)

The optic chiasm is variably situated near the top of the diaphragm of the sella turcica (most often posteriorly, projecting over the dorsum sellae) and usually separated from it by several millimeters of subarachnoid space. Above, the lamina terminalis forms the anterior wall of the third ventricle. The internal carotid arteries lie just laterally, adjacent to the cavernous sinuses. The chiasm is made up of the junction of the 2 optic nerves and provides for crossing of the nasal fibers to the opposite optic tract and the passage of temporal fibers to the ipsilateral optic tract. The macular fibers are arranged similarly to the rest of the fibers except that their decussation is farther posteriorly. In general, lesions of the chiasm cause bitemporal hemianopic defects. These defects are typically incomplete and are often asymmetric. The nasal field may also be involved, and central visual acuity may be decreased.

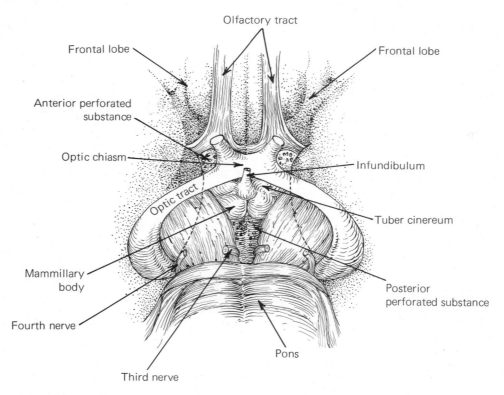

Figure 17–14. Relationship of optic chiasm from inferior aspect. (Redrawn and reproduced, with permission, from Duke-Elder WS: *System of Ophthalmology.* Vol 2. Mosby, 1961.)

INTRASELLAR PITUITARY TUMORS

The anterior lobe of the pituitary gland is the site of origin of pituitary tumors. Three types of cells are normally present (basophils, eosinophils, and neutrophils), and any one type can predominate in a tumor. Symptoms and signs include loss of vision and field changes (90%), x-ray evidence of bony erosion of the sella (80%), pituitary dysfunction (60%), and extraocular nerve palsies (10%).

Surgical removal is the usual method of treatment. Visual loss or endocrine dysfunction is an indication for treatment. Visual acuity and visual fields may improve dramatically after pressure has been removed from the chiasm. X-ray evidence of erosion of the sella is frequently seen as an incidental finding on skull films in patients over 50 with benign asymptomatic tumors. No treatment is indicated in such cases.

CRANIOPHARYNGIOMA

Craniopharyngiomas are a group of tumors arising from epithelial remnants of Rathke's pouch (80% of the population normally have such remnants) and characteristically are first seen between the ages of 10 and 25 years. They are usually suprasellar, occasionally intrasellar. The signs and symptoms vary tremendously with the age of the patient and the exact location of the tumor as well as its rate of growth. When a suprasellar tumor occurs, asymmetric chiasmal field defects are prominent. Papilledema is more common than in pituitary tumor. Pituitary deficiency may result, and involvement of the hypothalamus may cause disturbances such as diabetes insipidus or stunted growth. With the passage of years, calcification and ossification of parts of the tumor give a characteristic radiographic appearance. Treatment consists of surgical removal, if possible, but evacuation of the cystic contents and removal of cyst wall are often all that can be done.

SUPRASELLAR MENINGIOMAS

Suprasellar meningiomas arise from the meninges covering the tuberculum sella and the planum sphenoidale, with a high proportion of patients being female. The tumor is usually anterior and superior to the chiasm, and the visual field changes are characteristic. The optic nerves are often involved early (but asymmetrically) in the slowly progressive damage to the visual pathway. Skull x-rays may reveal hyperostosis or stippled calcification within the tumor, but the sella turcica is normal. Carotid arteriograms usually show displacement of the normal vessels and often filling of abnormal tumor vessels as well. Treatment consists of surgical removal.

GLIOMA OF THE OPTIC CHIASM

Optic chiasm glioma is a rare disorder, usually of children, that sometimes occurs as part of the clinical picture of neurofibromatosis. Onset may be sudden, with rapid loss of vision. Optic atrophy occurs, and visual field defects reveal a chiasmal syndrome. Orbital x-rays may reveal enlargement of the optic foramen; air contrast studies may reveal displacement of the third ventricle. Treatment is by irradiation, since surgical removal usually results in blindness.

THE RETROCHIASMAL VISUAL PATHWAYS

Anatomy

Each optic tract begins at the posterolateral angle of the chiasm and sweeps around the upper part of the cerebral peduncle to end in the lateral geniculate nucleus. Afferent pupillary fibers leave the tract just anterior to the nucleus and pass via the brachium of the superior colliculus to the midbrain. (The pupillary pathway is diagrammed in Fig 17–15). Afferent visual fibers terminate on cells in the lateral geniculate nucleus that give rise to the geniculocalcarine tract. This tract traverses the posterior limb of the internal capsule and then fans out into a broad bundle called the optic radiation. The fibers in this bundle curve backward around the anterior aspect of the temporal horn of the lateral ventricle and then medially to reach the calcarine cortex of the occipital lobe, where they terminate. The most inferior fibers, which carry the projections from the superior aspect of the contralateral half of the visual field, are displaced anteriorly into the temporal lobe in a configuration known as Meyer's loop. Lesions of the temporal lobe involving these fibers can produce superior quandrantanopic field defects.

The primary visual cortex (area 17) occupies the upper and lower lips and the depths of the posterior part of the calcarine sulcus on the medial aspect of the occipital lobe. Each lobe receives input from the 2 ipsilateral half-retinas, representing the contralateral half of the binocular visual field. The projection of the visual field onto the visual cortex occurs in a precise and orderly retinotopic pattern. The macula is represented at the posterior pole, and the peripheral parts of the retina project to the most anterior part of the calcarine cortex.

Lesions of the Retrochiasmal Pathways

Cerebrovascular disease and tumors are responsible for most lesions of the retrochiasmal visual pathways, although almost any intracranial disease process can involve these structures. The optic tracts and lateral geniculate nucleus are infrequently affected and, when involved, typically produce incongruous homonymous visual field defects. After several weeks,

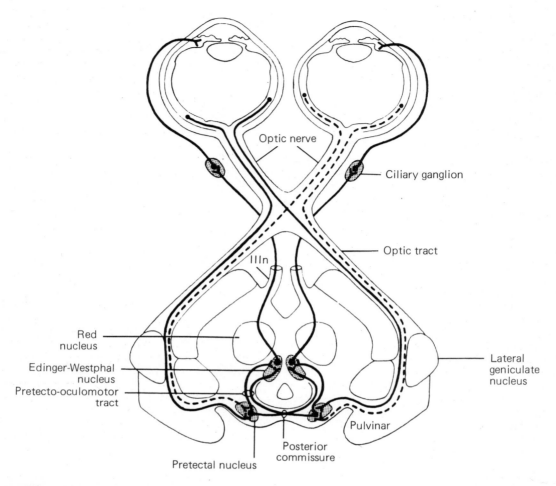

Figure 17–15. Diagram of the path of the pupillary light reflex. (Reproduced, with permission, from Walsh FB, Hoyt WF: *Clinical Neuro-ophthalmology,* 3rd ed. Vol 1. Williams & Wilkins, 1969.)

the disks may appear pale, and the retina nerve fiber layer is deficient.

Lesions involving the geniculocalcarine tract or occipital cortex produce homonymous field defects but do not result in optic atrophy. Generally, the more posterior a lesion is located, the more congruous the homonymous visual field defect. Tumors occur more frequently in temporal and parietal lobes, while occipital lobe lesions are overwhelmingly vascular. Lesions of the temporal and parietal lobes usually result in multiple neurologic deficits, and isolated visual loss is rare. Vascular lesions of the occipital lobe, on the other hand, are common and account for over 80% of isolated homonymous visual field loss in patients over age 50.

THE PUPIL

The size of the normal pupil varies at different ages and from person to person. The normal pupillary diameter is usually about 3–4 mm, tending to be larger in childhood and progressively smaller with advancing age. Many normal persons have a slight difference in pupil size (physiologic anisocoria). Occasionally there is a marked difference in pupil size in otherwise normal eyes. Mydriatic and cycloplegic drugs work more effectively on blue eyes than on brown eyes. The function of the pupil is to control the amount of light entering the eye to give best visual function under the various degrees of light intensity normally encountered. The pathways controlling this purely reflex function are described below and are diagrammed in Fig 17–1.

THE PUPILLARY PATHWAYS

The evaluation of the pupillary reactions is important in localizing lesions involving the optic pathways. A knowledge of the neuroanatomy of the pathway for reaction of the pupil to light and the miosis associated with accommodation is very important.

Neuroanatomy of the Pupillary Pathways

A. Light Reflex: The pathway for the light reflex is entirely subcortical. The afferent pupillary fibers are included within the optic nerve and pathway until they leave the optic tract just before the visual fibers synapse in the lateral geniculate body. They go to the pretectal area of the midbrain and synapse. Impulses are then relayed by crossed fibers through the posterior commissure to the opposite Edinger-Westphal nucleus. Some fibers also go directly ventral to the ipsilateral Edinger-Westphal nucleus. The efferent pathway is via the third nerve to the ciliary ganglion within the retrobulbar extraocular muscle cone. The postganglionic fiber goes via the short ciliary nerves to innervate the sphincter muscle of the iris.

B. The Near Reflex: When the eyes look at a near object, 3 reactions occur: accommodation, convergence, and constriction of the pupil, bringing a sharp image into focus on corresponding retinal points. There is convincing evidence that the final common pathway is mediated through the oculomotor nerve with a synapse in the ciliary ganglion. The afferent pathway has not been worked out, but there is evidence that it enters the midbrain ventral to the Edinger-Westphal nucleus and sends fibers to both sides of the cortex. Although the 3 components are closely associated, it cannot be considered a pure reflex as each component can be neutralized while leaving the other 2 intact—ie, by prism (neutralizing convergence), by lenses (neutralizing accommodation), and by weak mydriatic drugs (neutralizing miosis).

ARGYLL ROBERTSON PUPIL

A typical Argyll Robertson pupil is very suggestive of central nervous system syphilis associated with tabes dorsalis or general paresis. The pupil is less than 3 mm in diameter (miotic) and does not respond to light stimulation. The pupil does constrict with accommodation. The finding is nearly always bilateral. The pupils are commonly irregular and eccentric and dilate poorly with mydriatics. Less commonly, the sign is incomplete (slow response to light) or unilateral. Some degree of Argyll Robertson pupil is present in over 50% of patients with central nervous system syphilis. A wide variety of other central nervous system diseases infrequently cause incomplete Argyll Robertson pupil. These include diabetes, chronic alcoholism, encephalitis, multiple sclerosis, central nervous system degenerative disease, and tumors of the midbrain. The site or sites of the central nervous system lesion are not definitely known.

TONIC PUPIL

This not uncommon entity is characterized by a delayed or diminished direct and consensual reaction to light (80% unilateral) in a pupil larger than normal. It may be associated with loss of tendon reflexes (Adie's syndrome). It results from damage to the ciliary ganglion and aberrant regeneration of nerve flow. The cause is obscure but definitely is not syphilis, and it is important that tonic pupil be differentiated from Argyll Robertson pupil. It is most frequently seen in young adult women. It may come on abruptly and be noticeable to the patient because of increased sensitivity to light. A weak (0.25%) solution of pilocarpine instilled into the conjunctival sac causes a tonic pupil to constrict; normal pupils are not affected. The tonic pupil dilates slowly in the dark and reacts promptly to mydriatics.

HORNER'S SYNDROME

Horner's syndrome is caused by a lesion of the sympathetic pathway in the brain stem, upper spinal cord, or peripheral sympathetic chain. Unilateral miosis, ptosis, enophthalmos, and absence of sweating on the ipsilateral face and neck make up the complete syndrome. Causes of Horner's syndrome include cervical vertebral fractures, tabes dorsalis, syringomyelia, cervical cord tumor, apical tuberculosis, goiter, enlarged cervical lymph glands, apical bronchogenic carcinoma, mediastinal tumor, and aneurysm of the carotid or subclavian artery.

EXTRAOCULAR MOVEMENTS

This section deals with the neural apparatus that controls the movements of the eyes and causes them to move simultaneously in tandem up or down and side to side as well as in convergence or divergence.

SUPRANUCLEAR PATHWAYS

The supranuclear neural pathways of the extraocular muscles innervate conjugate lateral and vertical gaze as well as the disjunctive movements of convergence and divergence. They consist of central nervous system connections to the nuclei of cranial nerves III, IV, and VI located in the midbrain. The highest centers for these functions are located in the frontal lobe (voluntary or command movement) and the occipital lobe (involuntary or fixation movement).

Anatomy of Voluntary Conjugate Movements

A. Horizontal: The location of the cortical center that controls horizontal conjugate movements of the eyes is situated in the frontal lobe. The pathway de-

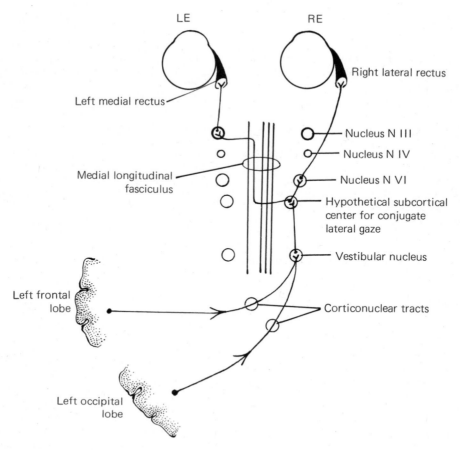

Figure 17–16. Conjugate gaze. The impulses for voluntary conjugate movements in right lateral gaze are initiated in the left frontal lobe. Involuntary conjugate movements in right lateral gaze are initiated in the left occipital lobe or, according to recent reports, the ipsilateral occipital lobe. (After Spiegel and Sommer. Redrawn with modifications and reproduced, with permission, from Moses R: *Adler's Physiology of the Eye,* 5th ed. Mosby, 1970.)

scends through the basal ganglia into the brain stem and crosses to the opposite side of the pons. Impulses enter the paramedian pontine reticular formation. The ipsilateral lateral rectus and the contralateral medial rectus muscles are stimulated to produce conjugate movement via the medial longitudinal fasciculus (Fig 17–16).

B. Vertical: The centers and pathways are probably the same as for horizontal movement, except that the subcortical pathway terminates in the pretectal area. The impulses then go to the medial longitudinal fasciculus and are distributed to the appropriate oculomotor nuclei to effect vertical gaze.

C. Convergence: It is probable that the supranuclear impulses for convergence travel much the same pathway as do those for conjugate horizontal and vertical gaze, arriving at a midbrain synapse near or in the oculomotor nucleus. From this synapse, stimulating impulses go to each medial rectus, and inhibitory impulses go to each lateral rectus via the medial longitudinal fasciculus.

D. Divergence: Electromyography has estab-

lished divergence as an active process (not a relaxation of convergence, as was once thought). The supranuclear pathway is probably more or less the same as for convergence, arriving at a midbrain center near the sixth nerve nuclei. Stimulating impulses go to each lateral rectus and inhibitory impulses to each medial rectus via the medial longitudinal fasciculus as the eyes undergo divergence.

Anatomy of Pursuit Horizontal & Vertical Conjugate Movements

The cortical center is a large ill-defined area of the occipital lobe. The descending pathway is not definitely known, but in general it follows a route similar to the voluntary pathway into the internal capsule, midbrain, and medial longitudinal fasciculus. This pathway carries the impulses of the "following movement" as demonstrated by optokinetic nystagmus. The eyes will "follow" a slowly moving object even when the voluntary pathway is nonfunctioning. When both pathways are intact, the voluntary influence dominates the pursuit influence.

1. LESIONS OF SUPRANUCLEAR PATHWAYS

Frontal Lobe

A seizure focus in the frontal lobe may cause involuntary turning of the eyes to the opposite side. Destructive lesions cause transient deviation to the same side, and the eyes cannot be turned voluntarily to the opposite side. This is termed a frontal gaze palsy. Ocular pursuit to the opposite side is retained. There is no diplopia. Exaggerated end point nystagmus can be the first sign of a frontal gaze palsy or may occur as a residuum of a clearing gaze palsy.

Occipital Lobe

Smooth ocular pursuit may be lost with posterior lesions of the hemispheres. The patient is unable to follow a slowly moving object in the direction of the gaze palsy. The command movement is not lost.

2. PARINAUD'S SYNDROME
(Pretectal Syndrome)

This syndrome is characterized by loss of voluntary upward gaze and (frequently) loss of the pupillary light response with retention of miosis in response to the near reflex. Nystagmus retractorius, which consists of convergent retraction movements of the globe on attempted upward gaze, is also a feature. There may also be accommodative spasm, a loss of conjugate voluntary downward gaze associated with loss of convergence and accommodation, ptosis or lid retraction, papilledema, or third nerve palsy. Surrounding structures may also be involved depending upon the size and location of the lesion. Conjugate horizontal ocular movements are usually not affected. The syndrome results from tectal or pretectal lesions affecting the periaqueductal area. Pinealomas, infiltrating gliomas, vascular lesions, and trauma may produce this picture.

3. LESIONS OF THE BRAIN STEM

Lesions of the brain stem are the most common causes of gaze palsies. The lesions most often encountered (in order of frequency) are vascular accidents, multiple sclerosis, tumors, and encephalitis.

4. SUPRANUCLEAR SYNDROMES INVOLVING DISJUNCTIVE OCULAR MOVEMENTS

Spasm of the Near Reflex

The near reflex consists of 3 components: convergence, accommodation, and constriction of the pupil. Spasm of the near reflex is usually caused by hysteria, although encephalitis, tabes dorsalis, and meningitis may cause spasm by irritation of the supranuclear pathway. It is characterized by convergent strabismus with diplopia, miotic pupils, and spasm of accommodation.

If hysteria is the cause, atropine, 1%, 2 drops in each eye twice daily, or minus (concave) lenses may give temporary relief. Psychiatric consultation is indicated for treatment of an underlying mental cause.

Convergence Paralysis

Convergence paralysis is characterized by a sudden onset of diplopia for near vision, with absence of any individual extraocular muscle palsy. It is caused by hysteria or destructive lesions of the supranuclear pathway for convergence. Multiple sclerosis, encephalitis, tabes dorsalis, tumors, aneurysms, minor cerebrovascular accidents, and Parkinson's disease are the most common organic causes.

5. SUPRANUCLEAR LESIONS & STRABISMUS

Strabismus is dealt with in Chapter 15, but it should be mentioned here that idiopathic esotropias and exotropias with onset early in life may result from cerebral developmental abnormalities of the supranuclear mechanisms regulating divergence and convergence.

NUCLEAR & INFRANUCLEAR CONNECTIONS

Peripheral & Intermediate Connections of the Nuclei of Cranial Nerves III, IV, & VI

A. Oculomotor (III): The motor fibers arise from a group of nuclei in the central gray matter ventral to the cerebral aqueduct at the level of the superior colliculus. Mainly uncrossed fibers course through the red nucleus and the inner side of the substantia nigra to emerge on the medial side of the cerebral peduncles. The nerve runs alongside the sella turcica, in the outer wall of the cavernous sinus, and through the superior orbital fissure to supply the medial, superior, and inferior rectus muscles and the inferior oblique and levator palpebrae muscles.

The parasympathetics arise from the Edinger-Westphal nucleus just rostrad to the motor nucleus of the third nerve and pass via the inferior division of the third nerve to the ciliary ganglion. From there the short ciliary nerves are distributed to the sphincter muscle of the iris and to the ciliary muscle, which controls the shape of the lens during accommodation.

B. Trochlear (IV): Motor (entirely crossed) fibers arise from the trochlear nucleus just caudad to the third nerve at the level of the inferior colliculus, run posteriorly, decussate in the anterior medullary velum, and wind around the cerebral peduncles. From here the fourth nerve follows the third nerve along the cavernous sinus to the orbit, where it supplies the superior oblique muscle.

C. Abducens (VI): Motor (entirely uncrossed)

fibers arise from the nucleus in the floor of the fourth
ventricle in the lower portion of the pons near the
internal genu of the facial nerve. Piercing the pons, the
fibers emerge anteriorly, the nerve running a long
course over the tip of the petrous portion of the temporal bone to the outer wall of the cavernous sinus. It
enters the orbit with the third and fourth nerves to
supply the lateral rectus muscle.

Central Reflex Connections of the Nuclei of Cranial Nerves III, IV, & VI

The central reflex connections of these nuclei
originate in 5 areas: (1) From the pretectal region via
the posterior commissure to the Edinger-Westphal nuclei for mediation of ipsilateral and consensual light
reflexes. Interruption of this pathway may cause an
Argyll Robertson pupil. (2) From the superior colliculi
via the tectobulbar tract to the nuclei of cranial nerves
III, IV, and VI for the mediation of miosis associated
with accommodation. (3) From the inferior colliculi
via the tectobulbar tract to the eye muscle nuclei for
reflexes correlated with hearing. (4) From the vestibular nuclei via the medial longitudinal fasciculus for
reflex gaze movement correlated with equilibrium. (5)
From the cortex through the corticobulbar tract for
mediation of voluntary and involuntary conjugate
movements of the eyes.

•   •   •

SUMMARY OF DISORDERS OF CRANIAL NERVES III, IV, & VI

Oculomotor Paralysis (Cranial Nerve III)

A. Complete Oculomotor Paralysis: The lesion
involves the third nerve anywhere from the nucleus
(midbrain) to the peripheral branches in the orbit. It
causes divergent strabismus since the eye is turned out
by the intact lateral rectus muscle and slightly depressed by the intact superior oblique muscle. There is
a dilated fixed pupil, absent accommodation, and
ptosis of the upper lid, often severe enough to cover the
pupil. The eye may only be moved laterally. Trauma,
carotid aneurysm, and diabetes are the most common
causes. In diabetes, the pupillary responses are usually
intact; in carotid aneurysm, they almost never are
spared.

B. Complete Internal Ophthalmoplegia: This
consists of a dilated and fixed pupil and paralysis of
accommodation. The lesion is nearly always peripheral in the ciliary ganglion and often results in tonic
pupil.

Trochlear Paralysis (Cranial Nerve IV)

Lesions of the fourth nerve are usually traumatic.
The nerve is vulnerable to injury at the site of exit from
the dorsal aspect of the posterior mid brain stem. Both
nerves may be damaged as they decussate in the anterior medullary velum, resulting in bilateral superior
oblique palsies. Superior oblique palsy results in upward deviation (hypertropia) of the eye. The hypertropia increases when the patient looks down and
with adduction. In addition, there is excyclotropia, and
one of the diplopic images will be tilted with respect to
the other. Tilting the head toward the involved side
increases the deviation. Tilting the head away from the
side of the involved eye may relieve the diplopia, and
patients frequently present with a head tilt.

Abducens Paralysis (Cranial Nerve VI)

This is the most common single muscle palsy,
since one nerve with a long intracranial course supplies
one extraocular muscle. Abduction of the eye is absent; esotropia is present in the primary position and
increases upon gaze to the affected side. Movement of
the eye to the opposite side is normal. Cerebrovascular
accidents are a common cause; basilar artery disease,
increased intracranial pressure, tumors at the base of
the skull, meningitis, diabetes, and trauma are other
frequent causes.

Duane's Syndrome

See p 229.

Symptoms & Signs of Extraocular Muscle Palsies

Diplopia occurs when the visual axes are not
aligned. This is especially true when the onset of
strabismus is after age 6 (suppression and abnormal
retinal correspondence do not develop). Dizziness is
often associated. Head tilt occurs, especially in paresis
of the superior oblique muscle, when the head tilt is to
the opposite side to avoid diplopia by moving the eye
out of the field of action of the paralyzed muscle.

Ptosis is caused by weakness or paralysis of the
levator muscle.

SYNDROMES AFFECTING CRANIAL NERVES III, IV, & VI

Peripheral Involvement of Cranial Nerves III, IV, & VI

A. Gradenigo's Syndrome: This is characterized by pain in the face (from irritation of the trigeminal nerve) and abducens palsy. The syndrome is produced by meningitis at the tip of the petrous bone and
most often occurs as a rare complication of otitis
media.

B. Cavernous Sinus Syndrome: See p 200.

C. Orbital Fissure Syndrome: All extraocular
peripheral nerves pass through the orbital fissure and
can be involved by a traumatic bone fracture in this
area or by tumor encroaching on the fissure from the
orbital or cranial side.

D. Orbital Apex Syndrome: This is similar to
the orbital fissure syndrome with the addition of optic
nerve signs. It is caused by an orbital tumor or trauma
that damages the optic and extraocular nerves.

Chronic Progressive External Ophthalmoplegia*

This rather rare disease involves all 3 extraocular nerves. It is characterized by a slowly progressive inability to move the eyes and very often is associated with severe early ptosis and normal pupillary reactions and accommodation. It may begin at any age and progresses over a period of 5–15 years to complete external ophthalmoplegia. This disease is frequently associated with other abnormalities such as pigmentary degeneration of the retina, deafness, cardiac conduction defects, and peripheral neuropathy. When it is part of a larger constellation of signs and symptoms, it is called **ophthalmoplegia plus,** or Kearns-Sayre syndrome. There is no effective treatment, although cosmetic surgery for strabismus or ptosis is often necessary. Myasthenia gravis is the major differential problem.

NYSTAGMUS

Nystagmus is defined as involuntary, rhythmically repeated oscillations of one or both eyes in any or all fields of gaze. The movements are either pendular, with undulatory movements of equal speed, amplitude, and duration in each direction; or jerky, with slower movements in one direction (slow component) followed by a rapid return to the original position (fast component). The full mechanism is unknown, and the location of the defect cannot usually be specified.

Nystagmus is classified as grade I, present only with the eyes directed toward the fast component; grade II, present also with the eyes in primary position; or grade III, present even with the eyes directed toward the slow component. The movements may be horizontal, vertical, oblique, rotatory, circular, or a combination of these. The direction may change depending upon the direction of gaze. Amplitude refers to the extent of the movement; rate refers to the frequency of oscillation. Generally, the faster the rate, the smaller the amplitude and vice versa.

Known factors relating to ocular movements, malfunction of which can cause nystagmus, are as follows. The labyrinth exerts influence on eye movements by 2 mechanisms: (1) The otolith apparatus influences torsional eye movements in response to head position; (2) the semicircular canals influence eye movements in response to acceleration and deceleration. The gaze mechanism influences the supraconnections of extraocular muscle function (see pp 215–219). These complicated pathways are known in a general but not a complete way. The fixation mechanism also

*"External ophthalmoplegia" is a general term that denotes inability to move the eyes normally as a result of any nuclear or infranuclear involvement of cranial nerves III, IV, or VI; the pupillary reaction and accommodation are normal.

is not completely understood but undoubtedly involves the retina, visual pathways, brain stem, and cerebellum.

Physiology of Symptoms

Reduced visual acuity is caused by inability to maintain steady fixation. False projection is evident in vestibular nystagmus, where past-pointing is present. Head tilting is usually involuntary, to decrease the nystagmus. The head is turned toward the fast components in jerky nystagmus, or set so that the eyes are in a position which minimizes ocular movement in pendular nystagmus. The patient sometimes complains of illusory movements of objects (oscillopsia). This is more apt to be present in nystagmus due to lesions of lower centers, such as the labyrinth, or associated with the sudden arrest of nystagmus in an adult. The apparent movement of the environment occurs during the slow component and causes an extremely distressing vertigo, so that the patient is unable to stand. Head nodding is most apt to accompany congenital nystagmus, spasmus nutans, and miner's nystagmus. Nystagmus is noticeable and cosmetically disturbing except when excursions of the eye are very small.

Classification of Nystagmus
A. Physiologic Nystagmus:
  1. End point.
  2. Optokinetic.
  3. Stimulation of semicircular canals.

B. Pathologic Nystagmus:
  1. Congenital–
     a. Sensory defect type.
     b. Motor defect type.
     c. Latent.
  2. Spasmus nutans.
  3. Nystagmus due to neurologic disturbances–
     a. Acquired pendular or jerky nystagmus.
     b. Ocular flutter.
     c. See-saw nystagmus.
     d. Nystagmus retractorius.
  4. Vestibular nystagmus.
  5. Gaze nystagmus.
  6. Voluntary and hysterical nystagmus.

PHYSIOLOGIC NYSTAGMUS

The following 3 types of nystagmus can be elicited in the normal person. Alteration of normal response may be helpful diagnostically.

End Point Nystagmus

A jerky type of nystagmus of small amplitude with the fast component in the direction of gaze commonly occurs in extreme lateral gaze after a latent period of not more than 30 seconds. The nystagmus appears earlier and is of larger amplitude in general fatigue states.

Optokinetic Nystagmus

This is a jerky type of nystagmus which may be elicited in all normal individuals, most easily by means of a rotating drum with alternating black and white lines. The slow component follows the object and the fast component moves rapidly counterwise to fixate each succeeding object. Unilateral or asymmetric horizontal response usually indicates a parietal lobe tumor. Anterior cerebral (ie, frontal lobe) lesions may inhibit this response only temporarily, which suggests the presence of a compensatory mechanism that is much greater than for lesions situated farther posteriorly. Asymmetry of response in the vertical plane suggests a brain stem lesion.

Nystagmus Elicited by Stimulation of Semicircular Canals

A. Bárány Rotating Chair: The horizontal canals are horizontal with the floor when the head is tilted 30 degrees forward. Rotation of the subject causes a jerky nystagmus in the direction of the turning. The slow component is in the opposite direction, the same as the flow of endolymph in the semicircular canals.

B. Caloric Stimulation: With the subject supine and the head flexed on the chest, cold water ear irrigation produces nystagmus with the fast component away from the side of irrigation while warm water produces nystagmus with the fast component toward the side of irrigation. (Mnemonic device is COWS: cold—opposite; warm—same.)

PATHOLOGIC NYSTAGMUS

1. CONGENITAL NYSTAGMUS

Sensory Defect Type

Congenital impairment of vision in any part of the eye or optic nerve can result in pendular nystagmus. Causes include corneal opacity, cataract, albinism, posterior polar chorioretinitis, aniridia, and optic atrophy. Oscillations of the head that are synchronous with the nystagmus but in the opposite direction often accompany sensory defect congenital nystagmus.

Motor Defect Nystagmus

This is manifested as a jerky nystagmus on gaze to either side with the fast component in the direction of gaze. The eyes are otherwise normal except when strabismus is associated (20%). There is always a position of relative rest. If this position is with the eyes deviated to one side, the head will be turned toward the opposite side to obtain the best possible vision. This condition shows some spontaneous improvement up to about age 10. The cause is not known, but a lesion of the brain stem is probably responsible. About 20% of cases are inherited as an autosomal recessive trait.

Latent Nystagmus

Latent nystagmus occurs upon occlusion of either eye. The nystagmus is conjugate and jerky, with the fast component toward the side of the covered eye. The condition has no known neurologic significance and is only of consequence when the affected individual loses one eye.

2. SPASMUS NUTANS

This uncommon condition of unknown cause occurs in infants 4–12 months of age. The nystagmus is of the dissociated vertical or asymmetric horizontal pendular type and is often associated with nonsynchronous head nodding. The prognosis is good; recovery occurs within a few months to 2 years.

3. NYSTAGMUS DUE TO NEUROLOGIC DISTURBANCES

Pendular or Jerky Nystagmus

Acquired pendular or jerky nystagmus is usually horizontal (occasionally vertical) and causes oscillopsia. It is frequently seen in demyelinating disease (occasionally in vascular disease) and is due to a lesion of the brain stem.

Ocular Flutter

Ocular flutter is a sign of cerebellar disease. It consists of a series of oscillating horizontal saccadic movements while fixating an object.

See-Saw Nystagmus

This rare type of nystagmus consists of regular reciprocating oscillations in which one eye rises while the other falls. Tumors in the region of the optic chiasm and diencephalon are the most frequent cause.

Nystagmus Retractorius

On attempted upward gaze, convergent nystagmus associated with retraction of the eyes occurs. It is diagnostic of a lesion of the rostral midbrain and is associated with signs of lid retraction, loss of upward gaze (Parinaud's syndrome), and abnormal pupillary reactions.

4. VESTIBULAR NYSTAGMUS

Vestibular nystagmus is always of the jerky type. The slow component is considered to be a response to impulses originating in the semicircular canals; the fast component is a corrective movement. Vestibular nystagmus is not dependent upon visual stimuli, ie, it is present with the lids closed as well as open and can be elicited in blind individuals also. It is inhibited or damped by visual fixation. Rotatory movements are especially characteristic of vestibular nystagmus, but horizontal or vertical vestibular nystagmus also occurs.

Physiologic nystagmus elicited by stimulation of the semicircular canals by means of the Bárány chair or caloric stimulation depends upon normal vestibular function.

The following characteristics of vestibular nystagmus demonstrate its origin in labyrinthine and vestibular nerve disease: (1) Vertigo, tinnitus, and deafness are apt to be associated. (2) Nystagmus is maximal early in the disease, and tends to improve or disappear in 2–3 weeks (unless the vestibular nuclei are affected directly, in which case nystagmus may be permanent). (3) The lesion is always destructive, and its direction (fast component) is away from the side the lesion is on.

Specific Lesions Causing Vestibular Nystagmus

Vestibular nystagmus may be due to labyrinthitis, Meniere's disease, traumatic (including surgical) destruction of one labyrinth; vascular, inflammatory, or neoplastic lesions of the vestibular nerves; lesions of the vestibular nuclei (encephalitis, multiple sclerosis, syringobulbia, poliomyelitis, thrombosis of the posteroinferior cerebellar artery); or cerebellar tumors and abscesses (probably as a result of pressure on the vestibular pathways). (*Note:* There is some dispute about whether a cerebellar lesion per se can cause nystagmus. Evidence suggests that nystagmus in such cases results from pressure on the vestibular structures. An alternative explanation is that the cerebellar hemispheres exert an inhibitory influence on nystagmus on its own side through the cerebellobulbar tract. Thus a lesion on one side causes nystagmus toward the lesion.)

5. GAZE NYSTAGMUS

Gaze nystagmus is probably the most common nystagmus and often represents the first sign or the residuum of a gaze palsy. These patients have no nystagmus on forward gaze but develop nystagmus in one or more fields of gaze with the fast component in the direction of gaze.

The causes vary and include drug toxicity (especially phenytoin, but barbiturates also) and demyelinating, degenerative, neoplastic, or vascular disease. Gaze nystagmus is of no specific localizing value except that it is suggestive of lesions of the posterior fossa.

6. VOLUNTARY & HYSTERICAL NYSTAGMUS

Voluntary nystagmus is an uncommon "parlor trick." The individual "wills" a rapid horizontal nystagmus of high frequency and low amplitude that can be maintained only a few seconds.

Hysterical nystagmus is similar to voluntary nystagmus. It is particularly common in anxiety neuroses.

CENTRAL NERVOUS SYSTEM TUMORS OF NEURO-OPHTHALMOLOGIC IMPORTANCE

CEREBRAL TUMORS

Frontal Lobe Tumors

Mental changes (depression, euphoria, or mental deficiency) and contralateral hemiparesis are the most frequent signs of frontal lobe tumors. Pressure upon the olfactory tracts may cause anosmia. Ophthalmologic signs include the following:

A. Papilledema (50%): Due to increased intracranial pressure.

B. Visual Field Changes (30%): These are not characteristic. Almost any defect is possible as a result of pressure upon the optic pathway.

C. Irregular Nystagmus (5–10%): This is of no localizing value.

D. Gaze Palsies: Irritative lesions cause the eyes to deviate to the opposite side. Destructive lesions cause deviation to the same side. These gaze palsies are usually incomplete and last only a few weeks or may be manifested by an end point nystagmus only.

Temporal Lobe Tumors

Gliomas are the most common type. Meningiomas are next most common and angiomas are rare.

Temporal lobe tumors may cause psychomotor convulsions and uncinate fits, sometimes preceded by an aura of abnormal smell. Formed visual hallucinations may occur, in contrast to occipital lobe tumors. A generalized or localized convulsion (chewing, sucking, or smacking movements) follows. Auditory disturbances are not common. Ophthalmologic signs include papilledema (often) and incongruous visual field changes (usually). The typical visual field change is an incongruous contralateral homonymous hemianopia of the upper quadrants.

Occipital Lobe Tumors

The occipital lobe is only rarely involved by tumor. Gliomas, meningiomas, and metastatic tumors may occur. Epileptic attacks (grand or petit mal) as well as mild mental abnormalities may be present. Papilledema can be extreme (up to 6 or 8 diopters). Contralateral homonymous hemianopia occurs in 85% of cases. It tends to be congruous with sparing of the macula. Loss of involuntary conjugate eye movements is due to a lesion of the supranuclear pathway. Visual agnosia occurs as a result of involvement of the visual association areas.

CEREBELLAR TUMORS

Cerebellar tumors are the most common brain tumors before age 15. Gliomas are common, and about one-fourth of these are the very malignant medulloblastomas of the roof of the fourth ventricle. Astrocytomas of the cerebellar hemisphere also occur, mainly in children. Papilledema due to increased intracranial pressure and abducens palsy due to pressure on the sixth nerve at the base of the brain are common findings. Vestibular nystagmus also occurs. Systemic signs of cerebellar tumor include ataxia, hypotonia, and tremor.

BRAIN STEM TUMORS

Tumors of the Midbrain

Lesions of the upper part of the midbrain (near the quadrigeminal bodies) cause Parinaud's syndrome, sometimes associated with retraction of the lids or ptosis. Lesions of the lower midbrain produce paralysis of downward gaze, paralysis of convergence, loss of pupillary reaction to light or accommodation (or both), and unequal pupil size. Increased intracranial pressure is often present as a result of obstruction of the cerebral aqueduct. Papilledema may be an early or a late sign. Gliomas and pinealomas are the most common tumors, especially in children.

Lesions involving the red nucleus produce Benedikt's syndrome and Weber's syndrome. Cerebellar signs (ataxia, hypotonia, and nystagmus) due to pressure on or direct involvement of the cerebellum may also be present.

Tumors of the Pons

Gliomas are the most common pontine tumors. Multiple nuclear palsies (particularly in childhood) involve principally the fifth, sixth, seventh, and eighth cranial nerves in combination with motor and sensory long tract signs in the limbs. Increased intracranial pressure develops late. Foville's syndrome is sometimes present. The course is usually chronic and progressive.

Tumors of the Medulla

Early manifestations include vertigo, cardiac irregularities, swallowing difficulties, and hoarseness. Paralysis of the tongue and papilledema develop later. Eye signs are not prominent. Death usually occurs early.

OTHER INTRACRANIAL TUMORS OF NEURO-OPHTHALMOLOGIC IMPORTANCE

Meningioma of Sphenoidal Ridge

The tumor arises from the small wing of the sphenoid bone. Ipsilateral slight (occasionally severe) progressive exophthalmos is present in about 40% of cases and is often the presenting sign. Visual field changes are at first unilateral and later bilateral and are not characteristic. Headache is common. All changes occur gradually over many years, since the tumor grows quite slowly.

Tumors of the Cerebellopontine Angle

Neurofibroma (or neurinoma) of the acoustic nerve sometimes occurs as part of Recklinghausen's disease. More often, the tumor occurs alone. A cerebellopontine angle tumor may also be a meningioma. Cerebellar signs include hypotonia, ataxia, and unsteady gait. Vestibular nystagmus is common as a result of pressure on the brain stem. Increased intracranial pressure causes papilledema. Cranial nerve palsies include facial paresis (seventh nerve), tinnitus, deafness, vertigo (eighth nerve), loss of corneal sensation and sneeze reflex (fifth nerve), and dysphagia (tenth nerve). Motor involvement produces contralateral hemiplegia (pyramidal).

Complete or partial excision of the tumor is usually possible.

Pineal Tumor

This rare tumor (2% of all gliomas) may occur at any age. Papilledema occurs early as a result of blockage of the cerebral aqueduct. Parinaud's syndrome develops later. Pressure on adjacent structures commonly occurs, causing cerebellar signs, extraocular muscle palsies, deafness, and pupillary signs.

These tumors are treated surgically with or without radiation.

CEREBROVASCULAR DISORDERS OF OPHTHALMOLOGIC IMPORTANCE

Vascular Insufficiency & Occlusion of the Internal Carotid Artery

Episodes of amaurosis fugax frequently occur as a result of atherosclerotic lesions of the ipsilateral internal carotid artery. Cerebral and retinal disturbances occur as a result of small emboli breaking loose from the sclerotic plaque and lodging in cerebral or retinal arterioles (occlusion of the central retinal artery or a major branch can occur). These small plaques (Hollenhorst plaques) may be visible with the ophthalmoscope as small glistening yellow spots situated at bifurcations of the retinal arteries. A finding of reduced ophthalmic artery pressure—as determined by ophthalmodynamometry, bruits over the internal carotid artery, and angiography—helps to confirm the diagnosis.

Removal of the plaque by carotid endarterectomy is frequently indicated and may prevent a major stroke or a central retinal artery occlusion.

Occlusion of the Middle Cerebral Artery

This disorder may produce severe contralateral hemiplegia, hemianesthesia, and homonymous hemianopia. The lower quadrants of the visual fields (upper radiations) are most apt to be involved. Aphasia may be present.

Vascular Insufficiency of the Vertebral-Basilar Arterial System

Brief episodes of transient bilateral blurring of vision commonly precede a basilar artery stroke. An attack seldom leaves any residual visual impairment, and the episode may be so minimal that the patient or doctor does not heed the warning. The blurring is described as a graying of vision just as if the house lights were being turned down at a theater. The change seldom lasts more than 5 minutes (often only a few seconds) and may be associated with other transient symptoms of vertebral-basilar insufficiency. Such episodes of visual loss are termed amaurosis fugax.

Occlusion of the Basilar Artery

Complete or extensive thrombosis of the basilar artery nearly always causes death. With partial occlusion of basilar "insufficiency" due to arteriosclerosis, a wide variety of brain stem and cerebellar signs may be present. These include nystagmus, supranuclear oculomotor signs, and involvement of cranial nerves III, IV, VI, and VII.

Prolonged anticoagulant therapy has become the accepted treatment of partial basilar artery occlusion or "insufficiency," but transluminal angioplasty may soon become a common form of therapy.

Occlusion of the Posterior Cerebral Artery

Occlusion of the posterior cerebral artery seldom causes death. Occlusion of the cortical branches (most common) causes homonymous hemianopia, usually superior quadrantic (the artery supplies primarily the visual cortex). Lesions on the left in right-handed persons can cause aphasia and dyslexia. Occlusion of the proximal branches may produce the thalamic syndrome (thalamic pain, hemiparesis, hemianesthesia, choreoathetoid movements) and cerebellar ataxia. Weber's, Benedikt's, or Parinaud's syndrome may result.

Cavernous Sinus Thrombosis

See p 200.

Subdural Hemorrhage

Subdural hemorrhage results from tearing or shearing of the veins bridging the subdural space from the pia mater to the dural sinus. It leads to an encapsulated accumulation of blood in the subdural space, usually over one cerebral hemisphere. It is nearly always caused by trauma to the head. The trauma may be minimal and may precede the onset of neurologic signs by weeks or even months.

In infants, subdural hemorrhage produces progressive enlargement of the head with bulging fontanelles. The diagnosis is established by the finding of bloody spinal fluid on tapping the subdural space and by enlarged head measurements. Ocular signs include strabismus, pupillary changes, papilledema, and retinal hemorrhages.

In adults, the symptoms of chronic subdural hematoma are severe headache, drowsiness, and mental confusion, usually appearing hours to weeks (or even months) after trauma. Symptomatology is similar to that of cerebral tumors. Papilledema is present in 30–50% of cases. Retinal hemorrhages occur in association with papilledema. Ipsilateral dilatation of the pupil is the most common and most serious pupillary sign and is an urgent indication for immediate surgical evacuation of blood. Unequal, miotic, or mydriatic pupils can occur, or there may be no pupillary signs. Other signs, including vestibular nystagmus and cranial nerve palsies, also occur. Many of these signs result from herniation and compression of the brain stem, and hence often appear late with stupor and coma.

Skull films may show a shift of a calcified pineal gland. Carotid arteriography frequently confirms the diagnosis.

Treatment of acute subdural hematoma consists of surgical evacuation of the blood. Without treatment, the course is progressively downhill to coma and death. With early and adequate treatment, the prognosis is good except for infants, in whom repeated subdural taps may be only temporarily lifesaving or may result in residual damage (convulsions, low mentality, motor and sensory defects).

Subarachnoid Hemorrhage

Subarachnoid hemorrhage most commonly results from ruptured congenital berry aneurysms of the circle of Willis in the subarachnoid space. It may also result from trauma, birth injuries, intracranial hemorrhage, hemorrhage associated with tumors, arteriovenous malformations, or systemic bleeding disorders.

The most prominent symptom of subarachnoid hemorrhage is sudden, severe headache, usually occipital and often associated with signs of meningeal irrita-

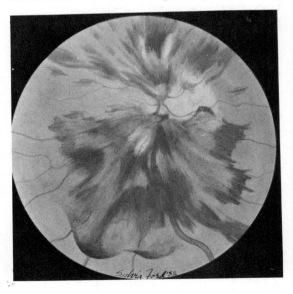

Figure 17–17. Subhyaloid hemorrhage around optic disk associated with subarachnoid hemorrhage. (Drawing.)

tion (eg, stiff neck). Drowsiness, loss of consciousness, coma, and death may occur rapidly. Ocular symptoms are not always present. Extraocular muscle palsies are the most common single ocular sign. An oculomotor palsy with associated numbness and pain in the distribution of the ipsilateral trigeminal nerve is pathognomonic of a supraclinoid, internal carotid, or posterior communicating artery aneurysm. Papilledema usually appears late when it does occur. Various types of retinal hemorrhage occur infrequently (preretinal hemorrhages are the most common). Exophthalmos may occur as a result of extravasation of blood into orbital tissues. Pressure of an aneurysm on the optic nerve may cause blindness in one eye.

Arteriography following injection of radiopaque substances may help to demonstrate and localize the aneurysms. Blood is present in the cerebrospinal fluid.

Ligation of aneurysmal vessels or of parent arterial trunks may be advisable. Supportive treatment, including control of blood pressure, is at times all that can be done.

Migraine

Migraine is a common episodic illness of unknown cause and varied symptomatology characterized by severe unilateral headache, visual disturbances, nausea, and vomiting. It is associated with dilatation and constriction of the external carotid artery and its branches. The neurologic symptoms that usually precede the headache occur in the vasoconstrictor phase; the headache follows in the vasodilative phase. There is usually a family history of a similar disorder. The disease usually becomes manifest between ages 15 and 30. It is more common and more severe in women. Many factors, particularly emotional ones, may predispose or contribute to attacks. Prodromal symptoms are common and include drowsiness, paresthesias, ''scintillating'' scotomas, blurred vision, and other symptoms. In some patients, homonymous hemianopia can be accurately recorded on the tangent screen during attacks. There are no other objective findings. The visual symptoms usually last no longer than 15–30 minutes.

Ergotamine tartrate, when given early in an attack, is often effective. Once the attack is well under way, treatment is of little value. The headaches last from several hours to several days. Bed rest is often helpful if not essential.

INTRACRANIAL INFECTIONS OF OPHTHALMOLOGIC IMPORTANCE

MENINGITIS

Acute Bacterial Meningitis

Acute meningitis may be due to *Neisseria meningitidis, Streptococcus pneumoniae, Haemophilus in-* *fluenzae, Staphylococcus aureus, Streptococcus viridans,* or other bacterial agents. There are many ocular manifestations of general meningeal irritation, depending upon the main area of associated inflammation. Basal meningitis causes oculomotor palsies (abducens palsy is the most common). Ptosis and pupillary changes, including sluggish light reaction and anisocoria, are also frequent. Papilledema indicative of increased intracranial pressure may be prominent. Locally the disease may be complicated by chemosis of the conjunctiva and edema of the lids, with photophobia a common symptom. Metastatic uveitis with resulting endophthalmitis and loss of all function occurs at times, especially in children. Treatment consists of massive systemic administration of sulfonamides and antibiotics (and intrathecal antiinfectives administered by lumbar puncture). Culture of the spinal fluid nearly always establishes the etiologic diagnosis.

Tuberculous Meningitis

Tuberculous meningitis is a more chronic form of bacterial meningitis. It occurs rarely, and usually in children. The general symptomatology is the same as outlined above for acute bacterial meningitis. When miliary lesions can be seen ophthalmoscopically as small oval yellowish lesions in the choroid, the prognosis for life is very bad. In the past, tuberculous meningitis was uniformly fatal. Long-term systemic administration of isoniazid, rifampin, ethambutol, and streptomycin has reduced the mortality rate significantly.

Syphilitic Meningitis

Acute syphilitic meningitis may be quite similar to acute infectious meningitis. The cranial nerves—particularly the oculomotor nerves—are often involved, causing diplopia. Papilledema and visual field changes, indicating chiasmal arachnoiditis (bitemporal hemianopia), are also common. All manifestations of meningitis clear well following antisyphilitic therapy.

Encephalomyelitides Associated With Infectious Diseases

Measles, mumps, vaccinia, chickenpox, herpes simplex, and smallpox are the most common viral diseases with neurologic complications. Complications may be due to activation of a neurotropic virus, a toxin, or an allergic phenomenon. There is no treatment.

Neurologic signs result from cerebral, cerebellar, or cord involvement as well as from optic neuritis. Most patients recover completely, but permanent sequelae and death do occur, especially following smallpox, vaccinia, and herpes simplex.

BRAIN ABSCESS

Abscesses form in the brain by direct extension of infection from the nasal sinuses (frontal lobe) and middle ear (temporal lobe or cerebellum). Penetrating head wounds and septicemia may also produce brain abscesses. Symptoms include persistent headache, fever, and vomiting. Increased intracranial pressure may develop rapidly. Papilledema is present. Localizing cerebral signs of cerebral abscess are the same as for cerebral tumors. Diagnosis is more difficult today because of the masking effect of inadequate antibiotic therapy. Treatment consists of systemic antibiotics and surgical drainage of the abscess.

• • •

THE PHAKOMATOSES

These 4 disease entities are logically grouped together because they are characterized by a combination of skin and central nervous system lesions with frequent ocular involvement. All are genetically determined as autosomal dominants.

Neurofibromatosis (Recklinghausen's Disease)

Neurofibromatosis is a generalized hereditary disease characterized by multiple tumors of the skin, central nervous system, peripheral nerves, and nerve sheaths. Other developmental anomalies, particularly of the bones, may be associated. Inheritance is autosomal dominant with incomplete penetrance. Thus, the disease can be quite mild in one generation and appear as a full-blown debilitating disease in the next.

Neurofibromas are made up of randomly oriented or palisaded cells of either fibroplastic or Schwann cell origin. Nerve fibers often course through or over the tumor. The tumors are discrete and benign but may undergo sarcomatous degeneration.

Tumors may occur anywhere in the body, including the eye. Café au lait spots (small pigmented areas of skin) tend to enlarge and darken with age. Tumors of the lids are often present. Tumors of the orbital portion of the optic nerve are particularly common, causing papilledema and retrobulbar neuritis early and optic atrophy later in the disease. There may be iris nodules and corneal nerve changes.

Neurofibromatosis of the lid is associated rarely with unilateral infantile glaucoma.

Intracranial gliomas may be associated with neurofibromatosis. Spinal cord neurofibromas frequently occur. The acoustic nerve is the cranial nerve most commonly involved and produces the syndrome of the cerebellopontine angle.

Bone development is affected when the tumor involves periosteum. Pulsating exophthalmos occasionally occurs when an osseous defect of the posterior orbit is present.

Orbital or intracranial surgery may be needed to remove tumors for functional or cosmetic reasons.

When lesions are confined to the skin, the prognosis is good. Intracranial and intraspinal lesions are usually multiple and have a bad prognosis. The disease tends to be fairly stationary, with only slow progression over long periods of time.

Angiomatosis Retinae
(Von Hippel-Lindau Disease)

This rare disease occurs most commonly in men in the third decade but can appear at any age up to 60. The earliest signs are dilatation and tortuosity of the retinal vessels, which later develop into an angiomatous formation with hemorrhages and exudates. A stage of massive exudation, retinal detachment, and absolute glaucoma occurs later, and usually destroys the eye within 5–15 years after onset. The disease is unilateral in 65% of cases. In 25% of cases the retinal angiomatosis is associated with a similar generalized process, most often affecting the cerebellum and less commonly the pancreas, kidney, adrenal gland, and other organs. The evidence at present suggests that this is all one genetically determined disease showing autosomal dominant inheritance with variable expression. Several reports of abnormal chromosomal patterns have been reported.

Early treatment of retinal lesions with photocoagulation and cryotherapy has been effective in some cases. Cerebral and cerebellar tumors have been successfully removed, but if the central nervous system is involved the prognosis for life is poor. A downhill course and death, usually by middle age, are the rule.

Sturge-Weber Syndrome

This uncommon disease is recognizable at birth by a characteristic nevus flammeus (port wine stain type of angioma) on one side of the face following the distribution of one or more branches of the fifth cranial nerve. Unilateral infantile glaucoma on the affected side frequently develops if there is extensive involvement of the eye with hemangioma of the choroid. Lid and conjunctival involvement nearly always implies ultimate intraocular involvement and glaucoma. Extensive venous aneurysms in the meningeal sheaths extending into the brain substance account for the high incidence of central nervous system disturbances, of which jacksonian convulsive seizures are the most common. These cranial lesions are on the same side as the skin lesions and usually become manifest within the first decade. Radiographically, calcification in the cerebral cortex is usually present. The disease follows an autosomal dominant hereditary pattern with variable expression. There is at least one study reporting a 22 trisomy on cytogenic study.

There is no effective treatment of Sturge-Weber syndrome, although the glaucoma can be controlled in rare cases by cyclodiathermy. Other glaucoma operations have been unsuccessful.

The prognosis for life as well as for sight is poor, with death before age 30 the rule.

Tuberous Sclerosis (Bourneville's Disease)

This is a generalized disease whose manifestations include adenoma sebaceum (85%), central nervous system tumors, retinal tumors (50%), renal tumors (50%), and multiple lung cysts. The signs may be present at birth or may develop within the first few years of life. Onset is with convulsive seizures and mental retardation. The large papular skin lesions have the appearance of overgrown "blackheads" and are often the earliest sign of the disease. The retinal tumors appear as oval or circular white areas in the peripheral fundus and characteristically have a mulberrylike appearance (Fig 22–12). Histologically, the retinal tumors are composed of hyaline material with areas of calcification.

The disease is inherited as an autosomal dominant with high penetrance. No treatment is available. The prognosis is very poor, with a progressive downhill course and death in adolescence the rule.

CEREBROMACULAR DEGENERATION

Genetically determined (autosomal recessive) neuronal lipid storage diseases of the brain may affect the neural elements of the retina as well. The clinical forms are classified mainly by the age at onset. The pathologic changes are present prenatally, with clinical manifestations occurring as a critical level of intraneuronal lipidosis is reached. A definite diagnosis can be established readily by rectal biopsy or appendectomy showing ganglioside accumulation even before clinical signs are present. Five forms of cerebromacular degeneration (ganglioside lipidosis) are recognized: congenital, infantile (Tay-Sachs), late infantile, juvenile (Spielmeyer-Vogt), and adult.

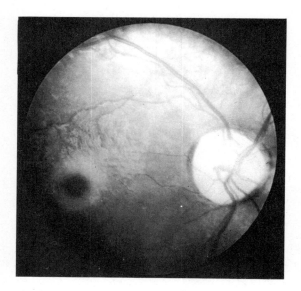

Figure 17–18. Cherry-red spot of Tay-Sachs disease in an 18-month-old child.

Severe mental and physical deterioration occurs, usually causing death within a few years. The later the onset, the milder the disease. The liver and spleen show increased gangliosides. The striking ocular finding of a cherry-red spot in the macula is seen in congenital and infantile cases (Fig 17–18). Optic atrophy and retinal pigmentary changes are frequently present in the juvenile and adult forms. Extraocular muscle dysfunction is a less frequent finding in all forms.

The exact enzymatic abnormalities are still not known, but a deficiency of serum fructose-1-phosphate aldolase is present in carriers as well as affected persons with Tay-Sachs disease.

NIEMANN-PICK DISEASE
(Sphingomyelin-Sterol Lipidosis)

This entity is quite similar to the ganglioside lipidoses. There is a deposition of glycolipid in the ganglion cells of the brain and retina. The spleen, liver, and other reticuloendothelial organs are massively infiltrated with glycolipid. Inheritance is autosomal recessive, and 2 clinical forms are recognized. The infantile form is the most common and most severe, with death usually occurring in 2 or 3 years. A cherry-red spot in the macula may be present. The juvenile or adult form is much more benign and usually without eye findings.

MISCELLANEOUS DISEASES OF NEURO-OPHTHALMOLOGIC IMPORTANCE

AMBLYOPIA DUE TO METHANOL POISONING

Methanol (methyl alcohol, wood alcohol) has long been used as an intoxicating drink, either by mistake or because ethyl alcohol was not available. It may be mixed either accidentally or purposely with ethyl alcohol. Its breakdown product, formaldehyde, can cause severe poisoning marked by gastroenteritis, pulmonary edema, cerebral edema, and extensive retinal damage. There are great individual variations in tolerance; small amounts (30 mL) may cause profound effects in some persons while much larger amounts cause no poisonous effects in others. Significant systemic absorption has been reported from inhaled fumes and, very rarely, through the skin.

There is a marked destruction of the ganglion cells of the retina as well as degeneration of nerve fibers in the optic nerve, occasionally extending well past the optic chiasm in severe cases.

Clinical Findings

A. Symptoms and Signs: Acute symptoms appear within 18 hours of ingestion. Weakness, anorexia, nausea, vomiting, headache, dizziness, Kussmaul respiration, and pain in the back, extremities, and abdomen may occur in succession or almost simultaneously. Extensive exposure will lead to delirium, convulsions, coma, and death.

Visual disturbances range from ''spots before the eyes'' to complete blindness. The field defects are quite extensive and nearly always include the centrocecal area (Fig 17–19).

Hyperemia of the disk is the first ophthalmoscopic finding. Within the first 2 days a whitish, striated edema of the disk margins and nearby retina appears. Papilledema can last up to 2 months and is followed by optic atrophy of mild to severe degree.

Decreased pupillary response to light occurs in proportion to the amount of visual loss. In severe cases the pupils become dilated and fixed. Extraocular muscle palsies and ptosis may also occur.

B. Laboratory Findings: Severe metabolic acidosis results from conversion of methanol→formaldehyde→formic acid. Bicarbonate in extracellular fluid is displaced by the organic acid. Analysis of arterial blood shows a low pH, low bicarbonate, and low P_{CO_2} (from compensatory hyperpnea).

Treatment

If ethanol and methanol are ingested or inhaled simultaneously, the effects of methanol will not become evident until most of the ethanol is excreted. If the patient is seen soon after exposure, gastric lavage should be performed. Acidosis should be controlled with large and repeated doses of bicarbonate. Ethanol inhibits the metabolic oxidation of methanol; therefore, a blood ethanol concentration of 100 mg/dL blood should be maintained until all methanol has been excreted.

Course & Prognosis

Patients with dilated, fixed pupils during the acute attack usually die. If they survive, they have severe visual loss. Patients with retinal edema usually have moderate to marked permanent visual loss. The initial loss of vision shows an early improvement that may be only transitory. Visual improvement occurs only during the first week; if little or no immediate improvement occurs, eventual optic atrophy with very low visual acuity is the rule. Only in mild cases is normal visual function regained.

NUTRITIONAL AMBLYOPIA
(Tobacco-Alcohol Amblyopia)

Nutritional amblyopia is the preferred term for the entity sometimes referred to as tobacco-alcohol amblyopia, tobacco amblyopia, or alcohol amblyopia since they are all the same entity. Persons with poor dietary habits, particularly if the diet is deficient in thiamine, may develop centrocecal scotomas that are usually of constant density. When density of the scotoma varies, the most dense portion usually lies between fixation and the blind spot.

Heavy drinking with or without heavy smoking is most often associated with the poor nutritional state. Occasionally, there is a history of heavy smoking without drinking.

Bilateral loss of central vision is present in over 50% of patients, reducing visual acuity below 6/60 (20/200). Most of the others have severe central loss in one eye with some deficit, often about 6/15 (20/50) visual acuity, in the better eye. Central visual fields reveal scotomas that nearly always include both fixation and the blind spot (centrocecal scotoma) (Fig

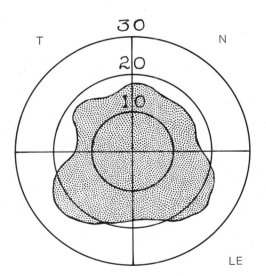

Figure 17–19. Methyl alcohol amblyopia showing very large centrocecal scotoma. VA = hand movements only.

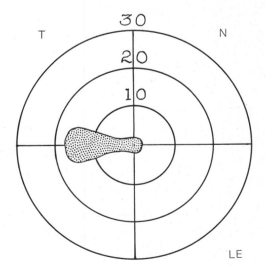

Figure 17–20. Nutritional amblyopia showing centrocecal scotoma. VA = 6/60 (20/200).

17–20). Pallor of the optic disks may be present. Loss of the ganglion cells of the macula and destruction of myelinated fibers of the optic nerve, and sometimes of the chiasm as well, are the main histologic changes.

Chiasmal lesions can cause similar visual field changes, but the scotomas generally stop at the midline, allowing differentiation. Rarely, multiple sclerosis, pernicious anemia, methanol poisoning, retrobulbar neuritis, or macular degeneration may cause diagnostic confusion.

Adequate diet plus thiamine, folic acid, and vitamin B_{12} is nearly always effective in completely curing the disease if it is recognized early. Withdrawal of tobacco and alcohol is advisable and may hasten the cure, but innumerable cases are known in which adequate nutrition alone effected the cure despite continued excessive intake of alcohol or tobacco or both. Improvement usually begins within 1–2 months, although occasionally significant improvement may not occur for a year. Visual function may not return to normal; permanent optic atrophy can occur depending upon the stage of disease at the time treatment was started. If there has been neuronal degeneration, permanent dysfunction results.

AMBLYOPIA DUE TO QUININE & RELATED COMPOUNDS

Quinine and quinacrine, used primarily in the treatment and prevention of malaria, occasionally cause visual disturbances on an idiosyncratic basis. The onset is acute, most often following a single dose. Other symptoms are a feeling of fullness in the head, ringing in the ears, and deafness. There is constriction of the visual field (Fig 17–21) and, rarely, total blind-

ness. The tendency is toward partial recovery, with permanent peripheral field defects the rule. The ganglion cells of the retina are affected first, presumably as a result of marked vasoconstriction of the retinal arterioles, easily visible with an ophthalmoscope. Varying degrees of retinal edema early, and optic atrophy later, occur bilaterally.

The most important treatment is drug withdrawal, after which there may be some improvement, no change, or gradual continued deterioration of visual function. Vasodilators such as amyl nitrite, acetylcholine, and sodium nitrite may favorably influence some cases in the acute phase.

AMBLYOPIA DUE TO ORGANIC ARSENIC COMPOUNDS

Sudden permanent visual loss sometimes resulted from organic arsenic compounds used in the treatment of syphilis. Peripheral field contraction and general field depression were followed by optic atrophy with no tendency toward recovery. In some cases, despite stopping the medication, complete blindness occurred.

AMBLYOPIA DUE TO SALICYLATES

Salicylic acid derivatives in very large doses cause a clinical picture of toxicity that is quite similar to that caused by quinine. Constriction of the visual field like that seen in quinine amblyopia (Fig 17–21), dilated pupils, tinnitus, and deafness may all be present. Upon withdrawal of the drug, visual function usually improves, but complete recovery is rare.

HERPES ZOSTER
(Shingles)

Infection with herpes zoster virus is characterized by the appearance of vesicles upon the skin along the course of a nerve. The virus has a predilection for the gasserian ganglion and the first 2 divisions of the fifth cranial nerve. Severe pain over one side of the face may precede by several days the eruption of vesicles on the forehead and eyelids on one side. The vesicles contain clear fluid that rapidly becomes purulent. These rupture, leaving ulcers that usually become secondarily infected and form crusts. Some permanent scarring always results. The eyelids become red and edematous, and there is tearing with scanty discharge. The conjunctiva is red and the cornea shows discrete white subepithelial opacities (involvement of the nasociliary branch of the first division of the fifth cranial nerve). Fine dendritic lesions may occur. Corneal sensitivity is markedly decreased, favoring exposure and secondary infection. The keratopathy lasts several months and may clear with minimal scarring. Complications include secondary glaucoma, iritis, and scleritis. Corneal opacity may persist and

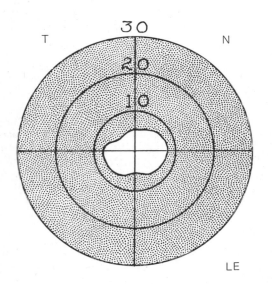

Figure 17–21. Quinine amblyopia showing only a central cone of field remaining. VA = 6/7.5 (20/25).

markedly reduce vision. Severe, persistent neuralgia may be a late manifestation.

Complete internal and external ophthalmoplegia occurs rarely. Incomplete palsy of the third nerve is the most common type of involvement. Optic neuritis is rare but quite serious, as recovery of function is minimal. Gaze palsies and encephalitis seldom occur.

There is no specific therapy for shingles. Ophthalmologic treatment is directed toward protecting the exposed cornea, combating secondary infection, and lowering the intraocular pressure if there is secondary glaucoma. Antibiotic ointments are used locally. Dilatation of the pupil with homatropine, 2–5%, puts the eye at rest and is particularly useful if iritis is present. Systemic corticosteroids do not help, and there are several reports of death following their administration. Postherpetic neuralgia has been treated with a variety of agents, including the major tranquilizers, with variable reports of success.

The prognosis is good, and recurrences are rare.

NEUROPARALYTIC KERATITIS

Loss of function of the sensory nerve to the cornea (nasociliary branch of the ophthalmic division of the fifth cranial nerve) can lead to trophic changes in the cornea. Punctate epithelial lesions appear first, usually as small vesicles that lead to irritation, photophobia, and ciliary injection. If the process continues, epithelium is lost and a corneal ulcer may develop with secondary infection. Iritis, hypopyon, and, at times, an overwhelming endophthalmitis with loss of the eye can occur.

Neuroparalytic keratitis usually occurs as a complication of section of the sensory fifth nerve root in the treatment of tic douloureux, and it also occurs following herpes zoster keratitis, posterior fossa tumor extirpations, and other rarer conditions.

Protection of the cornea and treatment of secondary infection are the only available measures. Antibiotic ointments should be applied locally, particularly at night. Protective eye shields may be necessary. In well-established cases, suturing the lids together temporarily may be the best way to control keratitis.

MARCUS GUNN PHENOMENON
(Jaw Winking)

This rare congenital condition consists of elevation of a ptotic eyelid upon movement of the jaw. Acquired cases occur after damage to the oculomotor nerve with subsequent abnormal regeneration of nerve fibers. Muscular palsies may be present.

Treatment is surgical. The best results have been obtained by severing the levator muscle completely and then doing a ptosis operation later, utilizing the frontalis muscle.

DUANE'S SYNDROME

This uncommon congenital, stationary, nearly always unilateral condition consists of deficient horizontal ocular motility originally thought to be due to fibrous rectus muscles. Recent evidence based on pathologic studies has determined that Duane's syndrome is a result of congenital absence of the sixth nerve. The lateral rectus is innervated by a branch of the third nerve. Attempted adduction movements result in retraction of the globe and narrowing of the lid fissure. The visual handicap is seldom severe. Visual acuity is normal, and the eye is otherwise normal. Unless the deviation is very large, strabismus surgery is best avoided.

CRANIOSYNOSTOSIS

Under this general heading are grouped a number of rare dysostoses causing distortion of the face and head and having recessive or irregular dominant inheritance. In oxycephaly the sutures of the bones of the face and head close before the brain growth is complete. Continued growth of frontal bone allows for brain expansion, leading to tower skull or other abnormal shapes of the skull. At times the sphenoid bone does not develop properly, leaving an inadequate optic canal and constricting the optic nerve and causing optic atrophy. Increased intracranial pressure may result from the inadequate cranial vault volume. One variant of particular note is gargoylism (Hurler's disease), a form of dwarfism with oxycephaly and hypertelorism (widely spaced eyes). Gargoylism is an autosomal recessive disease due to overproduction of mucopolysaccharides. Acid mucopolysaccharides and glycoproteins are deposited in the cornea, abdominal organs, and central nervous system, causing death before age 20.

MANDIBULOFACIAL DYSOSTOSIS
(Franceschetti's Syndrome)

Patients with this rare disorder have a characteristic antimongoloid facies with a temporally placed notch in the lower lids, hypoplasia of some facial bones, high palate, and other less striking facial changes. The disease is genetically determined as an irregular dominant.

WAARDENBURG'S SYNDROME

This rare entity, inherited as an irregular dominant, is distinguished by wide separation of the inner canthi, broad nasal root, heavy eyebrows, heterochromia of the iris, white forelock, and congenital deafness.

MYASTHENIA GRAVIS

This disease, characterized by ease of fatigability of the striated muscles, often is first manifested by weakness of extraocular muscles. Unilateral ptosis is a frequent first sign, with subsequent bilateral involvement of extraocular muscles so that diplopia is often an early symptom. Generalized weakness of the arms and legs, difficulty in swallowing, weakness of jaw muscles, and difficulty in breathing may follow rapidly in untreated cases. There are no sensory changes. The disease is not rare. It usually affects young adults age 20–40, though it may occur at any age.

The onset may follow an upper respiratory infection or an injury and has been noted as a transitory condition in newborn infants of myasthenic mothers. The disease has been associated with hyperthyroidism, collagen disease, and diffuse metastatic carcinoma. Accumulating evidence suggests that an autoimmune mechanism is a significant factor.

The differential diagnosis includes progressive nuclear ophthalmoplegia, brain stem lesions, epidemic encephalitis, bulbar and pseudobulbar palsy, and post-diphtheritic paralysis.

Although substantial neurophysiologic evidence indicates that the site of the disorder is the neuromuscular junction, convincing evidence of morphologic changes has not been presented. It is known that there is insufficient utilization of acetylcholine at the motor end plate. Thymomas have been reported in 25% of myasthenic persons over age 35. About half of patients with thymomas have myasthenia gravis. The 2 diseases must be related, but the mechanism remains obscure.

Cholinesterase destroys acetylcholine at the myoneural junction, and cholinesterase-inhibiting drugs (neostigmine) markedly improve the condition. The edrophonium chloride (Tensilon) test is used in addition to the neostigmine-atropine diagnostic test. Edrophonium, 2 mg (0.2 mL), is given intravenously over 15 seconds. Relief of ptosis constitutes a positive response and confirms the diagnosis of myasthenia gravis. If no response occurs in 30 seconds, an additional 8 mg (0.8 mL) are given. The test is most critical when marked ptosis is present. It is best performed with the patient looking upward, as this most effec-tively demonstrates improvement in levator action (30–60 seconds after injection).

Neostigmine bromide (Prostigmin) remains the drug of choice in most cases. A typical dose is 15 mg 4 times daily. Pyridostigmine (Mestinon) is also widely used. Topical anticholinesterase drops, especially demecarium bromide (Humorsol), sometimes help with ocular signs, which are often particularly resistant to systemic therapy. Ptosis usually does respond to treatment, but extraocular muscle weakness often does not respond. Thymectomy appears to be of benefit for patients with generalized muscle weakness.

The course of this chronic disease is not steady, and remissions are frequent. During a severe exacerbation, the patient may die from paralysis of respiration.

The prognosis depends to a great extent upon the patients' response to medication and their ability to regulate medication. An intelligent patient, well oriented to his or her disease, can live a normal life span.

CENTRAL NERVOUS SYSTEM COMPLICATIONS OF USE OF ORAL CONTRACEPTIVES

Since 1964, a number of reports have appeared of cerebrovascular accidents in younger women taking birth control pills of all types. The sudden onset of homonymous hemianopia, hemiplegia, convulsions, and other signs and symptoms has occurred in persons in good health receiving no other medication. Warnings against the use of such drugs in persons with a history of thrombophlebitis or other vascular problems were issued by the drug industry prior to issuing oral contraceptives. Migraine has also been noted to develop in persons taking oral contraceptives, and migraine sufferers should be advised against using such drugs. The central nervous system effects have cleared in some cases and have resulted in permanent neurologic deficits in others. While the percentage of complications reported so far is very low, there is no longer any question about the relationship. It is important for physicians to be aware of the possibility of the complications that can occur with such a widely used group of drugs.

●   ●   ●

References

Asbury AK et al: Oculomotor palsy in diabetes mellitus: A clinicopathological study. *Brain* 1970;**93(Part 3):**555.

Carroll FD: Nutritional amblyopia. *Arch Ophthalmol* 1966; **76:**406.

Chizek J, Franceschetti T: Oral contraceptives: Their side-effects and ophthalmological manifestations. *Surv Ophthalmol* 1969; **14:**90.

Chusid JG: *Correlative Neuroanatomy & Functional Neurology,* 18th ed. Lange, 1982.

Cogan DG: *Neurology of the Ocular Muscles,* 4th ed. Thomas, 1978.

Cogan DG: Ocular correlates of inborn metabolic defects. *Can Med Assoc J* 1966;**95:**1055.

Cogan DG, Lessell S: Neuro-ophthalmology and medical ophthalmology: A dialogue. *Arch Ophthalmol* 1976;**94:**393.

Feinsod M et al: Visually evoked response. *Arch Ophthalmol* 1976;**94:**237.

Frisén L: Swelling of the optic nerve head: A staging scheme. *J*

Neurol Neurosurg Psychiatry 1982;**45**:13.

Glaser JS: *Neuro-ophthalmology*. Harper & Row, 1978.

Gould ES et al: Treatment of optic neuritis by retrobulbar injection of triamcinolone. *Br Med J* 1977;**1**:1495.

Harrington DO: *The Visual Fields: A Textbook and Atlas of Clinical Perimetry*, 5th ed. Mosby, 1981.

Hayreh MS et al: Methyl alcohol poisoning. 3. Ocular toxicity. *Arch Ophthalmol* 1977;**95**:1851.

Hayreh SS: Anterior ischemic optic neuropathy: Treatment, prophylaxis, and differential diagnosis. *Br J Ophthalmol* 1974;**58**:981.

Hayreh SS: Optic disc edema in raised intracranial pressure. 5. Pathogenesis. *Arch Ophthalmol* 1977;**95**:1553.

Hedges TR III, Albert DM: The progression of the ocular abnormalities of herpes zoster: Histopathologic observations of nine cases. *Ophthalmology* 1982;**89**:165.

Henkind P, Benjamin JV: Vascular anomalies and neoplasms of the optic nerve head. *Trans Ophthalmol Soc UK* 1976;**96**:418.

Hepler RS: Therapeutic review: Management of optic neuritis. *Surv Ophthalmol* 1976;**20**:350.

Hollenhorst RW: Vascular status of patients who have cholesterol emboli in the retina. *Am J Ophthalmol* 1966;**61**:1159.

Hotchkiss MG et al: Bilateral Duane's retraction syndrome: A clinical-pathologic case report. *Arch Ophthalmol 1980;* **98**:870.

Hoyt WF: Ophthalmoscopy of the retinal nerve fibre layer in neuro-ophthalmologic diagnosis. *Aust J Ophthalmol* 1976; **4**:14.

Huber A: *Eye Signs and Symptoms in Brain Tumors*, 3rd ed. Mosby, 1976.

Keane JR: Bilateral sixth nerve palsy: Analysis of 125 cases. *Arch Neurol* 1976;**33**:681.

Knight CL et al: Syndrome of incipient prechiasmal optic nerve compressions: Progress toward early diagnosis and surgical management. *Arch Ophthalmol* 1972;**87**:1.

Knox DL: Optic nerve manifestations of systemic disease. *Trans Am Acad Ophthalmol Otolaryngol* 1977;**83**:743.

Lessell S: Current concepts in ophthalmology: Optic neuropathies. *N Engl J Med* 1978;**299**:533.

Libert J, Toussaint D, Guiselings R: Ocular findings in Niemann-Pick disease. *Am J Ophthalmol* 1975;**80**:991.

Lindenberg R, Walsh FB, Sacks JG: *Neuropathology of Vision: An Atlas*. Lea & Febiger, 1973.

Lowenfeld ID: The Argyll Robertson pupil, 1869–1969: A critical survey of the literature. *Surv Ophthalmol* 1969;**14**:199.

Miller NR (editor): *Walsh & Hoyt's Clinical Neuro-ophthalmology*, 4th ed. Vol 1. Williams & Wilkins, 1982.

Moses RA: *Adler's Physiology of the Eye: Clinical Application*, 7th ed. Mosby, 1981.

Nikoskelainen E, Frey H, Salmi A: Prognosis of optic neuritis with special reference to cerebrospinal fluid immunoglobulins and measles virus antibodies. *Ann Neurol* 1981;**9**:545.

O'Brien JF: The lysosomal storage diseases. *Mayo Clin Proc* 1982;**57**:192.

Paul TO, Hoyt WF: Funduscopic appearance of papilledema with optic tract atrophy. *Arch Ophthalmol* 1976;**94**:467.

Percy AK et al: Optic neuritis and multiple sclerosis: An epidemiologic study. *Arch Ophthalmol* 1972;**87**:135.

Quigley HA, Addicks EM: Quantitative studies of retinal nerve fiber layer defects. *Arch Ophthalmol* 1982;**100**:807.

Rush JA, Younge BR: Paralysis of cranial nerves III, IV, and VI: Cause and prognosis in 1,000 cases. *Arch Ophthalmol* 1981;**99**:76.

Sakalas R et al: Chronic sixth nerve palsy: An initial sign of basisphenoid tumors. *Arch Ophthalmol* 1975;**93**:186.

Selhorst JB et al: Disorders in cerebellar ocular motor control. 1. Saccadic overshoot dysmetria: An oculographic, control system and clinico-anatomical analysis. *Brain* 1976;**99**:497.

Spector RH, Troost BT: The ocular motor system. *Ann Neurol* 1981;**9**:517.

Thompson HS: Pupil in clinical diagnosis. (Symposium.) *Trans Am Acad Ophthalmol Otolaryngol* 1977;**83**:847.

Thompson HS: Pupillary signs in the diagnosis of optic nerve disease. *Trans Ophthalmol Soc UK* 1976;**96**:377.

Thompson HS et al: (editors): *Topics in Neuro-ophthalmology*. Williams & Wilkins, 1979.

Walsh FB, Hoyt WF: *Clinical Neuro-ophthalmology*, 3rd ed. 3 vols. Williams & Wilkins, 1969.

Young BR, Sulta F: Analysis of trochlear nerve palsies: Diagnosis, etiology and treatment. *Mayo Clin Proc* 1977;**52**:11.

18 | Ocular Disorders Associated With Systemic Diseases

Examination of the eye provides the ophthalmologist an opportunity to make a unique contribution to the diagnosis of systemic disease. Nowhere else in the body can a microcirculatory system be investigated with such precision, and nowhere else are the results of minute focal lesions so devastating. Most systemic diseases involve the eyes, and therapy demands some knowledge of the vascular, rheologic, and immunologic nature of these diseases.

VASCULAR DISEASE

NORMAL ANATOMY & PHYSIOLOGY

The blood supply to the eye is from the ophthalmic artery, which in turn is the first branch of the internal carotid artery. The first branches of the ophthalmic artery are the central retinal artery and the long posterior ciliary arteries. The retina is therefore perfused by retinal and choroidal vessels that provide contrasting anatomic and physiologic circulations. The retinal arteries correspond to arterioles in the systemic circulation but are thin-walled, with several layers of medial muscle cells. They function as end arteries and feed a capillary bed consisting of small capillaries (7 μm) with tight endothelial junctions. Dependent on this anatomic arrangement is the maintenance of the blood-retina barrier, and this system is autoregulated as there are no autonomic nerve fibers. Most of the blood within the eye, however, is in the choroidal circulation, which is characterized by a high flow rate, autonomic regulation, and an anatomic arrangement with collateral branching and large capillaries (30 μm), all of which have fenestrations in juxtaposition to Bruch's membrane. Clinical examination of the retinal vessels is facilitated by the use of red-free light, and fluorescein angiography enables us to obtain information about the dynamic and functional aspects of this circulation.

PATHOLOGIC APPEARANCES IN RETINAL VASCULAR DISEASE

Hemorrhages

Retinal hemorrhages result from diapedeses from veins or capillaries, and the morphologic appearances depend upon the size, site, and extent of damage to the vessel (Fig 18–1). Hemorrhages may be caused by any condition that alters the integrity of the endothelial cells. They usually indicate some abnormality of the retinal vascular system, and systemic factors should be considered in relation to (1) vessel wall disease (eg, hypertension, diabetes), (2) blood disorders (eg, leukemia, polycythemia), and (3) reduced perfusion (eg, carotid cavernous fistula, acute blood loss).

A. Preretinal Hemorrhages: These result from damage to the superficial disk or retinal vessels and are usually large, producing a gravity-dependent fluid level.

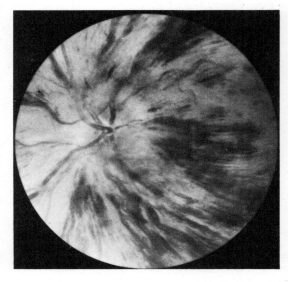

Figure 18–1. Flame-shaped retinal hemorrhages in the nerve fiber layer radiate out from the optic disk. Three days before the photograph was taken, the patient experienced sudden loss of vision, which left him with light perception only.

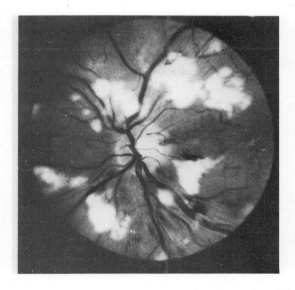

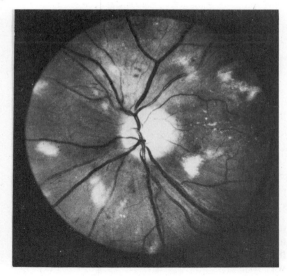

Figure 18–2. Cotton wool spots. *A:* Numerous cotton wool spots are seen in the posterior pole in a patient with accelerated hypertension. *B:* One month after hypotensive treatment. Note resolution of the infarcts.

B. Linear Hemorrhages: These usually small hemorrhages lie in the superficial nerve fiber layers and hence have a characteristic linear appearance, conforming to the alignment of nerve fibers in any particular area of the fundus.

C. Punctate Hemorrhages: Hemorrhages situated deeper in the substance of the retina are punctate and derived from capillaries and smaller venules. The circular appearance is related to the anatomic arrangement of structures in the retina.

D. Subretinal Hemorrhages: These hemorrhages are less common because normally there are no blood vessels between the retina and the choroid. Such hemorrhages are large and red, with a well-defined margin and no fluid level. They are seen in relation to the disk and in any condition where abnormal vessels pass from the choroidal circulation into the retina.

E. Hemorrhages Under the Pigment Epithelium: Hemorrhages situated under the pigment epithelium are usually dark and large, so that they must be differentiated from choroidal melanomas and hemangiomas.

F. White Central Hemorrhages (Roth's Spots): Superficial retinal hemorrhages with pale or white centers are not pathognomonic of any disease process but may arise in a variety of circumstances: (1) retinal infarction (cotton wool spot) with surrounding hemorrhage; (2) retinal hemorrhage in combination with extravasation of white corpuscles (eg, leukemia); and (3) retinal hemorrhage with central resolution.

Neuronal Effects of Focal Retinal Ischemia

The funduscopic appearance of arteriolar occlusion depends on the size of the vessel occluded, the duration of occlusion, and the time course. Occlusion of major arterioles produces a total, hemispheric, or segmental pallid swelling of the retina. Occlusion of a precapillary retinal arteriole produces the pathognomonic appearance of a cotton wool spot (Figs 18–2A and 18–2B). This consists of a pale, slightly elevated swelling usually one-fourth to one-half the size of the optic disk. Pathologic examination shows distention of neurons, with cytoid bodies (Fig 18–3); electron microscopy shows the accumulation of axoplasm and organelles. Occlusion of arterioles, whether due to intrinsic vessel wall disease or to intramural factors, may produce these pathognomonic signs.

A. Optic Disk Infarction (Ischemic Optic Neuropathy): Impairment of the blood supply to the optic disk produces sudden visual loss, usually with an altitudinal field defect and pallid swelling of the optic disk. The primary abnormality is complete or partial interruption of the choroidal blood supply to the disk,

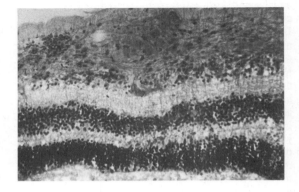

Figure 18–3. Cotton wool spot. Histologic examination shows cytoid bodies and distended neurons in the superficial retinal layers. Deeper retinal layers are normal. (Courtesy of Professor N Ashton.)

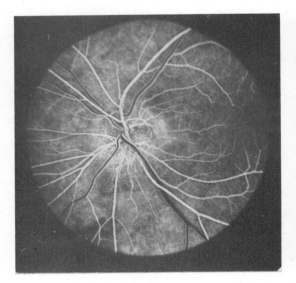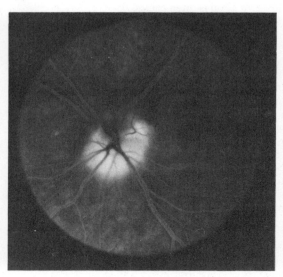

Figure 18–4. Ischemic optic neuropathy. Sudden visual loss in a 48-year-old man produced a complete inferior altitudinal field loss. *A:* Fluorescein angiography shows impaired filling of the upper part of the disk with dilatation of retinal capillaries at the lower part of the disk. *B:* Photograph 10 minutes after injection shows leakage of dye mainly at the lower part of the disk.

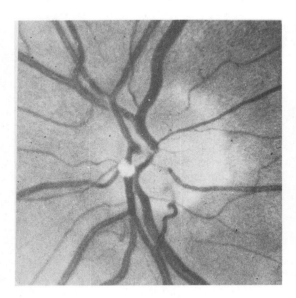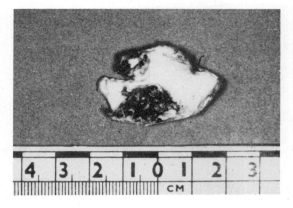

Figure 18–5. Cholesterol embolus (Hollenhorst plaque). *A:* A cholesterol embolus at the optic disk, which is refractile and appears larger than the vessel that contains it. A collateral vessel is seen at the lower border of the disk. *B:* Surgical specimen from a patient with a similar embolus shows an atheromatous ulcer at the bifurcation of the common carotid artery.

while the retinal capillaries on the surface of the disk appear dilated. Fluorescein angiography confirms the circulatory alterations (Figs 18–4A and 18–4B). Optic disk infarction is often caused by giant cell arteritis in old age and by arteriosclerotic disease in middle age.

Investigations should include serum lipids, blood glucose, serologic tests for syphilis, and assessment of blood viscosity by hemoglobin, hematocrit, and fibrinogen determinations. Giant cell arteritis merits measurement of the erythrocyte sedimentation rate and temporal artery biopsy on an urgent basis. Corticosteroids are essential in the management of giant cell arteritis, but the results of use of these drugs are equivocal in nonarteritic disorders.

B. Choroidal Infarction: Though the connection has rarely been recognized, certain clinical appearances have been attributed to ciliary vessel occlusion. These include small pale areas in the equatorial region which resolve to leave mottled pigmentary areas (Elschnig's spots). Elschnig's spots are called Siegrist's streaks when they are arranged in a linear manner.

C. Retinal Emboli: Transient episodes of monocular visual loss lasting 5–10 minutes are characteristic of amaurosis fugax. Patients often describe a curtain coming down from above or across their vision, usually with complete return of vision within seconds or minutes. Paresthesias in the contralateral limbs localize the disorder to the carotid artery and suggest involvement of the ophthalmic artery and middle cerebral artery. It is important for the ophthalmologist to auscultate the carotid for a systolic bruit and to search the fundus for emboli. Retinal emboli are of 3 main types:

1. Cholesterol emboli (Hollenhorst plaques)– These usually arise from an atheromatous plaque in the carotid artery and consist of cholesterol and fibrin. They lodge at the bifurcation of retinal arterioles, are refractile, and may appear larger than the vessel that contains them (Figs 18–5A and 18–5B).

2. Calcific emboli–Originating from damaged cardiac valves, these emboli lodge within the arteriole, producing complete occlusion and infarction of the distal retina. They are solid and calcified and occur in younger patients with a variety of cardiac lesions.

3. Platelet/fibrin emboli–Most cases of amaurosis fugax are probably due to the transit of platelet aggregates through the retinal and choroidal circulations. The emboli are usually broken up as they traverse the retinal circulation and hence are rarely seen, though occasionally they produce retinal infarction. Arising from abnormalities of the heart or great vessels, they may be reduced by drugs like aspirin or dipyridamole (Persantin), which reduce platelet coagulability.

D. Other Causes: There are several other causes of amaurosis fugax, including factors that induce temporary reduction in ocular perfusion, eg, arterial disease, cardiac disorders, hematologic disorders, and, rarely, elevation of intraocular pressure (see Table 18–1).

Table 18–1. Causes of amaurosis fugax.

Arterial disease	(1) Carotid artery stenosis
	(2) Carotid artery ulceration
	(a) Bifurcation
	(b) Carotid siphon
	(3) Ophthalmic artery stenosis
Cardiac disease	(1) Dysrhythmia
	(2) Valvular disease, eg, mitral leaflet prolapse
	(3) Left ventricular aneurysm or mural thrombus secondary to myocardial infarction
Hematologic disease	(1) Anemia
	(2) Polycythemia
	(3) Macroglobulinemia
	(4) Sickle cell disease
Other	(1) Mechanical compression of vertebral or carotid arteries
	(2) Hypertensive episode
	(3) Hypotensive episode
	(a) Drugs
	(b) Spontaneous (eg, diabetes mellitus, Addison's disease)
	(4) Arteritis
	(5) Raised intraocular pressure

Central Retinal Vein Occlusion (Fig 18–6)

Central retinal vein occlusion is an important cause of blindness in elderly people, particularly those with hypertension or glaucoma.

Fundus examination shows dilated tortuous veins with retinal and macular edema, hemorrhages all over the posterior pole, and soft exudates. The arterioles are usually attenuated, indicating generalized microvascular disease.

The prognosis for vision is poor. Fluorescein angiography demonstrates 2 types of response: a nonischemic type, with dilatation of retinal vessels and edema; and an ischemic type, which may be followed by the blinding complications of thrombotic glaucoma and retinal neovascularization.

Central retinal vein occlusion has an increased incidence in certain systemic conditions such as diabetes mellitus, hypertension, collagen vascular diseases, and hyperviscosity syndromes (eg, Waldenström's macroglobulinemia, angioimmunoblastic lymphadenopathy). Investigations include measurement of serum lipids, plasma proteins, a glucose load test, and assessment of blood viscosity by hemoglobin, hematocrit, and fibrinogen estimations. If hypertension is present, simple renal function tests, including urea and electrolytes, estimation of creatinine clearance, microscopic examination of the urine, and intravenous urography are indicated.

Treatment of retinal vein occlusion is unsatisfactory. Trials with anticoagulants and fibrinolytic agents have not been successful.

Occasionally, central retinal vein occlusion occurs in young people and may be associated with cells in the vitreous, suggesting an inflammatory cause. Rheologic investigations are usually negative.

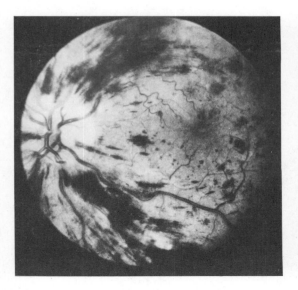

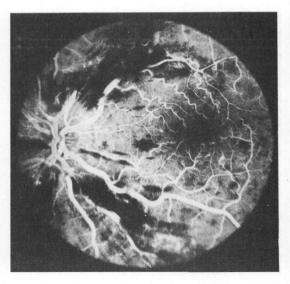

Figure 18–6. Central retinal vein occlusion. *Left:* Photograph shows linear hemorrhages in the nerve fiber layer and punctate hemorrhages in the deeper retinal layers. *Right:* Fluorescein angiogram shows dilatation of the veins.

Retinal Branch Vein Occlusion (Fig 18–7)

Occlusion of a branch vein should be viewed as part of the spectrum of central retinal vein occlusion. Investigations are similar in the 2 conditions, but arterial disease—particularly hypertension—is found more commonly in patients with retinal branch vein occlusion than in those presenting with central retinal vein occlusion.

ATHEROSCLEROSIS & ARTERIOSCLEROSIS

The process of atherosclerosis occurs in larger arteries and is due to fatty infiltration of a patchy nature occurring in the intima and associated with fibrosis. Involvement of smaller vessels (ie, less than 300 μm) by diffuse fibrosis and hyalinization is termed arteriosclerosis. The retinal vessels beyond the disk are

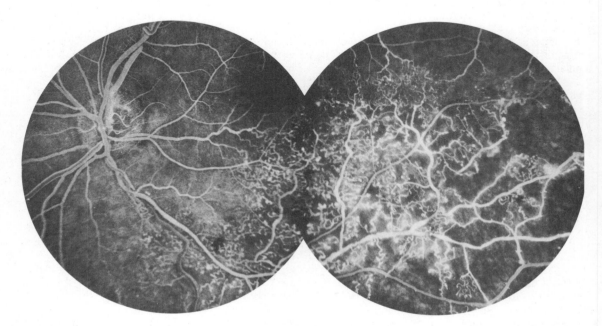

Figure 18–7. Retinal branch vein occlusion. The affected segment of retina shows changes of reduced perfusion. This results in irregularity of the arterioles and veins, areas of capillary closure, and dilated capillaries with microaneurysms.

less than 30 μm; therefore, involvement of the retinal arterioles should be termed arteriosclerosis, whereas involvement of the central retinal artery is properly termed atherosclerosis.

Atherosclerosis is a progressive change developing in the second decade, with lipid streaks in larger vessels, progressing to a fibrous plaque in the third decade. In the fourth and fifth decades, ulceration, hemorrhages, and thrombosis occur, and the lesion may be calcified. Destruction of the elastic and muscular elements of the media produces ectasia and rupture of the large vessels, though in smaller vessels obstruction is usually seen. The clinical results of atherosclerosis are seen several decades after the onset of the process. Contributing factors to atheroma include hyperlipidemia, hypertension, and obesity.

Arteriosclerosis is characterized by an enhanced light reflex, focal attenuation, and irregularity of caliber. These signs may also be seen in the arterioles of normotensive individuals in middle age. These findings are due to fibrosis and hyalinization as confirmed by fluorescein angiography and histologic examination. In elderly individuals with arteriosclerosis and associated mild hypertension, it is difficult to differentiate the changes of arteriosclerosis from those of hypertension.

Appearance of Retinal Vessels

A normal arteriolar wall is transparent, so that what is actually seen is the column of blood within the vessel. A thin, central light reflection in the center of the blood column appears as a yellow refractile line about one-fifth the width of the column. As the walls of the arterioles become infiltrated with lipids and cholesterol, the vessels become sclerotic. As this process continues, the vessel wall gradually loses its transparency and becomes visible; the blood column appears wider than normal, and the thin light reflex becomes broader. The grayish yellow fat products in the vessel wall blend with the red of the blood column to produce

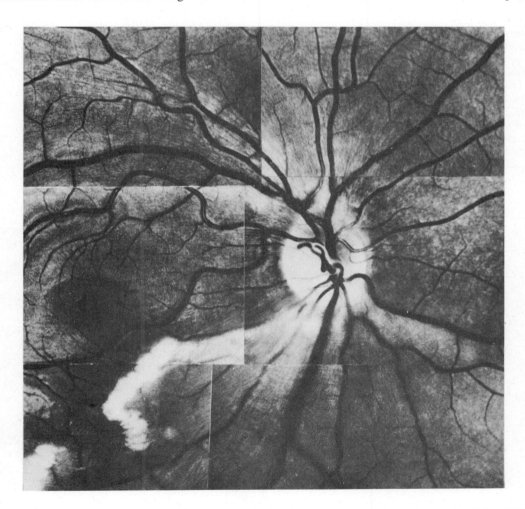

Figure 18–8. Acute retinal infarction. Red-free photograph shows acute arterial occlusion in a congenitally anomalous vessel at the disk. The inferior retina is infarcted, but axoplasm has accumulated beneath the fovea in an irregular pattern owing to preserved neuronal function of the distal ganglion cells.

a typical "copper wire" appearance. This indicates moderate arteriosclerosis. As sclerosis proceeds, the blood column–vessel wall light reflection resembles "silver wire," which indicates severe arteriosclerosis; at times, even occlusion of an arteriolar branch may occur.

Red-free light (a white light with a green filter) allows details of hemorrhages, focal irregularity of blood vessels, and nerve fibers to be seen more clearly (Fig 18–8).

HYPERTENSIVE RETINOPATHY

A major contribution to the study of hypertensive retinopathy was made by Wagener and Keith in 1939. They placed patients with hypertensive retinopathy into 4 groups (Figs 18–9, 18–10, 18–11, and 18–12). Stages I and II were restricted to arteriolar changes with attenuation and an increased light reflex ("copper" or "silver" wiring). The changes are mild, and subsequent observers have experienced difficulty in differentiating between these 2 groups. More emphasis has been placed on stages III and IV, which include cotton wool spots, hard exudates, hemorrhages, and extensive microvascular changes.

Stage IV is differentiated by the additional feature of edema of the optic disk. This was initially termed papilledema, but clinical and experimental evidence shows that the disk edema is due to infarction and hypoxia of the optic disk (the term papilledema being reserved for disk edema associated with elevated cerebrospinal fluid pressures).

The classification has been of particular value in assessing the prognosis of patients with hypertension.

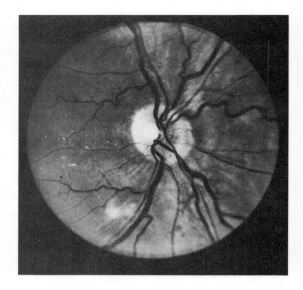

Figure 18–10. Keith-Wagener retinopathy stage II. There is irregularity of caliber of the arterioles and focal attenuation. Signs of retinal vascular disease include hard exudates at the macula, a cotton wool patch below the macula, and grooves in the nerve fiber layer beneath the disk, suggesting previous microinfarcts.

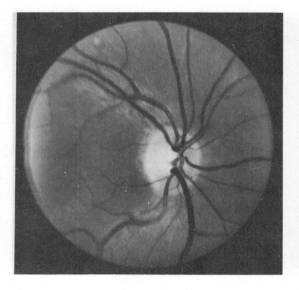

Figure 18–9. Keith-Wagener retinopathy stage I. Minimal vascular changes; a nearly normal fundus.

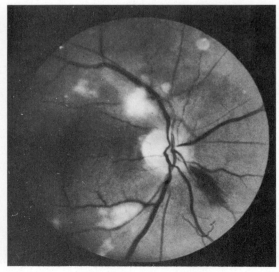

Figure 18–11. Keith-Wagener retinopathy stage III. Marked attenuation of retinal arterioles is apparent, with numerous microinfarcts and a large retinal hemorrhage.

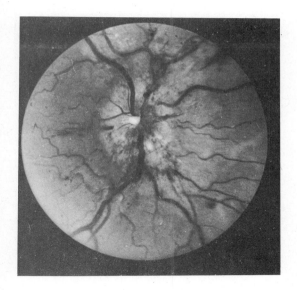

Figure 18–12. Keith-Wagener retinopathy stage IV. This may include the same retinal changes as stage III, but in addition there is disk swelling.

The 5-year survival rate of patients in group I is about 70%; in group IV it is about 1%.

The appearance of the fundus in hypertensive retinopathy is determined by the degree of elevation of the blood pressure and the state of the retinal arterioles. Thus, in young patients with accelerated hypertension, an extensive retinopathy is seen, with hemorrhages, retinal infarcts (cotton wool spots), choroidal infarcts (Elschnig's spots), and occasionally serous detachment of the retina (Fig 18–13). Experimental work on

monkeys made hypertensive suggests that ateriolar spasm initially occurs as a response to the high blood pressure and that this is followed by degeneration of the muscle of the blood vessel, with subsequent breakdown of the endothelial cells lining the vessel lumen. Secondary closure of the vessels occurs as a result of infiltration of the wall by plasma and fibrinogen to produce fibrinoid necrosis. The vascular damage is often associated with fibrin degradation products in the plasma, and this may play a part in the vascular changes of accelerated hypertension.

In contrast, elderly patients with arteriosclerotic vessels are unable to respond in this manner, and their vessels are thus protected by the arteriosclerosis. It is for this reason that elderly patients seldom exhibit florid hypertensive retinopathy (Fig 18–14).

Fluorescein angiography has made possible accurate documentation of these microcirculatory changes. In young patients with hypertension, arteriolar attenuation and occlusion are seen, and capillary nonperfusion can be verified in relation to a cotton wool spot, which is surrounded by abnormal dilated capillaries and microaneurysms and demonstrates increased permeability on fluorescein angiography.

Resolution of the cotton wool spots and the arteriolar changes occurs with successful hypotensive therapy. In elderly patients, the underlying arteriosclerotic changes are irreversible.

Other Forms of Hypertensive Retinopathy

A severe retinopathy may be seen in advanced renal disease, in patients with pheochromocytoma, and in toxemia of pregnancy. All such patients should receive a complete medical work-up to establish the nature of the hypertension, including measurement of

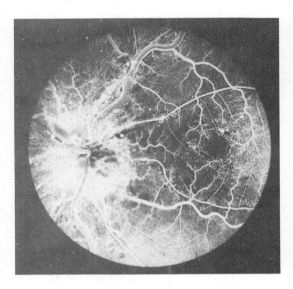

Figure 18–13. Accelerated hypertension. Fluorescein angiogram in a young man showing arteriolar constriction, dilatation of capillaries with microaneurysms, and areas of closure. Marked disk edema is present.

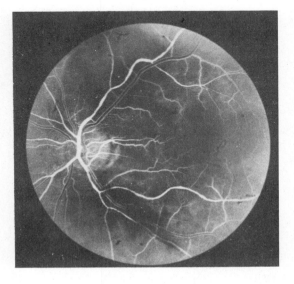

Figure 18–14. Accelerated hypertension. Fluorescein angiogram in an elderly woman showing marked arteriolar constriction and irregularity but few signs of florid retinopathy.

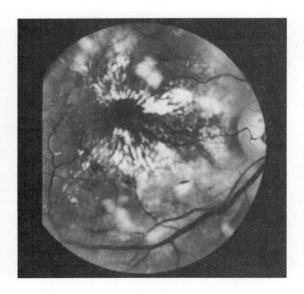

Figure 18–15. Pheochromocytoma. Marked circinate retinopathy with signs of recent retinal infarction and hemorrhages.

24-hour urinary vanilmandelic acid excretion and occasionally measurement of blood levels of norepinephrine and selective adrenal angiography in cases of suspected pheochromocytoma (Fig 18–15).

BENIGN INTRACRANIAL HYPERTENSION

Benign intracranial hypertension is a term used to indicate raised intracranial pressure in the presence of normal radiologic studies and normal cerebrospinal fluid. Patients present with headache, tinnitus, and dizziness; blurred vision and diplopia are the ophthalmologic features. Etiological factors include (1) drug therapy, particularly oral contraceptives, nalidixic acid, tetracyclines, sulfonamides, vitamin A, and prolonged steroid therapy or steroid withdrawal in children; (2) endocrine abnormalities (thyroid or parathyroid); (3) blood dyscrasia; (4) trauma; and (5) middle ear disease. Frequently there is no obvious cause and in this (idiopathic) group the patients are usually young overweight women with irregular menstrual periods. Benign intracranial hypertension is very rare in men, and a thorough search for a precipitating cause is mandatory in these women.

The cause of the intracranial pressure increase is unknown, although both diminished absorption of cerebrospinal fluid and cerebral edema secondary to abnormality of the cerebral vessels have been suggested.

On examination, visual fields are normal with enlarged blind spots due to gross papilledema. Cerebrospinal fluid pressure is raised and may be as high as 500 mm of water. The aims of treatment are to reduce spinal fluid pressure and prevent permanent visual loss and optic atrophy, which occurs in up to 25% of patients. Treatment includes strict diet, serial lumbar punctures, diuretics (eg, acetazolamide), and occasionally optic nerve sheath decompression or lumboperitoneal shunt procedures.

SUBACUTE INFECTIVE ENDOCARDITIS

Inflammatory changes on the cardiac valves may produce multiple embolization with frequent ocular manifestations. The emboli may arise from vegetations on the cardiac valves and may be composed of platelet and fibrinogen aggregates or calcified endocardial vegetations. Ocular changes therefore are related to transit or obstruction of emboli in the conjunctival, retinal, or choroidal circulatory systems (Fig 18–16). Focal vasculitis due to circulating immune complexes has been demonstrated in the kidney, and similar changes can presumably occur in the eye.

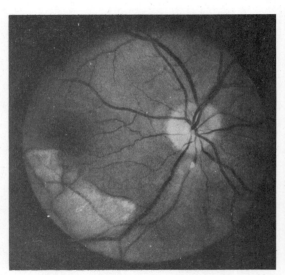

Figure 18–16. Subacute bacterial endocarditis. Calcific embolus impacted in arteriole below the disk, producing a distal area of retinal infarction.

HEMATOLOGIC & LYMPHATIC DISORDERS

PERNICIOUS ANEMIA

Pernicious anemia occurs when lack of intrinsic factor prevents absorption of vitamin B_{12}; the normal intake is 2 μg daily, and normal blood levels are 350 μg/L.

Macrocytic anemia with thrombocytopenia is the classic hematologic abnormality.

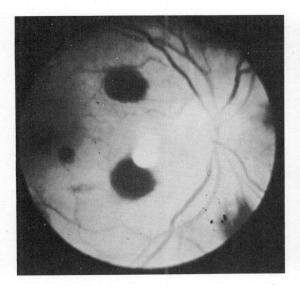

Figure 18–17. Retinal hemorrhages associated with severe pernicious anemia. (Woman, age 54.) Hemoglobin, 3 g/dL. Red cell count, 900,000/μL.

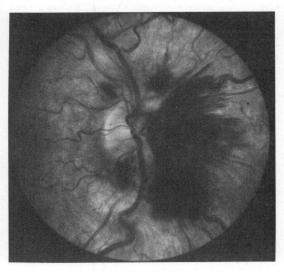

Figure 18–18. Flame-shaped hemorrhages radiating from the optic disk in a case of acute leukemia. Hemorrhages are in the nerve fiber layer of the retina. (Photo by Dennis Cordan.)

Ocular involvement is rare. Retinal and choroidal hemorrhages can occur as a result of platelet deficiency or if the red blood cell count is less than 2.5 million/μL (Fig 18–17). The paucity of red cells may produce characteristic pallor of the conjunctiva. Optic neuropathy is present in 5% of cases. Ophthalmoplegia occurs rarely.

Treatment is by intramuscular injection of hydroxocobalamin (vitamin B_{12}), 1000 μg weekly for 2 months and monthly thereafter for life.

ACUTE MASSIVE HEMORRHAGE

Complete and sudden, permanent blindness occurs rarely following acute massive hemorrhage, most commonly if bleeding is from the gastrointestinal tract or uterus. Such loss of vision is usually due to ischemic optic neuropathy (infarction of the disk). Though common prior to the use of blood transfusion, it is rarely seen today.

HEMORRHAGIC DISORDERS

Retinal and choroidal hemorrhage may occur in many types of hemorrhagic disorders; it is commonly associated with recurrent systemic hemorrhage (eg, thrombocytopenic purpura). Retinal edema, especially about the optic disk, may also be present. Following recovery or during remissions, the fundus is normal.

LEUKEMIA

The ocular changes of leukemia occur primarily in those structures with a good blood supply, including the retina, the choroid, and the optic disk. Changes are most common in the acute leukemias, where hemorrhages are seen in the nerve fiber (Fig 18–18) and preretinal layers. Visual loss may occur when the hemorrhage occurs at the macula, and some hemorrhages may have white centers. If the white blood cell count is excessively elevated, retinal evidence of the hyperviscosity syndrome (see below) may occur, with dilatation of the retinal arteries and veins, microaneurysms, and deep punctate hemorrhages.

Infiltration by leukemic cells may also occur in the retina, producing irregular pale areas, or in the choroid, causing pigmentary mottling. Infiltration at the optic disk is characteristic of acute lymphoblastic leukemia of infancy, in which blindness usually results.

HYPERVISCOSITY SYNDROMES

Increased viscosity results in a reduced flow of blood through the eye. This produces a characteristic appearance in the fundus of dilatation of the arteries and veins, which appear darker than normal, and retinal hemorrhages, microaneurysms, and areas of capillary closure (Fig 18–19). The main factors that contribute to blood viscosity are the red blood cells and plasma constituents, notably fibrinogen and the immunoglobulins. Polycythemia (high red cell count), either primary or secondary, may produce a hyperviscosity syndrome; the other main causes are mac-

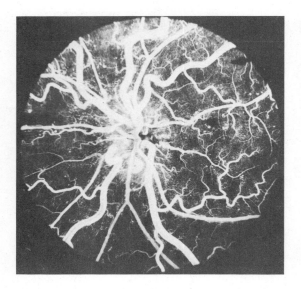

Figure 18 –19. Hyperviscosity syndromes. Dilated arteries and veins, with hemorrhages and microaneurysms in a patient with hyperviscosity due to elevated IgM levels.

roglobulinemia (high IgM concentration) and multiple myeloma. Reduction of the abnormalities producing hyperviscosity can reverse the retinal changes.

SICKLE CELL DISEASE

Sickle cell hemoglobinopathies are heritable disorders in which the normal adult hemoglobin is replaced by sickle hemoglobin in the red cell. This

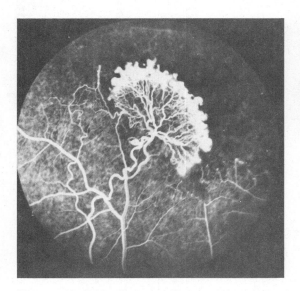

Figure 18 –20. Sickle cell disease. Fluorescein angiogram of equatorial "sea fan" with extensive capillary closure peripheral to the fan.

causes "sickle-shaped" deformity of the red cell on deoxygenation. Various types of sickling are described: sickle cell anemia (SS), sickle cell hemoglobin C (SC), and sickle cell thalassemia.

Ocular abnormalities include conjunctival changes, with "comma-shaped capillaries," and retinal changes, including arterial occlusions, neovascular patterns (sea fan), and extensive capillary closure (Fig 18–20). Vitreous hemorrhage may result from bleeding arising from neovascular membranes, and choroidal occlusive phenomena have also been reported.

LYMPHOMA

Orbital involvement with lymphosarcoma or Hodgkin's disease is not uncommon. Such a tumor may be the only sign of the lymphoma. It is usually present beneath the conjunctiva of the upper cul-de-sac and will readily respond to local radiation therapy.

Retinal hemorrhages such as those seen in severe anemia also occur (Fig 18–21).

Recently, patients have been described who have reticulum cell sarcoma with uveitis, abnormal cells in the vitreous, and infiltration of the optic disk.

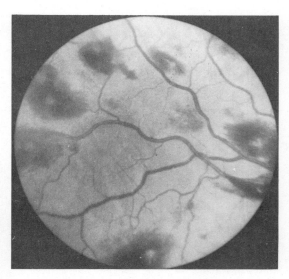

Figure 18–21. Retinal hemorrhages with white centers in an advanced case of Hodgkin's disease. (Courtesy of L Raymond.)

NEOPLASTIC DISEASE*
(Fig 18–22)

Increasing age is associated with an increasing incidence of malignant disease. Thus, the ophthalmologist encounters these diseases more frequently in

*Lymphoma is discussed above.

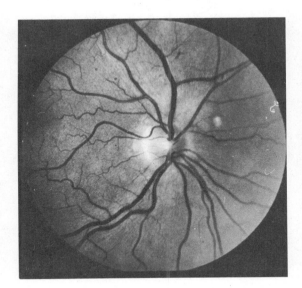

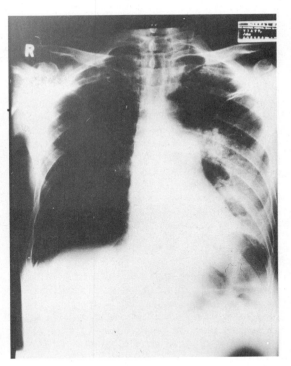

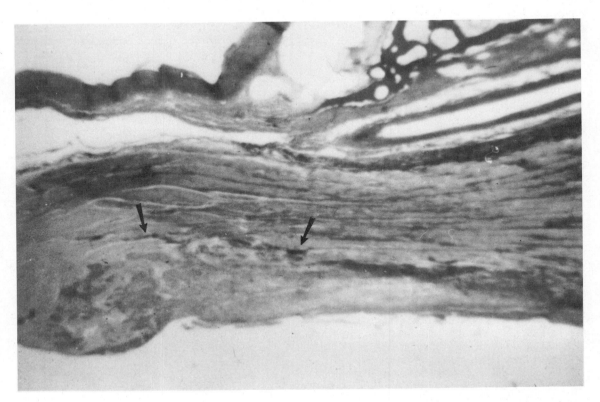

Figure 18–22. Neoplastic disease. *Top left:* Normal fundus of a patient with rapid visual loss in his only eye. *Top right:* Chest x-ray showed left lower lobe consolidation and a hilar mass. *Bottom:* Carcinoma of the bronchus was confirmed at autopsy, and metastasis was found in the optic nerve in the region of the canal (arrows).

elderly people and must be familiar with the broad spectrum of their manifestations.

Neoplastic disease may involve the eye and optic pathways by direct spread or by metastatic effects.

The effect of the metastases depends upon the size and site of the metastasis and the site of the primary lesion. The most frequent primary tumor metastasizing to the eye is carcinoma of the breast in women and bronchial carcinoma in men, followed by neoplasms of the genitourinary and intestinal tracts and, less frequently, tumors of the kidney, thyroid, and prostate and malignant melanoma.

Metastatic Effects

A. Conjunctiva: Direct spread may occur from an iris or ciliary body melanoma. Subconjunctival hemorrhage occurs with bleeding disorders secondary to neoplasia (eg, liver failure, disseminated intravascular coagulopathy).

B. Sclera: Metastatic deposits are rare. Jaundice indicates biliary obstruction (eg, due to carcinoma of the head of the pancreas).

C. Iris, Ciliary Body, and Choroid: Melanoma deposits are common in all of these structures, and metastases from primary breast tumors are often seen in the choroid. These are often multiple, bilateral, and asymptomatic unless situated near the macula. Choroidal metastases probably represent the commonest choroidal neoplasm.

Uveitis sometimes occurs secondary to these metastases.

D. Vitreous: Neoplastic disease associated with immunologic disturbance (eg, reticulum cell sarcoma, carcinoma, lymphoma) may present in patients with posterior uveitis.

Vitreous hemorrhage may occur directly from choroidal or retinal neoplasm or secondary to retinal neovascularization.

Amyloidosis, which may follow slow-growing tumors, produces strands in the vitreous.

E. Retina: Retinal detachment is a complication of choroidal metastases. Retinal vascular occlusion occurs secondary to hematologic abnormalities resulting from distant carcinomas (eg, pancreas, renal cell carcinoma); more rarely, photoreceptor degeneration may occur.

F. Orbit: Direct invasion from lacrimal adenocarcinoma or from carcinoma of the paranasal sinuses and nasopharynx will produce proptosis and painful ophthalmoplegia (known as the orbital apex syndrome due to involvement at the orbital fissure of cranial nerves II, III, IV, and VI). Compression of the optic nerve may produce central scotomas with disk edema or optic atrophy.

G. Extraocular Muscles: Orbital apex syndrome is discussed above. Discrete metastases of the extraocular muscles are rare. Meningeal carcinomatosis may produce nuclear palsies of the extraocular muscles or sixth nerve palsy secondary to raised intracranial pressure.

H. Optic Nerve: Direct infiltration or compression of the optic nerve sheath from metastases or meningiomas results in progressive visual loss and optic atrophy. A carcinomatous optic neuropathy is reported in association with meningeal carcinomatosis when the visual loss is thought to have a vascular cause.

I. Optic Chiasm: Metastatic deposits characteristically present in patients with diabetes insipidus, because the highly vascular posterior pituitary is more susceptible to hematogenous spread of tumor cells. These patients therefore present with bitemporal field defects in addition to polyuria and polydipsia. Symptoms of dysfunction of the anterior pituitary or suprasellar extension to the chiasm may occur later.

J. Optic Tract, Optic Radiation, and Optic Cortex: Neoplasms in this area produce characteristic hemianopic field defects (see Chapter 17). These are associated with different symptoms (eg, temporal lobe epilepsy) according to the site of the neoplasm.

Nonmetastatic Effects

Uveitis occurs in patients with immunologic disturbances.

The myasthenic (Eaton-Lambert) syndrome occurs in patients with bronchial carcinoma and is characterized by fatigable weakness of skeletal muscles and, very rarely, ptosis and ophthalmoplegia. The electromyographic findings are diagnostic: The action potential of the motor unit is reduced in the resting muscle after a single maximal stimulus but increases after 4 seconds of tetanic stimulation.

Cerebellar degeneration occurs most commonly in women with ovarian carcinoma. The characteristic features include ataxia, dysarthria, and nystagmus.

METABOLIC DISORDERS

DIABETES MELLITUS

Diabetes mellitus is a complex metabolic disorder that also involves the small blood vessels, often caus-

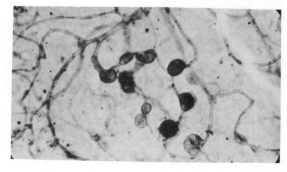

Figure 18–23. Diabetic retinopathy stage I. Trypsin-digested whole mount showing microaneurysms of the retinal capillaries.

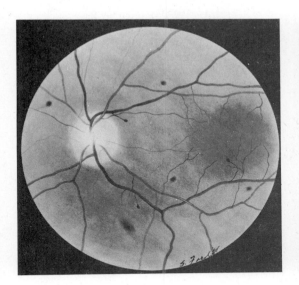

Figure 18–24. Diabetic retinopathy. Punctate hemorrhages and capillary aneurysms. All hemorrhages are essentially round in form.

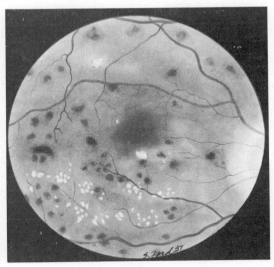

Figure 18–25. Diabetic retinopathy. Round hemorrhages are more prominent, and some small waxy exudates are present.

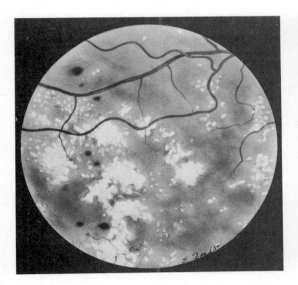

Figure 18–26. Diabetic retinopathy. Exudates coalesced into larger masses.

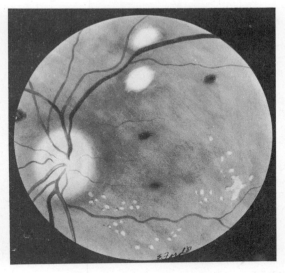

Figure 18–27. Nonproliferative diabetic retinopathy. Cotton wool patches have been added to hemorrhages and exudates.

(Figs 18–24 to 18–27 courtesy of F Cordes.)

ing widespread damage to many body tissues, including the eyes.

The ocular complications of diabetes are dependent not only upon impaired carbohydrate metabolism but also upon as yet undefined complexes of factors, and these may occur before the characteristic findings of glycosuria, hyperglycemia, polyuria, and polydipsia become manifest. The ocular complications occur approximately 20 years after onset despite apparently adequate diabetic control. Improved treatment measures (eg, improved insulins, antibiotics) that have lengthened the life span of diabetics have actually resulted in a marked increase in incidence of retinopathy and other ocular complications. Diabetes has become the most common cause of blindness in younger people throughout the world. The visual outlook for adult (maturity onset) diabetics is considerably better than for juvenile diabetics.

The possibility of diabetes should be considered in all patients with unexplained retinopathy, cataract, extraocular muscle palsy, optic neuropathy, or sudden changes in refractive error. Absence of glycosuria or a normal fasting blood glucose level does not exclude a diagnosis of diabetes. Postprandial blood glucose determinations and glucose tolerance tests may be required. Rarely, the diabetic ocular change may become evident before there is demonstrable evidence of impaired glucose tolerance.

Retinopathy (Figs 18–23 to 18–30)

Diabetic retinopathy is a common cause of blindness and now accounts for almost one-fourth of blind registrations in the western world.

Metabolic and hematologic factors are important in the development of diabetic retinopathy. Atheroma may be associated, and higher triglyceride and insulin

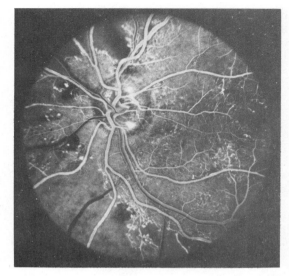

Figure 18–29. Diabetic retinopathy. Fluorescein angiogram shows florid retinopathy of diabetes with extensive areas of capillary closure, dilated capillaries with microaneurysms, and early new vessel formation at the optic disk.

levels are found in diabetics with atherosclerosis. Contributory rheologic factors include elevated blood viscosity and abnormal leukocyte and platelet function. The glycosylated hemoglobin HbA_{1c} increases the affinity of the blood for oxygen and is increased in diabetics to 12% from the normal level of 3.6% of total hemoglobin. The level of HbA_{1c} can be correlated with blood lipid concentrations and provides a measure of the efficacy of treatment.

HLA typing may be important in detecting dia-

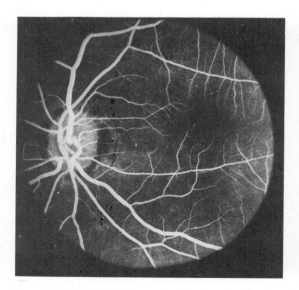

Figure 18–28. Diabetic retinopathy. Fluorescein angiogram shows earliest stage with microaneurysm in the macular region.

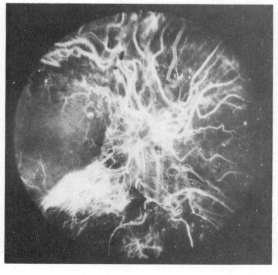

Figure 18–30. Proliferative diabetic retinopathy. Fluorescein angiogram shows extensive growth of vessels into the vitreous with marked fluorescein leakage.

betics who are vulnerable to severe diabetic retinopathy: (1) Increased incidence of HLA-A1 and HLA-B8 occurs in juvenile diabetes with microangiopathy; (2) HLA-B8, when occurring alone, is associated with severe diabetic retinopathy.

The presence and degree of retinopathy seem to be more closely related to the duration of the disease than to its severity. Control plays only a minor role (if any) in the onset, once the process is well under way.

The juvenile diabetic develops a severe form of retinopathy within 20 years in 60–75% of cases, even if under good control. The retinopathy often begins in stage IV and progresses to stage V. In older diabetic patients, retinopathy usually begins in stage I and seldom progresses beyond stage III. Macular degeneration may reduce the central visual acuity markedly in the later stages.

The details of characteristics and treatment of diabetic retinopathy are presented in Chapter 13.

Lens Changes

A. True Diabetic Cataract (Rare): Bilateral cataracts occasionally occur with a rapid onset in severe juvenile diabetes. The lens may become completely opaque in several weeks. The process starts as snow-white areas in the cortex—posterior subcapsular and some anterior subcapsular opacities that progressively involve more and more cortex—which finally become confluent to make the entire lens opaque.

B. Senile Cataract in the Diabetic (Common): Typical senile nuclear sclerosis, posterior subcapsular changes, and cortical opacities occur earlier and more frequently in diabetics.

C. Sudden Changes in the Refraction of the Lens: Especially when diabetes is not well controlled, changes in blood glucose levels cause changes in sugar alcohols of the lens that in turn cause changes in refractive power by as much as 3 or 4 diopters. This results in blurred vision. Such changes do not occur when the disease is well controlled.

Iris Changes

Glycogen infiltration of the pigment epithelium and sphincter and dilator muscles of the iris may cause diminished pupillary responses. The reflexes may also be altered by the autonomic neuropathy of diabetes.

Rubeosis iridis is common in severe juvenile diabetes. Numerous small intertwining blood vessels develop on the anterior surface of the iris. Spontaneous hyphema may occur. The formation of peripheral anterior synechiae is aided by the vascularization of anterior chamber structures, eventually blocking aqueous outflow sufficiently to cause secondary glaucoma.

Extraocular Muscle Palsy (Fig 18–31)

This common occurrence in diabetes is manifested by a sudden onset of diplopia caused by paresis of an extraocular muscle. This may be the presenting sign and is due to infarction of the nerve. When the third nerve is involved, pain may be a prominent symptom. Differentiation from a posterior communicating

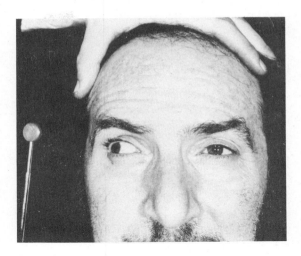

Figure 18–31. Pupil sparing third nerve palsy in diabetes mellitus. Sudden painful ophthalmoplegia, left ptosis, failure of adduction, and normal pupillary responses.

aneurysm is important, and in diabetic third nerve palsy the pupil is usually spared. Recovery of ocular motor function usually occurs within a year, frequently within 6–8 weeks. The fourth and sixth nerves may be similarly involved.

Iridocyclitis

This is particularly common in juvenile diabetes and nearly always responds well to standard treatment with topical corticosteroids and cycloplegics.

Optic Neuropathy

Visual loss may occur in diabetes. It is usually due to infarction of the optic disk or nerve. There is also a form of optic neuropathy that is associated with juvenile diabetes.

GOUT

Inflammatory changes in the eye, as in the joints, are due to the deposition of monosodium urate. This usually occurs in the conjunctiva and episclera, presenting as an acute and uncomfortable red eye. Less frequently, the sclera may be involved, and this can be associated with anterior uveitis, which is responsive to topical corticosteroid and cycloplegic therapy.

ENDOCRINE DISEASES

Disturbances of the endocrine glands have a number of important ocular manifestations. By far the most important of these are due to disturbances of the thyroid gland, although parathyroid and pituitary abnormalities also produce significant ocular changes.

THYROID GLAND DISORDERS

1. GRAVES'S DISEASE

The general term Graves's disease has been used to describe patients with hyperthyroidism due to an autoimmune process. Patients with the eye signs of Graves's disease but without clinical evidence of hyperthyroidism are referred to as having ophthalmic Graves's disease. Apart from signs of hyperthyroidism, patients may have pretibial myxedema and clubbing of the fingers, and this, in combination with the ocular signs, is termed thyroid acropachy.

The availability of more sophisticated diagnostic tests has now made possible accurate diagnosis of thyroid disease. These include the ability to recognize T_3 toxicosis and the ability to assess the hypothalamopituitary axis with the use of the TRH test.

Clinical Findings

Patients may present with nonspecific complaints such as dryness of the eyes, discomfort, or prominence of the eyes. The American Thyroid Association has graded the ocular signs in order of increasing severity:*

Class	Signs
0	No signs or symptoms
1	Only signs, which include upper lid retraction, with or without lid lag, or proptosis to 22 mm. No symptoms.
2	Soft tissue involvement
3	Proptosis > 22 mm
4	Extraocular muscle involvement
5	Corneal involvement
6	Sight loss due to optic nerve involvement

Lid retraction may be unilateral or bilateral and may be accompanied by impaired elevation of the eyes. Lid retraction appears to be pathognomonic of thyroid disease, particularly when associated with exophthalmos. The pathogenesis of lid retraction is not completely understood. Some features suggest overactivity of the sympathetic system, particularly the reversal of the retraction following administration of guanethidine eye drops. However, the absence of any pupillary dilatation has led to alternative explanations,

*Abridged classification of the eye signs of Graves's disease (after Werner).

Table 18–2. Thyroid function tests.

	Hyper-thyroid	Hypo-thyroid	Comments
Plasma T_4	+	−	
T_3 resin uptake	−	+	Thyopac technique. Other tests may vary.
Free thyroxine index	+	−	
Plasma TSH levels	−	+	In pituitary hypothyroidism, TSH is reduced.
Response to TRH	Absent	Exaggerated	Absent in pituitary hypothyroidism.
Autoantibodies	May be present	May be present (Hashimoto's)	

T_3 assay: A patient who is clinically hyperthyroid but with normal plasma T_4 may have T_3 thyrotoxicosis and raised plasma T_3 levels; the TRH test will show a hypothyroid response.

and spasm of the striated levator palpebrae superioris muscle has been suggested.

A. Exophthalmos (Fig 18–32): The degree of exophthalmos may be extremely variable. Measurements using the Hertel or Krahn exophthalmometer range from minimal (20 mm) to excessive (28 mm or more). The condition is usually asymmetric and may be unilateral, and it is important clinically to assess the resistance to manual retropulsion of the globe. The increase in orbital contents that produces the exophthalmos is largely due to an increase in the bulk of the ocular muscles. Visualization of the ocular muscles is now possible with the advent of the CT scan (Fig 18–32), which enables us to differentiate exophthalmos from an intraconal orbital tumor. In some cases, thickening of the ocular muscles may be restricted to certain muscles only (eg, medial or inferior rectus muscles).

B. Ophthalmoplegia: This is seen more commonly in ophthalmic Graves's disease, which usually affects older people and may be grossly asymmetric. Limitation of elevation is the most frequent finding, and this is mainly due to adhesions between the inferior rectus and inferior oblique muscles. Confirmation may be gained by measuring the intraocular pressure on elevation, when a substantial increase in the intraocular pressure suggests tethering. Often there is mild limitation of ocular movements in all positions of gaze. Patients complain of diplopia, which may be relieved by corticosteroid treatment, may spontaneously return to normal, or, if it remains static for 6–12 months, can frequently be relieved by surgical correction of one or more extraocular muscles.

C. Retinal and Optic Nerve Changes: Compression of the globe by the orbital contents may produce elevation of the intraocular pressure and retinal or choroidal striae. The optic disk may become swollen and progress to visual loss from optic atrophy. Optic neuropathy associated with Graves's disease occasionally occurs as a result of compression and ischemia of the optic nerve as it traverses the tense orbit.

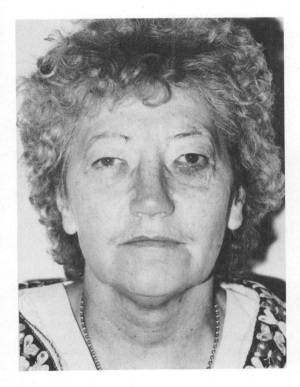
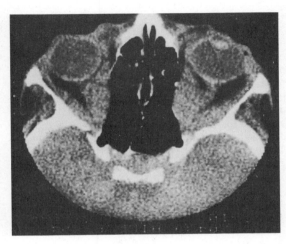

Figure 18–32. Thyroid ophthalmopathy. *Left:* Proptosis, visual loss, and ophthalmoplegia occurred in this elderly woman with a history of thyroid disease. *Right:* CT scans showed gross thickening of the ocular muscles, particularly in relation to the orbital apex. The increased intraorbital pressure is producing convexity of the medial orbital wall.

D. Corneal Changes: In some patients, a superior limbic keratoconjunctivitis may be seen, though this is not specific for thyroid disease. In severe exophthalmos, corneal exposure and ulceration may occur.

Pathogenesis of the Ocular Signs

The main feature is gross distention of the ocular muscles due to the deposition of mucopolysaccharides. The mucopolysaccharides are strongly hygroscopic, which accounts for the increased water content of the orbits. There is an increase in the orbital connective tissue, with numerous fibroblasts, and the tissues are infiltrated by lymphocytes and plasma cells.

The pathogenesis of Graves's disease remains unknown, though an immunologic disorder involving both cellular and humoral elements has been implicated. Long-acting thyroid stimulator (LATS) is unlikely to be of significance in humans as it is not always found in patients with ocular signs. There has, however, been good correlation between hyperthyroidism and human-specific thyroid stimulator, previously known as LATS protector, although this correlation is not seen in patients with Graves's disease. Thyroid autoantibodies against thyroglobulin and the microsome fraction of thyroid cells are frequently found in Hashimoto's disease and less often in Graves's disease. There are now thought to be 2 pathogenetic components to Graves's disease: (1) immune complexes of thyroglobulin-antithyroglobulin bind to extraocular muscles and produce a myositis; and (2) exophthalmos-producing substance acts with ophthalmic immunoglobulins to displace thyroid-stimulating hormones from the retro-orbital membranes, which results in the increase of retro-orbital fat.

Cellular immunity is also abnormal in Graves's disease. Lymphocytes from patients show increased migration inhibition. The total T lymphocyte count in peripheral blood may be abnormal, and there may be differences in the subpopulations of T cells. Patients with reduced T lymphocyte counts respond well to treatment with corticosteroids, but those with increased counts failed to improve with steroids. The finding of thyroid autoantibodies in a number of patients adds further credence to the immunologic theory of pathogenesis of this disorder.

Treatment

A. Medical Treatment: Medical treatment includes adequate control of the hyperthyroidism as a primary measure. However, thyroid ophthalmopathy may occur in the euthyroid or hypothyroid states. Severe cases with visual loss, disk edema, or corneal ulceration merit urgent medical treatment with corticosteroids in high doses (eg, prednisolone, 100 mg), as low doses are ineffective. Plasmapheresis is occasionally used with good results in the treatment of refractory cases of malignant exophthalmos, but full immunosuppression must follow plasmapheresis to prevent rebound increase of immunoglobulins and recurrence of disease. Immunosuppressive agents (eg, azathioprine) may play a supportive role and allow a lower maintenance dose of corticosteroids. In most cases, medical treatment produces adequate control, and surgical decompression is now performed less frequently. Guanethidine (Ismelin) eye drops, 10%, may produce temporary resolution of the lid retraction, which may be useful for cosmetic reasons.

B. Surgical Treatment: The lid retraction may be cosmetically improved by section of Müller's muscle (Henderson's operation) or by a lateral tarsorrhaphy. The latter may also provide some protection for the cornea. Decompression of the orbit may be performed from an intracranial approach (Krönlein's operation) with removal of the superior and lateral walls of the orbit. Currently in favor is the antral decompression (O'Gouras procedure), in which the inferior and medial walls of the orbit are removed. Finally, if troublesome diplopia persists, ocular muscle surgery is often effective.

2. HYPOTHYROIDISM
(Myxedema)

Significant ocular signs are not common in myxedema. Edema of the lids and periorbital tissue is commonly encountered. Thin superficial corneal opacities and small, flaky, white opacities in the lens cortex, neither of which seriously interferes with vision, may be present. Optic neuritis, with eventual optic atrophy and serious visual disability, occurs very rarely.

PARATHYROID GLAND DISORDERS

1. HYPOPARATHYROIDISM

Occasionally at thyroidectomy the parathyroid glands are removed inadvertently, causing hypoparathyroidism. Spontaneous cases, although rare, should be suspected in young patients with cataracts. The blood calcium decreases, and serum phosphates are increased. Tetany may ensue and can be severe enough to cause generalized convulsions. The ocular manifestations consist of blepharospasm and twitching eyelids. Small, discrete, punctate opacities of the lens cortex develop that may eventually require lens extraction. Treatment with calcium salts, calciferol, and dihydrotachysterol usually prevents further development of lens opacities, but any that have occurred prior to treatment remain.

2. HYPERPARATHYROIDISM

In hyperparathyroidism, deposition of calcium may rarely occur in soft tissue. "Metastatic" calcification of the cornea and conjunctiva may be an early sign of the hypercalcemia encountered in this disorder.

VITAMINS & EYE DISEASE

Vitamins are organic complexes that are essential for normal growth and maintenance of life. Vitamins A, D, and K are fat-soluble; vitamins B and E are water-soluble. Abnormal intake may produce systemic effects and ocular manifestations.

AVITAMINOSIS A

Vitamin A is found in fish oil and liver, and its precursor (carotene) is found in plants, vegetables, and cream. The normal daily requirement is 5000–7000 IU, and the normal blood level is 50–70 IU/L.

Symptoms and signs of vitamin A deficiency do not occur until the blood level drops below 50 IU/L. Vitamin A is essential for the maintenance of epithelium throughout the body, and deficiency produces changes in the epithelium around the eye **(xerophthalmia)** (Fig 18–33) and in retinal function. Deficiency is due to dietary factors in underdeveloped countries (eg, seasonal, pregnancy), although in developed countries malabsorption is more common (eg, blind loop syndrome, massive gut resection).

Pathology

The conjunctival and corneal epithelium become dry and thickened; under the microscope, keratinized epithelium has replaced the normal columnar epithelium.

In the cornea, there is degeneration of Bowman's membrane and infiltration of the stroma with inflam-

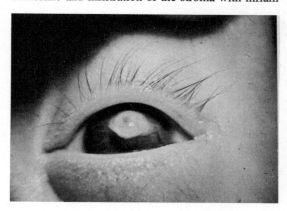

Figure 18–33. Keratomalacia. Case of xerophthalmia in a 5-month-old child.

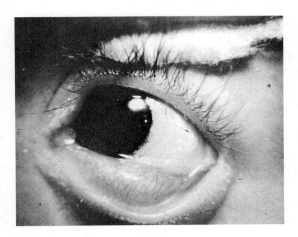

Figure 18–34. Xerophthalmia. Bitot's spot is seen as a foamy, white, wedge-shaped area with the base at the limbus.

matory cells and fluid. Yellow spots form in the cornea, and progression may result in hypopyon or perforation.

Clinical Findings

The damaged epithelium may produce dry, irritable eyes and blurred or distorted vision in severe cases. On examination, there are white foamy areas in the conjunctival tissue exposed by the palpebral apertures called Bitot's spots (Fig 18–34).

Xerosis of the corneal epithelium occurs in 2 stages: **prexerosis,** a loss of luster and reduction in corneal sensitivity; and **true xerosis,** an extension of conjunctival xerosis onto the cornea. Microscopic study of the scrapings from Bitot's spots shows large, keratinized epithelial cells with pale, indistinct cytoplasm and fragmented nuclei. The normal columnar conjunctival epithelium is keratinized and squamous. Xerosis bacilli (nonpathogenic diphtheroids originally thought to be the cause of xerosis) are numerous.

Complications & Sequelae

In severe cases, perforation of the cornea and subsequent loss of the eye can occur. Bilateral corneal scarring is common.

Night blindness is an early symptom and rarely severe. The fundi are normal, showing no pigmentary change, although yellow spots are occasionally seen in the retinal periphery. The mechanism of any relationship between vitamin A deficiency and retinitis pigmentosa is not known.

Treatment

Both night blindness and xerophthalmia can be cured with adequate doses of vitamin A (eg, 20,000 IU/d). Local antibiotic drops may be indicated.

HYPERVITAMINOSIS A

Vitamin A intoxication has produced benign intracranial hypertension. These patients present with bilateral papilledema that may resolve months after ceasing ingestion.

HYPERVITAMINOSIS D

Calcium deposits in the cornea (forming band keratopathy) and in the conjunctiva are the most common ocular changes. Strabismus, epicanthal folds, osteosclerosis of orbital bones, nystagmus, papilledema, sluggish pupillary reaction, iritis, and cataract are less common ocular findings. The incidence of these changes has declined substantially, since the content of vitamin D in milk and other foodstuffs has been subject to government regulation.

VITAMIN B

The vitamin B complex is subdivided into 8 groups, but only vitamin B_1 and vitamin B_2 will be discussed here. Pernicious anemia (vitamin B_{12} deficiency) is discussed on p 240.

Vitamin B_1 (thiamine) is found in animal and vegetable matter. The normal daily requirement is 1 mg, and the normal plasma levels are 21 μg/L.

Deficiency produces **beriberi,** characterized by high-output cardiac failure resulting in pleural and peritoneal effusions; in addition, peripheral neuritis is seen.

Seventy percent of patients have ocular abnormalities. Epithelial changes in the conjunctiva and cornea produce dry eyes and blurred vision. Visual loss with centrocecal scotomas may also be due to optic atrophy, and ocular motor palsies may be seen.

Treatment is by correction of dietary deficiency with liver, whole wheat bread, cereals, eggs, and yeast, or with parenteral injection of thiamine, 50 mg, or parenteral multivitamin preparation. **Wernicke's syndrome** of ophthalmoplegia, ptosis, and nystagmus is usually due to thiamine deficiency associated with alcoholism, although it can occur in other malnutrition states.

Vitamin B_2 (nicotinic acid and riboflavin) is found in animals and vegetables, particularly liver, yeast, and wheat germ. The minimal daily requirement is 12–15 mg.

Nicotinic acid deficiency (pellagra) is quite common in alcoholics and is characterized by dermatitis, diarrhea, and dementia. Ocular involvement is rare, and optic neuritis or retinitis may develop.

Riboflavin deficiency has been said to cause a number of ocular changes. Rosacea keratitis, vascularization of the limbal cornea, seborrheic blepharitis, and secondary conjunctivitis have all been attributed to riboflavin deficiency, but these conditions seldom respond to riboflavin therapy. Optic atrophy is at times caused by ariboflavinosis. Definite riboflavin-deficient conditions respond well to dried (brewer's) yeast, 25–30 g 3 times daily.

AVITAMINOSIS C
(Scurvy)

Vitamin C (ascorbic acid) is found in fresh citrus fruits and green vegetables. The daily requirement is 50–100 mg, and the normal plasma level is 6.32 mg/L.

In scurvy, hemorrhages may develop in a variety of sites, eg, skin, mucous membranes, body cavities, the orbits, and subperiosteally in the joints. Hemorrhages may also occur into the lids, subconjunctival space, anterior chamber, vitreous cavity, and retina.

Treatment of vitamin C deficiency is with proper diet, particularly adequate amounts of citrus juice. Supplements of ascorbic acid, 200–300 mg/d orally, or sodium ascorbate injection, 0.5–1 g intravenously or intramuscularly daily in divided doses, will help correct vitamin C deficiency rapidly.

GRANULOMATOUS DISEASES

Many of the so-called granulomatous infectious diseases, including tuberculosis, sarcoidosis, brucellosis, leprosy, and toxoplasmosis, undergo a chronic course with frequent exacerbations and remissions. The eye is often involved, particularly by anterior uveitis. The following paragraphs deal with other ocular complications of these systemic diseases.

TUBERCULOSIS

Ocular tuberculosis results from endogenous spread from systemic foci. The incidence of eye involvement is less than 1% in known cases of pulmonary tuberculosis.

Tuberculosis of the Uveal Tract
A. Iritis (Anterior Uveitis): Many cases of granulomatous uveitis are said to be tuberculous, although very few cases have been established. At times only the anterior segment of the eye is involved. A few patients develop cells in the vitreous cavity with the picture of central retinal vein thrombosis. This may be associated with a high platelet count and may represent a hypersensitivity "erythema nodosum" reaction in the retina. Local treatment of iritis with mydriatics and corticosteroids is indicated. Systemic tuberculosis therapy is useful in the treatment of established cases of tuberculous uveitis.

B. Miliary Tuberculosis: In this usually fatal form of tuberculosis, many small discrete yellowish nodules are visible ophthalmoscopically in the posterior pole of the eye.

C. Solitary Tubercles: These occur as gray isolated masses about the size of the optic disk in the posterior fundus and usually cause minimal functional disturbance. The tubercles may be the first sign of an impending generalized uveitis. Solitary tubercles are occasionally seen in the iris or ciliary body.

Occasionally, orbital periostitis has occurred because of a tubercle.

Tuberculosis of the Retina
Choroidal involvement usually causes associated retinitis as the pigmented epithelial layer is broken down. This process is spoken of as tuberculous chorioretinitis.

SARCOIDOSIS
(Fig 18–35)

Sarcoidosis is a multisystem disease, with pulmonary, ocular, cutaneous, and reticuloendothelial system manifestations. The pulmonary changes include hilar lymphadenopathy, although pulmonary fibrosis may occur in the later stages. Erythema nodosum is seen in some cases, and sarcoid infiltration of the skin also occurs. Hepatosplenomegaly and lymphadenopathy are important signs of generalized systemic involvement.

Clinical Findings
Enlargement of the parotid glands occurs and, when associated with uveitis, is called Heerfordt's syndrome. Enlargement of lacrimal and salivary glands (Mikulicz's syndrome) also occurs.

A granulomatous uveitis with large mutton fat keratic precipitates and posterior synechiae is the commonest ocular manifestation. Sarcoid follicles may also be seen in the conjunctiva. Recent reports have suggested that granulomatous involvement of the retina, choroid, and optic disk may be seen more frequently than heretofore recognized. There are also reports that vitreous inflammation and involvement of the pars plana may be due to sarcoidosis. Neurologic sarcoidosis may produce visual loss from optic nerve involvement, and ocular motor and other cranial nerve palsies may be seen.

Pathogenesis & Diagnosis
The immunologic basis of sarcoidosis is not fully understood, but there is a depression of cell-mediated immunity and hyperactivity of humoral immunity. Lymphopenia is common, and the distribution of T lymphocytes is abnormal. The T cell count in peripheral blood is reduced, although there is some evidence that it is raised in other organs (eg, lungs). There is no correlation between immunologic abnormalities and clinical status. The diagnosis depends on clinical suspicion and confirmation by biopsy. Tissue that has been biopsied includes the conjunctiva, liver, and scalene lymph node. Transbronchial biopsy is a useful technique that confirms the diagnosis in 85% of cases.

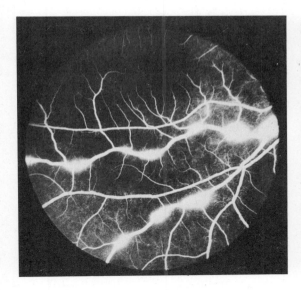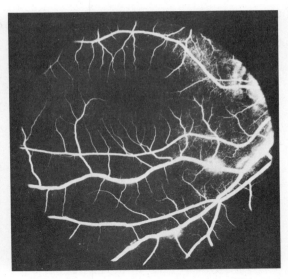

Figure 18–35. Sarcoidosis. Focal periphlebitis is a feature of ocular sarcoid and responds dramatically to corticosteroids. *Left:* Before treatment. *Right:* After treatment.

If biopsy confirmation is not available, the Kveim test should be performed. This test consists of the intradermal injection of sarcoid material and then, after a period of 6 weeks, biopsy of the area, which, if positive, shows a granulomatous reaction with giant cells. Unfortunately, this test is less specific than transbronchial biopsy and is positive in only 20% of patients presenting with uveitis who later develop sarcoidosis. The Mantoux test should also be performed, although it is usually negative. Serum angiotensin-converting enzyme is produced by epithelioid cells, and raised levels may be found in sarcoidosis. This is an excellent test for assessing disease activity but not for diagnosis. Angiotensin-converting enzyme levels may also be high in tuberculosis, leprosy, primary biliary cirrhosis, experimental allergic alveolitis, and Hodgkin's disease.

Treatment

The uveitis is controlled by corticosteroids and mydriatics applied topically. The development of new vessels in the retina merits photocoagulation in view of their propensity to cause vitreous hemorrhages. The systemic disease is controlled by the administration of oral corticosteroids.

EALES'S DISEASE

This disease was originally reported to occur in young men in a poor general state of health who experienced recurrent vitreous hemorrhages from areas of retinal neovascularization. However, such symptoms are also known to occur in sarcoidosis, systemic lupus erythematosus, sickle cell disease, and diabetes. Extensive investigations are therefore indicated to exclude these conditions in patients with consistent clinical features. If test results are negative, the term Eales's disease is then appropriate as a diagnosis arrived at by exclusion. Photocoagulation of the new vessels can reduce the chance of further vitreous hemorrhage.

LEPROSY
(Hansen's Disease)

Leprosy is a chronic granulomatous disorder caused by *Mycobacterium leprae*, an acid-fast bacillus. It is estimated that 12–15 million people in the world have leprosy and that of this number 20–50% (2.4 to 6 or 7 million) have ocular involvement. In tropical countries, the infection is endemic.

Three major types of leprosy are recognized: lepromatous, tuberculoid, and dimorphous. The type any

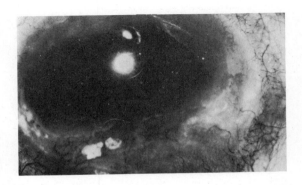

Figure 18–36. Leprosy keratitis, left eye. (Courtesy of W Richards.)

given patient will develop depends upon the individual's immunity to the organism and the number of invading organisms. Thus, a person with minimal or no cell-mediated immunity and in whom the organisms are numerous (multibacillary) develops lepromatous leprosy, whereas a person with strong resistance and few organisms (paucibacillary) develops tuberculoid leprosy. The eye may be affected in any type of leprosy, but ocular involvement is more common in the lepromatous type. Ocular lesions are due to direct invasion by *M leprae* of the ocular tissues or of the nerves supplying the eye and adnexa. Since the organism appears to grow better at lower temperatures, infection is more apt to involve the anterior segment of the eye than the posterior segment.

The early clinical signs of ocular leprosy are lagophthalmos, loss of the lateral portions of the eyebrows and eyelashes (madarosis), conjunctival hyperemia, and superficial keratitis (Fig 18–36), with interstitial keratitis—beginning typically in the superior temporal quadrant of the cornea—often supervening.

Scarring of the cornea from interstitial or exposure keratitis (or both) causes blurred vision and often blindness. Granulomatous iritis with lepromas (iris pearls) is common, and a low-grade iritis associated with iris atrophy and a pinpoint pupil may also occur. Hypertrophy of the eyebrows with deformities of the lids and trichiasis are late changes, and exposure keratitis, typically in the inferior and central cornea, can result from facial nerve palsy and absence of corneal sensation.

Ocular leprosy can be diagnosed on the basis of characteristic signs combined with a characteristic skin biopsy.

The best drugs for treating leprosy are the sulfones, which are bacteriostatic, and clofazamine and rifampin, which are bactericidal. In multibacillary infections, it is now recommended that the 2 types of drugs be used together. Since the host may harbor the organisms for years, long-term therapy is necessary. Drug reactions such as erythema nodosum leprosum may require thalidomide, corticosteroids, or clofazimine for adequate control. Granulomatous iritis may be benefited by topical atropine and corticosteroids; low-grade iritis with iris atrophy is benefited by topical phenylephrine and epinephrine.

SYPHILIS

Congenital Syphilis

Manifestations of syphilis acquired in utero or at birth include mental deficiency, saddle nose, rhinitis, Hutchinson's teeth, alopecia, exanthemas, deafness, and bone lesions. The most common eye lesion is interstitial keratitis (see p 102). Chorioretinitis unassociated with interstitial keratitis occurs fairly often. There are many small yellow dots and pigment clumps in the peripheral fundus, giving the typical "salt and pepper" appearance. In other cases, the chorioretinitis

occurs as larger isolated patches or may have the appearance of retinitis pigmentosa. Syphilitic conjunctivitis or dacryoadenitis is rare.

Congenital syphilis is treated with large doses of penicillin.

Acquired Syphilis

Ocular chancre (primary lesion) occurs rarely on the lid margins and follows the same course as a genital chancre.

Iritis and iridocyclitis occur in the secondary stage of syphilis along with the rash in about 5% of cases. The iritis is acute, with fibrous exudates in the anterior chamber. Posterior synechiae are common if care is not taken to keep the pupil dilated.

Other less common ocular manifestations of acquired syphilis are interstitial keratitis and chorioretinitis, which occur much less frequently in acquired than in congenital syphilis; chorioretinitis usually is widespread and often destroys useful vision. Syphilitic chorioretinitis may resemble retinitis pigmentosa in clinical appearance; however, unlike the genetically determined disease, it can be unilateral (Fig 18–37).

Most cases of syphilis can now be diagnosed by the Venereal Disease Research Laboratory (VDRL) or *Treponema pallidum* hemagglutination (TPHA) tests. Further tests include the *T pallidum* immobilization (TPI) test and the fluorescent treponemal antibody (FTA-ABS) test. The latter test can indicate whether a recent infection has occurred. The increasing incidence of syphilis requires the use of these tests in all patients with unexplained uveitis, vitritis, retinal vasculitis, ischemic optic neuropathy, or ocular motor nerve palsies. Treatment consists of systemic penicillin in very high dosage.

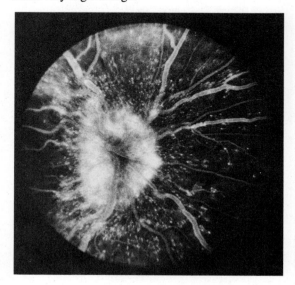

Figure 18–37. Secondary syphilis. Bilateral visual loss occurred in a 24-year-old man. Late fluorescein photographs showed disk leakage with dilatation and leakage of peripapillary capillaries.

Neuro-ophthalmologic Considerations

Argyll Robertson pupil is particularly common in tabes and paresis. Syphilis often causes complete internal ophthalmoplegia. Optic neuritis is usually due to basal meningitis and may resemble retrobulbar neuritis. Visual fields show marked peripheral constriction. Optic atrophy follows severe chorioretinitis or optic neuritis. A gumma occasionally involves the optic nerve, causing optic atrophy. The third cranial nerve is most commonly involved, causing individual extraocular muscle palsies. The sixth nerve is less frequently involved; the fourth nerve is rarely affected. Of the other cranial nerves, the seventh and eighth are most likely to be affected. Spinal fluid examination is required in all cases of neurologic syphilis.

BRUCELLOSIS

During the chronic stage of this disease, ocular involvement by the endogenous route is fairly common. Iritis is the most frequent ocular complication. The uveitis is not always granulomatous; if nongranulomatous, the inflammation tends to subside in a short time. Less common complications include choroiditis, generalized uveitis, and nummular keratitis, which has the same clinical appearance as epidemic keratoconjunctivitis. These lesions usually heal well but occasionally ulcerate, and they can develop into chronic keratitis with periodic exacerbations and remissions.

Other ocular complications of brucellosis, including scleritis, are rarely seen. Some cases of ocular brucellosis respond to systemic sulfadiazine and streptomycin, although the organism develops resistance easily. The iritis is treated locally by mydriatics. Corticosteroids are sometimes of value locally but are contraindicated systemically.

TOXOPLASMOSIS

This disease is of great ocular importance. The organism is a protozoal parasite that infects a great number of animals and birds and has worldwide distribution. Although there have not been a great many proved human cases, toxoplasmosis is probably the most common cause of posterior chorioretinitis.

Congenital Toxoplasmosis (Fig 18–38)

Infection occurs in utero, and one-third of infants born to mothers who acquired toxoplasmosis during pregnancy—particularly during the third trimester—will be affected.

The disease is recognized after birth by the typical posterior polar chorioretinitis, which is usually seen in the inactive stage. A number of cases also show cerebral or cerebellar calcification by x-ray, although only a minority show signs of central nervous system

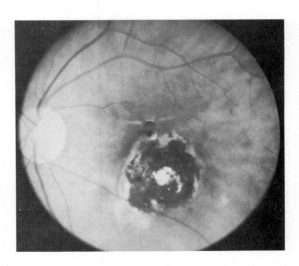

Figure 18–38. Healed toxoplasmic chorioretinitis. Note scarring in left macular area.

disease such as convulsions, mental deficiency, hemiplegia, or paraplegia. The congenital form is nearly always arrested by the time it can be diagnosed.

Congenital toxoplasmosis is perhaps the most common cause of posterior uveitis. A focal choroiditis is seen, usually in the posterior pole, and an active lesion is often related to an old healed lesion. Episodes of posterior uveitis and chorioretinitis usually represent a reactivation of a congenital infection. Rarely, panuveitis may occur, or papillitis progressing to optic atrophy. Isolated anterior uveitis does not occur. Peripheral vision is preserved, but because the macula is involved in at least 50% of cases, central vision is reduced.

Treatment with systemic corticosteroids reduces inflammation but does not prevent scar formation. Subconjunctival or retrobulbar injection of steroids is contraindicated, because it may cause severe exacerbation of disease.

Acquired Toxoplasmosis

Acquired toxoplasmosis affects young adults and is characterized by general malaise, lymphadenopathy, sore throat, and hepatosplenomegaly similar to that seen in infectious mononucleosis. Uveitis or chorioretinitis does not occur in this disease. Acquired ocular toxoplasmosis may occur in immunosuppressed patients.

VIRAL DISEASES*

HERPES SIMPLEX

The most common manifestation of herpes simplex is fever blisters on the lips. The most common and serious eye lesion is herpes simplex (dendritic) keratitis (see p 92). Vesicular skin lesions can also appear on the skin of the lids and the lid margins. Herpes simplex may cause iridocyclitis and may rarely cause severe encephalitis. (Corticosteroids should not be employed in early stages.)

There are 2 morphologic strains of the virus: type 1 and type 2. Ocular infections are usually produced by type 1, whereas genital infections are caused by type 2.

POLIOMYELITIS

Bulbar poliomyelitis severe enough to cause lesions of the third, fourth, or sixth cranial nerve is usually fatal. Any type of internal or external ophthalmoplegia may result in survivors. Supranuclear abnormalities ("gaze" palsies, paralysis of convergence or divergence) are rare residual defects. Optic neuritis is rarely present. Treatment is purely symptomatic, although occasionally a residual extraocular muscle imbalance can be greatly improved by strabismus surgery.

GERMAN MEASLES
(Rubella)

Maternal rubella during the first trimester of pregnancy causes congenital anomalies, including serious heart disease, genitourinary disorders, and many serious ocular diseases, in about 10% of infants. The most common eye complication is cataract, which is bilateral in 75% of cases. The embryonal and fetal nuclei of the lens are usually opaque, and visual acuity is often below 6/60 (20/200). Other congenital ocular anomalies are frequently associated with the cataracts, eg, uveal colobomas, searching nystagmus, microphthalmos, strabismus, retinopathy, and infantile glaucoma. Congenital cataract, especially if bilateral, may require surgical removal, but the prognosis is always guarded, since other ocular anomalies are often present that may not be recognized until the cataract is removed. Many physicians have felt that therapeutic abortion is advisable if rubella occurs during the first trimester of pregnancy, since the rate of serious congenital anomalies is so high.

Cataract surgery should be delayed until at least age 2, since the live virus is present in ocular tissues for many months after birth. The results of early surgery are unsatisfactory in a very high percentage of cases.

MEASLES
(Rubeola)

Acute conjunctivitis is common early in the course of measles. Koplik's spots can occur on the conjunctiva. There may also be an associated epithelial keratitis.

Interest has recently been shown in the slow virus of measles, which produces an encephalitis (Dawson's subacute sclerosing panencephalitis). Ocular signs include disk edema and macular changes due to neuroretinal involvement. The prognosis is extremely poor.

The treatment of the eye complications of measles is symptomatic unless there is secondary infection, in which case local antibiotic ointment is used.

MUMPS

The most common ocular complication of mumps is dacryoadenitis. A diffuse keratitis with corneal edema resembling the disciform keratitis of herpes simplex occurs rarely. It usually clears completely within 2–3 weeks. Other less common eye complications of mumps include episcleritis, iridocyclitis, choroiditis, and optic neuritis, all of which tend to heal with little or no residual damage. Mumps encephalitis can cause a wide variety of neuro-ophthalmologic abnormalities that may be permanent, including internal and external ophthalmoplegia, pupillary abnormalities, and gaze palsies. Convalescent serum and gamma globulin may help to modify the disease; otherwise, treatment is symptomatic.

CHICKENPOX
(Varicella)

Swollen lids, conjunctivitis, and, rarely, vesicular conjunctival lesions may occur as part of the clinical picture of chickenpox.

INFECTIOUS MONONUCLEOSIS

Although this fairly common disease is often looked upon as benign and self-limited, there is increasing evidence that significant complications are not rare. The disease process can affect the eye directly, causing nongranulomatous uveitis, scleritis, conjunctivitis, retinitis, or papillitis. Complete recovery is usual, but residual visual loss can result. The central nervous system may also be involved, causing infranuclear muscle palsies, nystagmus, and pupillary abnormalities. No specific therapy is available, although gamma globulin has been used with questionable benefit.

*Herpes zoster: See p 228.

CYTOMEGALIC INCLUSION DISEASE

Infection with cytomegalovirus, a member of the herpesvirus group, may range from a subclinical infection to classical manifestations of cytomegalic inclusion disease. The virus most frequently affects newborn infants and compromised hosts, and the disease can be acquired or congenital. The clinical findings in the newborn infant may include prematurity, hepatosplenomegaly, jaundice, and microcephaly. The ocular findings include focal necrotizing retinitis and choroiditis with perivascular infiltrates and retinal hemorrhages. Other reported ocular findings include microphthalmia, cataract, optic atrophy, and optic disk malformation.

Histopathologic examination of the retinal and choroidal lesion shows large inclusion-bearing cells characteristic of cytomegalovirus infections. There is disruption of the normal architecture of the retina and choroid, with evidence of necrosis and mononuclear and perivascular infiltration. Calcifications in the retina may be observed.

Laboratory studies include isolation of the virus from a fresh urine specimen, from a throat swab, or from a liver biopsy. Serologic tests, complement-fixing antibodies, and indirect FA tests may become positive. The evaluation of cord serum IgM and IgA in newborn infants is helpful as a nonspecific aid in the diagnosis of congenital cytomegalic inclusion disease.

The differential diagnosis in the congenital disease should include toxoplasmosis, rubella, herpesvirus hominis or herpes simplex infection, and syphilis.

No specific therapy has been shown to be effective against this virus. Some agents such as adenosine arabinoside (vidarabine) and interferon-inducers (poly I:C) may induce a decrease in viruria but do not cure the disease.

CANDIDIASIS

The introduction of modern surgical and immunosuppressive methods of treatment to clinical medicine has resulted in a marked increase in the number of people with compromised immune systems and, therefore, an increase in the susceptibility of these patients to a large number of opportunistic pathogens that were previously considered saprophytes. *Candida albicans* is one of the most important opportunistic fungi.

Many factors are responsible for this apparent emergence of *Candida* as an important opportunistic organism. These factors include the increasing long-term use of corticosteroids and cytotoxic agents, widespread use of antibiotics, abdominal surgery, prolonged use of indwelling intravenous catheters and hyperalimentation, widespread abuse of intravenous narcotic drugs, infusion of glucose solutions, diabetes, debilitating diseases, malnutrition, and malignant diseases.

The ocular involvement accompanies systemic *Candida* infection and candidemia in approximately two-thirds of cases. The initial *Candida* lesion is a focal necrotizing granulomatous retinitis with or without choroiditis, characterized by fluffy white exudative lesions associated with cells in the vitreous overlying the lesion. Such lesions may spread to involve the optic nerve and other ocular structures. Endophthalmitis, panophthalmitis, Roth's spots, papillitis, and exudative retinal detachment may occur. Spread into the vitreous cavity may result in the formation of a vitreous abscess. Anterior uveitis occurs with cells and flare in the anterior chamber, and a hypopyon may form.

Treatment consists of systemic administration of amphotericin B, flucytosine, or both. Successful treatment with a combination of amphotericin B and certain antibiotics such as rifampin has been reported.

MULTISYSTEM AUTOIMMUNE DISEASES

This ill-defined group of diseases is characterized by widespread inflammatory damage of connective tissue with deposition of fibrinoid tissue in the ground substance. There is evidence that an autoantibody reaction against normal tissue antigens produces tissue damage. Ocular involvement is frequent in most collagen diseases.

SYSTEMIC LUPUS ERYTHEMATOSUS

Discoid lupus erythematosus is localized to the skin region on either side of the nose, conforming to the characteristic "butterfly" distribution. There are no generalized features.

Systemic or disseminated lupus erythematosus is a multisystem disease including "butterfly skin lesions," pericarditis, Raynaud's phenomenon, renal involvement, arthritis, anemia, and central nervous system signs. Almost any ocular structure can be involved, but scleritis, conjunctivitis, and keratoconjunctivitis sicca (in 25% of cases) are predominant. Uveitis rarely occurs, and retinal involvement produces signs of arteriolar occlusion, probably a manifestation of arteritis. The fundus picture may be complicated by a hypertensive retinopathy, which in severe cases can cause capillary occlusion or even proliferative retinopathy.

Pathogenesis & Diagnosis

The disease is an immunologic disorder marked by the presence of circulating immune complexes. Diagnostic tests include anti-DNA antibodies and mitochondrial type V antibodies. Active disease is associated with raised circulating immune complexes and reduced fractions of complement.

Treatment

Systemic steroids and sometimes immunosuppressives may be very effective therapeutically.

DERMATOMYOSITIS

This rare disease occurs frequently in children. Characteristically there is a degenerative subacute inflammation of the muscles, sometimes including the extraocular muscles. The lids are commonly a part of the generalized dermal involvement and may show marked swelling and erythema. Retinopathy—consisting of multiple white, irregular opacities appearing much like cotton wool patches—as well as flame-shaped hemorrhages may occur. High doses of systemic corticosteroids will frequently effect a remission that continues even after cessation of therapy. The ultimate prognosis is poor, however.

SCLERODERMA

This rare chronic disease is characterized by widespread alterations in the collagenous tissues of the mucosa, bones, muscles, skin, and internal organs. Men and women between 15 and 45 years of age are affected. The skin in local areas becomes tense and "leathery," and the process may spread to involve large areas of the limbs, rendering them virtually immobile. The skin of the eyelids is often involved. Iritis and cataract occur less frequently. Retinopathy similar to lupus erythematosus and dermatomyositis may be present. Systemic corticosteroid treatment has improved the prognosis substantially, and retinopathy usually improves or disappears.

POLYARTERITIS NODOSA

This collagen disease affects the medium-sized arteries, most commonly in men. There is intense inflammation of all the muscle layers of the arteries, with fibrinoid necrosis. The main clinical features are fever of unknown origin, weight loss, nephritis, hypertension, acute abdominal symptoms, pulmonary signs, peripheral neuropathy, and muscle pain with wasting. Cardiac involvement is common, although death is usually caused by renal dysfunction.

Ocular changes are seen in 20% of cases and consist of episcleritis and scleritis. When the limbal vessels are involved, guttering of the peripheral cornea may occur. The commonest ocular signs are seen in the retinal circulation, where cotton wool spots and hemorrhages reflect retinal arteritis. The central artery

may be involved, and if the disk vessels are affected, disk edema results. Ophthalmoplegia may result from arteritis of the vasa nervorum (Fig 18–39). Systemic corticosteroids are of some value, but the long-term prognosis is uniformly bad.

WEGENER'S GRANULOMATOSIS

This granulomatous process shares certain clinical features with polyarteritis nodosa. The 3 diagnostic criteria are (1) necrotizing granulomatous lesions of the respiratory tract, (2) generalized necrotizing arteritis, and (3) renal involvement with necrotizing glomerulitis.

There is a spectrum of disease ranging from classic Wegener's granulomatosis, with the 3 features described above, to a more benign form, termed necrotizing sarcoidal granulomatosis.

Ocular complications occur in 50% of cases, and proptosis owing to orbital granulomatous involvement occurs with associated ocular muscle or optic nerve involvement (Fig 18–40). If the vasculitis affects the eye, conjunctivitis, episcleritis, scleritis, uveitis, and retinal vasculitis may occur. Nasolacrimal duct obstruction is a rare complication.

It has been suggested that there is a partial cell-mediated immunodeficiency, and therapy with combined corticosteroids and immunosuppressives (particularly cyclophosphamide) often produces a satisfactory response.

RHEUMATOID ARTHRITIS

Rheumatoid arthritis is a disease of middle and old age and is 3 times more common in women than in men. Uveitis is a rare complication, but scleritis and episcleritis are comparatively common. The scleritis may herald exacerbation of the systemic disease, tends to occur with widespread vasculitis, and may lead to scleromalacia perforans.

Corticosteroid drops are helpful in episcleritis or anterior uveitis, but systemic treatment (corticosteroids plus indomethacin or phenylbutazone) is necessary for scleritis. Operative procedures (subconjunctival injection, scleral biopsy) on the sclera are contraindicated, since risks are involved. Keratoconjunctivitis sicca is present in 15% of cases.

JUVENILE RHEUMATOID ARTHRITIS
(Still's Disease)

Ocular complications occur 3 times more frequently in girls, and particularly when few joints are affected, of which the knee is the most common. The systemic disease appears to be disproportionately mild

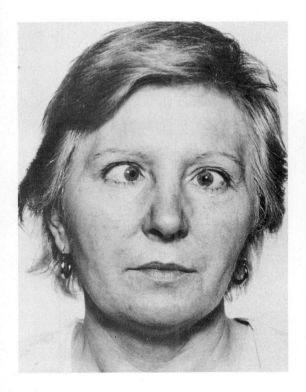

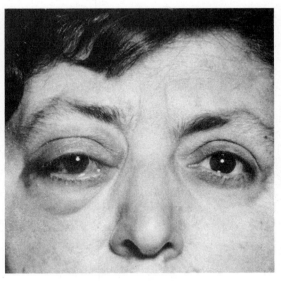

Figure 18–39. Polyarteritis nodosa. Bilateral sixth nerve palsies.

Figure 18–40. Classic Wegener's granulomatosis with proptosis, ptosis, and ophthalmoplegia. The condition has remained static for 10 years on corticosteroids and cyclophosphamide.

in children with severe visual loss, and diagnosis and treatment may therefore be delayed. Ocular involvement may occur before joint involvement. A chronic insidious uveitis with a high incidence of anterior segment complications develops (eg, posterior synechiae, cataract, secondary glaucoma, band-shaped keratopathy). Antinuclear antibodies are positive in 88% of patients with juvenile rheumatoid arthritis who develop uveitis, whereas it is positive in only 30% of the group as a whole.

SJÖGREN'S SYNDROME

Sjögren's syndrome is a systemic disorder with diverse features. The disease is characterized by the clinical triad of keratoconjunctivitis sicca (see p 53), xerostomia or dryness of the mouth, and a connective tissue disease, usually rheumatoid arthritis. It is more common in females. The onset of ocular symptoms occurs most frequently during the fourth, fifth, and sixth decades. Lymphoid proliferation is a prominent feature of Sjögren's syndrome and may involve the kidneys, the lungs, or the liver, causing renal tubular acidosis, pulmonary fibrosis, or liver cirrhosis. Lymphoreticular malignancy such as reticulum cell sar-

coma may complicate the benign course of Sjögren's syndrome many years after the onset.

The histopathologic changes of the lacrimal glands consist of lymphocytic infiltration and occasional plasma cells leading to atrophy and destruction of the glandular structures. These changes are part of the generalized polyglandular affection in Sjögren's syndrome, resulting in dryness of the eyes, mouth, skin, and mucous membranes.

Because of the relative inaccessibility of the lacrimal gland, the labial salivary gland biopsy serves as an important diagnostic procedure in patients with suspected Sjögren's syndrome.

The tear lysozyme level is absent or reduced in over 90% of patients.

Tubuloreticular viruslike structures resembling the unenveloped nucleocapsids of paramyxovirus have been observed in the renal biopsy and in the capillary endothelial cells and infiltrating lymphocytes of the labial salivary glands in patients with Sjögren's syndrome (Fig 18–42). Although the pathogenesis is not yet clear, there is increasing evidence that immunologic and viral factors interact in a susceptible host to account for the disease process.

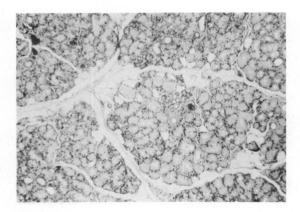

Figure 18–41. Normal labial salivary gland tissue. (Courtesy of T Daniels.)

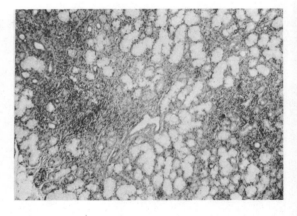

Figure 18–42. Labial salivary gland tissue of a patient with Sjögren's syndrome showing extensive lymphocytic infiltration. (Courtesy of T Daniels.)

ANKYLOSING SPONDYLITIS

Ankylosing spondylitis is a disease occurring mainly in men 16–40 years of age. There is almost always uveitis occurring at some stage in the disease, which is intermittent, exudative, and may be accompanied by scleritis. There is a strong association with HLA-B27. There is an antigenic cross-reactivity between HLA-B27 and *Klebsiella pneumoniae*, and active uveitis in ankylosing spondylitis patients is associated with the presence of this organism in the feces.

REITER'S DISEASE

The diagnosis of Reiter's disease is based on a triad of signs that includes urethritis, conjunctivitis, and arthritis. Scleritis, keratitis, and uveitis may also be seen in addition to conjunctivitis. The disease has a high correlation with HLA-B27 antigen.

BEHCET'S DISEASE

Behçet's disease consists of the clinical triad of relapsing iritis and aphthous and genital ulceration (Fig 18–43). Ocular signs occur in 75% of cases; the uveitis is severe, occasionally associated with hypopyon. Posterior uveitis is common, and retinal periphlebitis and papillitis may occur. Treatment is difficult, and the prognosis is poor. Systemic corticosteroids and azathioprine or chlorambucil constitute the most satisfactory regimen, but the immunostimulant levamisole may also be beneficial.

Exacerbation of the disease coincides with a raised erythrocyte sedimentation rate, raised IgG (with fall in IgA in the acute phase and a later rise of IgA in the convalescent phase), and raised C9 levels with C-reactive protein. Fibrinolytic studies may also be

abnormal, particularly in patients developing major vein thrombosis and retinal vein thrombosis.

UVEITIS WITH INFLAMMATORY BOWEL DISEASE

Scleral, episcleral, and uveal tract involvement may be seen in both ulcerative colitis and Crohn's disease. Conversely, bowel symptoms may be seen in patients with ankylosing spondylitis.

HUMAN LEUKOCYTE ANTIGENS

Histocompatability antigens are unique markers on the surfaces of all nucleated cells. The human leukocyte A system is the major group of such antigens.

The genes responsible for the formation of these antigens are found in 5 adjacent loci on each of the pair of chromosome 6. Therefore, each cell in a heterozygous individual can contain up to 10 different antigens.

The 5 loci are named locus A, B, C, D, and DR. Humoral antibodies that can be detected by serologic methods are bound to antigens at loci A, B, and C. Cross-reactivity occurs when an antiserum to one particular antigen reacts weakly with another antiserum. This may account for some of the associations of specific disorders with different HLA antigens. The antigen controlled by locus D can be detected by mixed lymphocyte culture when donor lymphocytes are incubated with lymphocytes of the proposed recipient and blastic transformation and division occur.

Some groups of HLA appear to be inherited together, eg, HLA-A8, HLA-B1, and HLA-Dw3, and are called haplotypes. This occurs because the different antigens are close together on a gene and therefore inherited "en bloc." This phenomenon is called link-

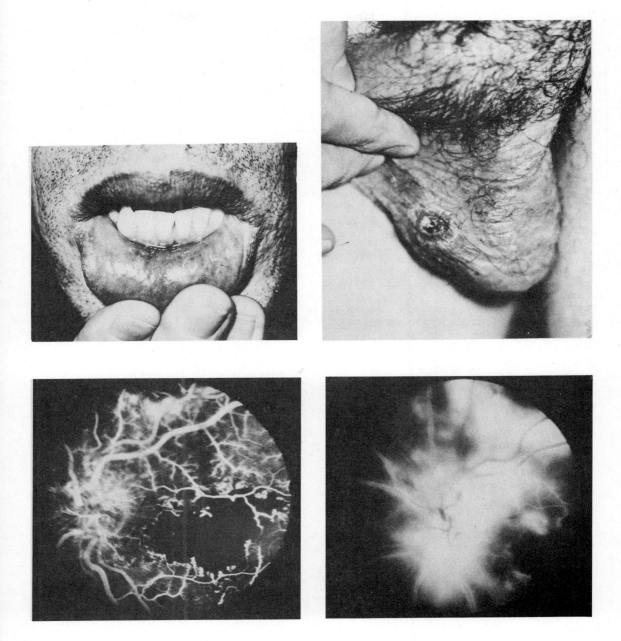

Figure 18–43. Behçet's disease. Clinical features include oral and genital ulcers. Ocular features include increased capillary permeability and areas of retinal ischemia and infiltration. Marked leakage of capillaries is seen in the late stages of fluorescein angiography (bottom right).

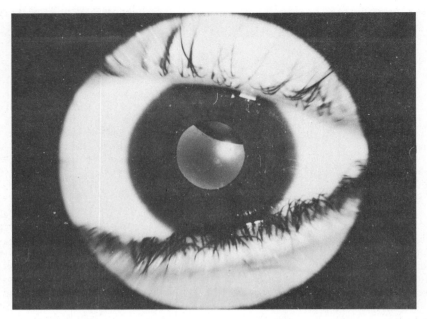

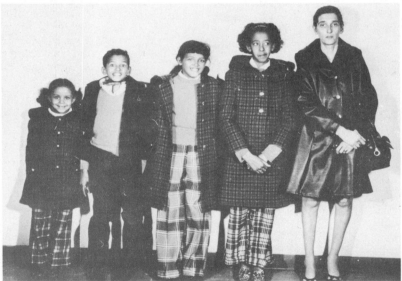

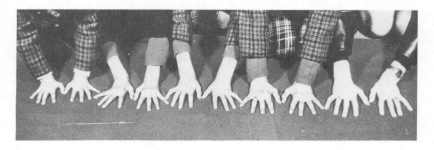

Figure 18–44. Marfan's syndrome. Familial expression of arachnodactyly and upward dislocation of the lens.

Table 18–3. Association of HLA types with systemic diseases.

Behçet's disease	HLA-B5
Juvenile diabetic retinopathy	HLA-B8 (without A1)
Myasthenia gravis	HLA-DR3
	HLA-B8
Thyrotoxicosis	HLA-Dw3
	HLA-B8
Multiple sclerosis	HLA-DR3
	HLA-Dw2
Ankylosing spondylitis	HLA-B27
Reiter's disease	HLA-B27
Acute anterior uveitis	HLA-B27
Rheumatoid arthritis	HLA-DR4
	HLA-Dw4

age disequilibrium, because there is a reduction in the normal genetic transfer that occurs during meiosis.

The association between different HLA haplotypes (ie, different HLA groups inherited together) and specific diseases is well known. Ninety percent of people with ankylosing spondylitis have HLA-B27. A person with HLA-B27 is 100 times more likely to develop ankylosing spondylitis than a person without this haplotype. However, only 5% of people who do possess HLA-B27 actually develop ankylosing spondylitis.

Other associations are listed in Table 18–3.

HERITABLE CONNECTIVE TISSUE DISEASES

MARFAN'S SYNDROME
(Arachnodactyly)
(Fig 18–44)

The most striking feature of this rare syndrome is increased length of the long bones, particularly of the fingers and toes. Other characteristics include scanty subcutaneous fat, relaxed ligaments, and, less commonly, other associated developmental anomalies, including congenital heart disease and deformities of the spine and joints. Ocular complications are often seen—in particular, dislocation of the lenses, usually superiorly and nasally. Less common ocular anomalies include severe refractive errors, megalocornea, cataract, uveal colobomas, and secondary glaucoma. There is a high infant mortality rate. Removal of a dislocated lens may be necessary. The disease is genetically determined, nearly always as an autosomal dominant, often with incomplete expression, so that mild, incomplete forms of the syndrome are seen. Several reports have correlated cytogenetic changes with Marfan's syndrome.

MARCHESANI'S SYNDROME

This is a rare hereditary disorder characterized by multiple skeletal and ocular abnormalities which is transmitted as an autosomal recessive trait. Patients are short and stocky, with well-developed muscles. The hands and feet are characteristically spade-shaped; in childhood, x-rays show delayed carpal and tarsal ossification. Ocular complications include spherophakia and ectopia lentis, which give rise to lenticular myopia, iridodonesis, and glaucoma. The prognosis for vision is usually poor because the glaucoma resists all forms of treatment.

OSTEOGENESIS IMPERFECTA
(Brittle Bones & Blue Scleras)

This rare autosomal dominant syndrome is characterized by multiple fractures, blue scleras, and, less commonly, deafness. The disease is usually manifest soon after birth. The long bones are very fragile, fracturing easily and often healing with fibrous bony union. The bones become more fragile with age. The very thin sclera allows the blue color imparted by the underlying uveal tract to show through. There is often no visual functional impairment. Occasionally, abnormalities such as keratoconus, megalocornea, and corneal or lecticular opacities are also present that do interfere with visual function.

Ophthalmologic treatment is seldom necessary.

HEREDITARY METABOLIC DISORDERS

MUCOPOLYSACCHARIDOSES

Mucopolysaccharides are long glycoside polymers consisting of a chain of 100 sugar residues attached to a protein core. The polymers are either dermatan or heparan sulfate, and in the mucopolysaccharidoses there is defective breakdown of those polymers due to enzyme deficiency, resulting in the deposition of mucopolysaccharide in the tissues and an elevated urinary excretion.

There are 6 clearly defined disorders of mucopolysaccharide metabolism (I–VI) that all used to be grouped together and called **gargoylism.**

Corneal clouding occurs in **Hurler's syndrome** (type I) (Fig 18–45), **Scheie's syndrome** (type I), **Morquio's disease** (type IV), and **Maroteaux-Lamy** syndrome (type V A+B) and noticeably not in **Hunter's syndrome** (type I), the only X-linked inherited variety; the others are all autosomal recessive. Other ocular features are megalocornea, buphthalmos, pigmentary retinopathy, and optic atrophy.

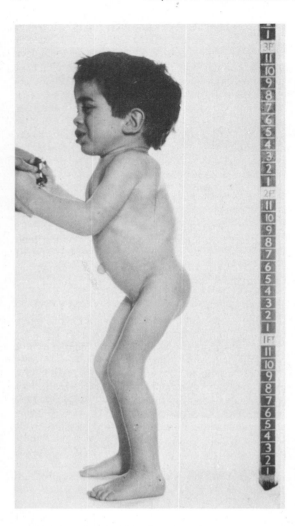

Figure 18–45. Clinical features of Hurler's syndrome include gargoylism, gibbus, and umbilical hernia.

HEPATOLENTICULAR DEGENERATION
(Wilson's Disease)

This rare autosomal recessive disease of young adults, characterized by abnormal copper metabolism, causes changes in the basal nuclei, cirrhosis of the liver, and a pathognomonic corneal pigmentation called the Kayser-Fleischer ring. The ring appears as a green or brown band peripherally and deep in the stroma near Descemet's membrane and may only be visible with a slit lamp. The disease is progressive and often results in death by age 40.

Treatment with dimercaprol (BAL) and penicillamine has resulted in sustained clinical improvement in some cases.

CYSTINOSIS

This rare autosomal recessive derangement of amino acid metabolism causes widespread deposition of cystine crystals throughout the body. Dwarfism, nephropathy, and death in childhood from renal failure are the rule. Cystine crystals can be readily seen in the conjunctiva and cornea, where fine particles are seen predominantly in the outer third of the corneal stroma.

There is no treatment.

ALBINISM

Generalized albinism is a disease affecting the metabolism of melanin and is inherited as an autosomal recessive trait. The skin and hair are white, and there is a generalized lack of pigment throughout the body that is apparent from birth. The eyebrows and lashes are white. The irides appear reddish, and the pupil appears red. The fundus is red, with a prominent choroidal vessel pattern, since the pigment epithelium of the retina is deficient. Photophobia is prominent. The macula is often poorly developed, greatly impairing visual function, and this often causes an associated searching nystagmus that reduces visual acuity to about 6/60 (20/200).

HOMOCYSTINURIA

Homocystinuria is a rare autosomal recessive disorder of amino acid metabolism characterized clinically by mental retardation, downward dislocation of the lenses of the eyes, and genu valgum. The plasma homocystine and methionine levels are elevated. Urinary excretion of homocystine is increased, and the nitroprusside test of the urine is positive. Thrombosis of medium-sized arteries is common, often resulting in early death from cerebrovascular, coronary, or renal vascular occlusions. These are relatively common during general anesthesia and are due to excess platelet aggregation. Dietary therapy is possible with either a high-pyridoxine diet or a low-methionine diet with added cystine, or a combination of these two.

GALACTOSEMIA

Galactosemia is a rare autosomal recessive disorder of carbohydrate metabolism that becomes clinically manifest soon after birth by feeding problems, vomiting, diarrhea, abdominal distention, hepatomegaly, jaundice, ascites, cataracts, mental retardation, and elevated blood and urine galactose levels. Dietary exclusion of milk and all foods containing galactose and lactose for the first 3 years of life will prevent the clinical manifestations and will result in improvement of existing abnormalities. Even the cataract changes, which are characterized by vacuoles of the cortex, are reversible in the early stage.

Identification of the carrier state is possible by finding a 50% reduction of galactose-6-phosphatase.

MISCELLANEOUS SYSTEMIC DISEASES WITH OCULAR MANIFESTATIONS

VOGT-KOYANAGI-HARADA SYNDROME

Bilateral uveitis associated with alopecia, poliosis, vitiligo, and hearing defects, usually in young adults, has been termed Vogt-Koyanagi disease. When the choroiditis is more exudative, serous retinal detachment occurs and the complex is known as Harada's syndrome. Japanese and Italians are affected more commonly than other groups, but even among these the disease is rare. There is a tendency toward recovery of visual function, but this is not always complete. Corticosteroids have been reported to have a favorable effect upon the disease. Local corticosteroids and mydriatics are indicated. There have been a few reports of isolation of a virus from these cases, but a viral cause has not yet been definitely established.

ERYTHEMA MULTIFORME
(Stevens-Johnson Syndrome)

Erythema multiforme is a serious mucocutaneous disease that occurs as a hypersensitivity reaction to drugs or food. Children are most susceptible. The manifestations consist of generalized maculopapular rash, severe stomatitis, and purulent conjunctivitis, sometimes leading to symblepharon and occlusion of the lacrimal gland ducts (**dry eye syndrome**). In severe cases corneal ulcers, perforations, and panophthalmitis can destroy all visual function. Systemic corticosteroid treatment often favorably influences the course of the disease and usually preserves useful visual function. Secondary infection with *Staphylococcus aureus* is common and must be vigorously treated by local antibiotics instilled into the conjunctival sac. Frequently there is marked reduction of tear formation that can be helped by instillation of artificial tears.

GIANT CELL ARTERITIS
(Including Temporal or Cranial Arteritis)

This is a disease of elderly patients (over age 60). Medium-sized arteries are involved, particularly the intima of the vessels. Branches of the external carotid system are frequently involved, though pathologic studies have shown more diffuse arterial involvement. Polymyalgia rheumatica may precede or accompany the disease. Patients feel ill and have excruciating pain over the temporal or occipital arteries. Visual loss due to an ischemic optic neuropathy is frequent, and a few cases have a central retinal artery occlusion. Visual loss may also be due to cortical blindness. Other central nervous system signs include cranial nerve palsies and signs referable to brain stem lesions. The diagnosis is confirmed by a high erythrocyte sedimentation rate (ESR) and a positive temporal artery biopsy. In early stages of the disease, the ESR may be normal, but usually it is 80–100 mm in the first hour. It is important to make the diagnosis early, because immediate systemic corticosteroids produce dramatic improvement. The disease activity is monitored by the erythrocyte sedimentation rate and the clinical state. The corticosteroid dose may have to be maintained for several years and should be kept below 5 mg prednisolone daily if possible, since with higher doses the survival rate is markedly reduced.

IDIOPATHIC ARTERITIS OF TAKAYASU
(Pulseless Disease)

This disease, found most frequently in young women and occasionally in children, is a polyarteritis of unknown cause with increased predilection for the aorta and its branches. Manifestations may include evidence of cerebrovascular insufficiency, syncope, absence of pulsations in the upper extremities, and ophthalmologic changes compatible with chronic hypoxia of the ocular structures. Ophthalmodynamometry may be of value by demonstrating decreased carotid blood flow on one or both sides. The disease is sometimes associated with rheumatoid arthritis, which supports the idea that it is a collagen disease.

Thromboendarterectomy, prosthetic graft, and systemic corticosteroid therapy have been reported to be successful.

WERNER'S SYNDROME

Werner's syndrome is a rare hereditary disorder characterized ocularly by juvenile cataracts, glaucoma, and corneal opacities. It is probably transmitted as a recessive trait. The onset is usually between age 20 and 30, with graying and thinning of the hair of the scalp, genital region, and axillas. Atrophic skin changes may occur on the face, limbs, hands, and feet.

LAURENCE-MOON-BIEDL SYNDROME

Obesity, mental deficiency, polydactyly, hypogenitalism, and retinitis pigmentosa form the complete syndrome. The retinal changes are not always typical of retinitis pigmentosa and may be present soon after birth or develop during adolescence. This rare syndrome is genetically determined and follows an autosomal recessive pattern with a high rate of consanguinity. The heterozygous state may be identified by mild incomplete evidences of the disease. It is interesting that a single abnormal gene can account for such a multiplicity of clinical findings.

ROSACEA
(Acne Rosacea)

This disease of unknown cause is primarily dermatologic, beginning as a hyperemia of the face associated with acneiform lesions and eventually causing hypertrophy of tissues (such as rhinophyma). Chronic blepharitis due to staphylococcal infection or seborrhea is often present. Rosacea keratitis develops in about 5% of cases. Episcleritis, scleritis, and nongranulomatous iridocyclitis are rare ocular complications.

Topical corticosteroids are helpful in controlling keratitis or iridocyclitis, but there is no specific therapy.

LOWE'S SYNDROME

This rare syndrome consists of cerebral defects, mental retardation, and ocular anomalies associated with dwarfism due to renal dysfunction (a congenital defect of reabsorption in the renal tubules, causing aminoaciduria). The eye findings include congenital cataract, infantile glaucoma, and nystagmus. All cases reported to date have occurred in males, suggesting X-linked inheritance. There is a high early mortality rate.

OCULAR COMPLICATIONS OF CERTAIN SYSTEMICALLY ADMINISTERED DRUGS

AMIODARONE

Amiodarone is a benzofuran derivative used to treat cardiac dysrhythmias, particularly Wolff-Parkinson-White syndrome, and angina pectoris. Most patients develop small punctate deposits in the basal cell layer of the corneal epithelium. The severity of keratopathy is related to the total daily dose and is mild at a dose of less than 200 mg daily. The deposits rarely interfere with vision, and although they progress with continued treatment, even in low dosage, they always resolve completely when treatment is stopped (Fig 18–46).

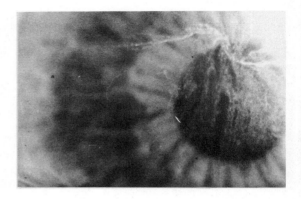

Figure 18–46. Amiodarone keratopathy. (Courtesy of DJ Spalton.)

ANTICHOLINERGICS
(Atropine & Related Synthetic Drugs)

All of these drugs, when given preoperatively or for gastrointestinal disorders, may cause blurred vision in presbyopic patients because of a direct action on accommodation. They also tend to dilate the pupils, so that in patients with narrow anterior chamber angles there is the added threat of angle-closure glaucoma. This is the cause of angle-closure glaucoma (frequently attributed to "nervousness") occasionally seen in patients hospitalized for general surgery.

ANTIDEPRESSANTS

Tricyclic antidepressants and monoamine oxidase inhibitors have an anticholinergic effect and theoretically may exacerbate open-angle glaucoma or provoke an attack of angle-closure glaucoma. However, this is rare in clinical practice, and if a patient is already receiving treatment for open-angle glaucoma, the medication will overcome any effect of the antidepressants.

CHLORAMPHENICOL

Chloramphenicol, in addition to the possibility of causing severe blood dyscrasias, hepatic and renal disease, and gastrointestinal disturbances, can sometimes cause optic neuritis. This is especially true in children. Bilateral blurred vision with central scotomas occurs. Stopping the drug does not always restore vision.

Despite the possibility of toxic optic neuropathy, chloramphenicol may still be required for the treatment of bacterial endophthalmitis. The drug is generally not administered for more than 1 week.

CHLOROQUINE

Originally employed as an antimalarial drug, chloroquine has also been widely used in the treatment of many collagen diseases, especially systemic lupus erythematosus and rheumatoid arthritis, and skin diseases, including discoid lupus erythematosus and sarcoidosis. With high dosage—often 250–750 mg daily administered for months or years—serious ocular toxicity has occurred. Corneal changes were described first and consisted of diffuse haziness of the epithelium and subepithelial area, occasionally sufficient to simulate an epithelial dystrophy. These changes cause only mild blurring of vision and are reversible upon drug withdrawal. Similar changes have been described in patients receiving quinacrine. Minimal corneal involvement is not necessarily an indication for discontinuance of chloroquine therapy. Corneal changes have been reported in about 30% of patients on long-term chloroquine treatment.

A less common but more serious ocular complication of long-term chloroquine therapy is retinal damage, causing loss of central vision as well as constriction of peripheral visual fields. Pigmentary changes and edema of the macula, marked alteration of the retinal vessels, and in some cases peripheral pigmentary changes can be seen ophthalmoscopically. Fluorescein fundus photography aids greatly in establishing early diagnosis or evaluating the extent of macular involvement. Visual field examination reveals central scotomas and peripheral field constriction. There are also changes in the electroretinogram, dark adaptation, and color vision. The damage is always bilateral and is usually equal in both eyes. The visual loss is irreversible and may even progress after cessation of therapy. No treatment is of any value.

Long-term chloroquine therapy must be undertaken only upon urgent indications. These patients should be examined by an ophthalmologist every 3–4 months. Between examinations, patients should make a rough test of visual acuity once weekly.

CHLOROTHIAZIDE

Xanthopsia (yellow vision) has been reported in patients taking this oral diuretic.

CONTRACEPTIVES, ORAL

Although numerous reports suggest that in predisposed individuals oral contraceptives can provoke or precipitate ophthalmic vascular occlusive disease or optic nerve damage, it is difficult to establish a definite cause and effect relationship. Optic neuritis, retinal arterial or venous thrombosis, and pseudotumor cerebri have been described in patients taking oral contraceptives. Since there is some uncertainty regarding the possibility of such ocular complications, oral contraceptives should be used only by healthy women with no history of vascular, neurologic, or ocular disease.

CORTICOSTEROIDS

It has been clearly demonstrated that long-term systemic corticosteroid therapy can cause chronic open-angle glaucoma and cataracts and can provoke and worsen attacks of herpes simplex keratitis. Locally administered corticosteroids are much more potent in this respect and have the added disadvantage of causing fungal overgrowth if the corneal epithelium is not intact. Steroid-induced subcapsular lens opacities cause some impairment of visual function but usually do not progress to advanced cataract. Cessation of therapy will arrest progression of the lenticular opacities, but the changes are irreversible.

Systemic corticosteroids may also cause papilledema associated with pseudotumor cerebri, both during administration and shortly after withdrawal.

DIGITALIS

Blurred vision and disturbed color vision are said to be the most common ocular complications of digitalis toxicity, although the actual incidence of such symptoms in patients receiving digitalis is extremely low. The purified glycosides of digitalis probably produce fewer of the toxic ocular symptoms than the whole leaf.

Visual acuity may be decreased. Objects may appear yellow (xanthopsia) or, less commonly, green, brown, red, "snowy," or white. The patient may complain of photophobia and flashes of light. Scotomas and, very rarely, transient and permanent amblyopia have been described. The toxic effects of digitalis may be due to direct effects on the retinal reception cells or retrobulbar neuritis, or they may be of central origin.

ETHAMBUTOL

Ocular complications are rare unless the daily dose is greater than 25 mg/kg, but they do occur because the drug is often used in resistant cases of tuberculosis. Optic neuropathy affecting the papillomacular bundle produces centrocecal scotoma and reduced color vision. A chiasmal pattern of involvement may also be seen. Visual loss is dose-dependent and may improve over 6 months after cessation of the drug.

OXYGEN

Any concentration of oxygen in excess of that in air may lead to retrolental fibroplasia in premature infants. Premature infants should receive only the amount of oxygen necessary for survival. The concentration should not exceed 40% for brief periods as indicated. In adults, administration of hyperbaric oxygen (3 atmospheres) can cause constriction of the retinal arterioles. In one reported case, a patient with an old inactive retrobulbar neuritis exposed to 100% oxygen at 2 atmospheres of pressure developed almost complete loss of visual field in 2 hours.

PHENOBARBITAL & PHENYTOIN

Ocular complications relate to oculomotor involvement, producing nystagmus and weakness of convergence and accommodation. The nystagmus may persist for many months after cessation of the drug, and the degree of oculomotor abnormality is related to drug dosage. Early abnormalities include disturbance of smooth pursuit.

PHENOTHIAZINES

The phenothiazines usually exert an atropinelike effect on the eye so that the pupils may be dilated, especially with large dosages. Of greater clinical significance, however, are the pigmentary ocular changes, which include pigmentary retinopathy and pigment deposits on the corneal endothelium and anterior lens capsule. The corneal and lens pigmentation may cause blurring of vision, but the pigment deposits usually disappear several months after the drug is discontinued. In pigmentary retinopathy, there is a diminution of central vision, night blindness, diffuse narrowing of the retinal arteries, and occasionally severe blindness.

The piperidine group (eg, thioridazine) has a higher risk of causing pigmentary retinopathy, and the maximum daily dose should not exceed 600 mg. The retinal changes are partly reversible under normal circumstances, but in some patients more severe irreversible changes occur at the "safe" dosage level.

The dimethylamine group (eg, chlorpromazine) rarely produces retinal pigmentary changes.

The piperazine group (eg, trifluoperazine) does not produce these retinal complications.

All of these drugs can produce an extrapyramidal syndrome that may involve eye movements. Large doses can provoke profound hypotension, which may produce ischemic optic neuropathy.

Patients receiving large dosages or prolonged treatment with phenothiazines should be questioned regarding visual disturbances and should have periodic ophthalmoscopic examinations.

QUININE & QUINACRINE

Quinine and quinacrine, when used in the treatment of malaria, may cause bilateral blurred vision, sometimes following a single dose. There is constriction of the visual field and, rarely, total blindness. The tendency is toward partial recovery, although usually there are permanent peripheral field defects. The ganglion cells of the retina are affected first, presumably as a result of vasoconstriction of the retinal arterioles. Varying degrees of retinal edema occur early. Optic atrophy is a late finding.

SALICYLATES

Hypersensitivity reactions are common with aspirin taken at therapeutic dosage levels, producing angioneurotic edema and conjunctivitis. Withdrawal of the drug usually results in improved visual function, but complete recovery is rare.

SEDATIVE TRANQUILIZERS

When taken regularly, the so-called minor tranquilizers can decrease tear production by the lacrimal gland, thus resulting in ocular irritation because of dry eyes. Tear production returns to normal when the tranquilizers are discontinued.

The principal drugs in this group are meprobamate, chlordiazepoxide, and diazepam.

FETAL EFFECTS OF DRUGS

The visual pathways of the fetus are occasionally affected by drugs taken by the mother during pregnancy.

Phenytoin may cause optic nerve hypoplasia.

Pigmentary retinopathy has been reported in a child of a mother taking **busulfan** for acute myeloid leukemia.

Warfarin is teratogenic and may produce a hypoplastic nose, stippled epiphyses, and skeletal abnormalities. Affected children may present with recurrent sticky eyes from obstruction of the nasolacrimal duct secondary to malformation of the nose. Other ocular abnormalities include optic atrophy, microphthalmia, and lens opacities. (**Heparin** does not produce these abnormalities, since it is a large molecule that does not cross the placenta.)

• • •

References

Asbury AK et al: Oculomotor palsy in diabetes mellitus: A clinico-pathological study. *Brain* 1970;**93(Part 3):**555.

Astle JN, Ellis PP: Ocular complications in renal transplant patients. *Ann Ophthalmol* 1974;**6:**1269.

Bachman DM et al: Culture proven cytomegalovirus retinitis in a homosexual man with the acquired immunodeficiency syndrome. *J Am Acad Ophthalmol* 1982;**89:**797.

Bergsma D, Bron AJ, Cotlier E (editors): *The Eye and Inborn Errors of Metabolism.* AR Liss, Inc, 1976.

Brewerton DA: The histocompatibility antigen (HLA 27) and acute anterior uveitis. *Trans Ophthalmol Soc UK* 1974; **94:**735.

Cant JS: *Vision and Circulation.* Mosby, 1976.

Cogan DG: *Ophthalmic Manifestations of Systemic Vascular Disease.* Saunders, 1974.

De Venecia G et al: Cytomegalic inclusion retinitis in an adult. *Arch Ophthalmol* 1971;**86:**44.

Diabetic Retinopathy Study Group: Preliminary report on effects of photocoagulation therapy. *Am J Ophthalmol* 1976;**81:**383.

Dunlap EA (editor): *Gordon's Medical Management of Ocular Disease,* 2nd ed. Harper & Row, 1976.

Edwards JE Jr et al: Ocular manifestations of Candida septicemia: Review of seventy-six cases of hematogenous Candida endophthalmitis. *Medicine* 1974;**53:**47.

Elliot AJ: 30-year observation of patients with Eales's disease. *Am J Ophthalmol* 1975;**80:**404.

Eva PR, Pascoe PT, Vaughan DG: Refractive change in hyperglycaemia: Hyperopia, not myopia. *Br J Ophthalmol* 1982; **66:**500.

Ferry AP, Font RL: Carcinoma metastatic to the eye and orbit. *Arch Ophthalmol* 1975;**93:**472.

Fraunfelder FT: *Drug-Induced Ocular Side-Effects and Drug Interactions.* Lea & Febiger, 1976.

Garner LL, Wang RIH, Hieb E: Ocular effects of phenothiazines. *Med Lett Drugs Ther* (Dec) 1974;**4:**30.

Gass JDM, Olson CL: Sarcoidosis with optic nerve and retinal involvement. *Arch Ophthalmol* 1976;**94:**945.

Goldberg MF: Retinal vaso-occlusion in sickling hemoglobinopathies. In: *The Eye and Inborn Errors of Metabolism.* Bergsma D, Bron AJ, Cotlier E (editors). Vol 12 of: *Birth Defects* (original article series). AR Liss, Inc, 1976.

Griffin JR et al: Blood-borne candida endophthalmitis. *Arch Ophthalmol* 1973;**89:**450.

Hall R: The eye signs of Graves' disease. In: *Medical Ophthalmology.* Rose FC. Chapman & Hall, 1976.

Hanshaw JB: Congenital cytomegalovirus infection. *N Engl J Med* 1973;**288:**1406.

Hart PD, Russell E Jr, Remington JS: The compromised host and infection. 2. Deep fungal infections. *J Infect Dis* 1969; **120:**169.

James DG, Spiteri MA: Behçet's disease. *J Am Acad Ophthalmol* 1982;**89:**1279.

Keltner JL: Giant-cell arteritis: Signs and symptoms. *J Am Acad Ophthalmol* 1982;**89:**1101.

Mason EO Jr, South AM, Montgomery JR: Cord serum IgA in congenital cytomegalovirus infection. *J Pediatr* 1976; **89:**945.

Mausolf FA: *The Eye and Systemic Disease.* Mosby, 1975.

Rahi AHS, Garner A: *Immunopathology of the Eye.* Blackwell, 1976.

Rose FC: *Medical Ophthalmology.* Chapman & Hall, 1976.

Rosenman RH et al: Relation of corneal arcus to cardiovascular risk factors and the incidence of coronary disease. *N Engl J Med* 1974;**291:**1322.

Salvaggio JE (editor): Primer on allergic and immunologic diseases. *JAMA* 1982;**248:**2579. [Special issue.]

Svardsudd K et al: Hypertensive eye ground changes. *Acta Med Scand* 1978;**204:**159.

Walsh JB: Hypertensive retinopathy: Description, classification, and prognosis. *J Am Acad Ophthalmol* 1982;**89:**1279.

Wise GN, Dollery CT, Henkind P: *The Retinal Circulation.* Harper & Row, 1971.

19 | Immunologic Diseases of the Eye

The eye is frequently considered to be a special target of immunologic disease processes, but proof of the causative role of these processes is lacking in all but a few disorders. In this sense, the immunopathology of the eye is much less clearly delineated than that of the kidney, the testis, or the thyroid gland. Because the eye is a highly vascularized organ and because the rather labile vessels of the conjunctiva are embedded in a nearly transparent medium, inflammatory eye disorders are more obvious (and often more painful) than those of other organs such as the thyroid or the kidney. The iris, ciliary body, and choroid are the most highly vascularized tissues of the eye. The similarity of the vascular supply of the uvea to that of the kidney and the choroid plexus of the brain has given rise to justified speculation concerning the selection of these 3 tissues, among others, as targets of immune complex diseases (eg, serum sickness).

Immunologic diseases of the eye can be grossly divided into 2 major categories: antibody-mediated and cell-mediated diseases. As is the case in other organs, there is ample opportunity for the interaction of these 2 systems in the eye.

ANTIBODY-MEDIATED DISEASES

Before it can be concluded that a disease of the eye is antibody-dependent, the following criteria must be satisfied: (1) There must be evidence of specific antibody in the patient's serum or plasma cells. (2) The antigen must be identified and, if feasible, characterized. (3) The same antigen must be shown to produce an immunologic response in the eye of an experimental animal, and the pathologic changes produced in the experimental animal must be similar to those observed in the human disease. (4) It must be possible to produce similar lesions in animals passively sensitized with serum from an affected animal upon challenge with the specific antigen.

Unless all of the above criteria are satisfied, the disease may be thought of as *possibly* antibody-dependent. In such circumstances, the disease can be regarded as antibody-mediated if only one of the following criteria is met: (1) if antibody to an antigen is present in higher quantities in the ocular fluids than in the serum (after adjustments have been made for the total amounts of immunoglobulins in each fluid); (2) if abnormal accumulations of plasma cells are present in the ocular lesion; (3) if abnormal accumulations of immunoglobulins are present at the site of the disease; (4) if complement is fixed by immunoglobulins at the site of the disease; (5) if an accumulation of eosinophils is present at the site of the disease; or (6) if the ocular disease is associated with an inflammatory disease elsewhere in the body for which antibody dependency has been proved or strongly suggested.

HAY FEVER CONJUNCTIVITIS

This disease is characterized by edema and hyperemia of the conjunctiva and lids (Fig 19–1) and by itching and watering of the eyes. There is often an associated itching sensation in the nose as well as rhinorrhea. The conjunctiva appears pale and boggy because of the intense edema, which is often rapid in onset. There is a distinct seasonal incidence, some patients being able to establish the onset of their symp-

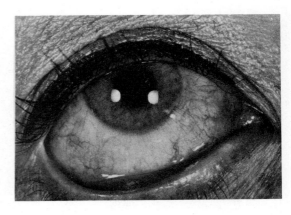

Figure 19–1. Hay fever conjunctivitis. Note edema and hyperemia of the conjunctiva. (Courtesy of M Allansmith and B McClellan.)

toms at precisely the same time each year. These times usually correspond to the release of pollens by specific grasses, trees, or weeds.

Immunologic Pathogenesis

Hay fever conjunctivitis is one of the few inflammatory eye disorders for which antibody dependence has been definitely established. It is recognized as a form of atopic disease with an implied hereditary susceptibility. IgE (reaginic antibody) in its dimeric form is believed to be attached to mast cells lying beneath the conjunctival epithelium. Contact of the offending antigen with IgE triggers the release of vasoactive amines, principally histamine, in this area, and this in turn results in vasodilatation and chemosis.

The role of circulating antibody to ragweed pollen in the pathogenesis of hay fever conjunctivitis has been demonstrated by passively transferring serum from a hypersensitive person to a nonsensitive one. When exposed to the offending pollen, the previously nonsensitive individual reacted with the typical signs of hay fever conjunctivitis.

Immunologic Diagnosis

Victims of hay fever conjunctivitis show many eosinophils in Giemsa-stained scrapings of conjunctival epithelium. They show the **immediate** type of response, with wheal and flare, when tested by scratch tests of the skin with extracts of pollens or other offending antigens. Biopsies of the skin test sites have occasionally shown the full-blown picture of an **Arthus reaction,** with deposition of immune complexes in the walls of the dermal vessels. Passive cutaneous anaphylaxis can also be used to demonstrate the presence of circulating antibody.

Treatment

Systemically administered antihistaminics such as diphenhydramine or tripelennamine are effective, particularly when given prophylactically during the season of greatest exposure. Sustained-release capsules of antihistaminics such as Ornade (chlorpheniramine maleate) are preferred by some. Locally applied antihistaminics such as Prefrin-A drops contain both an antihistaminic agent (pyrilamine) and a vasosconstrictor (phenylephrine). Where conjunctival edema is severe and of sudden onset, epinephrine drops (1:100,000) instilled into the conjunctival sac may help to reduce the edema quickly. Corticosteroids applied locally offer some relief. Topical use of cromolyn (disodium cromoglycate; Cromoptic), a stabilizer of the mast cell, is still being evaluated in clinical experiments and appears to be a promising method of treatment.

Hyposensitization with gradually increasing doses of subcutaneously injected pollen extracts or other suspected allergens appears to reduce the severity of the disease in some individuals if started well in advance of the season. The mechanism is presumed to be production of blocking antibodies in response to the injection of small, graded doses of the antigen. This procedure cannot be recommended routinely, however, in view of the generally good results and relatively few complications of antihistamine therapy. Acute anaphylactoid reactions have occasionally resulted from overzealous hyposensitization therapy.

VERNAL CONJUNCTIVITIS & ATOPIC KERATOCONJUNCTIVITIS

These 2 diseases also belong to the group of atopic disorders. Both are characterized by itching and lacrimation of the eyes but are more chronic than hay fever conjunctivitis. Furthermore, both ultimately result in structural modifications of the lids and conjunctiva.

Vernal conjunctivitis characteristically affects children and adolescents; the incidence decreases sharply after the second decade of life. Like hay fever conjunctivitis, vernal conjunctivitis occurs only in the warm months of the year. Most of its victims live in hot, dry climates. The disease characteristically produces giant (''cobblestone'') papillae of the tarsal conjunctiva (Fig 19–2). The keratinized epithelium from these papillae may abrade the underlying cornea, giving rise to complaints of foreign body sensation.

Atopic keratoconjunctivitis affects individuals of all ages and has no specific seasonal incidence. The skin of the lids has a characteristic dry, scaly appearance. The conjunctiva is pale and boggy. Both the conjunctiva and the cornea may develop scarring in the later stages of the disease. Atopic cataract has also been described. Staphylococcal blepharitis, manifested by scales and crusts on the lids, commonly complicates this disease.

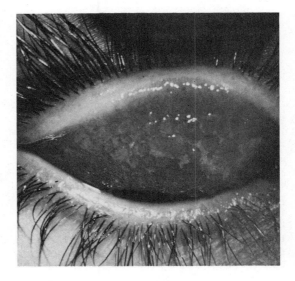

Figure 19–2. Giant papillae (''cobblestones'') in the tarsal conjunctiva of a patient with vernal conjunctivitis.

Immunologic Pathogenesis

Reaginic antibody (IgE) is fixed to subepithelial mast cells in both of these conditions. Contact between the offending antigen and IgE is thought to trigger degranulation of the mast cell, which in turn allows for the release of vasoactive amines in the tissues. It is unlikely, however, that antibody action alone is responsible, since—at least in the case of the papillae of vernal conjunctivitis—there is heavy papillary infiltration by mononuclear cells. Hay fever and asthma occur much more frequently in patients with vernal conjunctivitis and atopic keratoconjunctivitis than in the general population. Of the criteria outlined above (see p 270) for demonstration of *possibly* antibody-mediated diseases, (2), (5), and (6) have been met by atopic keratoconjunctivitis.

Immunologic Diagnosis

As in hay fever conjunctivitis, patients with atopic keratoconjunctivitis and vernal conjunctivitis regularly show large numbers of eosinophils in conjunctival scrapings. Skin testing with food extracts, pollens, and various other antigens reveals a wheal-and-flare type of reaction within 1 hour of testing, but the significance of these reactions is not reliably established.

Treatment

Local instillations of corticosteroid drops or ointment relieve the symptoms. However, caution must be observed in the long-term use of these agents because of the possibility of steroid-induced glaucoma and cataract. Corticosteroids produce less dramatic relief in vernal conjunctivitis than in atopic keratoconjunctivitis, and the same can be said of the antihistamines. Cromolyn is currently being investigated for its usefulness in both vernal conjunctivitis and atopic disease. The initial results of clinical testing are encouraging.

Avoidance of known allergens is helpful; such objects as duck feathers, animal danders, and certain food proteins (egg albumin and others) are common offenders. Specific allergens have been much more difficult to demonstrate in the case of vernal disease, although some workers feel that such substances as rye grass pollens may play a causative role. Installation of air conditioning in the home or relocation to a cool, moist climate is useful in vernal conjunctivitis if economically feasible.

RHEUMATOID DISEASES AFFECTING THE EYE

The diseases in this category vary greatly in their clinical manifestations depending upon the specific disease entity and the age of the patient. Uveitis and scleritis are the principal ocular manifestations of the rheumatoid diseases. **Juvenile rheumatoid arthritis** affects females more frequently than males and is commonly accompanied by iridocyclitis of one or both

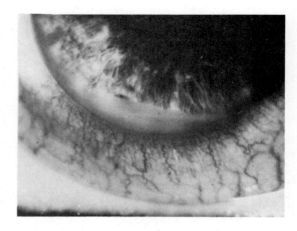

Figure 19–3. Acute iridocyclitis in a patient with ankylosing spondylitis. Note fibrin clot in anterior chamber.

eyes. The onset is often insidious, the patient having few or no complaints and the eye remaining white. Extensive synechia formation, cataract, and secondary glaucoma may be far-advanced before the parents notice that anything is wrong. The arthritis generally affects only one joint (eg, a knee) in cases with ocular involvement.

Ankylosing spondylitis affects males more frequently than females, and the onset is in the second to sixth decades. It may be accompanied by iridocyclitis of acute onset, often with fibrin in the anterior chamber (Fig 19–3). Pain, redness, and photophobia are the initial complaints, and synechia formation is common.

Rheumatoid arthritis of adult onset may be accompanied by acute scleritis or episcleritis (Fig 19–4). The ciliary body and choroid, lying adjacent to the sclera, are often involved secondarily with the inflammation. Rarely, serous detachment of the retina results. The onset is usually in the third to fifth decade, and women are affected more frequently than men.

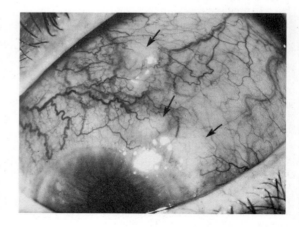

Figure 19–4. Scleral nodules in a patient with rheumatoid arthritis. (Courtesy of S Kimura.)

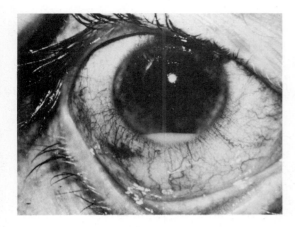

Figure 19–5. Acute iridocyclitis with hypopyon in a patient with Reiter's disease.

Reiter's disease affects men more frequently than women. The first attack of ocular inflammation usually consists of a self-limited papillary conjunctivitis. It follows, at a highly variable interval, the onset of nonspecific urethritis and the appearance of inflammation in one or more of the weight-bearing joints. Subsequent attacks of ocular inflammation may consist of acute iridocyclitis of one or both eyes, occasionally with hypopyon (Fig 19–5).

Immunologic Pathogenesis

Rheumatoid factor, an IgM autoantibody directed against the patient's own IgG, may play a major role in the pathogenesis of rheumatoid arthritis. The union of IgM antibody with IgG is followed by fixation of complement at the tissue site and the attraction of leukocytes and platelets to this area. An occlusive vasculitis, resulting from this train of events, is thought to be the cause of rheumatoid nodule formation in the sclera as well as elsewhere in the body. The occlusion of vessels supplying nutriments to the sclera is thought to be responsible for the "melting away" of the scleral collagen that is so characteristic of rheumatoid arthritis (Fig 19–6).

While this explanation may suffice for rheumatoid arthritis, patients with the ocular complications of juvenile rheumatoid arthritis, ankylosing spondylitis, and Reiter's syndrome usually have negative tests for rheumatoid factor, so other explanations must be sought.

Outside the eyeball itself, the lacrimal gland has been shown to be under attack by circulating antibodies. Destruction of acinar cells within the gland and invasion of the lacrimal gland (as well as the salivary glands) by mononuclear cells result in decreased tear secretion. The combination of dry eyes (keratoconjunctivitis sicca), dry mouth (xerostomia), and rheumatoid arthritis is known as Sjögren's syndrome (see Chapter 18).

A growing body of evidence indicates that the immunogenetic background of certain patients accounts for the expression of their ocular inflammatory disease in specific ways. Analysis of the HLA antigen system shows that the incidence of HLA-B27 is significantly greater in patients with ankylosing spondylitis and Reiter's syndrome than could be expected by chance alone. It is not known how this antigen controls specific inflammatory responses.

Immunologic Diagnosis

Rheumatoid factor can be detected in the serum by a number of standard tests involving the agglutination of IgG-coated erythrocytes or latex particles. Unfortunately, the test for rheumatoid factor is not positive in the majority of isolated rheumatoid afflictions of the eye.

The HLA types of individuals suspected of having ankylosing spondylitis and related diseases can be determined by standard cytotoxicity tests using highly specific antisera. This is generally done in tissue typing centers where work on organ transplantation necessitates such studies. X-ray of the sacroiliac area is a valuable screening procedure that may show evidence of spondylitis prior to the onset of low back pain in patients with the characteristic form of iridocyclitis.

Treatment

Patients with uveitis associated with rheumatoid disease respond well to local instillations of corticosteroid drops (eg, dexamethasone 0.1%) or ointments. Orally administered corticosteroids must occasionally be resorted to for brief periods. Salicylates given orally in divided doses with meals are thought to reduce the frequency and blunt the severity of recurrent attacks. Atropine drops (1%) are useful for the relief of photophobia during the acute attacks. Shorter-acting mydriatics such as phenylephrine 10% should be used in the subacute stages to prevent synechia formation. Corticosteroid-resistant cases, especially those causing progressive erosion of the sclera, have been treated successfully with immunosuppressive agents such as chlorambucil.

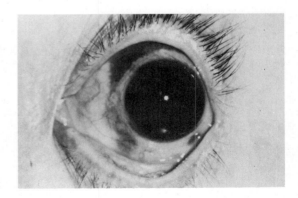

Figure 19–6. Scleral thinning in a patient with rheumatoid arthritis. Note dark color of the underlying uvea.

OTHER ANTIBODY-MEDIATED EYE DISEASES

The following antibody-mediated diseases are infrequently encountered by the practicing ophthalmologist.

Systemic lupus erythematosus, associated with the presence of circulating antibodies to DNA, produces an occlusive vasculitis of the nerve fiber layer of the retina. Such infarcts result in cytoid bodies or "cotton wool" spots in the retina (Fig 19–7).

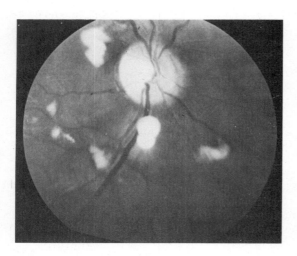

Figure 19–7. "Cotton wool" spots (cytoid bodies) in the retina of a patient with lupus erythematosus.

Pemphigus vulgaris produces painful intraepithelial bullae of the conjunctiva. It is associated with the presence of circulating antibodies to an intercellular antigen located between the deeper cells of the conjunctival epithelium.

Cicatricial pemphigoid is characterized by subepithelial bullae of the conjunctiva. In the chronic stages of this disease, cicatricial contraction of the conjunctiva may result in severe scarring of the cornea, dryness of the eyes, and ultimate blindness. Pemphigoid is associated with local deposits of tissue antibodies directed against one or more antigens located in the basement membrane of the epithelium.

Lens-induced uveitis is a rare condition that may be associated with circulating antibodies to lens proteins. It is seen in individuals whose lens capsules have become permeable to these proteins as a result of trauma or other disease. Interest in this field dates back to Uhlenhuth (1903), who first demonstrated the organ-specific nature of antibodies to the lens. Witmer showed in 1962 that antibody to lens tissue may be produced by lymphoid cells of the ciliary body.

CELL-MEDIATED DISEASES

This group of diseases appears to be associated with cell-mediated immunity or delayed hypersensitivity. Various structures of the eye are invaded by mononuclear cells, principally lymphocytes and macrophages, in response to one or more chronic antigenic stimuli. In the case of chronic infections such as tuberculosis, leprosy, toxoplasmosis, and herpes simplex, the antigenic stimulus has clearly been identified as an infectious agent in the ocular tissue. Such infections are often associated with delayed skin test reactivity following the intradermal injection of an extract of the organism.

More intriguing but less well understood are the granulomatous diseases of the eye for which no infectious cause has been found. Such diseases are thought to represent cell-mediated, possibly autoimmune processes, but their origin remains obscure.

OCULAR SARCOIDOSIS

Ocular sarcoidosis is characterized by a panuveitis with occasional inflammatory involvement of the optic nerve and retinal blood vessels. It often presents as iridocyclitis of insidious onset. Less frequently, it occurs as acute iridocyclitis, with pain, photophobia, and redness of the eye. Large precipitates resembling drops of solidified "mutton fat" are seen on the corneal endothelium. The anterior chamber contains a good deal of protein and numerous cells, mostly lymphocytes. Nodules are often seen on the iris, both at the pupillary margin and in the substance of the iris stroma. The latter are often vascularized. Synechiae are commonly encountered, particularly in patients with dark skin. Severe cases ultimately involve the posterior segment of the eye. Coarse clumps of cells ("snowballs") are seen in the vitreous, and exudates resembling candle drippings may be seen along the course of retinal vessels. Patchy infiltrations of the choroid or optic nerve may also be seen.

Infiltrations of the lacrimal gland and of the conjunctiva have been noted on occasion. When the latter are present, the diagnosis can easily be confirmed by biopsy of the small opaque nodules.

Immunologic Pathogenesis

Although many infectious or allergic causes of sarcoidosis have been suggested, none has been confirmed. Noncaseating granulomas are seen in the uvea, optic nerve, and adnexal structures of the eye as well as elsewhere in the body. The presence of macrophages and giant cells suggests that particulate matter is being phagocytosed, but this material has not been identified.

Patients with sarcoidosis are usually anergic to extracts of the common microbial antigens such as those of mumps, *Trichophyton, Candida,* and *Mycobacterium tuberculosis.* As in other lymphoproliferative disorders such as Hodgkin's disease and chronic lymphocytic leukemia, this may represent suppression of T cell activity such that the normal delayed hypersensitivity responses to common antigens cannot take place. Meanwhile, circulating immunoglobulins are usually detectable in the serum at higher than normal levels.

Immunologic Diagnosis

The diagnosis is largely inferential. Negative skin tests to a battery of antigens to which the patient is known to have been exposed are highly suggestive, and the same is true of the elevation of serum immunoglobulins. Biopsy of a conjunctival nodule or scalene lymph node may provide positive histologic evidence of the disease. X-rays of the chest reveal hilar adenopathy in many cases. Elevated levels of serum lysozyme or serum angiotensin converting enzyme may be detected.

Treatment

Sarcoid lesions of the eye respond well to corticosteroid therapy. Frequent instillations of dexamethasone 0.1% eye drops generally bring the anterior uveitis under control. Atropine drops should be prescribed in the acute phase of the disease for the relief of pain and photophobia; short-acting pupillary dilators such as phenylephrine should be given later to prevent synechia formation. Systemic corticosteroids are sometimes necessary to control severe attacks of anterior uveitis and are always necessary for the control of retinal vasculitis and optic neuritis. The latter condition often accompanies cerebral involvement and carries a grave prognosis.

SYMPATHETIC OPHTHALMIA & VOGT-KOYANAGI-HARADA SYNDROME

These 2 disorders are discussed together because they have certain common clinical features. Both are thought to represent autoimmune phenomena affecting pigmented structures of the eye and skin, and both may give rise to meningeal symptoms.

Clinical Features

Sympathetic ophthalmia is an inflammation in the second eye after the other has been damaged by penetrating injury. In most cases, some portion of the uvea of the injured eye has been exposed to the atmosphere for at least 1 hour. The uninjured or "sympathizing" eye develops minor signs of anterior uveitis after a period ranging from 2 weeks to several years. Floating spots and loss of the power of accommodation are among the earliest symptoms. The disease may progress to severe iridocyclitis with pain and photophobia. Usually, however, the eye remains relatively quiet and painless while the inflammatory disease spreads around the entire uvea. Despite the presence of panuveitis, the retina usually remains uninvolved ex-

cept for perivascular cuffing of the retinal vessels with inflammatory cells. Papilledema and secondary glaucoma may occur. The disease may be accompanied by vitiligo (patchy depigmentation of the skin) and poliosis (whitening) of the eyelashes.

Vogt-Koyanagi-Harada syndrome consists of inflammation of the uvea of one or both eyes characterized by acute iridocyclitis, patchy choroiditis, and serous detachment of the retina. It usually begins with an acute febrile episode with headache, dysacusis, and occasionally vertigo. Patchy loss or whitening of the scalp hair is described in the first few months of the disease. Vitiligo and poliosis are commonly present but are not essential for the diagnosis. Although the initial iridocyclitis may subside quickly, the course of the posterior disease is often indolent, with longstanding serous detachment of the retina and significant visual impairment.

Immunologic Pathogenesis

In both sympathetic ophthalmia and Vogt-Koyanagi-Harada syndrome, delayed hypersensitivity to melanin-containing structures is thought to occur. Although a viral cause has been suggested for both of these disorders, there is no convincing evidence of an infectious origin. It is postulated that some insult, infectious or otherwise, alters the pigmented structures of the eye, skin, and hair in such a way as to provoke delayed hypersensitivity responses to them. Soluble materials from the outer segments of the photoreceptor layer of the retina have recently been incriminated as possible autoantigens. Patients with Vogt-Koyanagi-Harada syndrome are usually Orientals, which suggests an immunogenetic predisposition to the disease.

Histologic sections of the traumatized eye from a patient with sympathetic ophthalmia may show uniform infiltration of most of the uvea by lymphocytes, epithelioid cells, and giant cells. The overlying retina is characteristically intact, but nests of epithelioid cells may protrude through the pigment epithelium of the retina, giving rise to **Dalen-Fuchs** nodules. The inflammation may destroy the architecture of the entire uvea, leaving an atrophic, shrunken globe.

Immunologic Diagnosis

Skin tests with soluble extracts of human or bovine uveal tissue are said to elicit delayed hypersensitivity responses in these patients. Several investigators have recently shown that cultured lymphocytes from patients with these 2 diseases undergo transformation to lymphoblasts in vitro when extracts of uvea or rod outer segments are added to the culture medium. Circulating antibodies to uveal antigens have been found in patients with these diseases, but such antibodies are to be found in any patient with longstanding uveitis, including those suffering from several infectious entities. The spinal fluid of patients with Vogt-Koyanagi-Harada syndrome may show increased numbers of mononuclear cells and elevated protein in the early stages.

Treatment

Mild cases of sympathetic ophthalmia may be treated satisfactorily with locally applied corticosteroid drops and pupillary dilators. The more severe or progressive cases require systemic corticosteroids, often in high doses, for months or years. An alternate-day regimen of oral corticosteroids is recommended for such patients in order to avoid adrenal suppression. The same applies to the treatment of patients with Vogt-Koyanagi-Harada disease. Occasionally, patients with long-standing progressive disease become resistant to corticosteroids or cannot take additional corticosteroid medication because of pathologic fractures, mental changes, or other reasons. Such patients may become candidates for immunosuppressive therapy. Chlorambucil has been used successfully for both conditions.

OTHER DISEASES OF CELL-MEDIATED IMMUNITY

Giant cell arteritis (temporal arteritis) (see Chapter 18) may have disastrous effects on the eye, particularly in elderly individuals. The condition is manifested by pain in the temples and orbit, blurred vision, and scotomas. Examination of the fundus may reveal extensive occlusive retinal vasculitis and choroidal infarcts. Atrophy of the optic nerve head is a frequent complication. Such patients have an elevated sedimentation rate. Biopsy of the temporal artery reveals extensive infiltration of the vessel wall with giant cells and mononuclear cells.

Polyarteritis nodosa (see Chapter 18) can affect both the anterior and posterior segments of the eye. The corneas of such patients may show peripheral thinning and cellular infiltration. The retinal vessels reveal extensive necrotizing inflammation characterized by eosinophil, plasma cell, and lymphocyte infiltration.

Behçet's disease (see Chapter 18) has an uncertain place in the classification of immunologic disorders. It is characterized by recurrent iridocyclitis with hypopyon and occlusive vasculitis of the retinal vessels. Although it has many of the features of a delayed hypersensitivity disease, dramatic alterations of serum complement levels at the very beginning of an attack suggest an immune complex disorder. Furthermore, high levels of circulating immune complexes have recently been detected in patients with this disease.

Contact dermatitis of the eyelids represents a significant though minor disease caused by delayed hypersensitivity. Atropine, perfumed cosmetics, materials contained in plastic spectacle frames, and other locally applied agents may act as the sensitizing hapten. The lower lid is more extensively involved than the upper lid when the sensitizing agent is applied in drop form. Periorbital involvement with erythematous, vesicular, pruritic lesions of the skin is characteristic.

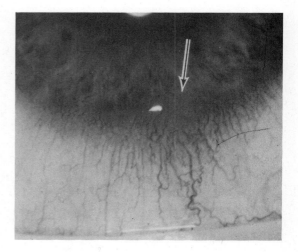

Figure 19–8. Phlyctenule (arrow) at the margin of the cornea. (Courtesy of P Thygeson.)

Phlyctenular keratoconjunctivitis (Fig 19–8) represents a delayed hypersensitivity response to certain microbial antigens, principally those of *M tuberculosis*. It is characterized by acute pain and photophobia in the affected eye, and perforation of the peripheral cornea has been known to result from it. The disease responds rapidly to locally applied corticosteroids. Since the advent of chemotherapy for pulmonary tuberculosis, phlyctenulosis is much less of a problem than it was 30 years ago. It is still encountered occasionally, however, particularly among American Indians and Alaskan Eskimos. Rarely, other pathogens such as *Staphylococcus aureus* and *Coccidioides immitis* have been implicated in phlyctenular disease.

CORNEAL GRAFT REACTIONS

Blindness due to opacity or distortion of the central portion of the cornea is a remediable disease. If all other structures of the eye are intact, a patient whose vision is impaired solely by corneal opacity can expect great improvement from a graft of clear cornea into the diseased area. Trauma, including chemical burns, is one of the most common causes of central corneal opacity. Others include scars from herpetic keratitis, endothelial cell dysfunction with chronic corneal edema (Fuchs's dystrophy), keratoconus, and opacities from previous graft failures. All of these conditions represent indications for penetrating corneal grafts, provided the patient's eye is no longer inflamed and the opacity has been allowed maximal time to undergo spontaneous resolution (usually 6–12 months). It is estimated that approximately 10,000 corneal grafts are performed in the USA annually. Of these, about 90% can be expected to produce a beneficial result.

The cornea was one of the first human tissues to be successfully grafted. The fact that recipients of corneal grafts generally tolerate them well can be attributed to (1) the absence of blood vessels or lymphatics in the normal cornea and (2) the lack of presensitization to tissue-specific antigens in most recipients. Reactions to corneal grafts do occur, however, particularly in individuals whose own corneas have been damaged by previous inflammatory disease. Such corneas may have developed both lymphatics and blood vessels, providing afferent and efferent channels for immunologic reactions in the engrafted cornea.

Although attempts have been made to transplant corneas from other species into human eyes (xenografts), particularly in countries where human material is not available for religious reasons, most corneal grafts have been taken from human eyes (allografts). Except in the case of identical twins, such grafts always represent the implantation of foreign tissue into a donor site; thus, the chance for a graft rejection due to an immune response to foreign antigens is virtually always present.

The cornea is a 3-layered structure composed of a surface epithelium, an oligocellular collagenous stroma, and a single-layered endothelium. Although the surface epithelium may be sloughed and later replaced by the recipient's epithelium, certain elements of the stroma and all of the donor's endothelium remain in place for the rest of the patient's life. This has been firmly established by sex chromosome markers in corneal cells when donor and recipient were of opposite sexes. The endothelium must remain healthy in order for the cornea to remain transparent, and an energy-dependent pump mechanism is required to keep the cornea from swelling with water. Since the recipient's endothelium is in most cases diseased, the central corneal endothelium must be replaced by healthy donor tissue.

A number of foreign elements exist in corneal grafts that might stimulate the immune system of the host to reject this tissue. In addition to those mentioned above, the corneal stroma is regularly perfused with IgG and serum albumin from the donor, although none—or only small amounts—of the other blood proteins are present. While these serum proteins of donor origin rapidly diffuse into the recipient stroma, these substances are theoretically immunogenic.

Although the ABO blood antigens have been shown to have no relationship to corneal graft rejection, the HLA antigen system probably plays a significant role in graft reactions. HLA incompatibility between donor and recipient has been shown by several authors to be significant in determining graft survival, particularly when the corneal bed is vascularized. It is known that most cells of the body possess these HLA antigens, including the endothelial cells of the corneal graft as well as certain stromal cells (keratocytes). The epithelium has been shown by Hall and others to possess a non-HLA antigen that diffuses into the anterior third of the stroma. Thus, while much foreign antigen may be eliminated by purposeful removal of the epithelium at the time of grafting, that amount of antigen which has already diffused into the

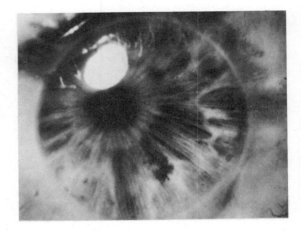

Figure 19–9. A cornea severely scarred by chronic atopic keratoconjunctivitis into which a central graft of clear cornea has been placed. Note how distinctly the iris landmarks are seen through the transparent graft. (Reproduced, with permission, from Stites DP et al [editors]: *Basic & Clinical Immunology,* 4th ed. Lange, 1982.)

stroma is automatically carried over into the recipient. Such antigens may be leached out by soaking the donor cornea in tissue culture for several weeks prior to engraftment.

Both humoral and cellular mechanisms have been implicated in corneal graft reactions. It is likely that early graft rejections (within 2 weeks) are cell-mediated reactions. Cytotoxic lymphocytes have been found in the limbal area and stroma of affected individuals, and phase microscopy in vivo has revealed an actual attack on the grafted endothelial cells by these lymphocytes. Such lymphocytes generally move inward from the periphery of the cornea, making what is known as a "rejection line" as they move centrally. The donor cornea becomes edematous as the endothelium becomes compromised by an accumulation of lymphoid cells.

Late rejection of a corneal graft may occur several weeks to many months after implantation of donor tissue into the recipient eye. Such reactions may be antibody-mediated, since cytotoxic antibodies have been isolated from the serum of patients with a history of multiple graft reactions in vascularized corneal beds. These antibody reactions are complement-dependent and attract polymorphonuclear leukocytes, which may form dense rings in the cornea at the sites of maximum deposition of immune complexes. In experimental animals, similar reactions have been produced by corneal xenografts, but the intensity of the reaction can be markedly reduced either by decomplementing the animal or by reducing its leukocyte population through mechlorethamine therapy.

Treatment

The mainstay of the treatment of corneal graft

reactions is corticosteroid therapy. This medication is generally given in the form of frequently applied eye drops (eg, prednisolone acetate, 1%, hourly) until the clinical signs abate. These clinical signs consist of conjunctival hyperemia in the perilimbal region, a cloudy cornea, cells and protein in the anterior chamber, and keratic precipitates on the corneal endothelium. The earlier treatment is applied, the more effective it is likely to be. Neglected cases may require systemic corticosteroids (80–150 mg prednisone daily) in addition to local eye drop therapy. Occasionally, vascularization and opacification of the cornea occur so rapidly as to make corticosteroid therapy useless, but even the most hopeless-appearing graft reactions have occasionally been reversed by corticosteroid therapy.

Patients known to have rejected many previous corneal grafts are managed somewhat differently, particularly if disease affects their only remaining eye. An attempt is made to find a close HLA match between donor and recipient. Pretreatment of the recipient with immunosuppressive agents such as azathioprine has also been resorted to in some cases. Although HLA testing of the recipient and the potential donor is indicated in cases of repeated corneal graft failure or in cases of severe corneal vascularization, such testing is not necessary or practicable in most cases requiring keratoplasty.

• • •

References

Allansmith MR, O'Connor GR: Immunoglobulins: Structure, function, and relation to the eye. *Surv Ophthalmol* 1970; **14**:367.

Cogan DG: Immunosuppression and eye disease. *Am J Ophthalmol* 1977;**83**:777.

Friedlaender MH: *Allergy and Immunology of the Eye.* Harper & Row, 1979.

Godfrey WA et al: The use of chlorambucil in intractable idiopathic uveitis. *Am J Ophthalmol* 1974;**78**:415.

Maumenee AE, Silverstein AM (editors): *Immunopathology of Uveitis.* Williams & Wilkins, 1964.

Nussenblatt RB: HLA and ocular disease. Proceedings of the Immunology of the Eye Workshop 1. Steinberg GM, Gery I, Nussenblatt RB (editors). *Immunology Abstracts* 1980;**Spr Suppl**:25.

O'Connor GR: Eye diseases. Pages 663–671 in: *Basic & Clinical Immunology,* 4th ed. Stites DP et al (editors). Lange, 1982.

Potts AM: The relation of immunology to the study of eye disease. Pages 335–338 in: *Year Book of Ophthalmology 1978.* Hughes WF (editor). Year Book, 1978.

Rahi AHS, Garner A: *Immunopathology of the Eye.* Blackwell, 1976.

Reed CE, Friedlaender R: Immunologic aspects of diseases of the eye. Chapter 12 in: Primer on allergic and immunologic diseases. Salvaggio JE (editor). *JAMA* 1982;**248**:2579. [Special issue.]

Sherman H, Feldman L, Walzer M: Studies in atopic hypersensitiveness of the ophthalmic mucous membranes. *J Allergy* 1933;**4**:437.

Silverstein AM, O'Connor GR (editors): *Immunology and Immunopathology of the Eye.* Masson, 1979.

Smolin G, O'Connor GR: *Ocular Immunology.* Lea & Febiger, 1981.

Theodore FH, Lewson AC: Bilateral iritis complicating serum sickness. *Arch Ophthalmol* 1939;**21**:828.

Theodore FH, Schlossman A: *Ocular Allergy.* Williams & Wilkins, 1958.

Witmer R: Phaco-antigenic uveitis. *Doc Ophthalmol* 1962;**16**:271.

Wong VG, Anderson RR, McMaster PRB: Endogenous immune uveitis. *Arch Ophthalmol* 1971;**85**:93.

The immediate examination of the newborn infant consists of a brief observation of color, responses, extremities, and digits, and a quick inspection of body surfaces. The more complete examination is done in the nursery.

Because the development of the eye often reflects organ and tissue development of the body as a whole, many congenital somatic defects are mirrored in the eye. A careful eye examination soon after birth may suggest the need for further investigative procedures. Subjective response is limited to the following response to a moving light. The only instruments required for the ocular examination of the newborn are a good hand light, an ophthalmoscope, and a loupe if necessary for magnification.

External Inspection

The eyelids are inspected for growths, deformities, lid notches, and symmetric movement with opening and closing of the eyes. The absolute and relative size of the eyeballs is noted, as well as position and alignment. The size and luster of the corneas are noted, and the anterior chambers are examined for clarity and iris configuration. The size, position, and light reaction of the pupils are also noted.

Ophthalmoscopic Examination

With undilated pupils, some information can be obtained by use of the ophthalmoscope in a dimly lighted room. Ideally, however, all newborns should be examined with an ophthalmoscope through dilated pupils. Ophthalmoscopic examination will demonstrate any corneal, lens, or vitreous opacities as well as abnormalities in the fundus. Neonatal retinal hemorrhages have been reported in 15% of newborns, usually clearing completely within a few weeks and leaving no permanent visual dysfunction.

THE NORMAL EYE IN INFANTS & CHILDREN

Eyeball

In the newborn, the eye is relatively larger in comparison with body size than in later life. However, the anteroposterior diameter, which determines the focusing of the eye, is relatively short (averaging about

---

Pediatric Eye Examination Schedule

Hospital Nursery

External eye examination and ophthalmoscopic examination through dilated pupils as outlined in the text. Two drops of sterile 5% homatropine and 2.5% phenylephrine in each eye are instilled 1 hour prior to examination. Special emphasis should be placed on the optic disks and maculas; detailed examination of the peripheral retinas is not necessary.

Age 4

Visual acuity test with illiterate "E" chart to rule out amblyopia. Visual acuity is normal (6/6 [20/20] to 6/9 [20/30]) by 4–5 years of age.

Age 5–16

Test visual acuity at age 5. If normal, test visual acuity with the Snellen chart every 2 years until age 16. Color vision should be tested at age 8–12. No other routine eye examination (eg, ophthalmoscopy) is necessary if visual acuity is normal and the eyes appear normal upon inspection.

17.3 mm). This would produce a marked hyperopia if it were not for the greater curvature of the lens at this time.

Cornea

The cornea of the newborn is also relatively large and reaches adult size by about 2 years of age. It is flatter than the adult cornea, however, and the curvature is greater at the periphery than in the center, whereas the opposite is true in the adult.

Lens

At birth the lens is more globular than in adulthood, and its greater refractive power compensates for the shortness of the eye. The lens grows throughout life as new fibers are added to the periphery, and this causes it to flatten. The consistency of the lens material changes throughout life from a soft plasticlike material to the glassy consistency seen in old age. This accounts for the gradual loss in power of accommodation with advancing age.

Refractive State

About 80% of children between the ages of 2 and 6 years are hyperopic, 5% myopic, and 15% emmetropic. About 10% have refractive errors that require correction before age 7 or 8. Hyperopia remains relatively static or gradually diminishes until 19 or 20 years of age. Myopia often develops between age 6–9 and increases throughout adolescence, with the greatest change at the time of puberty. Astigmatism is congenital and remains relatively constant throughout life. Transient refractive changes are well documented in the neonatal period.

Iris

At birth there is little or no pigment on the anterior surface of the iris. The posterior pigment layer shows through the translucent tissue, usually giving the effect of a bluish or slate-gray color. As the pigment begins to appear on the anterior surface, the iris assumes its definitive color. If considerable pigment is deposited, the eyes become brown. Less pigmentation results in blue, gray, hazel, or green eyes. It may take 1–2 years for the pigmentary deposits to occur; in the meantime it is impossible to ascertain the ultimate color of the eyes.

Pupil

In the newborn, the pupil is situated slightly to the nasal side of and below the center of the cornea. Because of the refractive power of the cornea in the neonatal period, the pupil appears larger than it actually is. The apparent diameter varies between 2.5 and 5.5 mm and averages about 4 mm. In infancy, the pupil is smaller than at birth. Congenital underdevelopment of the dilator muscle is common in children with congenital cataracts. The pupillary reflexes appear at about the fifth fetal month and are active by the sixth month. At about age 1 the pupil begins to widen, and it reaches its greatest diameter during adolescence. It again becomes smaller with advancing age. Myopes have larger pupils than hyperopes.

Normal pupils are round and regular and constantly move in response to changes in lighting and upon focusing. Anisocoria, a difference in the size of the 2 pupils, is often a normal finding; in the absence of neurologic abnormalities, it requires no further special diagnostic consideration.

Position

During the first month of life, eye movements may be poorly coordinated and there may be some doubt about the straightness of the eyes. By 3 months of age, however, the binocular reflexes are well developed; any deviation noted after that time should be investigated. Stereoacuity can be shown to develop in most infants beginning at 3 months of age.

Nasolacrimal System

The fetal development of the nasolacrimal passages begins as cords of cells that usually hollow out about the time of birth. Because there may normally be a few weeks' delay in duct formation, failure of tear production in the first few weeks does not necessarily indicate any difficulty; failure of the ducts to function by 6 months of age, however, needs attention.

Optic Nerve

By term, some fibers in the optic nerve near the globe begin to become myelinated, but the amount of myelin surrounding individual nerves increases dramatically during the ensuing months and may continue to increase up to the age of 2 years.

The Normal Ocular Fundus of Infants & Children

The ophthalmoscopic appearance of the normal fundus in an infant differs greatly from that of an adult. Most of the differences are due to the distribution of pigments.

In premature infants, remnants of the tunica vasculosa lentis are frequently visible with the ophthalmoscope, either in front of the lens, behind the lens, or in both positions. The remnants are usually absorbed by the time the infant has reached term, but rarely they remain permanently and appear as a complete or partial "cobweb" in the pupil. At other times remnants of the primitive hyaloid system fail to absorb completely, leaving a cone on the optic disk that projects into the vitreous and is called Bergmeister's papilla.

Physiologic cupping of the disk is usually not seen in premature infants and is rarely seen at term; if seen then, it is usually very slight. In such cases the optic disk will appear gray, resembling optic nerve atrophy. This relative pallor, however, gradually changes to the normal adult pink color at about 2 years of age.

The foveal light reflection is absent in infants. Instead, the macula has a bright "mother-of-pearl" appearance with a suggestion of elevation. This is more pronounced in black infants. At 3–4 months of age, the macula becomes slightly concave and the foveal light reflection appears.

The peripheral fundus in the infant is gray, in contrast to the orange-red fundus of the adult. In white infants the pigmentation is more pronounced near the posterior pole and gradually fades to almost white at the periphery. In black infants there is more pigment in the fundus and a gray-blue sheen is seen throughout the periphery. In white infants a white periphery is normal and should not be confused with retinoblastoma. During the next several months, pigment continues to be deposited in the retina, and usually at about 2 years of age the adult color is evident.

CONGENITAL EYE DEFECTS

Most congenital ocular defects are genetically determined. Examples include congenital ptosis, refractive errors, aniridia, strabismus, retinitis pigmentosa, and arachnodactyly (Marfan's syndrome). Absence of a positive family history is no proof that the defect is not in the germ plasm (see Chapter 21).

Other congenital defects may be caused by interference with the development of the embryo, such as the multiple defects associated with rubella infection of the mother during the first 3 months of pregnancy. In this instance the infant may suffer from any or all of the following: cataracts, heart disease, deafness, microcephaly, microphthalmos, and mental deficiency. Eye defects are common in cerebral palsy.

Anophthalmos

This is a rare condition in which one or both eyeballs are absent or rudimentary. There may be either a congenital absence of any ocular structure or an arrest of development to the point where only histologic evidence is present. The eyelids are usually present. They are often adherent at the margins but can be separated. Anophthalmos may be associated with a chromosomal variation and there may be associated intracranial anomalies.

Congenital Cystic Eye

This is a developmental abnormality resulting from complete or partial failure of invagination of the primary optic vesicle. The eye is variable in size and is usually associated with some degree of neuroglial proliferation. The malformation occurs at about the fourth week of embryonic life.

Cyclopia

Cyclopia, which is a rare midline fusion of developing eye structures together with generalized anterior brain and skull defects, is usually not compatible with life since it is transmitted by a recessive lethal gene.

Palpebral Colobomas

A unilateral cleft of one upper lid is the most common type of palpebral coloboma. Bilateral clefts or fissures can occur in lower as well as upper lids and may be associated with other malformations of the face or globe. No specific embryonic maldevelopment has been established as being causative.

Microphthalmos

In microphthalmos, one or both eyes are markedly smaller than normal. Many other ocular abnormalities may be present also, eg, cataract, glaucoma, aniridia, and coloboma. Somatic abnormalities are also often present, eg, polydactyly, syndactyly, clubfoot, polycystic kidneys, cystic liver, cleft palate, and meningoencephalocele. Microphthalmos is nearly always genetically determined—most frequently as a recessive but occasionally as a dominant trait.

Corneal Defects

There may be partial or complete opacity of the corneas such as is found in congenital glaucoma, faulty development of the cornea with persistent corneal-lens attachments, birth injuries, intrauterine inflammation, interstitial keratitis, and mucopolysaccharide depositions of the cornea as in Hurler's syndrome. The most frequent cause of opaque corneas in infants and young children is congenital glaucoma. In most instances, the eye is larger than normal (macrophthalmos, hydrophthalmos, buphthalmos). Birth injuries may cause extensive corneal opacities with edema as a result of rupture of Descemet's membrane. These usually clear spontaneously.

Megalocornea is an enlarged cornea with normal function usually transmitted as an X-linked recessive trait. It must be differentiated from infantile glaucoma. There are usually no associated defects.

Iris & Pupillary Defects

Misplaced or ectopic pupils are frequently observed. The usual displacement is upward and laterally (temporally) from the center of the cornea. Such displacement is occasionally associated with ectopic lens, congenital glaucoma, or microcornea. Multiple pupils are known as **polycoria.** A true pupil must constrict on exposure to light, indicating a sphincter muscle. Congenital miosis is due to a poorly developed dilator muscle. Little change in pupillary size is noted after instillation of a mydriatic. Congenital mydriasis is characterized by large and inactive pupils and underdeveloped sphincter muscles, and must be differentiated from mydriasis due to juvenile paresis and pineal tumor. **Coloboma of the iris** indicates incomplete closure of the fetal ocular cleft and usually occurs below and nasally. It may be associated with coloboma of the lens, choroid, and optic nerve. **Aniridia** (absence of the iris) is a rare abnormality, frequently associated with secondary glaucoma (see p 169) and due to an autosomal dominant hereditary pattern. Various abnormalities in the shape of the pupils have been described but are not necessarily significant. Persistent mesodermal remnants usually appear as threadlike bands running across the central pupillary space and attached to the lesser circle of the iris. They rarely have clinical significance or interfere with visual acuity.

The color of the iris is determined largely by heredity. Abnormalities in color include **albinism** (see p 264), due to the absence of normal pigmentation of the ocular structures and frequently associated with poor visual acuity and nystagmus; and **heterochromia,** which is a difference in color in the 2 eyes that may be a primary developmental defect with no functional loss or may be secondary to an inflammatory process.

Lens Abnormalities

The lens abnormalities most frequently noted are cataracts, although there may be faulty development, forming colobomas, or subluxation, as seen in Marfan's syndrome.

Any lens opacity that is present at birth is a congenital cataract, regardless of whether or not it interferes with visual acuity. Congenital cataracts are often associated with other conditions. Maternal rubella during the first trimester of pregnancy is a common cause of congenital cataract. Other congenital cataracts have a hereditary background.

If the opacity is small enough so that it does not occlude the pupil, adequate visual acuity is attained by focusing around the opacity. If the pupillary opening is entirely occluded, however, normal sight does not develop, and the poor fixation may lead to nystagmus and amblyopia. Good visual results have been reported with both monocular and binocular cataracts receiving early surgery and aphakic correction.

Choroid & Retina

Gross defects of the choroid and retina are visible with the ophthalmoscope. The choroidal structures may show congenital colobomas, usually in the lower nasal region, which may also include the iris and all or part of the optic nerve. Posterior polar chorioretinal scarring is a pigmentary disturbance often caused by intrauterine toxoplasmosis. Other congenital lesions of the choroid and retina include drusen, aneurysms, optic nerve malformations, medullated nerve fibers, and hereditary macular degeneration.

DEVELOPMENTAL BODY DEFECTS ASSOCIATED WITH OCULAR DEFECTS

Albinism

Congenital deficiency of pigment may involve the entire body (complete albinism) or a part of the body (incomplete albinism). When incomplete albinism involves only the eye, function may be normal or impaired. In complete ocular albinism, there is usually an abnormal development of the macula, a significant refractive error, nystagmus, and severe photophobia. The eyebrows and eyelashes are white, the conjunctiva is hyperemic, the irides are gray or red, and the pupil appears red. Treatment consists of relieving photophobia with tinted glasses or opaque contact lenses with a clear central area 2–3 mm in diameter.

Marfan's Syndrome

A congenital disorder of mesodermal origin that is nearly always transmitted as an autosomal dominant trait; the major features are (1) long, thin fingers and toes (arachnodactyly), (2) generalized relaxation of ligaments, (3) generalized muscular underdevelopment, (4) bilateral dislocation of the lenses (ectopia lentis), (5) abnormalities of the heart and, occasionally, aortic aneurysm, (6) high-arched palate, and (7) other deformities of the sternum, thorax, and joints.

The lenses are usually dislocated and visual acuity suffers because the patient is not seeing through the lens centers. Cataracts frequently develop in the subluxated lenses. Cataract surgery may become necessary but has a less favorable prognosis than routine cataract surgery.

Osteogenesis Imperfecta

This rare affliction is characterized by increased fragility of the bones and laxity of the ligaments, with frequent fractures and dislocations; dental defects, deafness, and blue scleras. The blue color is darker in the anterior parts of the scleras over the ciliary bodies. It is thought to be due to abnormal thinness of the sclera and remains unchanged throughout life. Cataracts, megalocornea, and keratoconus may also be present. It nearly always occurs as an autosomal dominant trait.

Gargoylism or Hurler's Syndrome

This is a rare condition due to autosomal recessive inheritance in which there is infiltration of mucopolysaccharides into the tissues, especially the liver, spleen, lymph nodes, pituitary gland, and corneas. Other ocular signs include slight ptosis, larger thickened eyelids, and strabismus (esotropia). The corneas show a diffuse haziness, which progresses to a milk-white opacity. Glaucoma may eventually develop. There is no satisfactory treatment.

Oxycephaly
(Acrocephaly, Tower Skull, Steeple Head)

This deformity is evident at birth but is often attributed to normal distortion during delivery and is seldom diagnosed at the time of delivery. It is characterized by a high, dome-shaped or pointed skull, high forehead, bulging temporal fossae, flattened cheekbones, shallow orbits, a high, narrow palatal arch, and synostosis of the cranial suture. Syndactyly may also be present. The ocular signs include exophthalmos (due to flatness of the orbits), wide separation of the eyes, and exotropia. Closure of the eyelids may be difficult or impossible. Loss of vision may follow increased intracranial pressure. Nystagmus is common. Various operative procedures have been devised for the relief of intracranial pressure. If vision is to be preserved, surgery must be performed before optic atrophy has progressed. The syndrome is due to an autosomal dominant gene of weak penetrance.

Acrobrachycephaly

In this abnormality the head is wide, whereas in oxycephaly it is narrow. Acrobrachycephaly is caused by premature closure of the coronal sutures. Growth occurs only laterally and vertically, and the anteroposterior diameter is short. The ocular signs are similar to those of oxycephaly.

Other abnormalities involving the development of the skull are scaphocephaly (increased anteroposterior diameter due to premature closure of the sagittal suture) and plagiocephaly (asymmetric flattening, usually due to premature closure of a single coronal suture).

Craniofacial Dysostosis (Crouzon's Disease)

This rare hereditary deformity, due to an autosomal dominant gene, is characterized by exophthalmos, atrophy of the maxilla, enlargement of the nasal bones, abnormal increase in the space between the eyes (ocular hypertelorism), optic atrophy, and bony abnormalities of the region of the perilongitudinal sinus. The palpebral fissures slant downward (in contrast to the upward slant of Down's syndrome). Strabismus and nystagmus are also present. The strabismus is secondary to both structural anomalies of the muscles and orbital angle anomalies.

Laurence-Moon-Biedl Syndrome

This syndrome includes retinitis pigmentosa, polydactyly, obesity, hypogenitalism, and mental retardation. It is inherited as an autosomal recessive.

POSTNATAL PROBLEMS

The most common ocular disorders of children are external infections of the conjunctiva and eyelids (bacterial conjunctivitis, sties, blepharitis), strabismus, ocular foreign bodies, allergic reactions of the conjunctiva and eyelids, refractive errors (particularly myopia), and congenital defects. Since it is more difficult to elicit an accurate history of causative factors and subjective complaints in children, it is not uncommon to overlook significant ocular disorders (especially in very young children). Aside from the altered frequency of occurrence of the types of ocular disorders, the causes, manifestations, and treatment of eye disorders are about the same for children as for adults. Certain special problems encountered more frequently in infants and children are discussed below.

Ophthalmia Neonatorum
(Conjunctivitis of the Newborn)

Conjunctivitis in the newborn may be of chemical, bacterial (including chlamydial), or viral origin. Differentiation is usually made according to age at onset and by appropriate smears and cultures. Chemical conjunctivitis caused by the silver nitrate drops instilled into the conjunctival sac at birth is the most common form. Inflammation is greatest during the first or second day of life. Bacterial conjunctivitis is usually of staphylococcal, pneumococcal, *Pseudomonas*, or gonococcal origin, the latter being the most serious because of potential corneal damage. The onset of bacterial conjunctivitis is between the second and fifth days of life; the diagnosis is confirmed by bacteriologic smear and culture. Inclusion blennorrhea has its onset between the fifth and tenth days. The presence of typical inclusion bodies in the epithelial cells confirms this diagnosis.

Silver nitrate conjunctivitis is usually self-limited. Bacterial conjunctivitis requires instillation of antibacterial agents such as sodium sulfacetamide, bacitracin, or tetracycline ointment for several days. Treatment should be instituted without waiting for the results of the culture. Inclusion conjunctivitis is treated with sulfonamide or tetracycline ointments.

Silver nitrate solution (1%) should be used in sealed, single-use, disposable containers. Some institutions advocate the use of antibiotic ophthalmic preparations in place of silver nitrate. Prenatal diagnosis and treatment of maternal gonorrhea will prevent many cases of neonatal gonococcal conjunctivitis; however, prophylactic medication of the newborn must not be neglected. Prevention of inclusion conjunctivitis is difficult, since it is carried in the mother's genitourinary tract. Instillation of silver nitrate or an antibiotic (usually penicillin) is required by law in most states.

Retrolental Fibroplasia

This condition, relatively common in the 1940s and 1950s, is described on p 144. With the recognition of its causative factor—excessively high oxygen therapy to premature babies in incubators—retrolental fibroplasia is seen with increasing frequency as a result of the greater survival of neonates weighing less than 1200 g at birth.

Congenital Glaucoma

Congenital glaucoma (see Chapter 14) may occur alone or in association with many other congenital lesions. Early recognition is essential to prevent permanent blindness. Involvement is often bilateral. The most striking symptom is extreme photophobia. Early signs are corneal haze or opacity, increased corneal diameter, and increased intraocular pressure. Since the outer coats of the eyeball are not as rigid in the child, the increased intraocular pressure expands the corneal and scleral tissues. Useful vision may be preserved by early diagnosis and medical and surgical treatment by an ophthalmologist.

Leukocoria (White Pupil)

Parents will occasionally see a white spot through the infant's pupil (leukocoria). Although retinoblastoma must be ruled out, the opacity is more often due to cataract, retrolental fibroplasia, persistence of the tunica vasculosa lentis, or corneal scarring.

Retinoblastoma

This rare malignant tumor of childhood is fatal if untreated. Two-thirds of cases occur before the end of the third year; rarely, cases have been reported in later childhood, adolescence, and even (very rarely) in adults. In about 30% of cases, retinoblastoma is bilateral. The tumor results from mutation of an autosomal dominant gene that is passed with high penetrance. Children of survivors therefore have a nearly 50% chance of having retinoblastoma. It is more apt to be bilateral in succeeding generations. Parents who have produced one child with retinoblastoma run a 4–7% risk of producing the disease in each subsequently born child. Retinoblastoma is usually not discovered until it has advanced far enough to produce an opaque pupil. Infants and children with presenting symptoms of strabismus should be examined carefully to rule out retinoblastoma, since a deviating eye may be the first sign of the tumor.

Enucleation is the treatment of choice in nearly all unilateral cases of retinoblastoma. Additional discussion, including other possible methods for treatment, is presented on p 298.

Juvenile Xanthogranuloma

This uncommon entity is most often diagnosed by spontaneous unilateral hyphema. The fellow eye is normal. Diffuse thickening and nodulation of the iris may be seen on slit lamp examination. The iris lesion is occasionally localized enough to be excised. Associated skin lesions or nevoxanthoendotheliomas are frequent. The small, elevated, yellowish nodules appear in the skin of infants and characteristically regress spontaneously. The ocular and dermal lesions are not neoplastic and microscopically are composed of multinucleated giant cells and eosinophils. Large, thin-walled capillaries frequently run through the lesions. They are easily ruptured, causing hyphema and possible secondary glaucoma.

Strabismus

Strabismus is present in about 2% of children. Its early recognition is often the responsibility of the pediatrician or the family physician. Occasionally, childhood strabismus has neurologic significance. Treatment of strabismus is best started at the age of 6 months to ensure development of the best possible visual acuity and a good cosmetic and functional result (binocular vision). The idea that a child may outgrow crossed eyes should be discouraged. Neglect in the treatment of strabismus may lead to undesirable cosmetic effects, psychic trauma, and permanent impairment of vision (see below) in the deviating eye. Strabismus is covered in depth in Chapter 15.

Amblyopia

Amblyopia is decreased visual acuity of one eye (uncorrectable with lenses) in the absence of organic eye disease. The most common causes are strabismus and anisometropia.

In strabismus, the image from the deviated eye is suppressed (which prevents diplopia). If treatment is not instituted before cessation of the visual maturing process (ie, before age 5 or 6), good vision cannot develop in the deviating eye. A similar situation exists when there is a great difference in refractive power of the 2 eyes (anisometropia). Even though the eyes may be correctly aligned, they are unable to focus together and the image of one eye is suppressed. If corrective measures are not instituted before age 5 or 6, amblyopia will result.

Early suspicion and prompt referral for treatment of the underlying condition are important in preventing amblyopia.

•   •   •

TESTS FOR VISUAL ACUITY

In the early years, visual acuity should be appraised as part of each general "well child" examination. It is best not to wait until the child is old enough to respond to visual charts, since these may not furnish accurate information until school age. Estimations of vision should be made in the first few days by ascertaining the pupillary responses to light, which rules out complete dysfunction of the eyes. In later weeks, light fixation reflexes can be elicited—single and bilateral reflexes first, and then binocular following and converging reflexes. A good response consists of prompt fixation and following reflexes, equal in each eye, with the light reflex centered in the pupil when the source is near the examiner's eyes. Although these indirect inferences about the status of the developing sensory systems are useful, newer techniques are both quantitative and qualitative in nature. Data beginning to accumulate with the use of at least 3 different techniques now suggest that visual acuity can be assessed. These techniques are optokinetic nystagmus, forced choice preferential looking, and visually evoked potentials.

During the growing years, the parents' observations of the child's clumsiness, awareness of surroundings, and apparent sharpness of vision are valuable aids. From about age 4 on, it becomes possible to elicit subjective responses by use of the illiterate "E" chart. Usually, at the first or second grade level, the regular Snellen chart may be employed.

The number of cases of amblyopia due to strabismus or anisometropia can be greatly decreased by the alert pediatrician or general physician who tests visual acuity at age 4. The parent's help can be solicited. The parent can be given an "E" card and asked to do the test at home and phone or mail the results to the doctor's office. The test will often be more accurate than when given by a nurse or physician because the parent has more time and has a paramount interest in the child's health.

Table 20–1. Development of visual acuity (approximate).

Age	Visual Acuity	
2 months	6/120	(20/400)
6 months	6/60	(20/200)
1 year	6/30	(20/100)
2 years	6/18	(20/60)
3 years	6/9	(20/30)
4–5 years	6/6	(20/20)

•   •   •

References

Banks MS: Infant refraction and accommodation. *Int Ophthalmol Clin* 1980;**20**:205.

Beller R: Good visual function after neonatal surgery for congenital monocular cataracts. *Am J Ophthalmol* 1981;**91**:559.

Cameron JH, Cameron M: Visual screening of pre-school children. *Br Med J* 1978;**2**:1693.

Dobson J, Teller DY: Visual acuity in human infants: A review of behavioral and electrophysiological studies. *Vision Res* 1978;**18**:1469.

Harley RD (editor): *Pediatric Ophthalmology.* Saunders, 1975.

Helveston EM: Strabismus: Annual review. *Arch Ophthalmol* 1975;**93**:1205.

Hoyt CS, Nickel BL, Billson FA: Ophthalmological examination of the infant. *Surv Ophthalmol* 1982;**26**:177.

Kalina RE: Examination of the premature infant. *Ophthalmology* 1980;**86**:1689.

Mohindra I et al: Astigmatism in infants. *Science* 1978;**202**:329.

Reinecke RD, Feman SS: *Handbook of Pediatric Ophthalmology.* Grune & Stratton, 1978.

Rice NSC: Congenital cataract: A cause of preventable blindness in children. *Br Med J* 1982;**285**:581.

Taylor D: The assessment of visual function in young children: An overview. *Clin Pediatr* 1978;**17**:226.

21 | Genetic Aspects

As genetic factors are proved responsible for more and more diseases, it becomes increasingly important to understand the principles of genetic transmission. Much of the background work in clinical medical genetics has been done in ophthalmology, since the eye seems unusually prone to genetically determined disease. Mainly because the cornea is a convenient window through which the inner eye can be observed, accurate diagnosis of ocular disease is the rule.

Clinicians can estimate the risk of occurrence of many genetically determined diseases (usually the rare but severe ones), but the familial incidence of many other diseases also known to be genetically determined still cannot be accurately predicted.

It is now possible to study the structure of individual chromosomes in some detail. It has been definitely established that there are 23 pairs of chromosomes in the nucleus of the normal human somatic cell. Twenty-two of these pairs are somewhat similar and therefore have been termed **autosomal.** Each pair is made up of 2 identical chromosomes. The twenty-third pair is composed of the sex chromosomes. Special staining methods have allowed classification of the chromosomes. Cytogenetic studies have shown abnormal chromosomal numbers in several syndromes such as Turner's syndrome and Down's syndrome that include ocular anomalies.

Newer techniques in the study of human chromosomes have recently been described. A number of agents (quinacrine mustard, trypsin, Giemsa's stain) have produced morphologic banding of the human chromosome that permits identification of each specific chromosome. These techniques have greatly contributed to the study of cytogenetics and are of great help in the investigation of chromosomal abnormalities.

The gametes (spermatozoon and ovum) are produced by a special type of cell division called reduction-division meiosis in which the 23 pairs of chromosomes dissociate; each chromosome of a pair separates and passes intact to a daughter cell to give it 23 unpaired chromosomes. At fertilization, each chromosome of the spermatozoon joins its corresponding chromosome of the ovum to produce a cell with 46 chromosomes. All cell divisions after fertilization (mitosis) involve duplication and separation of all the chromosomes to produce cells with the constant number of 46 chromosomes.

Each chromosome is composed of many small units termed **genes.** Genes are arranged in pairs and determine bodily characteristics. Paired genes are either similar (homozygous) or dissimilar (heterozygous). If dissimilar, one determines the bodily characteristic and is termed **dominant** while the other gene is unexpressed and is termed **recessive.** At fertilization the reassortment of chromosomes is purely by chance, so that either chromosome of a pair from one parent has an equal chance to combine with either chromosome of the same pair from the other parent. Normal characteristics are inherited in the same way as genetically determined disease, which is discussed under the headings of autosomal dominant, autosomal recessive, and X-linked (sex-linked) recessive inheritance.

AUTOSOMAL DOMINANT INHERITANCE

An abnormal dominant gene produces its specific abnormality even though its paired gene (allele) is

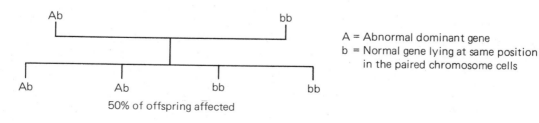

A = Abnormal dominant gene
b = Normal gene lying at same position in the paired chromosome cells

50% of offspring affected

Figure 21–1. Autosomal dominant inheritance.

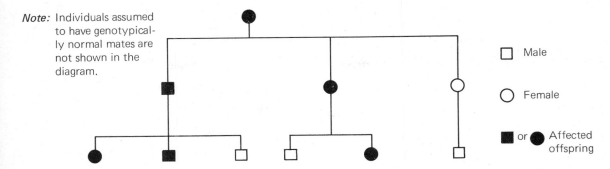

Note: Individuals assumed to have genotypically normal mates are not shown in the diagram.

☐ Male

○ Female

■ or ● Affected offspring

Figure 21–2. Pedigree of congenital stationary night blindness (abnormal dominant gene).

normal. Males and females are affected alike and have a theoretical 50% chance of passing along the affected gene (and therefore the abnormality) to each of their offspring, even when mated to genotypically normal individuals (Fig 21–1).

Given a particular group of pedigrees, autosomal dominant inheritance is established if the following conditions are met: (1) Males and females are equally affected. (2) Direct transmission has occurred over 2 or more generations. (3) About 50% of individuals in the pedigrees are affected.

Quite a large number of uncommon but serious diseases with ocular manifestations are transmitted in this way: forms of juvenile glaucoma, Marfan's syndrome, congenital stationary night blindness (Fig 21–2), osteogenesis imperfecta, and all the phakomatoses, which include neurofibromatosis, Lindau-Von Hippel disease, tuberous sclerosis, and Sturge-Weber syndrome. The process of natural selection tends to keep most of these serious diseases at a low incidence in the general population, since many of these people are unable to produce children even if they do manage to live to the age of reproduction.

Dominant disease may be more or less severe from generation to generation depending upon its **expression;** a disease with "variable expression" is one that can occur in a mild or severe form. An example is neurofibromatosis, in which genotypically affected individuals may have merely café au lait spots or may have many serious manifestations. One cannot predict if or when the disease will be more serious (with central nervous system tumors or optic nerve gliomas)

in a succeeding generation. If the genetic pattern is present but there is no evidence of the disease, one says that its **penetrance** is reduced. It may be quite difficult to differentiate dominant inheritance with reduced penetrance from recessive inheritance (see below). To quote Duke-Elder, "It may well be said that dominance and recessiveness are not two distinct antitheses but represent the two extremes of a continuous series of variable types of hereditary transmission, all of which are fundamentally the same." Those pedigrees which demonstrate neither a definite autosomal dominant nor a definite recessive pattern are properly classified as irregular dominants (dominant inheritance with variable expression) or incomplete recessives (carrier state identifiable clinically).

AUTOSOMAL RECESSIVE INHERITANCE

Abnormal recessive genes must lie in pairs (duplex state) to produce manifest abnormality. Thus, each parent must contribute one recessive abnormal gene. Each parent is clinically unaffected (genotypically affected but phenotypically normal), since a normal dominant gene makes the abnormal gene recessive (Fig 21–3).

It is difficult to establish that a given disease results from autosomal recessive inheritance. Some of the criteria used to establish recessive inheritance are the following:

(1) Occurrence of the same disease in collateral branches of the family.

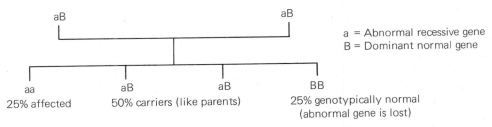

aB   aB

a = Abnormal recessive gene
B = Dominant normal gene

aa
25% affected

aB   aB
50% carriers (like parents)

BB
25% genotypically normal
(abnormal gene is lost)

Figure 21–3. Mating of 2 carriers.

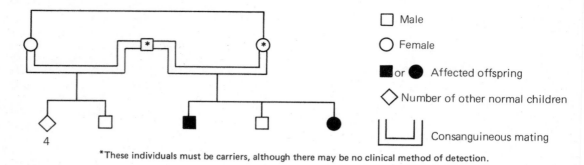

*These individuals must be carriers, although there may be no clinical method of detection.

Figure 21–4. Pedigree of oculocutaneous albinism. In this case a man married successively 2 sisters, his first cousins.

(2) History of consanguinity. The higher the rate of consanguinity in the pedigrees of a given disease, the more likely the disease is to be recessive and the rarer the occurrence of the disease in the general population. Consanguinity creates greater opportunities for the genes to lie in the duplex state, inasmuch as an individual with 2 related parents can receive the same affected gene from each, a common ancestor having originally passed on the affected gene.

(3) The occurrence of the disease in about 25% of siblings. This only holds for groups of pedigrees. There is a 25% chance that the 2 abnormal genes will be passed on to one individual. There is a 50% chance that a normal gene will modify the affected gene. In this case, the individual is a carrier of the disease (just like the parents) but is not affected with the disease (ie, genotypically affected but phenotypically normal). In the remaining 25% of siblings, 2 normal genes lie together and the abnormal gene is completely lost (ie, the individual is genotypically normal). Although a number of pedigrees are required to definitely establish recessive inheritance, even a single pedigree is suggestive if more than one sibling is similarly affected without antecedent history.

Many disease processes have been definitely established as resulting from autosomal recessive inheritance, and many others are suspected of having such a

genetic background. Included among the definite cases are Laurence-Moon-Biedl syndrome and inborn errors of metabolism such as oculocutaneous albinism (Fig 21–4), galactokinase deficiency, and Tay-Sachs disease.

X-LINKED (SEX-LINKED) RECESSIVE INHERITANCE

The sex chromosomes are one of the 23 pairs of human chromosomes. Identical chromosomes appear in females; these have been labeled with X chromosomes. One such chromosome appears with a dissimilar mate in the male; this smaller chromosome has been labeled the Y chromosome. Therefore, XX is female and XY is male.

The criteria for X-linked inheritance are (1) that only males are affected, (2) that the disease is transmitted through carrier females to half of the sons, and (3) that there is no father-to-son transmission.

Many of the genes of the X chromosome are unopposed by a gene of the Y chromosome. Abnormalities of these genes cause disease in the male, whereas in the female an abnormal recessive gene of the sex chromosome is masked by its normal allele. Therefore, nearly all of the X-linked diseases are man-

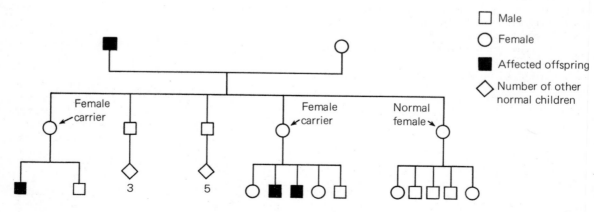

Figure 21–5. Pedigree of red-green color blindness.

ifested in males, whereas the disease is passed through the female. A male and his maternal grandfather are affected, and the intervening female is the carrier.

Among the important eye diseases with an X-linked genetic pattern are color blindness (Fig 21–5), ocular albinism, and one type of retinitis pigmentosa.

Females have a mosaic of somatic cells consisting of cell groups with one X chromosome functioning and cell groups with the other X chromosome functioning (Lyon hypothesis). When the female is a carrier of an X-linked disease, this mosaicism is occasionally detectable. Such is the case in female carriers of ocular albinism, in whom groups of pigmented and albino retinal pigment epithelial cells are visible ophthalmoscopically.

CYTOGENETIC ABNORMALITIES

When mitosis is interrupted in metaphase, the chromosomes can be spread on a slide, counted, and photographed. These cytogenetic studies have made possible the classification of chromosomes into 7 groups based upon characteristics such as size and the position of the centromere. The groups contain as few as 2 or as many as 7 chromosomes, with the chromosomes of any group being indistinguishable from each other. The study of cytogenetics has also established that some clinical states can be correlated with an abnormal number of chromosomes, most frequently one more (trisomy) or occasionally one less (monosomy) than the normal number of 46. A few of the more common syndromes are summarized briefly below. Since the addition or subtraction of an entire gene is obviously a major genetic abnormality, these syndromes are characterized by many and extensive deformities. Many such abnormal fertilizations result in early abortions and stillbirths.

SYNDROMES ASSOCIATED WITH AN ABNORMAL NUMBER OF CHROMOSOMES

Trisomy 13 (Patau's Syndrome)

Anophthalmos, microphthalmos, retinal dysplasia, optic atrophy, coloboma of the uvea, and cataracts are the major eye anomalies; cerebral defects, cleft palate, heart lesions, polydactyly, and hemangiomas are the more severe nonophthalmic changes. Cytogenetically, there is an extra chromosome indistinguishable from group 13–15. Death by age 6 months is the rule.

Trisomy 18 (Edward's Syndrome)

The main features of this rare syndrome are mental and physical retardation, congenital heart defects, and renal abnormalities. Corneal and lenticular opacities, unilateral ptosis, and optic atrophy have been described.

Trisomy 21 (Down's Syndrome)

Although Down's syndrome is a fairly common and well-known entity, the hereditary pattern was long ill-defined. Waardenburg originally suggested that Down's syndrome was a chromosomal problem in 1932. Cytogenetic studies in 1958 revealed an extra chromosome indistinguishable from chromosome 21. The principal manifestations are small stature, a flattened, round, mongoloid facies, saddle nose, thick lower lip, large tongue, soft, seborrheic skin, smooth hair, obesity, small genitalia, short fingers, a simian fold, congenital heart anomalies, mental retardation, and frequent psychic disturbances. The ocular signs include hyperplasia of the iris, narrow palpebral fissures with Oriental slant, frequent strabismus, epicanthus, frequent cataract, high myopia (33%), and Brushfield (silver-gray) spots on the iris.

The incidence of Down's syndrome is significantly increased in children born to older women, particularly those past age 35.

ABNORMALITIES INVOLVING SEX CHROMOSOMES

Turner's syndrome is a monosomy (45 chromosomes). For some reason, the affected female receives only one X chromosome. Clinically, growth retardation, rudimentary ovaries and female genitalia, amenorrhea, pterygium colli, epicanthus, cubitus valgus, and ptosis occur. Of particular ophthalmic interest is the high incidence of color blindness (8%). This is the same frequency as for males (female incidence, 0.4%) and is readily explained by the fact that the normally recessive gene is unopposed and is expressed just as in the male.

Klinefelter's syndrome is a trisomy involving the X chromosomes. These phenotypical males have 47 chromosomes: the normal 44 autosomes and 3 sex chromosomes, XXY. These individuals are sterile, with small testes, have a eunuchoid physique, and frequently gynecomastia. The ocular finding of interest is the very rare occurrence of color blindness, since the recessive X chromosome is masked by a normal dominant (as in the normal female).

OTHER GENETIC CONSIDERATIONS

Genetic Counseling

Valuable advice can often be given to families concerned with the possibilities of transmitting serious disease to future generations. This entails a working knowledge of basic genetic principles and sensitive counseling skills. A careful history of the pedigree in question is very important, as a single disease may have more than one mode of transmission (eg, retinitis pigmentosa has 3 or more basic patterns). On the other hand, careful inquiries about maternal health during pregnancy may suggest that the anomaly is developmental and therefore unrelated to the genes. The recognition of the genetic carrier state may enable the physician to give intelligent advice.

Consanguineous mating increases the risk of birth defects, since it is estimated that the average individual carries several undesirable recessive genes.

In some cases it is possible to offer families at risk for a specific hereditary disease the option of prenatal diagnosis. Prenatal diagnosis by testing amniotic fluid cells obtained by amniocentesis at 14–16 gestational weeks has become a safe and practical procedure. The list of hereditary diseases that can be diagnosed with this method is rapidly increasing.

Genetic Carrier State

Recognition of the genetic carrier state is most important. Detection is possible in many diseases. There are 3 types:

(1) Autosomal dominant diseases in which the disease appears in a mild or subclinical form (low expression). Because the offspring of such individuals still have the theoretical 50% chance of passing on the disease process, the recognition of this carrier state is important in genetic counseling.

(2) Autosomal recessive diseases with heterozygous manifestations. Affected genes that are normally balanced by a normal allele may cause minor subclinical abnormalities which disclose the presence of the abnormal gene. One can predict the 25% possibility of occurrence of some autosomal recessive diseases if the carrier state can be recognized in both potential mates.

(3) Female carrier in X-linked recessive disease. Subclinical evidence of the disease in daughters of affected fathers differentiates carriers from noncarriers in a number of X-linked recessive diseases (often quite obvious in tapetoretinal degenerative conditions).

Mutation

Mutation occurs when a gene undergoes alteration in the germ cell as a result of spontaneous chemical change within the gene and the change is manifested by a new characteristic. The causes of the change are now well understood, but such extrinsic environmental factors as heat, x-rays, and exposure to radioactive materials may induce it. Most often the new characteristic is unfavorable (ie, disease-producing), but some mutations are favorable and account for the evolution of species (Darwin).

Certain mutations occur repeatedly in specific genes and cause specific disease. Hemophilia, which follows an X-linked pattern, and retinoblastoma, which follows an autosomal dominant pattern, are examples of disease occurring as a result of mutation. Very few individuals with severe abnormalities reproduce, so that the incidence of such diseases is dependent almost entirely upon mutation. Mutations causing less severe diseases are inherited as dominant, recessive, or X-linked traits depending upon the type of mutated gene.

GLOSSARY OF GENETIC TERMS*

Abiotrophic disease: Genetically determined disease which is not evident at birth but which becomes manifest later in life.

Acquired: Not hereditary; contracted after birth or in utero.

Alleles: See Allelic genes, below.

Allelic genes: Paired genes or partner genes; genes occupying the same locus on homologous (paired) chromosomes and which, therefore, normally segregate from each other during the reduction-division of mitosis.

Autosomes: The chromosomes (22 pairs of autosomes in humans) other than the sex chromosomes.

Chromosome: A small threadlike or rodlike structure into which the nuclear chromatin separates during mitosis. The number of chromosomes is constant for any given species (23 pairs in humans: 22 pairs of autosomes and one pair of sex chromosomes).

Congenital: Existing at or before birth; not necessarily hereditary.

Dominant: Designating a gene whose phenotypic effect largely or entirely obscures that of its allele.

Familial: Pertaining to traits, either hereditary or acquired, which tend to occur in families.

Gamete (germ cell): A cell that is capable of uniting with another cell in sexual reproduction (ie, the ovum and spermatozoon).

Gene: A unit of heredity which occupies a specific locus in the chromosome which, either alone or in combination, produces a single characteristic. It is usually a single unit that is capable of self-duplication or mutation.

Genetic carrier state: A condition wherein a given hereditary characteristic is not manifest in one individual but may be genetically transmitted to the offspring of that individual.

Genotype: The hereditary constitution, or combination of genes, that characterizes a given individual or a group of genetically identical organisms.

Germ cells (gametes): Cells capable of uniting with other cells sexually in reproducing the organism; spermatozoa in the male and ova in the female.

Hereditary: Transmitted from ancestor to offspring through the germ plasm.

Heterozygous: Having 2 members of a given hereditary factor pair that are dissimilar, ie, the 2 genes of an allelic pair are not the same.

Homozygous: Having 2 members of a given hereditary factor pair that are similar, ie, the 2 genes of an allelic pair are identical.

Meiosis: A special type of cell division occurring during the maturation of sex cells, by which the normal diploid set of chromosomes is reduced to a

*Modified from Krupp MA et al: *Physician's Handbook*, 20th ed. Lange, 1982.

single (haploid) set, 2 successive nuclear divisions occurring, while the chromosomes divide only once.

Mutation: A transformation of a gene, often sudden and dramatic, with or without known cause, into a different gene occupying the same locus as the original gene on a particular chromosome; the new gene is allelic to the normal gene from which it has arisen.

Penetrance: The likelihood or probability that a gene will become morphologically (phenotypically) expressed. The degree of penetrance may depend upon acquired as well as genetic factors.

Phenotype: The visible characteristics of an individual or those which are common to a group of apparently identical individuals.

Recessive: Designating a gene whose phenotypic effect is largely or entirely obscured by the effect of its allele.

Sex chromosome: The chromosome or pair of chromosomes that determines the sex of the individual. (In the human female, the sex chromosome pair is homologous, XX; in the male, nonhomologous, XY.)

Sex linkage: See X linkage, below.

Somatic cells: Cells incapable of reproducing the organism.

Trisomy: The existence of 3 chromosomes of one variety, rather than the normal pair of chromosomes.

X linkage: The pattern of inheritance of genes located on the X chromosome.

Zygote: The cell formed by the union of 2 gametes in sexual reproduction.

● ● ●

References

Aherne GES, Roberts DF: Retinoblastoma: A clinical survey and its genetic implications. *Clin Genet* 1975;**8**:275.

Cotlier E et al: Aniridia, cataracts, and Wilms' tumor. *Am J Ophthamol* 1978;**86**:129.

Deutman AF: Genetically determined retinal and choroidal disease. *Trans Ophthalmol Soc UK* 1974;**94**:1014.

Duke-Elder S: *System of Ophthalmology.* Vol 7. Mosby, 1962.

François J: "Counseling" in ophthalmology. *Ann Ophthalmol* 1976;**8**:265.

François J: *Heredity in Ophthalmology.* Mosby, 1961.

Goldberg MF (editor): *Genetic and Metabolic Eye Disease.* Little, Brown, 1974.

Keith CG: *Genetics and Ophthalmology.* Churchill Livingstone, 1978.

Krupp MA et al: *Physician's Handbook,* 20th ed. Lange, 1982.

McKusick VA: *Human Genetics,* 2nd ed. Prentice-Hall, 1969.

Miller M: Fetal alcohol syndrome. *J Pediatr Ophthalmol Strabismus* 1981;**18**:5.

Newell F: *Hereditary Disorders of the Eye and Ocular Adnexa.* Ophthalmic Publishers, 1981.

Stanbury JB, Wyngaarden JB, Fredrickson DS: *The Metabolic Basis of Inherited Disease,* 4th ed. McGraw-Hill, 1978.

Waardenburg PJ, Franceschetti A, Klein D: *Genetics and Ophthalmology.* 2 vols. Thomas, 1961, 1963.

Whitwell J: Inherited eye diseases. *Practitioner* 1975;**214**:621.

22 | Tumors

Both benign and malignant tumors are encountered in the eye and its related structures. Most can be diagnosed early since they are visible, interfere with vision, or displace the eyeball. Care must be taken not to overlook the possibility of malignancy. Fluorescein angiography is helpful in the detection of intraocular tumors but may fail to differentiate benign from malignant lesions. Ultrasonography may be very useful in detecting orbital and intraocular masses, especially when visibility with an ophthalmoscope is poor, as occurs when cataract is present. Delay in diagnosis makes curative surgery technically more difficult and may result in loss of all useful vision. As far as possible, biopsies should be taken of all accessible suspicious lesions, excising completely the smaller lesions, since a positive diagnosis of malignancy can only be made by histologic examination. Accurate diagnosis of intraocular and retrobulbar tumors is difficult but vital, since curative therapy can only be given early; later, only palliation is possible.

Secondary (metastatic) ocular malignancies do occur but are less common. The most frequent site of metastasis is the choroid. The ophthalmoscopic appearance may be difficult to differentiate from that of primary malignancies of the choroid, and finding the primary tumor elsewhere is of the greatest diagnostic importance. X-ray or other treatment may relieve the ocular symptoms, but enucleation is sometimes necessary to relieve pain.

Physiology of Symptoms

Small tumors of the lids are asymptomatic except in the case of verrucae and molluscum contagiosum, which occasionally cause chemical conjunctivitis. Tumors of the conjunctiva are usually painless unless they have a rough, keratinized surface. A central corneal lesion causes decrease in vision. An intraocular lesion involving the macula causes blurring of vision as a presenting symptom. Extramacular tumors are not manifested until they become large enough to obstruct vision or produce secondary changes in the eye such as retinal detachment, a rise in intraocular pressure, or anterior uveitis. Retrobulbar tumors may be relatively asymptomatic until they are well-developed, at which time diplopia, displacement, or exophthalmos is likely to occur.

A history of recent change in size or appearance of an external ocular growth calls for careful observation, including photographs. If there is any suspicion of malignancy, biopsy or total removal is indicated for microscopic examination.

LID TUMORS

BENIGN TUMORS OF THE LIDS
(Nevus, Verruca, Molluscum Contagiosum, Xanthelasma, Hemangioma)

Nevus

Melanocytic nevi of the eyelids are common benign tumors with the same pathologic structure as nevi found elsewhere. They are usually congenital but may be relatively unpigmented at birth, enlarging and darkening during adolescence. Many never acquire visible pigment, and many resemble benign papillomas. Nevi rarely become malignant.

Nevi may be removed by shave excision if desired for cosmetic reasons.

Verrucae (Warts)

Warts commonly appear along the margins of the lids as fleshy, multilobulated, flat-based to pedunculated lesions. They are thought to be caused by viruses.

If treatment is indicated for cosmetic reasons, verrucae may be removed by excision with cauterization at the base of the lesion. Care must be exercised to avoid producing a marginal notch in the eyelid.

Molluscum Contagiosum (Fig 22–1)

The typical lesion of this unusual disorder is a small, flat, symmetric, centrally umbilicated growth along the lid margin. It is caused by a large virus and may produce toxic conjunctivitis and even keratitis if the lesion sheds into the conjunctival space.

Cure can usually be obtained by incising the lesion and allowing blood to permeate the central portion, by cautery, or by excision.

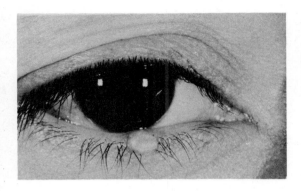

Figure 22–1. Molluscum contagiosum. Note central umbilication.

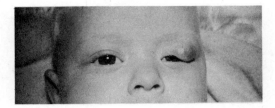

Figure 22–3. Cavernous hemangioma of left upper lid.

Xanthelasma (Fig 22–2)

Xanthelasma is a common disorder that occurs on the anterior surface of the eyelid, usually bilaterally near the inner angle of the eye. The lesions appear as yellow, wrinkled patches on the skin, and occur more often in elderly people. Xanthelasma represents lipid deposits in histiocytes in the dermis of the lid. Clinical evaluation of serum cholesterol levels is indicated, but only rarely is a direct relationship found.

Treatment is indicated for cosmetic reasons. Surgical removal is simple. Cauterization of the smaller lesions is sometimes effective. Recurrence following removal is not unusual.

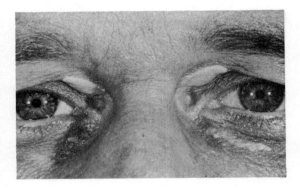

Figure 22–2. Xanthelasma. (Courtesy of M Quickert.)

Hemangioma (Fig 22–3)

Two main types of congenital vascular tumors occur in the lids: cavernous hemangiomas and capillary hemangiomas. Cavernous hemangiomas are composed of large venous channels lying in the subcutaneous tissue; they are bluish in color and change in size according to their distention with blood. Capillary (strawberry) hemangiomas are bright-red spots composed of dilated capillaries and proliferating endothelial cells. They are painless unless spontaneous hemorrhage causes marked swelling. They may show rapid

growth in the newborn period and frequently undergo involution later.

Treatment is usually not indicated in infancy or early childhood unless the defect is extensive enough to cause occlusion amblyopia. Various types of treatment have been used, including surgical excision of smaller lesions or freezing with CO_2. Radiation is not recommended because of the extensive scarring it causes.

PRIMARY MALIGNANT TUMORS OF THE LIDS
(Carcinoma, Xeroderma Pigmentosum, Sarcoma, Malignant Melanoma)

Carcinoma (Figs 22–4 and 22–5)

Carcinoma of the lids has the highest incidence of any malignant ocular tumor (42%). It is most frequent in men over 50 years of age.

The commonest site of the tumor is near the margin of the lower lid near the inner canthus. Ninety-five percent of lid carcinomas are of the basal cell type. The remaining 5% consist of squamous cell carcinomas and meibomian gland carcinomas. Keratoacanthomas and inverted follicular keratoses are benign lesions that resemble squamous cell carcinomas. In the past this was not recognized, and the

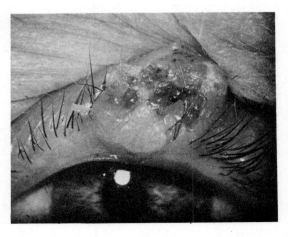

Figure 22–4. Squamous cell carcinoma of upper lid. (Courtesy of A Rosenberg.)

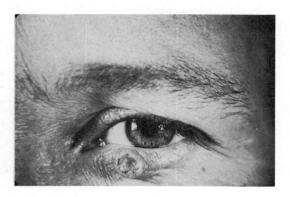

Figure 22–5. Basal cell carcinoma of left lower lid. (Courtesy of S Mettier, Jr.)

incidence of squamous cell carcinomas was thought to be higher than it actually is. Basal cell carcinoma is much more common in the lower lid; squamous cell carcinoma in the upper lid. Diagnosis is based upon clinical appearance and biopsy.

Squamous cell carcinoma may spread via the lymphatic system to the preauricular and submaxillary lymph nodes. Most do not spread if they are recognized and treated. Basal cell tumors grow very slowly, are locally invasive, and do not spread to the regional lymph nodes.

Squamous cell carcinoma grows slowly and painlessly, and it may be present for many months before it is noted. It usually begins as a small warty growth with a keratotic covering, gradually eroding and fissuring until an ulcer develops. The base of the ulcer is indurated and hyperemic and the edges hard. Unless the tumor is excised early it grows through the skin, connective tissue, cartilage, and bone until large areas are destroyed in a fungating crater that may eventually reach the cranial cavity. Pain then becomes severe and constant. When sensory nerves are involved, the pain may be excruciating. The patient may die of hemorrhage, meningitis, or general debility.

Basal cell carcinoma begins in a similar manner, eventually forming the typical rodent ulcer with a raised nodular border and indurated base. It eventually erodes the surrounding tissue in somewhat the same way as squamous cell carcinoma, but much more slowly. Biopsy of the tumor itself is a simple office procedure and is the only sure method of diagnosis.

Basal cell tumors of the lower lid near the inner canthus tend to invade the structures of the inner canthus and the orbit. Complete eradication of these tumors is important.

The sclerosing or morphealike basal cell carcinoma, an unusually aggressive variety of basal cell carcinoma, may lie beneath the skin surface and manifest its presence by subtle signs such as alopecia, lid notching, ectropion, or entropion.

Sebaceous gland carcinomas of the eyelid, most of which arise from the meibomian glands and the

glands of Zeis, are potentially fatal neoplasms; about half of them may resemble benign inflammatory diseases such as chalazions and chronic blepharitis.

Any suspicious growths on the lids should be submitted for pathologic examination.

The objective of treatment is complete destruction of the tumor. Surgery is an effective method, particularly if frozen sections are used to ensure complete excision. Radiotherapy can also be effective for basal cell carcinomas and squamous cell carcinomas; cryotherapy has been successful in the treatment of some basal cell carcinomas.

Carcinoma Associated With Xeroderma Pigmentosum

This rare, congenitally determined (usually autosomal recessive) disease is characterized by the appearance of a large number of freckles in the areas of the skin exposed to the sun. These are followed by telangiectases, atrophic patches, and eventually a warty growth that may undergo carcinomatous degeneration. The eyelids are frequently affected and may be the first area to show degenerative changes, causing atrophy and ectropion with secondary inflammatory changes of the conjunctiva, symblepharon, corneal ulceration, and carcinoma of the lids. Malignant tumors include basal cell carcinomas, squamous cell carcinomas, and malignant melanomas. This condition is inherited as an autosomal recessive trait. Carriers can often be identified by excessive freckling.

The disease appears early in life and in most cases is fatal by adolescence as a result of metastasis. Life may be prolonged by carefully protecting the skin from actinic rays and treating carcinomatous tumors as rapidly as they appear.

Sarcoma

Sarcoma of the lids is rare and usually represents an anterior extension of an orbital sarcoma. Rhabdomyosarcomas involving the orbit and lids represent the most common malignant tumor in these tissues in the first decade of life. Other sarcomas (usually named after the predominant type of cell) also occur. Most are radiosensitive, but a combination of surgery and radiation is often required. They may be associated with similar lesions elsewhere in the body.

Malignant Melanoma

Malignant melanomas of the eyelids are similar to those elsewhere in the skin and include 3 distinct varieties: superficial spreading melanoma, lentigo maligna melanoma, and nodular melanoma. Not all malignant melanomas are pigmented. Most pigmented lesions on the eyelid skin are not melanomas. Therefore, biopsy should be used to establish the diagnosis. The prognosis for melanomas of the skin depends upon the depth of invasion or the thickness of the lesion.

CONJUNCTIVAL TUMORS

PRIMARY BENIGN
TUMORS OF THE CONJUNCTIVA
(Nevus, Papilloma, Granuloma, Dermoid,
Dermolipoma, Lymphoma, Fibroma, Angioma)

Nevus (Fig 22–6)

One-third of melanocytic nevi of the conjunctiva lack pigment. Over half have cystic epithelial inclusions that can be seen clinically.

Histologically, conjunctival nevi are composed of nests or sheets of typical nevus cells. Conjunctival nevi, like other nevi, rarely become malignant. Many are excised because they are disfiguring.

Papilloma

Conjunctival papillomas are not rare, occurring most frequently near the limbus, on the caruncle, or at the lid margins. Those on the caruncle and lid margin are usually soft and pedunculated, with irregular surfaces. They frequently recur after removal.

Granuloma

Granulomas are seen as vascular fungating masses protruding from areas in which the palpebral conjunctiva (usually at the lid margins) has been broken or incised, as in draining chalazions, open conjunctival wounds, or conjunctival foreign bodies. Occasionally, specific etiologic agents such as the tubercle bacillus or cysts containing *Coccidioides immitis* are identified histologically. They can attain large size rapidly and may outgrow their blood supply and strangulate, with spontaneous recovery. Treatment is by surgical excision and cleansing of the base. The wound may have to be closed with sutures.

Dermoid Tumor (Fig 22–7)

This rare congenital tumor appears as a smooth, rounded, yellow elevated mass, frequently with hairs protruding. A dermoid tumor may remain quiescent, although it often increases in size during puberty.

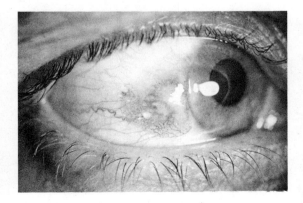

Figure 22–6. Conjunctival nevus. (Courtesy of A Irvine, Jr.)

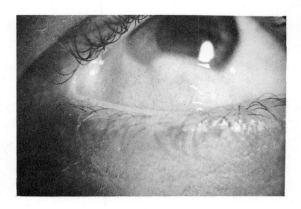

Figure 22–7. Dermoid tumor at the inferior limbus. (Courtesy of A Irvine, Jr.)

Removal is indicated only if cosmetic deformity is significant or if vision is impaired or threatened.

Dermolipoma

Dermolipoma is a common congenital tumor that usually appears as a smoothly rounded growth in the upper temporal quadrant of the bulbar conjunctiva near the lateral canthus. Treatment is usually not indicated, but at least partial removal should be done if the growth is enlarging or is cosmetically disfiguring. Posterior dissection must be undertaken with extreme care (if at all) since this lesion is frequently continuous with orbital fat; orbital derangement may cause scarring and complications far more serious than the original lesion.

Lymphoma & Lymphoid Hyperplasia

These are uncommon conjunctival lesions that may appear in adults without evidence of systemic disease or as part of the clinical picture of lymphosarcoma, lymphocytic leukemia, Hodgkin's disease, or other related conditions. Benign lymphoid hyperplasia can sometimes be distinguished by a pebbly appearance corresponding to follicle formation. However, the clinical appearance of benign lymphoid hyperplasia and malignant lymphoma can be similar; therefore, biopsy is essential to establish a diagnosis.

Treatment of both benign and malignant lesions is best accomplished with radiotherapy.

Fibroma

Fibromas are rare small, smooth, pedunculated, transparent growths that may appear anywhere in the conjunctival tissues but are most often seen in the lower fornix. Histologically, they consist of fibrous overgrowths covered by epithelium. Treatment is by excision.

Angioma

Conjunctival angiomas may take 2 forms: hemangioma or lymphangioma. The latter are rare and usually congenital. Conjunctival hemangiomas may appear as diffuse telangiectases or capillary nevi, or as encapsulated cavernous hemangiomas (more common). The latter consist of large communicating, fairly well encapsulated vascular spaces that tend to enlarge. Treatment is by excision or electrocoagulation.

PRIMARY MALIGNANT TUMORS OF THE BULBAR CONJUNCTIVA
(Epithelioma, Malignant Melanoma, Lymphosarcoma)

Carcinoma
Carcinoma of the conjunctiva arises most frequently at the limbus in the area of the palpebral fissure and less often in nonexposed areas of the conjunctiva. Some of these tumors may resemble pterygiums. Most have a gelatinous surface; sometimes, abnormal keratinization of the epithelium produces leukoplakia. Growth is slow, and deep invasion and metastases are extremely rare; therefore, complete excision is effective treatment. Recurrences are common if the lesion is incompletely excised; treatment consists of reexcision.

Conjunctival dysplasia, a benign condition that occurs as an isolated lesion or sometimes over pterygiums and pingueculas, can resemble carcinoma in situ (Fig 22–8) clinically and even histologically. An excisional biopsy will establish a diagnosis and result in cure of most of these lesions.

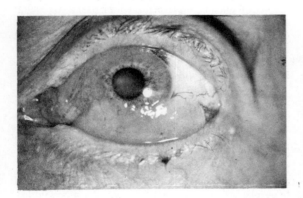

Figure 22–8. Intraepithelial epithelioma. (Courtesy of A Irvine, Jr.)

Malignant Melanoma
Malignant melanoma of the conjunctiva is rare. It may arise from a preexisting nevus, from an area of acquired melanosis, or de novo from formerly normal-appearing conjunctiva. Pigmentation may vary greatly, and the clinical course is often unpredictable.

Many can be locally excised. The value of more radical surgery (such as exenteration of the orbit) has still not been determined.

Lymphosarcoma
Malignant lymphomas of the conjunctiva are much rarer than benign lymphoid hyperplasia. Most also involve the orbit and are associated with systemic lymphoma. However, the conjunctival lesion may be the initial sign of a systemic problem.

CORNEAL TUMORS

PRIMARY MALIGNANT TUMORS OF THE CORNEA
(Epithelioma, Melanoma)

Carcinomas of the corneal epithelium are rare; extension of conjunctival carcinoma (especially at the limbus) onto the cornea is not uncommon. The same is true for melanomas in the corneal epithelium.

INTRAOCULAR TUMORS

PRIMARY BENIGN INTRAOCULAR TUMORS
(Nevus, Angioma, Tuberous Sclerosis, Hemangioma of Choroid)

Nevus
Nevi may occur on any of the 3 portions of the uvea: the iris, ciliary body, or choroid. They are usually flat pigmented lesions lying in the stroma of the tissue. On the anterior surface of the iris they may be noted as iris "freckles." Posteriorly in the choroid one may see flat pigmented areas. Large choroidal nevi are difficult to differentiate from malignant melanomas. Their unchanging slate-gray color and flat appearance and the lack of extension are important in the differential diagnosis from malignant melanoma.

Because of the difficulties in differentiation from

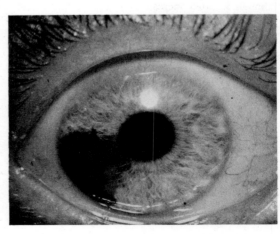

Figure 22–9. Nevus of the iris. (Courtesy of A Rosenberg.)

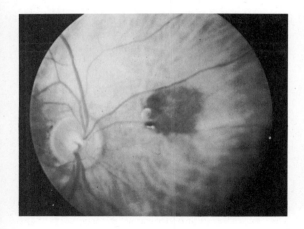

Figure 22-10. Nevus of the choroid. (Photo by Diane Beeston.)

near one of the pairs of enlarged retinal vessels. Angiomas may enlarge. Photocoagulation therapy (xenon or argon laser) and cryotherapy are currently utilized to eradicate these lesions.

Tuberous Sclerosis (Bourneville's Disease)

The rare intraocular tumor (glial hamartoma) associated with tuberous sclerosis in about half of cases varies in size and color but is most often a yellow or white nodular swelling, frequently mulberry in appearance, located in any portion of the posterior fundus but with a predilection for the area near the optic nerve. Other manifestations of tuberous sclerosis include skin changes (adenoma sebaceum), intracranial changes causing epilepsy and mental retardation, and other neurologic symptoms (see p 226).

There is no treatment. The prognosis is very poor, with 75% of patients dead by age 20.

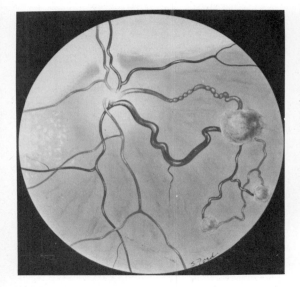

Figure 22-11. Angiomatosis retinae of Von Hippel-Lindau disease (drawing). (Courtesy of F Cordes.)

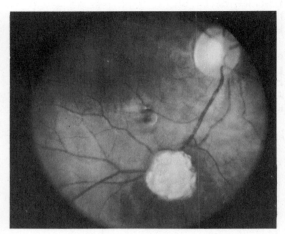

Figure 22-12. Tuberous sclerosis.

malignant melanomas, fundus photographs (including fluorescein angiography) or careful line drawings should be made of all suspicious lesions. Observations should be made periodically for changes.

Retinal Angioma*

Angioma of the retina is a rare congenital disorder. Blurring of vision may result if bleeding occurs or if the retina is secondarily detached. Occasionally, angioma is associated with angioma in the cerebral cortex (Lindau's disease). The tumor occurs in the posterior fundus, often in the lower temporal quadrant. It is globular in outline and may be located

*See also Angiomatosis Retinae in Chapter 17.

Hemangioma of the Choroid

Choroidal hemangioma occurs in most cases of Sturge-Weber syndrome associated with unilateral infantile glaucoma (see p 225). Cases occurring with no other signs of Sturge-Weber syndrome are frequently mistaken for malignant melanoma of the choroid (see below), and the mistaken diagnosis has often led to unnecessary removal of the affected eye. The tumor involves the posterior pole, usually near the optic disk and sometimes extending out to the equator, most often on the temporal side. It may produce a solid elevation or a serous detachment of the retina. The borders are irregular, and the tumor is never pigmented. Hemangiomas can produce arcuate field defects or localized scotomas.

Histologically, the tumor consists of endothelium-lined spaces engorged with blood separated by sparse connective tissue. Retinal degeneration over the tumor is common.

Secondary glaucoma, usually severe and refractory to any treatment, is associated with larger choroidal hemangiomas.

The differentiation from malignant melanoma is most important and frequently difficult.

There is no treatment, although eyes tolerate smaller hemangiomas very well. Enucleation may be necessary for intractable, painful secondary trauma.

PRIMARY MALIGNANT TUMORS OF THE INTRAOCULAR STRUCTURES
(Malignant Melanoma, Retinoblastoma, Diktyoma)

Malignant Melanoma

It has been estimated that intraocular malignant melanoma occurs in 0.02–0.06% of the total eye patient population in the USA. It is seen only in the uveal tract and is the most common intraocular malignant tumor in the white population. The average age of patients with this disorder is 50 years. It is almost always unilateral. Eighty-five percent appear in the choroid, 9% in the ciliary body, and 6% in the iris. Most of the choroidal tumors are in the posterior portion of the eye, especially on the temporal side. In the iris, the lower half is most often affected. Intraocular malignant melanoma is rare in blacks, although uveal nevi are common.

This tumor may be seen in its early stages only accidentally during routine ophthalmoscopic examination or because of blurring due to macular invasion. Blood-borne metastases may occur at any time, and death may occur before local spread or ocular symptoms appear. Glaucoma may be a late manifestation.

Histologically, these tumors are composed of spindle-shaped cells, with or without prominent nucleoli, and large epithelioid tumor cells. Tumors composed of the former have a good prognosis; tumors with the latter, a poor prognosis.

Intraocular malignant melanomas may spread directly through the sclera, by local invasion of intraocular structures, or by metastasis.

Clinical manifestations are usually absent unless the macula is involved. In the later stages, growth of the tumor may lead to retinal detachment with loss of a large amount of visual field. A tumor located in the iris may be large enough to change the color of the iris or deform the pupil. Pain does not occur in the absence of glaucoma.

The first step in diagnosis is to suspect the lesion. Most intraocular malignant melanomas can be seen ophthalmoscopically. Transillumination is of some value in differentiation from serous retinal detachment.

A high incidence of intraocular tumors has been found in the study of blind, painful, phthisic (atrophic) eyes, one writer reporting that 10% of such eyes contained previously unsuspected malignant melanomas.

Enucleation of an eye with a choroidal melanoma has been the traditional treatment. Recently, other forms of therapy, particularly radiotherapy with cobalt plaques or charged particles, has been used for eyes with small tumors and useful vision. Very small melanomas (less than 10 mm in diameter) have an excellent prognosis and are often impossible to differentiate from benign nevi; therefore, many authorities advocate not treating these tumors until unequivocal growth can be documented (usually with serial photographs or ultrasound measurements).

Small melanomas of the iris that have not invaded the iris root can be safely observed until growth is documented; then they can be removed by iridectomy. Lesions that invade the iris root and ciliary body can sometimes be treated with iridocyclectomy.

Retinoblastoma

Retinoblastoma is a rare but life-endangering tumor of childhood. Two-thirds of cases appear before the end of the third year; rare cases have been reported at almost every age. It is bilateral in about 30% of cases. The tumor results from mutation of an autosomal dominant gene, which is passed on with fairly high penetrance. About 94% of retinoblastomas arise

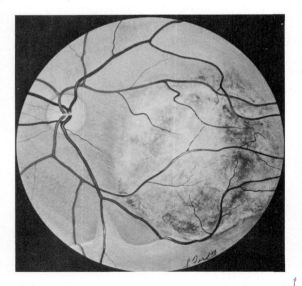

Figure 22–13. Malignant melanoma of the choroid, macular area, left eye (drawing). (Courtesy of F Cordes.)

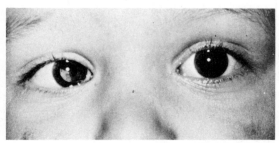

Figure 22–14. Retinoblastoma visible through pupil.

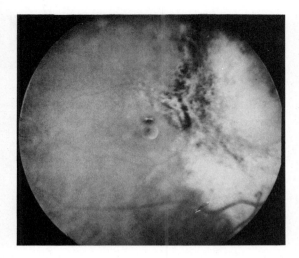

Figure 22–15. Retinoblastoma after x-ray radiation.

Retinoblastoma usually remains unnoticed until it has advanced far enough to produce a white pupil—unless strabismus has occurred, leading to earlier diagnosis. Otherwise, the tumor is usually seen in the early stages only when sought for, as in children having a hereditary background or where the other eye has been affected. In the early stages small, yellowish-white nodular masses may be seen protruding into the vitreous from the retina. Infants and children with esotropia should be examined to rule out retinoblastoma, since blind eyes of children will often turn inward.

Retrolental fibroplasia, persistence of the primary vitreous, retinal dysplasia, Coats's disease, and nematode endophthalmitis may simulate retinoblastoma.

In general, the earlier the discovery and treatment of the tumor, the better the chance to prevent spread through the optic nerve and orbital tissues.

Enucleation is the treatment of choice for large retinoblastomas; smaller ones in eyes with potentially useful vision can be effectively treated with radiotherapy, sometimes augmented by chemotherapy, cryotherapy, or photocoagulation.

Medulloepitheliomas ("Diktyoma") of the Ciliary Body

Benign and malignant medulloepitheliomas are rare tumors that may arise from the ciliary body epithelium. Those with one or more heteroplastic elements, such as hyaline cartilage, brain tissue, or rhabdomyoblasts, are called teratoid medulloepitheliomas. Those that arise near birth may infiltrate the area around the lens and produce a white pupillary reflex similar to that seen in eyes with retinoblastoma.

by mutation; therefore, only about 6% are familial. When the inheritance is familial, a retinoblastoma survivor has approximately a 50% chance of producing an affected child.

Retinoblastomas usually arise from the posterior retina. Growth tends to be nodular, with numerous satellite or seeding nodules that may produce multiple secondary tumors. They gradually fill the eye and extend through the optic nerve to the brain and along the emissary vessels and nerves in the sclera to the orbital tissues. Microscopically, most retinoblastomas are composed of small, closely packed, round or polygonal cells with large, darkly staining nuclei and scanty cytoplasm. They sometimes form characteristic Flexner-Wintersteiner rosettes indicative of photoreceptor differentiation. Degenerative changes are frequent, with necrosis and calcification. A few spontaneous cures have been reported.

ORBITAL TUMORS

Gradually enlarging orbital tumors may attain a diameter of 1 cm before any displacement of the eyeball is noted. The direction of displacement offers a

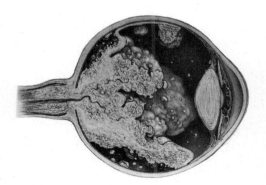

Figure 22–16. Retinoblastoma with multiple seedings and optic nerve invasion. (Courtesy of B Crawford and W Spencer.)

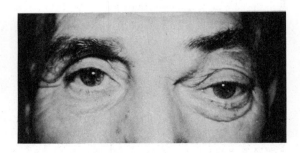

Figure 22–17. Orbital tumor displacing left eye.

clue to the location of the tumor—eg, posterior tumors tend to displace the eyeball anteriorly, whereas tumors between the eyeball and one of the walls of the orbit will cause lateral displacement. These observations indicate the site of exploration when biopsy is indicated.

With displacement of the eyeball, diplopia is a common symptom. Pressure resulting from marked exophthalmos may interfere with blood supply to the optic nerve and retina, causing blurred vision. Exposure of the eye due to inability to close the lids causes corneal epithelial damage with resultant pain and irritation.

The use of the CT scan and ultrasonography has helped resolve the diagnostic dilemma presented by many orbital tumors and can aid the surgeon in determining when and where to explore the orbit for these masses.

The common or otherwise important tumors from the following classification will be discussed below. References are given to discussions elsewhere in the text. The uncommon orbital tumors are briefly described or only listed.

Classification*
A. Primary in Orbit:
1. **Choristomas**–Dermoid cyst, epidermal cyst, teratoma.
2. **Hamartomas**–Hemangioma, neurofibroma.
3. **Mesenchymal**–
   a. **Adipose**–Lipoma, liposarcoma.
   b. **Fibrous**–Fibroma, fibrosarcoma.
   c. **Myomatous**–Rhabdomyosarcoma.
   d. **Cartilaginous**–Chondroma, chondrosarcoma.
   e. **Osseous**–Osteoma, osteosarcoma.
4. **Neural**–Neurofibroma, neurilemmoma, other rare tumors.
5. **Epithelial**–Lacrimal gland tumors.
6. **Lymphoid tumors**–Lymphomas, lymphoid hyperplasia, and other inflammatory infiltrates (granulomas, sarcoid, and others).
B. Secondary in Orbit From Adjacent Structures:
1. **Intraocular**–Malignant melanoma, retinoblastoma.
2. **Cornea and conjunctiva**–Malignant melanoma, epidermoid carcinoma.
3. **Eyelids and face**–Basal cell carcinoma, other rare malignant tumors.
4. **Upper respiratory tract**–Carcinoma of the upper respiratory epithelium, sarcoma, mucocele.
5. **Cranial**–Meningioma, other intracranial tumors.
C. Metastatic From Distant Sites: Carcinoma, sarcoma, neuroblastoma.

*Modified from Hogan MJ, Zimmerman LE: *Ophthalmic Pathology,* 2nd ed. Saunders, 1962.

D. Other Types:
1. **Reticuloendothelioses**–Juvenile xanthogranuloma (see p 284), eosinophilic granuloma, other rare entities.
2. **Metabolic disorders**–Thyroid exophthalmos (see p 248).
3. **Phakomatoses**–Neurofibromatosis (Recklinghausen's disease) (see p 225).

PRIMARY ORBITAL TUMORS

Choristomas
A choristoma is defined as a tumor composed of tissue elements not normally present in the area. For the orbit this includes dermoid cyst, epidermal cyst, and teratoma.

Dermoid cysts are most often found in the superior temporal portion of the orbit, usually anterior to the lacrimal gland. They are benign. They frequently contain particles of hair. Rupture of these cysts, either spontaneously or after trauma, may produce a granulomatous inflammatory reaction that is often the first sign of the tumor.

Hamartomas
A. Hemangiomas: These are the most common orbital tumors, usually appearing by early adulthood. They vary greatly in size, the larger ones causing marked proptosis. The tumor varies from small capillary-sized endothelium-lined channels (called capillary hemangiomas) to large vascular channels called cavernous hemangiomas. There is usually a mixture with additional inflammation or scarring. Malignant vascular tumors are very rare. Treatment is usually unnecessary unless significant proptosis exists, in which case surgical excision (partial or total) is indicated.

B. Neurofibroma: There is doubt that this tumor ever occurs as an isolated orbital tumor without other evidence of neurofibromatosis (Recklinghausen's disease—see p 225).

Mesenchymal Tumors
A. Lipoma: Rare. Usually minor or no clinical signs.

B. Liposarcoma: Very rare malignant orbital tumor.

C. Fibroma: Simple fibromas are rare, but they are more common in the upper and inner portions of the orbit than elsewhere. They are usually evident by the third decade. Exophthalmos, diplopia, and displacement of the eyeball are the first symptoms.

Fibromatous tumors are usually encapsulated, firm, and have a meager blood supply. Simple excision to relieve symptoms is feasible in many cases.

D. Rhabdomyosarcoma: This is the most common malignant tumor of mesenchymal origin in the orbit. These tumors occur most frequently in Caucasians prior to age 10, and there is a slight male preponderance. They usually cause proptosis downward and temporally and grow rapidly. Metastases to the brain and lungs are common. Irradiation has improved the prognosis of this highly malignant tumor. Exenteration may become necessary in some cases.

E. Cartilaginous: Chondromas and chondrosarcomas are very rare in the orbit. Chondrosarcoma is associated with osteosarcoma following radiation therapy for retinoblastoma.

F. Osseous: Osteoma and osteosarcoma are very rare.

Neural

Neurofibroma (see above) and other rare tumors.

Epithelial (Lacrimal Gland) Tumors

There are 3 main types of tumors of the lacrimal fossa: (1) epithelial tumors of the lacrimal gland (50%), (2) inflammatory pseudotumors (30%), and (3) lymphomas and lymphoid hyperplasias (20%). The latter 2 are classified below under inflammatory tumors (pseudotumors) of the orbit.

Lacrimal gland tumors are divided into benign and malignant mixed tumors and carcinomas unrelated to mixed tumors.

Most mixed tumors are benign but are locally invasive into adjacent periosteum and soft orbital tissue. Surgical removal is indicated, but recurrence frequently occurs as a consequence of incomplete removal.

Carcinoma not associated with mixed tumor is hard to differentiate clinically from other tumors of the lacrimal fossa. Frozen sections at the time of surgery are important because this tumor is highly invasive and requires radical surgical management, usually including exenteration.

Lymphoid Tumors

Benign lymphoid hyperplasia, sometimes erroneously called a pseudotumor, is a common orbital tumor of unknown cause composed of proliferating benign lymphoreticular elements. The clinical course may be quite varied, and inflammatory signs are often not evident. Proptosis may be marked, and ocular muscle abnormalities are common. High doses of systemic corticosteroids may effectively treat some of these lesions. However, the absence of a response to steroid therapy does not rule out an inflammatory tumor, and the presence of a response to steroid therapy does not prove that the tumor is a benign process. (Some malignant tumors, particularly those with an inflammatory component, can show an apparent temporary resolution with corticosteroid therapy.)

Malignant lymphomas of the orbit can occur as isolated tumors or can be part of a systemic malignant lymphoma. When confronted with these tumors, it is important to search for a malignant process elsewhere in the body.

Radiotherapy is usually the best treatment for malignant lymphomas and may be useful for treating benign lymphoid hyperplasia that does not respond satisfactorily to corticosteroid therapy.

SECONDARY ORBITAL TUMORS & METASTATIC TUMORS FROM DISTANT SITES

These are listed in the orbital tumor classification (see above).

All tumors from adjacent structures invade the orbit by direct extension and usually call for a radical surgical approach, including exenteration, unless the prognosis is already hopeless because of malignant tumor spread.

Metastatic orbital tumor masses are rarely removed surgically. Radiation is occasionally used in the orbit as a palliative measure. The orbit is a relatively uncommon site for blood-borne metastases.

● ● ●

References

Abramson DH et al: The management of unilateral retinoblastoma without primary enucleation. *Arch Ophthalmol* 1982;**100**:1249.

Beard C: Observations on treatment of basal cell carcinoma of eyelids. *Trans Am Acad Ophthalmol Otolaryngol* 1975;**79**:O664.

Bedford MA: *Color Atlas of Ocular Tumors.* Year Book, 1979.

Bedford MA, Bedotto C, Macfaul PA: Retinoblastoma. *Br J Ophthalmol* 1971;**55**:19.

Blodi FC: Ocular melanocytosis and melanoma. *Am J Ophthalmol* 1975;**80**:389.

Boniuk M, Zimmerman LE: Sebaceous carcinoma of the eyelid, eyebrow, caruncle and orbit. *Trans Am Acad Ophthalmol Otolaryngol* 1968;**72**:619.

Bullock JD, Beard C, Sullivan JH: Cryotherapy of basal cell carcinoma in oculoplastic surgery. *Am J Ophthalmol* 1976;**82**:841.

Char DH: The management of small choroidal melanomas. *Surv Ophthalmol* 1978;**22**:377.

Collin JRO: Basal cell carcinoma in the eyelid region. *Br J Ophthalmol* 1976;**60**:806.

Davidorf FH: Conservative management of malignant melanoma. 2. Transscleral diathermy as a method of treatment for malignant melanomas of the choroid. *Arch Ophthalmol* 1970;**82**:273.

Davidorf FH, Lang JR: The natural history of malignant melanoma of the choroid: Small vs large tumors. *Trans Am Acad Ophthalmol Otolaryngol* 1975;**79**:310.

Fraunfelder FT et al: The role of cryosurgery in external ocular and periocular disease. *Trans Am Acad Ophthalmol Otolaryngol* 1977;**83**:713.

Gass JDM: Problems in the differential diagnosis of choroidal nevi and malignant melanomas: The 33rd Edward Jackson memorial lecture. *Trans Am Acad Ophthalmol Otolaryngol* 1977;**83**:19.

Henderson JW: *Orbital Tumors.* Thieme-Stratton, 1980.

Hogan MJ, Zimmerman LE: *Ophthalmic Pathology,* 2nd ed. Saunders, 1962.

Jakobiec FA (editor): *Ocular and Adnexal Tumors.* Aesculapius, 1978.

Jensen RD, Miller RW: Retinoblastoma: Epidemiologic characteristics. *N Engl J Med* 1971;**285**:307.

Jones IS, Jakobiec FA: *Diseases of the Orbit.* Harper & Row, 1979.

Knowles DM II, Jakobiec FA: Orbital lymphoid neoplasms: A clinicopathologic study of 60 cases. *Cancer* 1980;**46**:576.

Knowles DM II, Jakobiec FA, Halper JP: Immunologic characterization of ocular adnexal lymphoid neoplasms. *Am J Ophthalmol* 1979;**87**:603.

Kopf AW, Bart RS, Rodriguez-Sains BA: Malignant melanoma: A review. *J Dermatol Surg Oncol* 1977;**3**:43.

McLean IW, Foster WD, Zimmerman LE: Prognostic factors in small malignant melanomas of choroid and ciliary body. *Arch Ophthalmol* 1977;**95**:48.

Reese AB: *Tumors of the Eye,* 3rd ed. Harper & Row, 1976.

Robins JH et al: Xeroderma pigmentosum. *Ann Intern Med* 1974;**80**:221.

Shields JA: *The Diagnosis and Management of Intraocular Tumors.* Mosby, 1982.

Sigelman J, Jakobiec FA: Lymphoid lesions of the conjunctiva: Relation of histopathology to clinical outcome. *Trans Am Acad Ophthalmol Otolaryngol* 1978;**85**:818.

Spencer WH: Optic nerve extension of intraocular neoplasms. *Am J Ophthalmol* 1975;**80**:465.

Thompson RW et al: Treatment of retinoblastoma. *Ophthalmol Digest* 1972;**34**:17.

Yanoff M, Fine BS: *Ocular Pathology,* 2nd ed. Harper & Row, 1982.

In spite of the protection afforded by the bony orbit, the cushioning effect of the retrobulbar fat, and the lids and lashes—and in spite of the great strides made in recent years in the development of protective devices, especially the use of safety goggles—the incidence of eye injuries remains high. Childhood eye injuries continue to occur as a result of air rifle, bow and arrow, catapult (slingshot), and throwing accidents.

Pain or photophobia caused by the injury may produce blepharospasm severe enough to prevent examination of the eye. If this happens, instill a sterile topical anesthetic. With the aid of a loupe and well-focused light, the anterior surface of the cornea is examined for foreign materials or wounds, regularity, and luster. The conjunctiva is inspected for hemorrhage, foreign material, or tears. The depth and clarity of the anterior chamber are noted. The size, shape, and light reaction of the pupil should be compared with those of the pupil of the uninjured eye. If the eyeball is intact, the lids are carefully inspected to the fornices, everting the upper lid. The lens, vitreous, and retina are examined with an ophthalmoscope for evidence of intraocular damage such as hemorrhage or retinal detachment.

If the patient complains of a foreign body sensation but none can be seen with oblique illumination, instill sterile fluorescein. This may demonstrate an irregularity of the corneal surface due to a minute abrasion, laceration, or foreign body.

A small child may be difficult to examine adequately. If a rupture or laceration of the eyeball is suspected, it is best not to struggle but to examine with the aid of a short-acting general anesthetic. If a severe injury is not suspected, the lids may be manually separated under topical anesthesia with the use of lid retracting forceps.

It is important to determine and record visual acuity (see p 16). Visual acuity should be tested again upon recovery from the injury, and a refraction performed if vision is below normal. This record may have legal significance.

In severe injuries it is important for the nonspecialist to bear in mind the possibility of causing further damage by unnecessary manipulation.

Caution: Topical anesthetics, dyes, and other medications placed in an injured eye *must be sterile.*

Both tetracaine and fluorescein can be autoclaved repeatedly without impairment of their pharmacologic properties. Most ophthalmic solutions are now available in individual disposable sterile units.

NONPENETRATING INJURIES OF THE EYEBALL
(Abrasions, Contusions, Rupture, Superficial Foreign Bodies, Burns)

Abrasions

Abrasions of the lids, cornea, or conjunctiva do not require surgical treatment. The wound should be cleansed of imbedded foreign material. In order to facilitate the examination, the pain associated with abrasions of the cornea and conjunctiva can be relieved by instillation of a topical anesthetic such as 0.5% tetracaine solution, but routine instillation of a topical anesthetic by the patient *must not be permitted* since it delays normal healing of the epithelium. Ophthalmic antibiotic ointment instilled into the eye lessens the chance of infection. An eye bandage applied with firm but gentle pressure lessens discomfort and promotes healing by preventing movement of the lids over the involved area. The dressing should be changed daily and the eye inspected for evidence of infection or corneal ulcer formation.

Corneal abrasions cause severe pain and may lead to recurrent corneal erosion, but they rarely become infected.

Contusions

Contusions of the eyeball and its surrounding tissues are commonly produced by traumatic contact with a blunt object. The results of such injury are variable and are often not obvious upon superficial examination. Careful study and adequate follow-up are indicated. The possible results of contusion injury are hemorrhage and swelling of the eyelids (ecchymosis, ''black eye''), subconjunctival hemorrhages, edema or rupture of the cornea, hemorrhage into the anterior chamber (hyphema), rupture of the root of the iris (iridodialysis), traumatic paralysis of the pupil (mydriasis), rupture of the iris sphincter, paralysis or spasm of the muscles of accommodation, anterior chamber angle recession with subsequent sec-

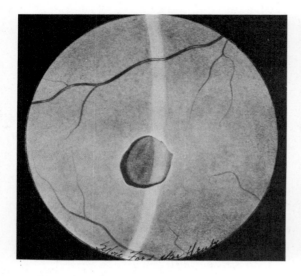

Figure 23–1. Hole in retina, macular area, posttraumatic.

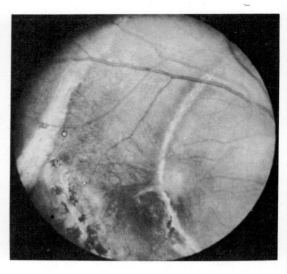

Figure 23–2. Choroidal tears. (Photo by Diane Beeston.)

ondary glaucoma (see p 170), traumatic cataract, dislocation of the lens (subluxation and luxation), vitreous hemorrhage, retinal hemorrhage and retinal edema (most common in the macular area, called commotio retinae, or Berlin's traumatic edema), detachment of the retina, rupture of the choroid, and optic nerve injury.

Many of these injuries cannot be seen on external observation. Some, such as cataract, may not develop for many days or weeks following the injury.

Except for injuries involving rupture of the eyeball itself (see below), most of the immediate effects of contusion of the eye do not require immediate definitive treatment. However, any injury severe enough to cause intraocular hemorrhage involves the danger of delayed secondary hemorrhage from a damaged uveal vessel, which may cause intractable glaucoma and permanent damage to the eyeball. Patients who show evidence of intraocular hemorrhage should be put at absolute bed rest for 4 or 5 days with both eyes bandaged to minimize the chance of further bleeding. Secondary hemorrhage rarely occurs after 72 hours. A short-acting cycloplegic such as 5% homatropine may be used. Acetazolamide, mannitol, or other systemically administered agents to lower intraocular pressure may be necessary.

Rupture of the Eyeball

Rupture of the eyeball may occur as a result of penetrating trauma or of contusion that causes a sudden increase in intraocular pressure, causing the wall of the eyeball to tear at one of the weaker points. The most common site of rupture is along the limbus; occasionally, rupture occurs around the optic nerve. Anterior ruptures can be repaired surgically by interrupted sutures unless intraocular contents are so deranged that

useful function of the eye is not possible, in which case enucleation is required.

Corneal & Conjunctival Foreign Bodies
(Fig 23–3)

Foreign bodies are the most frequent cause of eye injury. Small metallic or nonmetallic foreign bodies are frequently blown into the eye and may become lodged under the upper lid or be embedded in corneal epithelium. In removing corneal foreign bodies, a sterile topical anesthetic is essential. Minute corneal foreign bodies that are not readily visualized with the naked eye or loupe may be outlined with sterile fluorescein. If a foreign body containing iron has remained in the tissue for any length of time, rust pene-

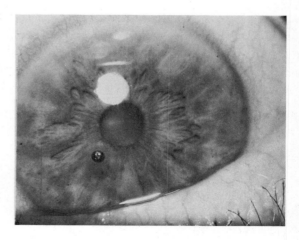

Figure 23–3. Metallic corneal foreign body. (Courtesy of A Rosenberg.)

trates the corneal tissue and must be removed to prevent further irritation.

Although foreign bodies may often be removed satisfactorily using a light and magnifying loupe, the most satisfactory method is under direct observation with the aid of the greater magnification and illumination of the slit lamp. Although the cornea is very tough, it is also thin (1 mm). Care must be taken not to penetrate the cornea in the process of removing a deeply imbedded foreign body. When in doubt, such deeply placed foreign bodies should be removed in the operating room where the anterior chamber can be re-formed (if necessary) under sterile conditions. Many types of instruments are used for removing superficial corneal foreign bodies, including special "hockey stick" or "golf club" spuds, scalpel blades, and the points of hypodermic needles. A dental drill of the burr type is often useful for removing an imbedded rust ring from the cornea.

Following removal of the foreign body, an antibiotic ointment such as polymyxin B–bacitracin or gentamicin should be instilled 3 times a day into the conjunctival sac to prevent infection. If the wound is extensive, an eye bandage can be used to minimize movement of the lid over the injured area. The wound should be inspected daily for evidence of infection until it is completely healed.

Burns

Thermal burns of the eye structures are treated as burns of skin structures elsewhere, as the tissues of the lids are most commonly involved. If the damage has been deep enough to cause sloughing of the corneal tissue, the eye is almost certainly lost by extensive scarring or perforation.

Ultraviolet irradiation, even in moderate doses, often produces a superficial keratitis that is quite painful, although recovery occurs within 12–36 hours without complications. Pain often comes on 6–12 hours after exposure. This type of injury occurs following exposure to an electric welding arc without the protection of a filter. Many "flash burns" are caused by careless exposure in the mistaken belief that the eyes can be burned in this way only when looking directly at the arc. A short circuit in a high-voltage line may cause the same type of injury.

In severe cases of "flash burn," instillation of a sterile topical anesthetic may be necessary for examination. A mydriatic (eg, homatropine hydrobromide, 2–5%) should be used. Systemic sedation or narcotics are preferable to topical anesthetics, which interfere with corneal healing. Patching and cold compresses are indicated to relieve discomfort.

Infrared exposure rarely produces an ocular reaction. ("Glassblower's cataract" is rare today but once was common among workers who were required to watch the color changes in molten glass in furnaces without proper filters.) Radiant energy from viewing the sun or an eclipse of the sun without an adequate filter, however, may produce a serious burn of the macula resulting in permanent impairment of vision.

Persons using hallucinogenic drugs such as LSD have been particularly prone to solar macular burns.

Excessive exposure to radiation (x-ray) produces cataractous changes that may not appear for many months after the exposure. The same risk is inherent in exposure to nuclear radiation.

PENETRATING INJURIES TO THE EYE
(Lacerations, Intraocular Foreign Bodies)

Note: Tetanus prophylaxis is indicated whenever penetrating eye injury occurs.

Lacerations (Fig 23–4)

Lacerations are usually caused by sharp objects (knives, scissors, a projecting portion of the dashboard of an automobile, etc). Such injuries are treated in different ways depending upon whether or not there is prolapse of tissue.

A. Lacerations Without Prolapse of Tissue: If the eyeball has been penetrated anteriorly without evidence of prolapse of intraocular contents, and if the wound is clean and apparently free from contamination, it can usually be repaired by direct interrupted sutures of fine silk or catgut. Blood clots can be gently removed from the anterior chamber by irrigation and the chamber re-formed after corneal repair by injection of normal saline solution or air. A mydriatic should be used and an antibiotic solution instilled in the conjunctival sac, and bilateral eye bandages applied. The patient should be placed at bed rest for a few days and systemic antibiotics given to minimize the chance of intraocular infection.

B. Lacerations With Prolapse: If only a small portion of the iris prolapses through the wound, this should be grasped with a forceps and excised at the level of the wound lip. Small amounts of uveal tissue can be removed in a similar way. The wound should then be closed in the same manner as a wound without prolapse, and the same follow-up care given. If uveal

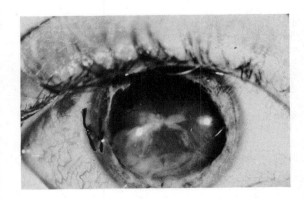

Figure 23–4. Corneal laceration with sutures in place. Note also traumatic cataract.

tissue has been injured, the possibility of sympathetic ophthalmia is always present.

If the wound has been extensive and loss of intraocular contents has been great enough that the prognosis for useful function is hopeless, evisceration or enucleation is indicated as the primary surgical procedure.

Intraocular Foreign Bodies (Fig 23–5)

Foreign bodies that have become lodged within the eye should be identified and localized as soon as possible. Particles of iron or copper must be removed to prevent later disorganization of ocular tissues by degenerative changes (siderosis from iron and chalcosis from copper). Some of the newer alloys are more inert and may be tolerated. Other kinds of particles, such as glass or porcelain, may be tolerated indefinitely and are usually better left alone.

A complaint of discomfort in the eye with blurred vision and a history of striking steel upon steel should arouse a strong suspicion of an intraocular foreign body. The anterior portion of the eye, including the cornea, iris, lens, and sclera, should be inspected with a loupe or slit lamp in an attempt to localize the wound of entry. Direct ophthalmoscopic visualization of an intraocular foreign body may be possible. An orbital soft tissue x-ray must be taken to verify the presence of a radiopaque foreign body as well as for medicolegal reasons.

Localizing x-rays can be obtained by several methods, usually by the method of Comberg, using a contact lens; or the method of Sweet, with a geometric calculation following accurate positioning of a guide post. By one of these special means the radiologist is able to plot the approximate position of the foreign body within the eye or orbit.

The Berman metal locator (see p 31) is an electronic instrument for detecting the presence of metals. It is useful in pinpointing an intraocular foreign body located near one of the accessible areas of the eyeball. The wand of the instrument can be sterilized and passed posteriorly over the exposed field at surgery.

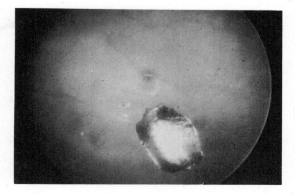

Figure 23–5. Ophthalmoscopic view of intraocular metallic (iron) foreign body in vitreous.

If the foreign body is anterior to the lens zonules, it should be removed through an incision into the anterior chamber at the limbus. If it is located behind the lens and anterior to the equator, it should be removed through the area of the pars plana that is nearest to the foreign body because less retinal damage is caused in that manner. If the foreign body is posterior to the equator, it should be removed directly through that point on the wall of the eyeball which is nearest to it, unless that area is at the macula.

If the foreign body has magnetic properties, the sterilized tip of a hand magnet (or giant magnet) near the area of exit can be used to facilitate its removal. If it is nonmagnetic and removal is essential, small forceps have been devised for introduction into the posterior portion of the eye with minimal displacement and trauma. A special instrument has been devised to grasp a spherical air rifle or shotgun pellet.

Any damaged area of the retina must be treated with diathermy or photocoagulation to prevent retinal detachment.

INJURIES TO THE LIDS

Many lacerations of the lid do not involve the margins and may be sutured in the same way as other lacerations of the skin. If the margin of the lid is involved, however, precautions must be taken to prevent marginal notching. The most effective technique is to freshen the lacerated edges by vertical incisions perpendicular to the lid margins through the full height of the tarsus. The incisions are then joined by a "V," thus forming a pentagonal wedge. The conjunctiva and tarsus are closed by interrupted gut sutures and the lid margin is carefully aligned with two 7-0 silk sutures: one in the posterior margin through the orifices of the meibomian glands and the other in the anterior lid margin through the lash line. The sutures are allowed to remain about 5 mm long and tied over the skin closure sutures to prevent their abrading the cornea.

If primary repair is not effected within 24 hours, edema may necessitate delayed closure. The wound should be cleansed well and antibiotics administered. After swelling has subsided, repair may be performed. Debridement should be minimized, especially if the skin is not lax.

Lacerations near the inner canthus frequently involve the canaliculi. Early repair is desirable, since the tissue becomes more difficult to identify with swelling. The upper canaliculus is rarely essential to lacrimal drainage and can often serve as the sole excretory path when the lower one has been destroyed. Nonetheless, it is preferable to repair such lacerations to prevent stricture. The Veirs rod is an effective canaliculus splint in some cases. The preferred method of repair is an encircling tube of silicone (Fig 23–6). A pigtail probe is used to identify the lumen of the severed canaliculus. Silicone tubing is threaded back through the common canaliculus and uninjured punctum. A nylon suture inside the silicone tubing is knotted and

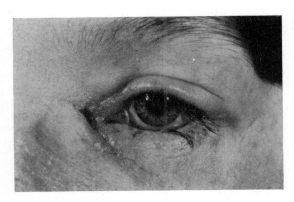

Figure 23–6. Laceration of upper and lower canaliculi and medial canthal region. Silicone tube encircling puncta: (Courtesy of J Sullivan.)

the encircling tube rotated to place the knot away from the palpebral opening. Alternatively, the 2 ends of the silicone tubing may be threaded from the 2 puncta with a Quickert probe through the nasolacrimal duct and knotted beneath the inferior turbinate in the nose. These tubes should be left in place for several weeks to months. They are easily removed without anesthetic.

INJURIES INVOLVING THE ORBIT & ITS CONTENTS

Bony Injury

Fractures of the walls of the orbit may be caused by direct blows or by extension of a fracture line from adjacent bones. The outer table of the frontal bone above the orbit may receive crushing injuries without damaging the orbital contents. Similarly, fractures and displacement of the zygomatic bone, nasal bone and accessory sinuses, and the medial wall of the orbit can be involved in depressed injuries of the face in automobile accidents. If a fracture involves the paranasal sinuses—most frequently the ethmoid bone—emphysema may be noted by crepitation on palpation. Such an involvement may be followed by the development of chronic osteomyelitis.

Blowout Fracture

Isolated orbital floor or "blowout" fracture, without concurrent orbital rim fracture, usually follows blunt injury to the eye. Orbital contents herniate into the maxillary sinus, and the inferior rectus or inferior oblique muscle may become incarcerated at the fracture site.

Signs and symptoms are pain and nausea at the time of injury and diplopia on looking up or down. The infraorbital nerve is frequently damaged and anesthesia is noted over the upper lip and gingiva. Enophthalmos (backward displacement of the eyeball) may not be present until the orbital edema subsides. The fracture site is best demonstrated by antral roof deformation on Waters' view x-rays or tomograms. There is limited movement of the eye even with forced ductions.

Prompt surgical reduction is indicated when a large bony defect can be demonstrated on radiography or is suspected because of enophthalmos and restricted upgaze. Forced duction is useful in distinguishing the vertical imbalance of entrapment from muscle contusion. If enophthalmos or restricted motility is not evident, surgical repair is not necessary even if a fracture can be demonstrated. Frequently, a decision cannot be made immediately after injury. There is little danger in waiting 7–10 days to evaluate surgical indications.

Two effective means of surgical treatment are available. A Caldwell-Luc antrostomy can be used for antral packing after direct reduction from below. Packing is generally left in place 2 weeks. Traction on the extraocular muscles by forceps or sling sutures will verify reduction. The fracture site may be approached through the lower lid along the orbital floor. In this instance, the prolapsed tissue is reduced and the orbital floor defect is bridged with a graft of bone, cartilage, or alloplastic material.

Penetrating Injury

Penetrating injuries of the orbital tissue may be produced by flying missiles or sharp instruments. Radiopaque foreign bodies can be localized by x-ray methods similar to those used in locating foreign bodies within the eye. Most orbital foreign bodies are best left alone.

Contusions

Contusion injuries to the orbital contents may result in hemorrhage or subsequent atrophy of the tissue, with enophthalmos. Traumatic paresis of the extraocular muscles occasionally occurs in this way but is usually transient.

Pulsating Exophthalmos

Pulsating exophthalmos occasionally follows a penetrating or contusion injury to the orbital contents that has caused a shunt between the arterial and venous channels so that the pulse is transmitted into the orbital tissues. (This condition may develop spontaneously but is more frequently traumatic in origin.) A common site of involvement is a fracture through the cavernous sinus.

Pulsating exophthalmos occasionally requires ligation of the carotid artery on the side of the aneurysm.

References

Benson WE, Machemer R: Severe perforating injuries treated with pars plana vitrectomy. *Am J Ophthalmol* 1976;**81**:728.

Brown SI, Rosen J: Scleral perforation. *Arch Ophthalmol* 1975;**93**:1047.

Brown SI et al: Treatment of the alkali-burned cornea. *Am J Ophthalmol* 1972;**74**:316.

Cinotti AA, Maltzman BA: Prognosis and treatment of perforating ocular injuries. *Ophthalmol Surg* 1975;**6**:54.

Coleman OJ: Early vitrectomy in the management of the severely traumatized eye. *Am J Ophthalmol* 1982;**93**:543.

Cullen GCR, Luce CM, Shannon GM: Blindness following blowout orbital fractures. *Ophthalmol Surg* 1977;**8**:60.

Dotan S, Oliver M: Shallow anterior chamber and uveal effusion after nonperforating trauma to the eye. *Am J Ophthalmol* 1982;**94**:782.

Eagling EM: Ocular damage after blunt trauma to the eye. *Br J Ophthalmol* 1974;**58**:126.

Eagling EM: Perforating injuries of the eye. *Br J Ophthalmol* 1976;**60**:732.

Edwards WC, Layden WE: Traumatic hyphema: A report of 184 consecutive cases. *Am J Ophthalmol* 1973;**75**:110.

Emery JM et al: Management of orbital floor fractures. *Am J Ophthalmol* 1972;**74**:299.

Grove AS: Computerized tomography in the management of orbital trauma ophthalmology. *Ophthalmology* 1982;**89**:433.

Helveston EM: Eye trauma in childhood. *Pediatr Clin North Am* 1975;**22**:501.

Hoefle FB: Initial treatment of eye injuries. *Arch Ophthalmol* 1968;**79**:33.

Holekamp TLR, Becker B: Ocular injuries from automobile batteries. *Trans Am Acad Ophthalmol Otolaryngol* 1977;**83**:805.

Jabaley ME, Lerman M, Sanders HJ: Ocular injuries in orbital fractures. *Plast Reconstr Surg* 1975;**56**:410.

McCord DW: Acute orbital trauma. In: *Oculoplastic Surgery.* Raven Press, 1981.

McKinlay RT, Cohen DN: Ophthalmic injuries: Handbook of initial evaluation and management. *Trans Am Acad Ophthalmol Otolaryngol* 1975;**79**:880.

Paton D, Goldberg MF: *Management of Ocular Injuries.* Saunders, 1976.

Percival SPB: A decade of intraocular foreign bodies. *Br J Ophthalmol* 1972;**56**:454.

Putterman AM: Late management of blowout fractures of the orbital floor. *Trans Am Acad Ophthalmol Otolaryngol* 1977;**83**:650.

Sanders N: Repair of corneal lacerations. *Ann Ophthalmol* 1975;**7**:1515.

Sutherland GR: B-scan echography in eye trauma. *Ophthalmol Digest,* April 15, 1976.

Sydnor CF et al: Traumatic superior oblique palsies. *Ophthalmology* 1982;**89**:134.

Yasuna E: Management of traumatic hyphema. *Arch Ophthalmol* 1974;**91**:190.

The science of optics may be divided into **physical** and **geometric.** Physical optics—the study of interference, diffraction, polarization, fluorescence, etc—is of little interest to the ophthalmologist and will not be discussed here. Geometric optics is the study of light rays as they are reflected or bent or changed as they pass through surfaces and media in which there is a change in their velocity, ie, a change of the index of refraction.

Geometric Optics

The laws of reflection and refraction were formulated in 1621 by the Dutch astronomer and mathematician Willebrord Snell at the University of Leyden. These, together with Fermat's principle (p 311), still form the basis of geometric optics. The laws can be stated as follows: (See Fig 24–1).

(1) Incident, reflected, and refracted rays all reside in a plane known as the plane of incidence, which is normal (at a right angle) to the interface.

(2) The angle of incidence equals the angle of reflection but has the opposite sign: $I = -I'$.

(3) Incident ray and refracted ray directions are related by the principle of **Snell's law:** The product of the index of refraction of the medium of the incident ray and the sine of the angle of incidence of the incident ray is equal to the product of the same terms of the refracted ray. The refracted ray is denoted by a prime: $n \sin I = n' \sin I'$.

Index of Refraction

The field of optics is replete with reciprocals. The 1/X key of calculators and computers is of great use in optics. The index of refraction, n, is no exception to this: it is the reciprocal of the speed of light in the substance compared to that in a vacuum (absolute index) or to air (relative index). The index of refraction of air varies with temperature, pressure, humidity, and frequency (color) of light but is about 1.00032 absolute. In optics, n is assumed to be relative to air unless otherwise stated. The slower the speed, the higher the index and the more potent the effect on refraction.

Thermal Coefficient of Index of Refraction

Temperature changes the index of refraction. It is higher when the substance is colder. This lability of n to temperature is different for different substances. The change in n per degree Celsius for the following substances (all to be multiplied by 10^{-7}) is as follows: glass 1, fluorite 10, plastics 140, water 185. This makes plastic undesirable for precision optical devices. (Plastic also has 8 times the thermal expansion of glass.) Water lenses date back to antiquity but are not practical because of their thermal instability, evaporation, freezing, and susceptibility to nonbiologic and biologic contamination. It is interesting that in the eye these objections nearly vanish, making the fluid lenses of the eye acceptable.

Dispersion

Fortunately, the speed of all frequencies (colors) of light is the same in a vacuum. Thus, in a vacuum, n is the same for all colors (1.00000). In all substances, n is different for each color or frequency, being larger at the blue end and smaller at the red end of the spectrum. A substance to be used with visual light is usually tested for n with yellow sodium light, giving n_d (index of refraction for yellow sodium light). It is then tested with light from a rarefied hydrogen discharge tube, which yields the blue f line and the red c line. This gives n_f (index of refraction for blue f line)

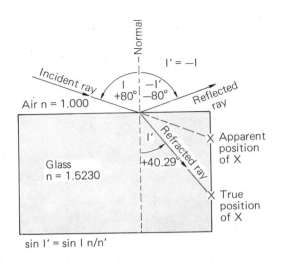

$\sin I' = \sin I \, n/n'$

Figure 24–1. Example of the laws of reflection and refraction.

Table 24—1. Indices of refraction and dispersion values of some substances of ophthalmologic interest.

	Indices of Refraction (n)	Dispersion Values (V)
Water 37 °C	1.33093	55.6
Water 20 °C	1.33299	
Polymethylmethacrylate	1.49166	57.37
Acrylonitrile styrene copolymer	1.56735	34.87
Polystyrene	1.59027	30.92
Fluorite	1.4338	95.2
Spectacle crown glass	1.5230	58.8
Flint glass	1.6170	36.6
Aqueous and vitreous	1.336	
Hydroxyethylmethacrylate (HEMA)	1.430	
Cellulose acetate butyrate (CAB)	1.470	
Silicone	1.439	

and n_c (index of refraction for red c line). The dispersion value, V, is

$$\frac{n_d - 1}{n_f - n_c}$$

The higher the value of V, the less the dispersion of colors. Table 24–1 gives the indices of refraction and some dispersion values for substances of ophthalmologic interest.

Transmittance

Optical materials vary in their transmittance or transparency to different frequencies. "Transparent" material such as glass is almost opaque to ultraviolet light. Red glass would be almost opaque to the green frequency. Special selections must be made for special purposes.

Speed, Frequency, & Wavelength of Light

In optical substances, speed and wavelength of light change but frequency is constant. Color depends on frequency, so that color is not changed by passing through optical media.

$$\text{Frequency} = \frac{\text{Speed}}{\text{Wavelength}}$$

is the relationship of the 3 values. The speed of light in a vacuum is 299,792.8 kilometers per second, or 186,282.4 statute miles per second. The frequency of the yellow d line is approximately 5.085×10^{14} Hz. The wavelength, λ in a vacuum of the blue f line is 0.4861 μm, of the d line is 0.5896 μm, and of the red c line is 0.6563 μm.

Critical Angle

In Fig 24–1, consider the ray in the more dense medium as the arriving ray. We see it is refracted into the less dense medium away from the normal. If we gradually increase the angle of incidence (Fig 24–2) in

the more dense medium until we reach the critical angle, a startling event takes place: None of the light escapes, but all is suddenly, totally, and perfectly reflected. This angle is reached as the sine of the incident ray in the more dense media reaches the value n'/n. This is one method used to determine the index of refraction. For water with an index of refraction of 1.330, the critical angle has the sine of 1/1.330, or 48.75 degrees.

Total Reflection

If the angle of incidence is greater than the critical angle, the sine becomes greater than 1. Sines over 1 are a "tilt" in mathematics and "not allowed"—another of the many examples of the way in which mathematics, as if by magic, corresponds to the real world. Prior to experiment, one would wonder what would happen to the "refracted" ray when its sine becomes greater than 1, as may occur. Incredibly, the refracted ray ceases to exist!

Total reflection obeys the laws of regular reflection, ie, $I = -I'$. This allows perfect reflection without coatings and is used extensively in prisms and fiberoptics.

In Fig 24–2, the shaded area is not visible from the surface. This is why the angle of the eye is invisible until the gonioscopic lens (Chapter 3) is used.

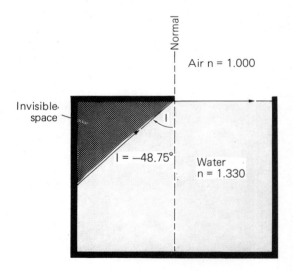

Figure 24–2. Example of the critical angle.

Prisms

In ophthalmology, prisms are used with the nearer face normal to the visual axis, which is not the classic minimal deviation angle of a symmetric prism usually given in texts on optics. Thus, prism equations are slightly different for ophthalmology. Fig 24–3 represents a prism as used in ophthalmology. The eye is to the left of the prism. This solution demonstrates an important point in optics: one may trace rays forward or backward with no change in results. In the example,

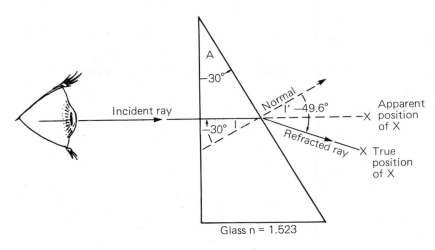

Figure 24–3. Example of the prism as used in ophthalmology.

it is easier to trace the ray as if it emanates from the eye to the object (as was once popularly believed). The ray strikes the prism and is not refracted by the first surface, as the ray is normal to this surface. At the second surface, the angle of incidence is seen to be the same as A, the vertex angle. From Snell's law, $\sin I' = n/n' \sin A$. For example, if the prism is of glass with $n = 1.523$ and $A = 30$ degrees, then $\sin I'$ is 1.523×0.5, or 0.7615. I' is 49.6 degrees. The angle of deviation is $I'-A$, or 19.6 degrees. An object seen through the prism appears deviated toward the apex A, or away from the base. The power of a prism is measured in prism diopters (Δ). One prism diopter deviates an image 1 cm at 1 m. The arc tangent of 1/100 is 0.57 degrees. So 1 Δ is almost one-half degree. The "rule of thumb" is that 2 Δ equals 1 degree.

Prism Use

Prisms are used in ophthalmology both to measure and to treat heterotropia and heterophoria (see Chapter 15). The prism is prescribed as magnitude in prism diopters and direction of the base, ie, "base-up right eye," "base-down left eye," "base-in," or "base-out." Prisms may be prescribed by the angle of the base in the usual mathematical way. Thus, we start at 0 degrees on the horizontal, nasally for the right eye (base-in) counterclockwise facing the patient to 360 degrees (Fig 24–4A). The zero axis begins with the left eye on the horizontal line temporally. Prisms obey vector laws. Thus, 4Δ base-out right eye (180 degrees) combined with 2Δ base-down right eye (270 degrees) will result by vector addition in 4.47Δ base 206 degrees. Vector addition is explained in the manual of any calculator capable of polar to rectangular and rectangular to polar operations. Conversely, if we change 206 degrees, 4.47Δ to its rectangular coordinates, we get X = –4 and Y = –2. This is our original 4-prism base-out right eye and 2 prism diopters base-down.

Fermat's Principle

In 1657, Pierre de Fermat restated Hero of Alexandria's 2000-year-old principle as follows: "A ray of light traversing a route from one point to another follows the path that takes the least time to negotiate." Optical path length is the index of refraction times the actual path length. This principle is used for other optical equations and by calculus confirms Snell's law.

Two Methods of Calculations Used in Optics

The study of geometric optics can be approached in 2 ways: the first is the meticulous method of **trigonometric ray tracing;** the second is the approximate **algebraic method.** Most courses in general physics, most books on physiologic optics, most books on refraction, most ophthalmology residency programs, and most postgraduate "continuing education" courses stress only the algebraic method. The trigonometric method, if mentioned at all, is usually dismissed as being too complicated for practical application. However, it must be emphasized here that *the optical problems the practicing ophthalmologist must confront—contact lenses, intraocular lenses, surgery that changes the shape of the eye, etc—cannot be dealt with using the algebraic method alone.* Fortunately, the tedium and complexity of ray tracing have been dramatically reduced in modern times by the ready availabilty of computers and programmable calculators. We shall discuss the algebraic method first, since this is "classic optics" in ophthalmology at present.

Algebraic Method

Correct trigonometric optical methods were well known in the time of the mathematician Karl Friedrich Gauss (1777–1855). The calculations were very time-consuming, as they involved multiple use of logarithm and trigonometry tables for each calculation. Gauss developed a method that in the beginning

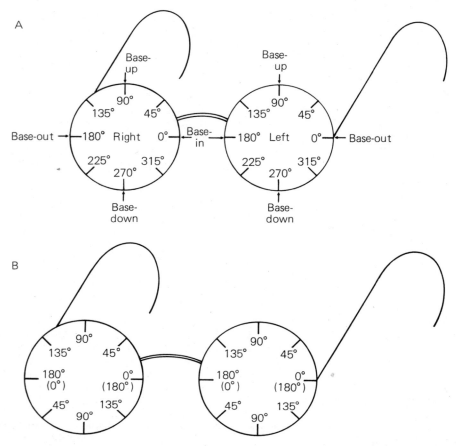

Figure 24–4. *A:* Illustration of prism base notation. *B:* Illustration of cylinder axis notation.

was far more simple and gave reasonable results if applied to very thin lenses with very small diameters placed very close together. In fact, the restrictions are for "infinitely thin lenses," etc. By assuming these mythical conditions, we rid the equations of sines and cosines and no longer must use the tables. The restraints allow one to assume that any angle involved will be so small, measured in radians, that it will have the same value as the sine of the angle. Also, the sine and the tangent of the angle will be close enough to be assumed to be the same. From this, Gauss derived the general thin lens equations, also called the "lensmaker's formulas," used by opticians to calculate curves for lenses. "Fudge factors" will be found at the bench of the optician and the "lathe man" for contact lenses to enter corrections shown by experience to help correct inaccuracies in the equations. These equations must not be used to calculate complicated thick lens systems such as those of the eye.

Fig 24–5 shows some of the important thin lens algebraic equations.

Vertex Change

If a lens of a given power at a given distance from the eye is changed to a different distance from the eye (vertex distance), it will have a different effect. To calculate a new lens that will have the same effect at the new distance, we may use the following equation:

$$Dio \simeq \frac{1}{\frac{1}{Dio_1} - (Dist_1 - Dist_2)}$$

Example 1: A +13 diopter lens at 11 mm (0.011 m) is to be replaced by a lens at 9 mm (0.009 m)

$$Dio_2 \simeq \frac{1}{\frac{1}{13} - (0.011 - 0.009)} \simeq 13.347 \text{ diopters}$$

Example 2: Same lens to be replaced by a contact lens

$$Dist_2 = 0$$

$$Dio \simeq \frac{1}{\frac{1}{13} - (0.011)} \simeq 15.169 \text{ diopters}$$

Remember that the vertex equation is also an approximate equation. It is used incorrectly for intraocular lens calculations, which partially explains why different authors using the equation arrive at different results.

The often-quoted statement that a lens at the "anterior focal plane" of the eye gives no magnification or minification is not valid. The anterior focal plane location has no more significance than any other location.

In an attempt to make the lensmaker's formula more accurate for thicker lenses, a "thick lens equation" (below) has been derived. It is still an algebraic approximation but will give more accurate results for making high plus contacts or thick spectacle lenses.

$$\text{Dio} \simeq \frac{1}{F} \simeq (n-1)\left[\frac{1}{R_1} - \frac{1}{R_2} - \frac{(n-1)d}{nR_1R_2}\right]$$

where F = focal length, R = radius, and d = thickness of lens, all measured in meters.

The sign convention for the radius of curvature varies from author to author. The above formulas agree with the sign convention as used by Conrady (an authority in the field) and will be described in our discussion of ray tracing. One other equation that may be of interest to the practicing ophthalmologist is the conversion of "diopters" to radius of curvature with contact lenses, since it is based on the above equations.

$$\text{Dio} \simeq \frac{(n-1)}{R} \simeq \frac{1.3375 - 1}{R} \simeq \frac{337.5}{Rmm} \text{ and } Rmm \simeq \frac{337.5}{\text{Dio}}$$

n of "cornea" is for this purpose assumed to be 1.3375. Rmm = radius in millimeters.

The algebraic equations of Gauss do not all remain simple (as above) but may become very complex. They may be used with complicated matrix methods. This may lead one to the erroneous conclusion that because of their complexity they are accurate. One may not want to spend hours of study on these complex methods if one is aware of their limitations. These are the equations that involve principal planes, principal points, nodal points, etc. When these terms are mentioned in works on optics, one knows that the algebraic method was employed and that the results are not reliable. Magnification by these equations also results in incorrect answers when the results are applied to ophthalmologic optics. Again, this can save hours of study. Sylvanus P. Thompson (1851–1916), an English physicist, called these calculations "examination optics," involving mathematical acrobatics, as opposed to "real optics." A caution is required at this point. Nearly all examinations given today in ophthalmology courses in medical school are based on thin lens algebraic methods. The student should be prepared to use algebra for examinations (at present) but should learn how to use trigonometric methods when seeking "right answers" in the spirit of the quotation of SP Thompson about 70 years ago.

Diopter

As indicated in the above equations, the diopter is a measure of lens power. It was first introduced in 1872 by Felix Monoyer, a French ophthalmologist. It is defined as the reciprocal of the focal length measured in air in meters. Diopters are supposedly additive, such that a +2 diopter lens combined with a +1 diopter lens results in almost a +3 diopter lens. Combine this pair with a −1 diopter lens, and the result is nearly 2 diopters, and so on. This breaks down for lenses of higher power. Thus, a "+20 diopter" lens plus a "+40 diopter" lens are not even close to a "+60 diopter" lens. The result also varies greatly with the separation distance and with thickness. The phrase "60-diopter lens" has almost no meaning, because the powers at the edge, middle, and center portions are vastly different. "Diopter" is also an algebraic approximation concept and not acceptable when calculating lens systems such as those that make up the eye. *Strong lenses must be described by 3 values:* (1) radii of curvatures, (2) index of refraction, and (3) thickness.

Curvature

Curvature *(c)* is a term used by optical engineers to express a function similar to diopters in that it increases with a lens power and is approximately additive. It is the reciprocal of radius. It is useful in "bending" lenses, which is frequently done to achieve a better image. "Bending" a lens changes both curves, keeping effective power the same. The effective power of the lens will remain about the same if curvature 1 minus curvature 2 is kept constant.

Trigonometric Ray Tracing

Not every ophthalmologist who does refractions will choose to acquire facility with ray tracing. However, every reader of this book should know of its existence and should know that *ray tracing is the correct method for calculating complex lens systems*. Those who become familiar with the technique of ray tracing will be rewarded with a powerful tool in optics: Complex lens systems can be "made" mathematically and tested without the expense of actual production, and many controversial questions can be resolved with minimal effort.

Object of Ray Tracing

In ray tracing, the important components of the calculations are the radius of curvature of each surface, the index of refraction of each substance, and the thickness, or the distance to the next surface. If these data are available, any ray can be traced through the system to the final image. The 3 rays most frequently traced are shown in Fig 24–6: the paraxial ray, very near the optical axis (center of the lens); the marginal ray, at the margin of the lens; and the zonal ray, which passes through the lens at the portion where the average luminous flux ("volume") of light passes. By finding where these rays "focus" or cross the optical axis, much is determined about the lens system. The spread indicates the spherical aberration. The spread for various colors indicates the chromatic aberration. The optical pathway, as mentioned previously, is the sum of the actual distances a ray passes through the

Algebraic Thin Lens Approximations
($\simeq$ indicates approximation) (all lengths in meters)

$$\text{Diopters} \simeq \frac{1}{\text{Focal length}} \simeq \frac{1}{\text{Distance of image}} - \frac{1}{\text{Distance of object}}$$

$$\text{Diopters} \simeq (n-1)\ \frac{1}{\text{Radius}_1} - \frac{1}{\text{Radius}_2}$$

$$\frac{\text{Size of image}}{\text{Distance of image}} \simeq \frac{\text{Size of object}}{\text{Distance of object}}$$

$$\text{Magnification} = \frac{\text{Size of image}}{\text{Size of object}} \simeq \frac{\text{Distance of image}}{\text{Distance of object}}$$

Power for Several Lenses Combined
(Diopters total $\simeq \text{Dio}_1 + \text{Dio}_2 + \text{Dio}_3$, etc)

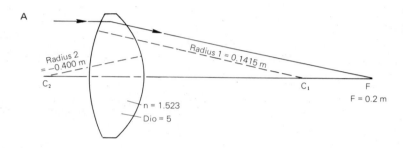

Example Figure 24–5A   Radius 1 = 0.1415
Radius 2 = −0.400
n = 1.523

$$\text{Dio} \simeq 0.523 \left(\frac{1}{0.1415} - \frac{1}{-0.4} \right) \simeq 5 \text{ diopters}$$

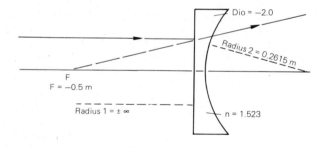

Example Figure 24–5B   Radius 1 = ∞
Radius 2 = 0.2615
n = 1.523

$$\text{Dio} \simeq 0.523 \left(\frac{1}{\infty} - \frac{1}{0.2615} \right) \simeq -2 \text{ diopters}$$

Example Figure 24–5A lens combined with Figure 24–5B lens

Diopters total $\simeq 5 - 2 \simeq 3$ diopters

Figure 24–5. A: Algebraic approximation to determine diopters power of biconvex lens. B: Algebraic approximation to determine diopters power of plano-concave lens.

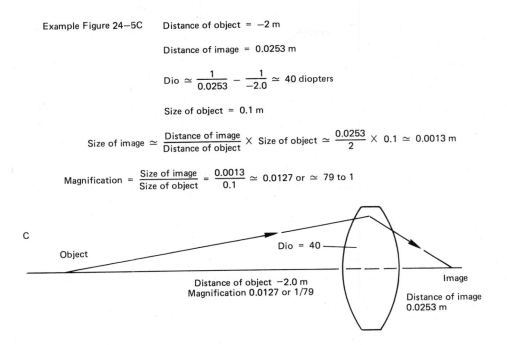

Example Figure 24—5C   Distance of object = −2 m

Distance of image = 0.0253 m

$$\text{Dio} \simeq \frac{1}{0.0253} - \frac{1}{-2.0} \simeq 40 \text{ diopters}$$

Size of object = 0.1 m

$$\text{Size of image} \simeq \frac{\text{Distance of image}}{\text{Distance of object}} \times \text{Size of object} \simeq \frac{0.0253}{2} \times 0.1 \simeq 0.0013 \text{ m}$$

$$\text{Magnification} = \frac{\text{Size of image}}{\text{Size of object}} = \frac{0.0013}{0.1} \simeq 0.0127 \text{ or} \simeq 79 \text{ to } 1$$

C

Object

Dio = 40

Distance of object −2.0 m
Magnification 0.0127 or 1/79

Image

Distance of image
0.0253 m

Figure 24—5 (cont'd). *C:* Algebraic approximation to determine diopters power and magnification of a biconvex lens.

substances multiplied by the index of refraction in the various substances through which it passes. If the optical pathways of the marginal ray and the paraxial ray have similar values, they give a bright image with good contrast. If the optical pathways differ by many wavelengths, they are out of phase and tend to cancel one another. By ray tracing, one may determine the "goodness" or "badness" of each surface relative to its contribution to the final image. Thus, an intraocular lens gives a better image with the convex surface forward and the flat surface closer to the retina. Lens parameters may be changed in various ways to improve the result. The precise focus of even complicated systems may be calculated by ray tracing. This point of

Marginal ray

Zonal ray

Paraxial ray

Axis

Figure 24—6. Illustration of 3 rays frequently traced.

focus could be changed by what ophthalmologists call refracting. *However, the distorted image caused by selecting an intraocular lens of improper shape cannot be repaired by refracting.* The use of algebraic methods will not indicate any of these features.

Method of Ray Tracing

The classic reference for ray tracing is *Applied Optics and Optical Design,* by Alexander Eugen Conrady, Volume 1, published in 1929. Volume 2 was delayed by the death of the author but was completed and published in 1960 by Conrady's son-in-law, Rudolf Kingslake. Kingslake studied under Conrady at the Imperial College in London, was Director of Optical Design at Eastman Kodak Company for 30 years, and taught lens design in the Institute of Optics at the University of Rochester for about 45 years. Kingslake's book, *Lens Design Fundamentals,* published in 1977, presents modern methods of ray tracing utilizing computers and programmable calculators that were of course not available at the time of the classic edition. The classic equations are still valid, however, and have been used many times by this author, yielding the same results as the modern edition equations. The modern equations will be utilized in the following discussion.

What follows is intended for those who choose to utilize ray tracing. It will be necessary to program a computer or calculator or obtain programs for the method. The signs and labels of the various functions are very important (Fig 24—7).

There is a graphic method of ray tracing that lacks the precision of the computer method but is precise enough, if done with care, to determine the correct

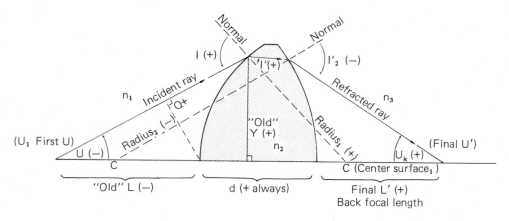

Figure 24–7. Ray tracing notation and signs.

power of an intraocular lens. It is therefore discussed under that heading later in this chapter.

As mentioned above, the 3 most important arriving rays are the marginal ray, which enters the first surface near its margin; the zonal ray, which enters the first surface at that distance from the center that equals the square root of 0.5 times the semidiameter of the lens; and the paraxial ray, near the axis. Any small value may be used for the paraxial ray, but 0.01 times the semidiameter of the lens is an acceptable value to use. Only English letters are used, and capitals are used for values except n, the index of refraction, and those values pertaining to the paraxial rays, for which small letters are used. Vowels are used for angles. Consonants are used for distances. Y is treated as a consonant. Solid lines are used before refraction and dashed lines after refraction. Regular letters are used before refraction and primed letters after refraction. This creates some small confusion, for the refracted ray at the first surface, which would have the prime, is the nonrefracted or arriving ray at the second (emerging) surface. The prime is dropped as a transfer for the second surface. Distances are measured from the intersection of the vertex of the surface and the optical axis, *measured along the optical axis*. Distances are minus to the left of this point. L is the distance of the arriving ray and was used in the old system. Q is now used as an opener instead of L. Q is a distance measured from a perpendicular to the arriving ray reaching the vertex. Its method of derivation will follow momentarily. U is the angle of the arriving ray relative to the optical axis. It was and still is an opener for the equations. U is positive if a ruler moves clockwise from the optical axis to the ray (converging ray if above the axis). Q is then defined as $L \sin U$. For infinite or parallel rays, L is infinite and $\sin U$ is zero. In this case, simply enter Q as the height of the ray (the Y of the old system). The radius of curvature of the surface is R. This is positive if the center of curvature is to the right of the surface. Therefore, the corneal curve would be positive, and the last curve of the lens of the eye would be negative. In the old system, R was used directly; in the new

system, curvature (c) is used. The reciprocal of R is c. The final L' is an important distance, as it is the final back focal length, ie, the distance of the focus from the last surface. The final U' is an important angle, for it determines magnification, as will be shown later. I is the angle of incidence, and I' is the angle of incidence of the refracted ray. I and I' are positive if a ruler must be turned clockwise from the ray to reach the normal (or radius). The sign of I is measured in an opposite fashion to that of U, which seems confusing, but efforts to avoid the confusion have created even worse confusion. U is the more important definition to remember. Think of I as the contrary one.

The old equations were less intimidating, but the new ones, set forth below, move faster through the computer. For the opening of the computation—given c of the first surface, n to the left of the first surface, n' to the right of the first surface, Q of the arriving ray, U of the arriving ray, and d, the distance to the next surface—we immediately calculate $\sin U$ and $\cos U$ and store them. The following equations are then programmed, using the results from the upper equations to fill in values in lower equations. G is an internal value to be stored and used. Its definition and the derivation of these equations may be found in the references cited. Initial $Q = L \sin U$.

(1) $\sin I = Qc - \sin U$
(2) $\cos I = (1 - \sin^2 I)^{1/2}$
(3) $\sin (U + I) = \sin U \cos I + \cos U \sin I$
(4) $\cos (U + I) = \cos U \cos I - \sin U \sin I$
(5) $\sin (-I') = -(n/n') \sin I$
(6) $\cos I' = [1 - \sin^2 (-I')]^{1/2}$
(7) $\sin U' = \sin (U + I) \cos (-I') + \cos (U + I) \sin (-I')$
(8) $\cos U' = \cos (U + I) \cos (-I') - \sin (U + I) \sin (-I')$
(9) $G = Q/(\cos U + \cos I)$
(10) $Q' = G (\cos U' + \cos I')$
(11) $Q_2 = Q_1 - d \sin U'_1$

Sin U' and the cos U' are carried over for the next surface as $\sin U$ and $\cos U$.

The lens system is methodically worked through for a ray from surface to surface. After the final surface, the final L' is desired for the back focal length. The equation for this is as follows:

$$\text{Final } L' = \frac{\text{Final } Q'}{\text{Final sin } U'}$$

If at any time the point of incidence is desired in X,Y coordinates measured from the vertex point, the following equations may be used:

$$Y = \frac{\sin (U + I)}{c} \text{ or } Y = G \ [1 + \cos (U + I)]$$

$$X = \frac{[1 - \cos (U + I)]}{c} \text{ or } X = G \sin (U + I)$$

If during any calculation sin I becomes greater than 1 (not allowed), it means the ray missed the lens surface. If the sin I' becomes greater than 1, it indicates total internal reflection.

The optical pathway equation for the marginal ray as compared with the paraxial ray for each surface is as follows:

$$OPD'_m = \frac{(Q - Q') \ n \ \sin \ I}{4 \ \cos \ \tfrac{1}{2}U \ \cos \ \tfrac{1}{2}I \ \cos \ \tfrac{1}{2}U' \ \cos \ \tfrac{1}{2}I'}$$

OPD'_m is in millimeters or in inches, depending on the units used. For wavelengths (λ), multiply this by 2000 for millimeters and by 50,000 for inches. The final OPD'_m is the sum of the OPD'_m for each surface. This is an excellent way to determine what help or hindrance each surface will contribute to the quality of the final image.

Proportionality Principle

Optics, unlike mechanics but like geometry and mathematics, follows the laws of proportionality. Thus, a well-designed lens will function just as well if all components are made many times larger or smaller. A model eye could be constructed the size of a swimming pool, with all structures relative and the quality of the image—eg, in aphakia with glasses, with contact lenses, or with intraocular lenses—studied, and the results would be valid.

Magnification

Linear magnification is the ratio of the height of the image to the height of the object. For an infinitely thin lens in air, this ratio is equal to the ratio of the distance of the image to the distance of the object. However, as usual, these relations are not valid for the eye. For real lens systems such as those of the eye, one must make use of the **LaGrange invariant.** LaGrange (1736–1813) found that the height, H, times the index of refraction, n, times the sine of the angle of the ray, sin U, results in a constant for any ray as it is traced through the system. The initial conditions at the object are noted by subscript 1, and subscript k represents the

final conditions at the image. The final magnification of the system is then derived by the following equation:

$$M = \frac{n_1 \ \sin \ U_1}{n_k \ \sin \ U_k}$$

Note that the index of refraction of the vitreous, n_k of 1.336, is involved.

The initial U_1 and final U_k are obtained from the ray tracing equations. In any system, only the initial and the final U and the initial and final n are required. Longitudinal magnification $\overline{M}$, which we are not as concerned with, has a different equation:

$$\overline{M} = \frac{n_1 \ (\sin \ U_1)^2}{n_k \ (\sin \ U_k)^2}$$

This explains the difference in perspective with a wide-angle lens and a telephoto lens. Portraits taken with a wide-angle lens are usually not flattering. The claim in the literature that, "$\overline{M} = M^2$," is not correct.

OPTICS & THE EYE

The ancients believed that some sort of sensory rays emanated from the eye and detected objects as if by feeling them. Then, before the time of Johannes Kepler (1571–1630), the eye was thought of as a miniature camera obscura. The camera obscura was usually a dark room with a small hole in one wall that cast an inverted image of the scene against the opposite wall. No lenses were used. Kepler suggested that the cornea and lens together refracted the rays and formed the image on the retina. Christopher Scheiner (1579–1650) made the first measurement of corneal curvature. He also demonstrated the small image of objects formed on the posterior surface of enucleated animal eyes. The concept that the image on the retina is focused by 2 lens elements, the cornea contributing about 43 diopters and the lens the remaining 19 diopters, is still widely entertained today. A little reflection and study of Fig 24–8 will show that a 3-lens system is a more realistic concept. All 3 lenses satisfy the thick lens definition: the aqueous lens, the lens lens, and the vitreous lens. In Fig 24–8, these 3 lenses are illustrated "prior to assembly" and then "assembled." The assembly is similar to a cemented system of lenses in cameras.

Contrary to popular belief, the cornea has almost no power of refraction in the optical system of the eye. Since the cornea has been regarded as the most important "lens" of the eye for over 300 years, some explanation and proof is in order. The cornea is important optically only in shaping the anterior curve of the aqueous lens. If the cornea is removed mathematically but the aqueous is kept in its former shape, ray tracing methods will reveal that the image location and quality are for all practical purposes the same. Further proof of this concept can be obtained by considering 3 glass

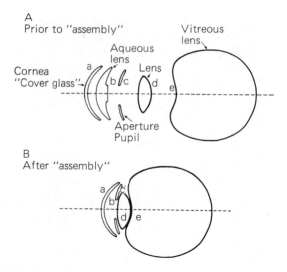

A
Prior to "assembly"

Vitreous lens

Aqueous lens

Cornea
"Cover glass"

Lens

a
b c
d
e

Aperture
Pupil

B
After "assembly"

a
b c
d e

Figure 24–8. The optical system of the eye illustrating the 3-lens concept.

flasks of almost spherical shape (Fig 24–9). Each flask is identical. The "empty" flask of air has almost no refractive power. The flask filled with water is a strong convex lens. The flask filled with carbon bisulfide is a very strong convex lens. The actual values by ray tracing are illustrated. The index of refraction of the glass container has almost no effect, whereas the index of refraction of the fluid content of the flask accounts almost entirely for the lens power of the flasks. In an analogous manner, the eye without the lens has almost no refractive power if filled with air. Its refractive power is then dependent on the filling fluid—just like the flasks. The index of refraction of the tears and the cornea has almost no importance to the refraction system of the eye.

The aqueous is a very powerful thick lens. If it is removed (replaced by air), the effect on refraction is striking. This also may be calculated by ray tracing techniques.

The lens lens (crystalline lens), the second lens of the ocular system, is the most baffling member of the

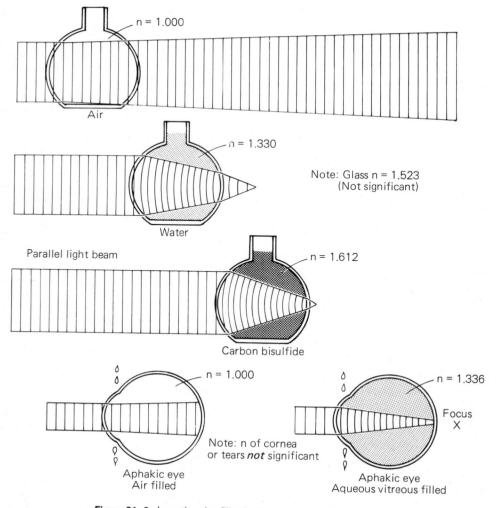

$n = 1.000$

Air

$n = 1.330$

Note: Glass $n = 1.523$
(Not significant)

Water

Parallel light beam

$n = 1.612$

Carbon bisulfide

$n = 1.000$

$n = 1.336$

Focus
X

Note: n of cornea
or tears **not** significant

Aphakic eye
Air filled

Aphakic eye
Aqueous vitreous filled

Figure 24–9. In optics the filler is significant, not the wrapper.

ocular refracting system. The equations used in optical calculations depend on a constant index of refraction for any one element. They also assume either spherical surfaces or surfaces with stable configurations and optical properties. The crystalline lens does not satisfy either of these requirements. The index of refraction of the lens changes like that of a syrup and water mixture, since the lens is more dense near the center. Various approximations have been made in an effort to create a hypothetical lens that might be used in ray tracing calculations. Once the lens is removed, as by cataract extraction, the mathematical curse vanishes and the aphakic eye may then be studied using conventional optical equations. Thus, aphakic correction by glasses, contact lenses, and intraocular lenses may be studied as to quality of image, magnification, and focus.

The third lens of the eye system is the vitreous lens. In a camera system, this would be the largest, heaviest, most expensive, and most important lens. When this lens is removed (replaced by air), there is a profound change in the refraction system of the eye. This too, of course, may be calculated by ray tracing. The vitreous has a major effect on magnification that is frequently ignored.

The reader must be cautioned again that the present examination system in medical school ophthalmology courses assumes the validity of the 2-lens theory, ie, the cornea as the main lens and the crystalline lens as the secondary lens.

Accommodation

The eye changes refractive power to focus on near objects by a process called accommodation. Thomas Young helped explain the principles of accommodation in 1801. Young himself had very prominent eyes. He was able to place one blade of a pair of calipers on his cornea and the other blade on the posterior pole of his eye. He claimed that he noted no increase in the size of the retinal scotoma from the caliper pressure when he accommodated. This discredited the theory that the eye accommodated by lengthening. Purkinje in 1823 described the various images reflected from the optical surfaces in the eye. Many observers have shown that the images from the lens change during accommodation. Contraction of the ciliary muscle results in thickening and increased curvature of the lens. This is probably due to relaxation of the elastic lens capsule. In the 3-lens concept, this causes a decrease in thickness and an increase in posterior curvature of the aqueous lens; an increase in thickness and both curvatures of the lens lens; and a slight decrease in thickness and an increase in anterior curvature of the vitreous lens. These peculiar changing fluid lenses are strangers to optical engineers.

Visual Acuity

Testing the function of the peripheral retina by visual field testing is described briefly in Chapter 3. Foveal vision is assessed by testing the ability to distinguish small objects. By tradition, Alcor, the second star in the handle of the Big Dipper, and its optical

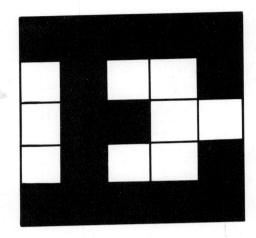

Figure 24–10. Snellen block E.

double, Mizar, have been used to determine "good vision." Since these stars are separated by 11.8 minutes of arc, they do not make a very demanding test of visual acuity. (This angle has not changed significantly during the history of the human race, as the 2 stars travel together.) Visual acuity is usually tested with the Snellen chart, also described in Chapter 3. The Snellen letters or block Es (Fig 24–10) are made from squares of 5 by 5 units. For "normal" vision, the eye should discriminate a letter with the total block size of 5 minutes of angle, or 1 minute angle per square of information. Thus, a person with "normal vision" could perceive a double star of 1 minute separation or could determine, for example, that an *F* is an *F* not a *P* if the whole letter is 5 minutes high or wide. Acuity is noted as a fraction: 6/6 (20/20), 6/12 (20/40), etc. Distance visual acuity is usually measured at 6 meters (or 20 feet); this is the numerator of the fraction. The denominator represents the distance at which a letter that size would make a visual angle of 5 minutes. Thus, a 6/6 (20/20) size letter has a visual angle of 5 minutes at 6 meters or 20 feet. A 6/12 (20/40) size letter has a visual angle of 10 minutes at 6 meters, etc. Another approach would be to say that a person with 6/12 (20/40) visual acuity can discriminate a size of letter at 6 meters (20 feet) that a person with 6/6 (20/20) vision could discriminate at 12 meters (40 feet). The letters must have good contrast and be illuminated by sufficient light (800 to 1000 lux or about 80 to 100 footcandles).

The 6/6 or 20/20 letter at 6 meters (20 feet) is about 8.7 mm or 0.35 inches high and wide. By ray tracing, one finds that the eye minifies an image at 6 meters (20 feet) by 351 times. Therefore, the size of the 6/6 (20/20) letter on the retina is 0.025 mm high and wide. Photographic films are often rated for resolution ability by lines per millimeter. Since it takes a line and a space to make each line, the size of the line and the space on the retina at 6/3 (20/10) visual acuity is 0.005 mm, or 200 lines per millimeter. Any lens system has a limit to the resolving power determined by diffraction. The sine of this limiting angle in radians is 0.61 times the wavelength of the light divided by the diameter of the aperture.

Remember that wavelength is smaller in the vitreous by a factor of $\lambda/1.336$. For a 6-mm pupil and the 0.00056-mm wavelength in air, the absolute limit is 0.29 seconds, or 345 lines per millimeter. The eye is an excellent optical instrument and comes close to its theoretical limit of resolving power.

REFRACTIVE ERRORS

The terms **emmetropia,** having no refractive error, and **ametropia,** having a refractive error, are used infrequently at present. Refractive errors are illustrated in Figs 24–11 and 24–12.

Presbyopia

The loss of accommodation that comes to all people is called presbyopia (Table 24–2). A person with emmetropic eyes (no refractive errors) will begin to notice an inability to read small print or discriminate fine close objects at about age 44–46. This is worse in dim light and usually worse early in the morning or when the subject is fatigued. Many people complain of a feeling of sleepiness when reading. These symptoms increase until about age 55, when they stabilize but persist. This is a major annoyance, but no more than that, whereas *before glasses became available, presbyopia had a devastating effect on the performance and well-being of the race.*

Presbyopia is corrected simply by use of a plus lens to make up for the lost automatic focusing power of the lens. This is analogous to the close-up lens of a camera. The plus lens may be used in several ways. Reading glasses have the near correction in the entire aperture of the glasses, making them fine for reading but blurred for distant objects. This requires putting them on for near vision and taking them off for far vision. Half-glasses can be worn to abate this nuisance by leaving the top open and uncorrected for distance vision. Bifocals do the same but allow correction of other refractive errors. Trifocals correct the distance vision by the top segment, the middle distance by the middle section, and the near distance by the lower segment.

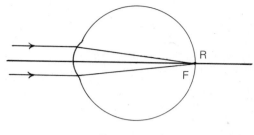

Emmetropia

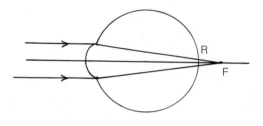

Hyperopia

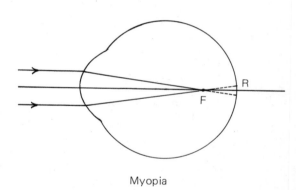

Myopia

Figure 24–11. Emmetropia, hyperopia, and myopia. F = focal point; R = retina.

Myopia

When the image of distant objects focuses in front of the retina in the unaccommodated eye, the eye is myopic or nearsighted. If the eye is longer than average, the error is called axial myopia. If the refractive elements are more refractive than average, the error is called curvature myopia or refractive myopia. As the object is brought closer than 6 meters, the image moves closer to the retina and comes into sharper focus. The point reached where the image is most sharply focused on the retina is called the "far point." One may estimate the extent of myopia by measuring the far point. Thus, a far point of 0.25 m would suggest a 4-diopter minus lens correction for distance. The myopic person has the advantage of being able to read at the far point without glasses even at the age of presbyopia.

Table 24–2. Table of accommodation.

Age (Years)	Mean Accommodation (Diopters)
8	13.8
25	9.9
35	7.3
40	5.8
45	3.6
50	1.9
55	1.3

Concave spherical (minus) lenses are used to correct the image in myopia. These lenses move the image back to the retina. One may detect a minus lens by looking through it 0.5 m (19 inches) or so from the eye and moving the lens at right angles to the visual axis. The image seen through the lens will tend to move *with* the minus lens. The same test with a convex or plus lens causes the image to tend to move *away from* the direction of motion. An astigmatic lens shows changing distortion of the image when the lens is rotated about the visual axis. Spherical lenses cause no change in the image when rotated about the visual axis.

A high degree of myopia results in greater susceptibility to degenerative retinal changes, including retinal detachment.

Hyperopia

Hyperopia (hypermetropia, farsightedness) is the state in which the unaccommodated eye would focus the image behind the retina. Hyperopia is a more difficult concept to explain than myopia. The term "farsighted" contributes to the difficulty, as does the prevalent misconception among laymen that presbyopia is farsightedness and that one who sees well far away is farsighted. If hyperopia is not too great, a young person may obtain a sharp distant image by accommodating, as a normal eye would to read. The young hyperopic person may also make a sharp near image by accommodating more—or much more than one without hyperopia. This extra effort may result in eye fatigue and is moreso for near work. The degree of hyperopia a person may have without symptoms is—like most clinical conditions—variable. However, the amount decreases with age as presbyopia (decrease in ability to accommodate) increases. Three diopters of hyperopia might be tolerated in a teenager but will require glasses later, even though the hyperopia has not increased. If the hyperopia is too high, the eye may be unable to correct the image by accommodation and is termed manifest hyperopia. This is one of the common causes of deprivation amblyopia in children and can be bilateral. There is a reflex correlation between accommodation and convergence of the 2 eyes. Hyperopia is therefore a frequent cause of esotropia (crossed eyes) and monocular amblyopia (see Chapter 15).

Latent Hyperopia

As explained above, a prepresbyopic person with hyperopia may obtain a clear retinal image by accommodation. This may become a "set condition." If one carries a heavy backpack all day, when the pack is removed the "set condition" remains for some time, and one has a peculiar feeling of lightness or jumping about, since muscular responses are still modified by the discarded extra weight. The ciliary muscle is no different. It is not unusual for an uncorrected hyperope to observe that any plus lens blurs the image. The diagnosis may thus be missed or the hyperopia greatly underestimated. When cycloplegic drops are instilled to extinguish accommodation, the full extent of the hyperopia may be found. This is "latent" (hidden) hyperopia, ie, hyperopia that is not demonstrated until cycloplegic refraction is done. Refraction with a cycloplegic is very important in young patients who complain of eyestrain when reading and is vital in esotropia, where full correction of hyperopia may achieve a cure.

Remember that a moderately "farsighted" person may see well for near or far when young. However, as presbyopia comes on, the hyperope first has trouble with close work and at an earlier age than the nonhyperope. Finally, the hyperope has blurred vision for near *and far* and requires glasses for both near and far.

Astigmatism

Astigmatism is a type of refractive error that occurs when some of the refractive components of the eye are "out of round" or "off center" or "tilted." Any of the refractive components may be defective in this way, but the cornea shaping the aqueous lens is the usual major cause of astigmatism. The lens may also contribute to astigmatic error. In contact lens terminology, lenticular astigmatism is called residual astigmatism, for it is not corrected by the usual spherical hard contact lens, which does correct "corneal astigmatism." Astigmatism can be at any angle from 0 to 180 degrees. The nature and extent of image distortion depend on the magnitude of the astigmatism and its angle (Fig 24–12). Astigmatism can make level objects appear slanted. All sorts of slanting may occur with the image of eyes being interpreted by the brain. The brain is very ingenious at correcting this "out of plumb" condition. (The brain cannot correct for the diminished visual acuity astigmatism causes.) When a patient has adapted to an uncorrected astigmatic error or if the correction has changed, the patient wearing new glasses that correct the error will still receive "aid" from the brain and for a week or so will have the impression of tilting. Finally, the "gyro" adjusts and levels are again correct. This is not always easy to explain to patients who are sure their glasses are incorrect because of slanting of the image.

Astigmatic errors can be corrected with cylindric lenses. Cylindric lenses may be positive or negative. They are frequently combined with spherical lenses. A typical prescription for nearsighted astigmatism might read as follows:

$$-3.00 +2.25 \times 175$$
$$-2.50 +1.75 \times 160$$

The top line refers to the right eye correction and the second line to the left eye. In the top line, -3.00 specifies the power of the spherical correction and $+2.25$ specifies diopters of magnitude of the cylindric correction to be combined with the sphere for the total correction. Most ophthalmologists use only plus or only minus cylinders; however, the same prescription may be written in either form. To change the form is called transposing. To transpose a prescription for

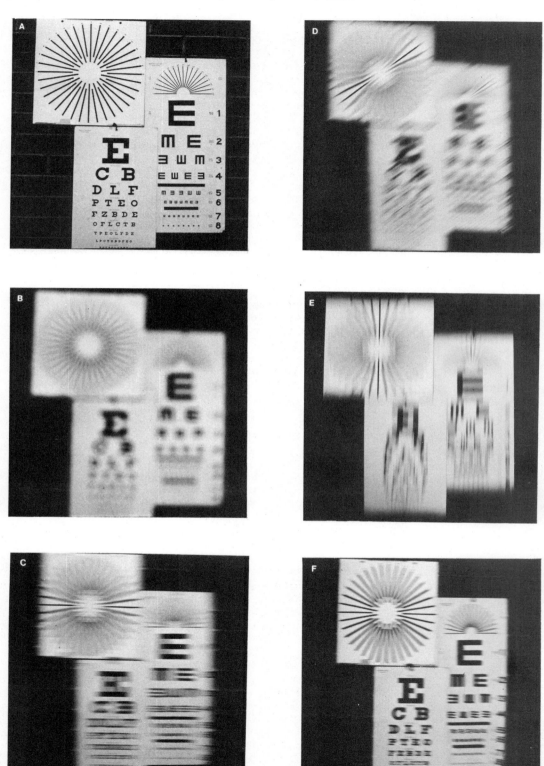

Figure 24–12. *A:* Emmetropia. *B:* Myopia or manifest hyperopia. *C, D, E, F:* Astigmatism.

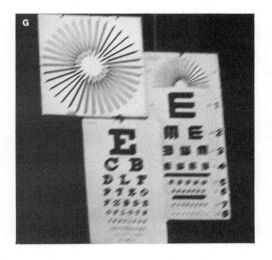

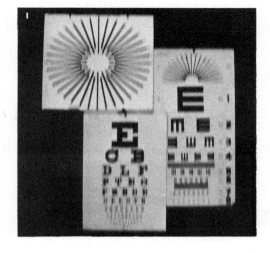

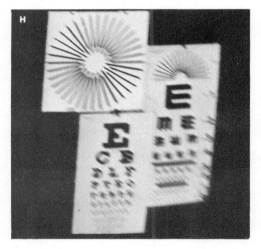

Figure 24–12 (cont'd). *G, H, I:* Astigmatism.

glasses, one algebraically adds the sphere and cylinder magnitudes to obtain the new sphere. Then one changes the sign of the cylinder and finally the axis by 90 degrees, keeping it between 0 and 180 degrees. For example, the former prescription transposed would read as follows:

$$-0.75 -2.25 \times 85$$
$$-0.75 -1.75 \times 70$$

The 2 prescriptions have the same meaning. The axis of the cylinder lens is the line of no refractive effect. Looking at the patient, zero degrees begins nasally in the right lens and temporally in the left lens and proceeds in a counterclockwise direction to 180 degrees (see Fig 24–4B, p 312). Further turning is a repetition. A cyclindric lens combined with one of the same magnitude at right angles to the first has the effect of a spherical lens of the same magnitude as either of the cylinders. The refractive power of a cylindric lens is 0 on axis and the nominal amount at 90 degrees from the axis. At other angles, the power is given by the sine squared of the angle off axis times the nominal value. The addition of 2 cylinders at oblique angles is a form of vector addition but is somewhat complex. Programmable calculators make this a simple task. Thus, overrefraction using spectacle addition and spectacle subtraction is now a practical aid to refraction, especially with strong lenses.

GRIN (Gradient-Index) Lenses

Having discussed the important 3-lens concept of the eye system, we must amplify the discussion of the unique and peculiar "lens" lens or crystalline lens. As previously mentioned, the index of refraction within the crystalline lens is not constant but is maximal at the center of the lens and decreases outwardly along the X, Y, and Z axes as a spherical gradient. James Clerk Maxwell over a century ago developed the theoretic mathematical properties of such lenses using the partial derivative and vector equations. Such a lens, a *gr*adient-*in*dex lens, is called a GRIN lens. In classic optics, a ray of light travels in straight lines until it

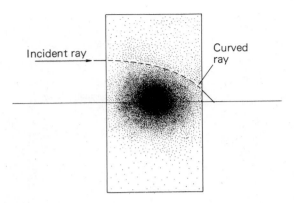

Figure 24–13. A noncurved GRIN lens simulating a convex lens.

meets an interface between 2 media with different indices of refraction, where it abruptly changes course along a new straight line until the next interface. Within a GRIN lens, the ray of light is bent along a gradient relative to the changing index of refraction and is therefore a curved line. A GRIN lens with parallel surfaces may function as a lens (Fig 24–13). A GRIN lens with curved surfaces such as the crystalline lens will be an even more effective lens (Fig 24–14). Earth's atmosphere is also a GRIN lens, and this may be the principal cause of sunset colors.

The optics of the eye submerged in seawater is of great importance in the phylogenesis of the eye. In submersion, the arriving incident ray is in water. This for all practical purposes cancels the effect of the aqueous lens and vitreous lens. The fish eye therefore has essentially one lens element—the crystalline lens, which is a GRIN lens. The full properties of GRIN lenses await further study. They should permit better transmission because there is less reflection from the surface. The lens may have the same *n* at the surface as the medium of the arriving ray. The effect on spherical aberration and chromatic aberration is unknown. To the author's knowledge, no investigator has yet produced a spherical gradient GRIN lens so that its

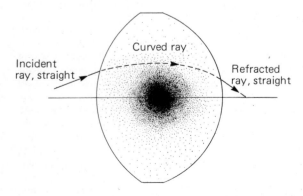

Figure 24–14. GRIN crystalline lens of the eye.

properties could be investigated. This type of GRIN lens could be easily made in zero gravity outer space.

As a nuclear cataract develops, it is common for the patient to develop myopia, which may be of high degree. At first, this may again allow reading without glasses and for that reason is called "second sight." The myopia is due to an increase in the gradient of the GRIN lens. High elevations of blood glucose may also cause either profound myopia or hyperopia, which is usually reversible, but the mechanism is not clearly established. (The increased index of refraction of the aqueous lens due to the increased glucose level is not of sufficient magnitude to explain the change.)

History of Spectacles

The history of the correction of refractive errors and presbyopia with spectacles is somewhat complex and vague, partly as a result of confusion about the definition of "spectacle." Bottles filled with water could be called one form of correction. However, plus lenses seemed to come into use during the 13th century. Minus lenses seem to date from the 15th or 16th century. The astronomer Sir George Biddell Airy corrected his own astigmatism in 1827, introducing this advance to humankind. Benjamin Franklin made the first bifocal spectacle lens in about 1775. It is a startling fact and unappreciated by most that *until very recently, the most common cause of functional blindness was refractive error, particularly presbyopia.*

Natural History of Refractive Status

Most babies are slightly hyperopic at birth. The hyperopia slowly decreases, with a slight acceleration in the teens, to approach emmetropia. Presbyopia becoming manifest in the fifth decade has been previously discussed.

Refractive errors are inherited. The mode of inheritance is complex, as it involves so many variables. The final result is the sum of the variables. Refractive errors, though inherited, need not be present at birth any more than tallness, which is also inherited, need be present at birth. For example, a child who reaches emmetropia at age 10 years will probably soon become myopic. Myopia usually increases during the teens. This should be expected, just as the need for larger shoes is expected, and not looked on with alarm by the patient and his or her parents. In a similar way, hyperopia usually decreases slightly during the teens. Myopia does not generally decrease with age, as is popularly believed, nor does farsightedness come with aging.

REFRACTION

Detailed discussion of refraction is better left to more specialized texts. However, some points are of general interest.

Patients over about 6 years of age can usually be refracted by eliciting subjective responses. Thus, the patient tells whether various steps are better or worse or the same until an end point is reached. One frequently begins with the correction of the patient's present glasses or with the correction indicated by the previous record and progresses from there to the new prescription. If one of these starting points is not available, the retinoscope can be used to make a preliminary reading. With patients unable to give subjective replies, the retinoscope is the key to refraction. Cycloplegic drops are used to place the eye in an unaccommodated rested state. The large pupil that results makes retinoscopy and ophthalmoscopy easier, but arrested accommodation is the main advantage of cycloplegia. Performing a refraction by retinoscopy in a young person without using cyclopegic drops has been likened to measuring a man for a suit of clothes while he is runniung down the street. The retinoscope casts a light through the pupil. The examiner moves the light back and forth and observes the direction of the light reflection from the retina (often called the shadow.) One adds plus or minus lenses depending on the character of the motion until a reversal occurs. This is the end point. The magnitude and axis of the cylinderic correction may also be determined using this technique. Thus, even day-old infants may be refracted. Early refraction is vital in strabismus. Opacity of the media of course makes retinoscopy impossible. Most ophthalmologists agree that subjective refraction, if possible, is more precise than retinoscopy alone.

Contact Lenses

A major stimulus to development of contact lenses was the problem of keratoconus, discussed in Chapter 8. In this condition, the cornea bulges forward progressively and irregularly, making the aqueous fluid lens cone-shaped. This creates an irregular astigmatism and, usually, increasing myopia that cannot be corrected by ordinary sphere-cylinder corrections. Before contact lenses became available, the next step was corneal transplant. It has long been known that if the cornea could be covered by a more perfectly curved substance, vision could be corrected. Leonardo da Vinci used a large bowl filled with water in which the eye was immersed. This in 1508 theoretically corrected the distorted vision. Thomas Young in 1801 immersed his prominent eye in a tube of water and, by adding lenses to the end of the tube, obtained a sharp image. Adolph Eugen Fick, a Zurich physician, first used glass contact lenses to correct irregular astigmatism in 1887. The Carl Zeiss Company of Jena manufactured a wide selection of glass fluid-filled scleral contact lenses. These were difficult to wear for extended periods and caused corneal edema and much ocular discomfort. Great efforts were made to perfect the fluid, without much success. In 1948, Kevin Tuohy made plastic corneal lenses that rested on the cornea with no added fluid. His lenses used the tears to fill the spaces between the lens and the cornea. These lenses have been made smaller and thinner, with various bevels and rounding and finishing of the edges, but they are basically the same today. This type of lens was

so successful that it gained wide use for cosmetic replacement of glasses as well as its first use as an optical aid for keratoconus. In aphakia, the contact lens gave a wider field than glasses and much less magnification of the image. This allowed most patients with monocular aphakia to fuse with the nonaphakic eye and achieve stereopsis—a major breakthrough in the treatment of aphakia.

A hard contact lens corrects refractive errors in 2 ways. The first may be explained by considering a contact lens as a shell with no refracting power per se. Assume that the cornea shapes the aqueous lens to a radius of 7.5 mm. Placing a shell contact lens on this eye with a steeper curvature of radius of 7.34 mm will increase the power of the aqueous lens by about 1 diopter. The vault or void under the contact is filled with tears, and there is some molding of the cornea to partially fill the void. This effect will be much the same no matter what the index of refraction of the cornea, tears, or contact lens. These substances are like cement in a cemented lens and largely cancel out. This you may prove if you have become familiar with ray tracing. Clinical experience proves the same point. The effect also rids the cornea of any astigmatic errors. There is much confusion about tear lenses, water lenses, or whether the index of refraction of the plastic suddenly makes the first lens system much stronger. These are all false concepts. In any event, the back curvature of this shell lens, called the base curve, makes the new curve of the aqueous lens.

The second way in which plastic contact lenses correct refractive error is inherent in the refractive power that exists when the front curvature is different from the back curvature. The gaussian equations may be used for these calculations without causing too great an error, especially if the thick lens modification is used. The index of refraction of the plastic is important here. This equation will tell the lathe man the radius of the front curve (knowing the base curve) so that the so-called power of the contact will be known. The actual power may be called the total power and is the sum of this power (that may be measured by the lensometer) and the power of the base curve converted into diopters. (The base curve may be measured by the radiuscope.) Remember that 337.5 divided by the base curve in millimeters gives power in diopters and, conversely, divided by diopters gives the base curve in millimeters. Thus, a 44-diopter base curve lens with no added refractive power (a shell) produces the same clinical effect as a 40-diopter base curve lens with +4 diopters of refractive power. The sum is 44 for both lenses. A lens of 46-diopter base curve with −2.00 refractive power is another twin. A reliable method of fitting contact lenses is to select a trial contact near the base curve desired with a refractive power near that estimated. Overrefraction is performed with spheres. These 3 values are added, ie, the base curve in diopters of the trial contact, the refractive power of the contact, and the power of the overrefraction, and called the total power. The base curve of the lens to be ordered is then determined. The sum of this base curve in diopters and its refractive power in diopters should equal the above total power found by the trial lens.

The selection of the base curve depends on the philosophy and training of the clinician. A significant clue is the keratometer reading of the corneal curve.

During overrefraction, one may determine the astigmatic correction along with the sphere used for the best power correction. This astigmatic correction represents the "residual astigmatism" (mostly in the lens of the eye). If a great deal of residual astigmatism is present, a clear image cannot be achieved with spherical contact lenses. Fewer than 10% of patients have this problem.

A contact lens should have the proper thickness, considering the front curve, the back curve, and the diameter, to ensure proper integrity of the center, the edge, and enough material on the edge to permit proper beveling and edging. These may all be programmed for the computer so that each order can be designed to perfection. Those who boast about making the "thinnest lens in town" apparently are not aware of the mathematics involved, for it takes little skill to make a lens too thin.

Soft Contact Lenses

Otto Wichterle of Czechoslovakia introduced a soft hydrophilic plastic and made the first soft contact lenses. Several companies make various types of soft lenses, and the field is in a state of flux. The lens has been declared a medical device and is therefore controlled by the Food and Drug Administration in the USA. Some of these lenses have a very high water content and can be worn for extended periods. They tend to follow the astigmatism of the cornea to some extent and are not as good with high astigmatism.

Other plastic materials are being used and have virtues, the total value of which must still be determined. Cellulose acetate butyrate is like a hard lens with increased gas permeability. Silicone lenses have superior oxygen and carbon dioxide permeability.

Intraocular Lenses

The principle of replacing a removed cataractous lens with a clear prosthesis of similar refracting power in or near the original position has obvious appeal. Harold Ridley of England observed that RAF pilots during World War II did rather well with retained intraocular foreign bodies of plexiglass windshields (polymethylmethacrylate). About 1949, he began using PMMA intraocular lens prostheses placed in the former lens position, ie, the posterior chamber. Many patients developed corneal edema, some several years later. Some of the patients had a remaining refractive error that was rather alarming. Cornelius Binkhorst of the Netherlands has for over 20 years used various types of lenses of his own design. At present, the intraocular lens has wide popularity. There are many styles, all with their devotees. The method has not been without severe complications. The hope is always that "this modification will prevent the complications." The lenses have been placed in the anterior chamber, at the iris plane, and in the posterior chamber. They have been supported by the iris, the angle, the ciliary body, and the capsular bag of cataract removed extracapsularly (the method that leaves the posterior capsule of the lens in the eye). Posts in the pupil (especially metal ones) caused some glare, and some iris-supported lenses may "jiggle," but most of the present lenses give an excellent optical result. The long-term safety of the lenses is still not fully known and is a worry to many ophthalmologists.

The optics of the intraocular lens are very interesting. Many equations have been devised to help determine beforehand the correct power for a given eye length measured by ultrasound and corneal curvature measured by the keratometer. The various equations result in various answers. Many ophthalmologists make an educated guess and claim they do better than the equations. One method used by some clinicians is to do many cases—a thousand with one style if possible. The results are then plotted for a best-fit regression. (The regression formulas use the least squares method to obtain constants for a best-fit equation.) Unfortunately, the constants differ for each lens style and for each manufacturer. The other equations advocated are all thin-lens gaussian approximations that are known not to be accurate with thick or solid lenses like the eye system. The accurate trigometric ray tracing equations discussed in the first portion of this chapter should give accurate solutions to this problem. One must know the radius of curvature, the thickness, and the index of refraction of the lens. These lenses are under strict government control in the USA. It is interesting that none of the 3 values were provided by the manufacturers to the surgeon, and only recently has the index of refraction been furnished on the lens inserts. When the other 2 values are furnished, one may start using the accurate method of calculation. There is a graphic method of ray tracing that also dates back to Snell. This may appeal to some more than the computer method. The drawing must be made carefully to achieve acceptable accuracy. The graphic method does not reveal the quality of the image, ie, it will not show a poorer image by reversing the intraocular lens nor indicate optimum form. This may be demonstrated by the full computer method. The graphic method will give the proper value of an intraocular lens for proper focus.

The graphic method is similar to nautical dead reckoning navigation (Fig 24–16). Parallel rulers, a long ruler, and a compass capable of making large circles are required. The method has other virtues in giving one an understanding of the importance of thickness, index of refraction, lens position, etc.

The cardboard paper should be at least 56 cm (22 inches) by about 30 cm (12 inches). Approximately 3 inches from the bottom, a line is drawn to represent the visual axis. This extends the full 56 cm of the paper. Toward the right end of this line, a vertical line represents the retinal "screen." On a scale of about 20:1, the cornea is drawn with the compass. This must have the proper corneal radius of curvature and must be placed to correspond with the axial length of the eye

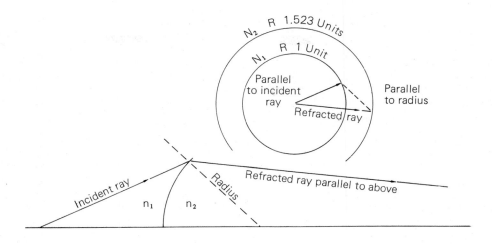

Figure 24–15. Graphical ray tracing.

(all 20:1). Next, the proposed intraocular lens is drawn in its proper position, using the radius of curvature (not given as of this publication date) and its thickness (also not furnished as of this date). The thickness may be about 0.6 mm, and the radius of curvature may be estimated by the following equation:

$$\text{Radius} \simeq \frac{[\text{n (Plastic)} - \text{n (Aqueous)}]}{\text{Diopters}}$$

Next, according to Snell's ingenious method, a portion of a circle is constructed that will be similar to a compass rose used in navigation.

The compass is extended so that its pin is near the left margin of the cardboard and the sharp pencil is near the right-hand side of the board, with this radius some multiple of the index of refraction of the plastic of the intraocular lens (1.491). To the same scale 2 more arcs are drawn. (A scale of 30 cm to 1 is suggested.) One arc is drawn with a radius of the index of refraction of air (1.000). (At 30 cm to 1, the air *n* arc is 30 cm radius.) The second arc is drawn with the radius of the index of refraction of aqueous (1.336). These use the

same scale multiplier as the first index arc of plastic. These are the concentric indices circles (or arcs, as the whole circle is not required for the intraocular lens calculation).

Now an arriving incident ray is drawn parallel to the optical axis and 2 mm above the axis to strike the cornea. (If the scale is 20:1, this will be 40 mm from the optical axis.) A ray is drawn on the index of refraction circles from their center parallel to the incident ray to strike the air index (1.000) circle. On the eye diagram, a radius is drawn from where the incident ray strikes the cornea to the center of curvature of the cornea. The parallel rulers carry this radius line to the index of air circle, where the incident ray met it, and carry it to the index circle of aqueous. A line from the index center to this point is then the direction of the incident refracted ray. This is transferred to the eye diagram with the parallel rulers. This will show where it strikes the intraocular lens. Similarly, the radius curve of the intraocular lens is transferred to the index drawing to connect the last intersection with the plastic index circle. A line from the index center to this point is the direction of the incident ray in the intraocular

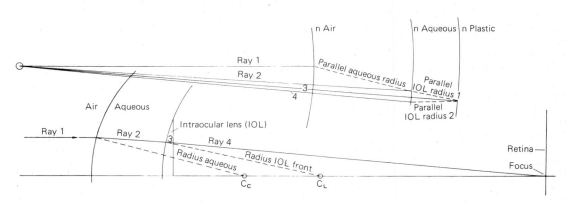

Figure 24–16. Intraocular lens graphical ray tracing calculation.

Table 24–3. Data for intraocular lens drawing of graphic or computer calculation.

Incident ray, Q = 2 mm (ray 2 mm from optical axis)
Incident ray, U = 0 degrees (parallel to axis)
Axial length of this eye = 23.28 mm
Distance, d = 3.5 mm. (The cornea may be ignored in the calculations if we subtract 0.3728 mm from d. The final calculated length of the eye is then adjusted by adding 0.3728 to determine the length of the eye including the cornea.)
Radius of aqueous lens = 7.85 mm
    Curvature, C = 0.12739 (1/R)
Index of refraction:
    air = 1.00
    aqueous = 1.336
Intraocular lens data:
    R = 8.1320 mm
    C = 0.12297 mm
    n = 1.491
    Thickness, d = 0.6 mm
Final vitreous surface data:
    R is infinite (flat)
    C = 0
    n = 1.336
Final L = 19.18196 mm. Add all d's plus final L for distance from aqueous lens, and add 0.3728 mm to this for distance focus from surface of cornea, 23.28196 mm. The image is on retina-lens proper.
Traditionally, lens calculations are carried to 5 places. Most of the data for the eye do not approach this degree of accuracy. However, it is best to use the full accuracy of the computer—10 places or whatever—for this helps in internal calculations of aberrations, etc.
Following are computer printouts of the above problem. Included is a reversed intraocular lens to show the degrading effect this causes in the image. Optic pathway difference of marginal ray in wavelengths of light is shown, but other aberrations confirm this.
At the retina, 1 diopter is 0.367 mm, and 1 mm is 2.72 diopters.

Intraocular Lens Convex Forward		Intraocular Lens Plano Forward
C= 0.12739		C= 0.12739
N= 1.00000		N= 1.00000
N/= 1.33600		N/= 1.33600
d= 3.12720		d= 3.12720
U= 0.00000		U= 0.00000
Q= 2.00000		Q= 2.00000
Q/= 2.01270		Q/= 2.01270
I= 14.76038		I= 14.76038
I/= 10.99372		I/= 10.99372
U/= 3.76666	Aqueous lens	U/= 3.76666
G= 1.01678		G= 1.01678
Y= 2.00000		Y= 2.00000
X= 0.25905		X= 0.25905
OPD λ-1.63947		OPD λ-1.63947
ΣOPD=-1.63947		ΣOPD=-1.63947
C= 0.12297		C= 0.00000
N= 1.33600		N= 1.33600
N/= 1.49100		N/= 1.49100
d= 0.60000		d= 0.60000
U= 3.76666		U= 3.76666
Q= 1.80726		Q= 1.80726
Q/= 1.80838		Q/= 1.80803
I= 9.00656		I=-3.76666
I/= 8.06366	Intraocular lens	I/=-3.37461
U/= 4.70955		U/=-3.37461
G= 0.91023		G= 0.90559
Y= 1.79793		Y= 1.81117
X= 0.20124		X= 0.00000
OPD λ-0.11753		OPD λ 0.03394
ΣOPD=-1.75700		ΣOPD=-1.60553
C= 0.00000		C=-0.12297
N= 1.49100		N= 1.49100
N/= 1.33600		N/= 1.33600
d= 0.00000		d= 0.00000
U= 4.70955		U= 3.37461
Q= 1.75912		Q= 1.77272
Q/= 1.75765		Q/= 1.76151
I=-4.70955		I=-16.07268
I/=-5.25740		I/=-17.99758
U/= 5.25740	Vitreous lens	U/= 5.29951
G= 0.88254		G= 0.90483
Y= 1.76507		Y= 1.78752
X= 8.82537-12		X=-0.19889
OPD λ-0.09008		OPD λ-2.36801
ΣOPD=-1.84708		ΣOPD=-3.97354
FIN L/= 19.18196		FIN L/= 19.07182
Σ d= 22.90916		Σ d= 22.79902
.37280 +		.37280 +
23.28196 ***		23.17182 ***

lens. The final radius of the intraocular lens is infinite (a flat) and therefore is parallel to the optic axis. This is transferred to the index drawing to connect the last intersection with the 1.491 arc back to the aqueous 1.336 arc. A final line from the index center to this point is the direction of the final ray. This line is transferred carefully with the parallel rulers to the eye drawing and extended until it meets the visual axis, ie, at the point of focus. If on the retina, all is well; if in front of the retina, the intraocular lens radius must be longer (a weaker intraocular lens), etc.

The numerical example is given so that the interested reader may draw the example. The "microsurgeon" should use the same care as in surgery to achieve an accurate result with the drawing. The accurate computer answer is included (Table 24–3).

This graphic method does not have the fallacies of the thin lens equations and will work for complex systems like the eye. The drawing must be very precise for accuracy. The computer method is preferable, as its accuracy is better than 5 places—much better than the most careful drawing.

There is no reason to think that proper data for correct calculations will not be released and furnished by the manufacturers of intraocular lens in the near future.

• • •

References

Conrady AE: *Applied Optics and Optical Design.* Vol 1. Oxford Univ Press, 1929. Dover Publications, Inc, 1957.

Conrady AE: *Applied Optics and Optical Design.* Vol 2. (Edited and completed by Kingslake R.) Dover Publications, Inc., 1960.

Duke-Elder S (editor): *System of Ophthalmology.* Vol 5. *Ophthalmic Optics and Refraction.* Mosby, 1970.

Eva PR, Pascoe PT, Vaughan DG: Refractive change in hyperglycaemia: Hyperopia, not myopia. *Br J Ophthalmol* 1982;**66**:500.

Hales RH: *Contact Lenses: A Clinical Approach to Fitting.* Williams & Wilkins, 1978.

Helmholtz H: *Helmholtz' Treatise on Physiological Optics, 1910.* Optical Society of America, 1925. [English edition.]

Kingslake R: *Lens Design Fundamentals.* Academic Press, 1978.

White O: Spectacle addition and spectacle subtraction. *Trans Pac Coast Otoophthalmol Soc* 1980;**61**:7.

Wyld J: The design of refractor objectives by ray tracing. In: *Amature Telescope Making.* Ingalls AG (editor). Vol 3. Kingsport Press/Scientific American, 1974.

25 | Preventive Ophthalmology

The decade of the 80s might be called the decade of preventive medicine. General medicine and all of the specialties have participated in this movement, and ophthalmology has been no exception. Prevention of ocular injuries in industry, in the schools, and in the home has had a long and successful history, but much remains to be done in the fields of infection, genetic disorders, iatrogenic disease, and other special areas.

Much of the responsibility for prevention of nontraumatic ocular disease rests with the pediatrician, the general practitioner, and the internist, but the ophthalmologist has a major role as disseminator of necessary information. Meanwhile, the nonophthalmologist practitioner must be aware of the eye problems that can be treated before visual loss has occurred if detected at an early stage.

Important problems fitting into this category are glaucoma, strabismus, and the complications of such systemic diseases as diabetes, tuberculosis, sarcoidosis, syphilis, and leprosy. It is indeed a tragedy to find hitherto undetected advanced ocular disease in a patient who has been receiving regular medical treatment for another illness. It is hoped that this chapter will give medical students, pediatricians, and general physicians—as well as young ophthalmology residents-in-training—a survey of preventive ophthalmology and that it will alert them to the huge opportunities available to them in sight conservation.

PREVENTION OF THE SEVERE CONSEQUENCES OF UNDIAGNOSED GLAUCOMA

About 1–2% of all people over 35 have glaucoma. In the USA alone it is estimated that there are at least 300,000 people with undetected glaucoma. About 90% of them have chronic open-angle glaucoma, which does not cause symptoms in the early stages but can ultimately lead to blindness. Patients often do not seek treatment until late in the disease, because there is no pain and the visual acuity (central vision) remains good even when the peripheral fields constrict.

The best way to detect glaucoma is to examine tonometrically all people over 20 every 3 years (or every year if there is a family history of glaucoma).

The next most important diagnostic steps are the visual field examination and the ophthalmoscopic examination for pathologic cupping of the optic disk. The visual field examination is normally done on the tangent screen; confrontation field testing in which the examiner's fingers are used as a target will pick up only gross visual field defects.

Tonometry and ophthalmoscopy should be part of every physical examination in the age group over 20. Unfortunately, the overdiagnosis of glaucoma is also a problem. It is also unfortunate that once a patient has been placed on miotics or other antiglaucomatous drugs, it is very difficult to establish the diagnosis of "nondisease."

PREVENTION OF AMBLYOPIA ("Lazy Eye")

Amblyopia can be defined for the purposes of this discussion as diminished visual acuity in one eye in the absence of organic eye disease. Central vision develops from birth to age 6 or 7; if vision has not developed by then, there is little or no chance that it will develop later. In the absence of eye disease, the 2 main abnormalities that will prevent a child from acquiring binocular vision are strabismus and anisometropia.

Strabismus
Esotropia or exotropia in a young child causes double vision. The child quickly learns to suppress the image in the deviating eye and learns to see normally with one eye. Unfortunately, vision does not develop in the unused eye; unless the good eye is patched, thus forcing the child to use the deviating eye, sight will never develop in that eye. The child will grow up with one perfectly normal eye that is essentially blind, since it has never developed a functional connection with the visual centers of the brain. This is more likely to occur with esotropia than with exotropia.

Anisometropia
Young children are more concerned with perception of near objects than with those at a distance. If one eye is nearsighted (myopic) and the other farsighted (hyperopic), the child will favor the nearsighted eye.

Thus, the farsighted eye will not be used even though it is straight. The result will be the same as in untreated strabismus, ie, monocular blindness due to failure of visual development in an unused eye. The incidence of anisometropia is about 0.75–1%.

Early Diagnosis

The best way to prevent amblyopia is to test the visual acuity of all preschool children. By the time a child reaches school, it is usually too late for occlusion therapy. The parents can perform the test at home with the illiterate "E" chart. This is sometimes known as the "Home Eye Test." Pediatricians and others responsible for the care of small children should test visual acuity no later than age 4.

PREVENTION OF CORNEAL INFECTION

In view of its exposure to the environment, the intact eye is remarkably resistant to infection; but once the epithelium of the cornea is breached, microorganisms find susceptible tissues, and even such opportunistic pathogens as *Pseudomonas aeruginosa* may proliferate. Protection of the corneal epithelium thus becomes all-important in the prevention of ocular infection. There are a few bacteria, particularly *Neisseria gonorrhoeae* and *Neisseria meningitidis,* that can proliferate on an intact epithelium, and it is of historical interest that Credé silver nitrate prophylaxis, introduced in 1881, has been responsible for saving thousands of eyes from total visual loss. Even viral infection such as herpes simplex virus infection (a cause of much ocular disability) is in large part dependent on corneal epithelial damage. It is safe to say that the majority of ocular infections, whether bacterial, fungal, chlamydial, or viral in origin, are preventable.

Ophthalmia neonatorum, especially inclusion blennorrhea, is still a problem despite the worldwide use of silver nitrate and other antimicrobial agents at birth. But recent research suggests that the antibiotic erythromycin, instilled in the eye of the newborn, may be effective in controlling not only gonococcal infection but chlamydial infection (inclusion blennorrhea) as well. In view of the high prevalence of gonococcal genital infection in this country and elsewhere, prophylaxis cannot be abandoned, but many state laws concerned with it are currently undergoing revision.

Corneal infections in general, particularly hypopyon ulcer, are a major cause of visual loss. It is therefore of first importance to realize that they are in large part preventable. Once the epithelial barrier is breached, the cornea is subject to infection with many pathogens, especially the pneumococcus, and with many opportunistic bacteria and fungi, especially *P aeruginosa, Candida* species, and *Fusarium* species.

P aeruginosa used to be a common contaminant of ophthalmic solutions, particularly fluorescein and physostigmine solutions, and was often responsible for the loss of an eye. Contaminated eye solutions should not be tolerated even for use in an eye with an intact epithelium. The responsibility for having only sterile solutions at hand should of course rest primarily with physicians, and pharmacists and pharmaceutical companies, but to a lesser extent it must also be the responsibility of nurses and of patients themselves.

The **injured eye** is particularly vulnerable to infection, and all emergency rooms should be equipped with small, single-use, disposable vials containing sterile ophthalmic solutions. The use of multiple-dose containers should be limited to the intact eye. If a solution in such a multiple-dose container *must* be used in an injured eye, its sterility can be assured by autoclaving or by sterile filtration.

As suggested above, the prevention of damage to the corneal epithelium is indisputably the key to the prevention of corneal infection. Fortunately, although direct trauma often occurs, minor abrasions heal so rapidly that infection can only follow a massive inoculation of bacteria or fungi. Such massive inoculations can come from (1) contaminated solutions, (2) dacryocystitis, (3) severe staphylococcal blepharitis, (4) a contaminated contact lens, etc, and all of these can be prevented or treated satisfactorily as called for.

Contact lenses can be contaminated by their carrying cases and can themselves cause epithelial damage by abrasion or oxygen deprivation. All contact lens wearers should be cautioned to report for examination at the first sign of inflammation. Pain, a helpful warning sign, may be absent, since partial corneal anesthesia develops characteristically in contact lens wearers.

Accidental epithelial injury incurred while participating in various sports is also common, and severe epithelial damage may be caused by (1) exposure during coma; (2) ultraviolet light while welding or skiing; or (3) desiccation associated with exophthalmos, facial nerve paralysis, or ectropion of the lower lid, eg, after a severe burn. Many of these damaged eyes have been lost as a result of infection when simple methods of protection have been omitted.

Temporary protection pending definitive therapy can be achieved by patching, tarsorrhaphy, or frequent instillations of ointment or artificial tears; exceptionally, the brief applications of soft contact lenses can be effective.

Prevention of intraocular infection arising from **penetrating foreign bodies** requires the common use, not only in industry but in the private sector, of protective lenses. Every individual should be encouraged to have a pair of protective lenses on hand for use around the house to prevent injuries from champagne and other corks, from power mowers, from power drills and other machines, and from hazardous chemicals such as may be used for opening drains or fertilizing crops with liquids containing ammonia.

Prevention of intraocular infection after **cataract extraction** or other intraocular surgery deserves much attention, since such infections are almost always avoidable. They should in fact never occur in a modern hospital, where committees on infections have the responsibility for preventing them. Fortunately, eye surgery requires such a brief stay in the hospital that colonization of an eye with so-called "hospital bacteria" is rare indeed.

Most intraocular infections come from (1) contaminated solutions; (2) chronic conjunctival or lid margin infections or chronic dacryocystitis; (3) rarely, aerosols from the noses and throats of surgeons and their assistants; and (4) prolonged surgery, vitreous loss, or ocular implants. All of these complications can be prevented or minimized. At the time of surgery, the susceptible tissues are exposed for only a short time, and the surgical wound seals rapidly. The eye's local defense mechanisms seem to be able to handle small numbers of microorganisms without difficulty unless compromised by topical corticosteroids or other immunosuppressive drugs.

Since most intraocular surgery is elective, the surgeon has time to assess the patient's immunologic status and to correct any immunodepression due to malnutrition, alcoholism, narcotic addiction, stress, etc. There is also time to make sure that the external eye is not compromised by blepharoconjunctivitis, overt or intermittent dacryocystitis and stenosis, or tear deficiency. Most of these conditions are correctable—or can at least be ameliorated—before surgery.

The bacterial flora of the lids and conjunctiva should be assessed prior to elective intraocular surgery, although not necessarily by means of preoperative cultures. If clinical examination shows normal lid margins and conjunctivas and if there is no history of exudate or gumming of the lids on waking, further examination is unnecessary. But if the external eye is *not* normal, the bacterial flora should be studied for potential pathogens, particularly gram-negative opportunistic pathogens such as *P aeruginosa* and *Proteus* species.

Elimination of such potential pathogens by suitable treatment is mandatory. Antibiotics or antibiotic mixtures used preoperatively cannot be relied upon, and the prolonged use of such agents before surgery tends to inhibit the growth of the normally harmless gram-positive flora. This unfortunately encourages the colonization of both gram-negative bacteria and fungi. There is no substitute for a careful preoperative clinical examination combined with a careful history of previous infection, particularly of intermittent dacryocystitis during the common cold.

If emergency intraocular surgery must be performed in the presence of external eye disease, careful irrigation of the conjunctiva to remove exudate and bacteria-containing mucous threads is indicated. If there is dacryocystitis to deal with, the puncta can be temporarily sealed by cautery.

PREVENTION OF RADIATION INJURY

Ultraviolet irradiation may cause superficial epithelial keratitis accompanied by pain, redness, and photophobia. The symptoms appear 6–12 hours after exposure to ultraviolet light, eg, while skiing or using an electric welding device. Prevention consists of avoidance of exposure or the wearing of appropriate protective sunglasses or goggles.

Solar retinitis (eclipse retinopathy) is a specific type of radiation injury that usually occurs after solar eclipses as a result of direct observation of the sun without an adequate filter. Under normal circumstances, sun-gazing is difficult because of the glare, but cases have been reported in young people who have suffered self-inflicted macular damage by deliberate sun-gazing, perhaps while under the influence of drugs.

The optical system of the eye behaves as a strong magnifying lens, focusing the light onto a small spot on the macula, usually in one eye only, and producing a thermal burn. The resulting edema of the retinal tissue may clear with minimal loss of function, or it may cause significant atrophy of the tissue and produce a defect that is visible ophthalmoscopically as a macular hole. In the latter event, a permanent central scotoma results.

Eclipse retinopathy can easily be prevented by the use of adequate filters when observing eclipses, but the surest way to prevent it is to watch the eclipse on television.

Workers with improperly screened nuclear materials face an increasingly important problem because of the frequent formation of cataracts.

Pterygium is an occupational disease of farmers, sheepherders, and others who live largely outdoors. It is presumably due to exposure (ultraviolet light, desiccation by wind, etc) and can be prevented by wearing protective lenses. This applies also to **basal cell carcinoma** and probably also to **melanoma** of the lids and lid margins. In patients with xeroderma pigmentosum, the eyelids and bulbar conjunctiva frequently develop carcinomas and melanomas, and their development can be minimized, if not prevented entirely, by protective lenses.

PREVENTION OF EXPOSURE KERATITIS

Patients in coma or under prolonged anesthesia who have lid retraction (eg, exophthalmos) or facial nerve paralysis may develop exposure keratitis. This condition can be prevented by patching the eyes, suturing the lids together (tarsorrhaphy), instilling artificial tears, or applying a soft contact lens.

PREVENTION OF XEROPHTHALMIA

Even in the USA, where it should now be all but unknown, occasional cases of xerophthalmia still occur, and in the underdeveloped areas the world over, where nutrition is often poor, it is still common. Vitamin A deficiency disease, in which the eye changes (xerophthalmia and keratomalacia) are the most damaging and often cause blindness (see Chapter 26), is usually the result of a deficient diet associated with poverty. It should be borne in mind, however, that it may also be associated with chronic alcoholism, weight-reducing diets, dietary management of food allergy, or poor absorption from the gastrointestinal tract due to the use of mineral oil or gastrointestinal disease such as chronic diarrhea.

In vitamin A–deficient children, measles may result in severe corneal disease. Because of the eye signs (ie, night blindness, Bitot's spots, or a lackluster corneal epithelium), the ophthalmologist may be the first to recognize vitamin A deficiency. Early recognition and treatment can prevent loss of vision or blindness due to secondary infection and corneal perforation. Treatment of the acute condition may require large intramuscular doses of vitamin A followed by corrective diet and careful analysis of all possible causes.

PREVENTION OF VISUAL LOSS DUE TO DRUGS & IATROGENIC DISEASE

All drugs can cause adverse reactions. It is the ophthalmologist's responsibility to prevent visual loss or major ocular disability from drugs used to treat eye diseases.

Ophthalmic drugs should be packaged and labeled so that mistakes are not made by elderly or poorly sighted patients. Atropine and other strong medications may call for color-labeling. On the first visit to a new ophthalmologist, the patient should be asked to bring along any previously prescribed medications in order to avoid duplication and possible overdosage.

Certain ophthalmic drugs have such frequently occurring and damaging side-effects that their use requires special monitoring and special warnings to the patient. Atropine and scopolamine, used to dilate the pupil in iridocyclitis, may precipitate acute glaucoma in certain patients with narrow anterior chamber angles. After prolonged use, they can also lead to conjunctivitis and allergic eczema of the eyelids. Many antiglaucoma drugs can product stenosis of the puncta and shrinkage of the conjunctiva.

Corticosteroids used locally in drop or ointment forms may depress the local defense mechanisms and precipitate corneal ulceration, often fungal. They may also worsen herpetic keratitis and other corneal infections, and on prolonged use may lead to open-angle glaucoma and to posterior polar cataract. Much of the severity of both herpes simplex virus and varicella-zoster virus corneal infections can be blamed on the unwise use of topical corticosteroids. In this situation, short-term improvement has beeen traded for long-term disaster. Fungal endophthalmitis after cataract surgery is usually the result of the unnecessary use of corticosteroids at the time of the operation and is therefore preventable.

Many drugs used **systemically** have serious ocular side-effects, eg, keratopathy, retrobulbar neuritis, retinopathy, and Stevens-Johnson syndrome (erythema multiforme). For this reason, the ophthalmologist must take a careful history of the patient's use of drugs as part of the initial examination. Of special interest are the keratopathy and retinopathy that often follow the use of chloroquine in discoid lupus erythematosus. It is the function of the consulting ophthalmologist to detect any early ocular changes and to inform the dermatologist of them so that he can substitute another medication.

Iatrogenic spread of adenoviral **epidemic keratoconjunctivitis** has been reported many times. It may be spread by the doctor's fingers, by contaminated tonometers, or by solutions contaminated by droppers accidentally rubbed against the infected conjunctiva or lid margin of a patient with epidemic keratoconjunctivitis. Office spread of this disease can be prevented by (1) handwashing between patients, (2) the sterilization of tonometers, and (3) the use of individual droppers for instilling topical solutions into the eyes.

Other infections can be similarly spread, but their occurrence is not generally recognized. The ophthalmologist should be alert to the possibility that if ophthalmic instruments are improperly sterilized (as by cold sterilization), they may be contaminated with hepatitis B virus.

PREVENTION OF METABOLIC & GENETIC DISEASES

Until recently, the prevention of metabolic and genetic disorders received little attention. Now, however, there are genetic counseling centers in many medical centers, and the genetic nature of the transmissibility of many genetic and metabolic traits that affect the eye is recognized and their transmission better understood than formerly. In conference with internists and pediatricians, it is up to the ophthalmologist to recommend genetic counseling for patients contemplating marriage and children. Patients with histories of childhood diabetes, retinitis pigmentosa, consanguineous mating, hemophilia, etc, need genetic counseling to prevent disaster for their offspring.

Some clinical conditions, eg, Down's syndrome (trisomy 21), are associated with an abnormal number of chromosomes or with abnormalities of the sex chromosomes. Prenatal diagnosis can now be made by testing amniotic fluid cells obtained by amniocentesis (a safe and practical procedure), and a positive diagnosis gives the patient the option of abortion.

Viral disease of the mother with resultant embryopathy may lead to such ocular anomalies in the offspring as retinopathy, infantile glaucoma, cataract, uveal tract coloboma, etc, and prevention may in some cases be possible. Two viruses, rubella and cytomegalovirus, can be extremely damaging to the infant, and one of them—rubella virus—can be prevented by vaccinations. Once a common childhood disease, rubella led to lifelong immunity, but vaccination is now indicated for susceptible young women approaching childbearing age. Susceptibility can be determined by assessing the antibody content of the young woman's blood. If a mother contracts rubella during early pregnancy, she should be informed of the likelihood of ocular and other abnormalities in her baby, and the arguments for and against abortion should be presented.

Unfortunately, cytomegalovirus (the other virus causing a high incidence of congenital anomalies) continues to be a serious and unsolved threat. No protective vaccine is currently available, though one is currently under study.

PREVENTION OF HERPES SIMPLEX & HERPES ZOSTER

Some progress has been made in the prevention of herpetic disease. The epidemiology of herpes simplex virus type 1 is such that protection of highly susceptible young children (under 5 years of age) from salivary exposure to relatives with labial herpes could conceivably prevent many cases of primary infection, labial or ocular. As for the recurrent disease, many cases can be prevented by modifying the trigger mechanisms—stress, fever, overexposure to sunlight, trauma, etc. Fever, the most frequent trigger, can be reduced by aspirin used at the onset of coryza or other upper respiratory infection, and stress can be minimized by office psychotherapy and, if necessary, by a tranquilizer. The patient with recurrent ocular herpes can

be taught to recognize his own trigger mechanisms and to modify them.

Primary infection of the newborn with herpesvirus type 2 can be prevented only by a change in the sexual mores of the population and by the cesarean delivery of mothers with vaginal or cervical herpetic infection.

Zoster ophthalmicus can be prevented by any means effective in preventing childhood varicella. There is as yet no effective vaccine, but varicella-zoster (VZ) immune globulin is available for immunosuppressed children (eg, with leukemia) who have been exposed to VZ virus. Recurrent infection (zoster) is known to have occurred only in patients immunosuppressed by Hodgkin's disease and other tumors, surgical shock, immunosuppressive drugs (eg, corticosteroids), extreme fatigue, advanced age, etc. Some of these trigger mechanisms, such as stress, may be preventable. Ways of measuring and reducing the immunosuppression of old age—the principal trigger for ophthalmic zoster—are currently under study.

PREVENTION OF RECURRENT UVEITIS

Some types of uveitis, notably toxoplasmic retinochoroiditis and acute anterior uveitis, have trigger mechanisms similar to those of recurrent herpes simplex keratitis. Stress is the trigger, and since fatigue is the principal cause of stress, this is one trigger that should be preventable. A familiar example of this sequence of events is the uveitis that is all too often precipitated by the stress of preparing for examinations.

In this chapter we shall discuss blindness as a worldwide health problem with emphasis on the preventable forms of this dread human affliction, ie, trachoma, leprosy, onchocerciasis, and xerophthalmia. There are at least 10 million totally blind people in the world today.

In the USA, the most widely used definition of partial blindness is that used by the Internal Revenue Service for the purpose of determining who is eligible for tax deductions on that basis: *Central visual acuity of 6/60 (20/200) or less in the better eye with best correction, or widest diameter of visual field subtending an angle of no greater than 20 degrees.* An alternative functional definition favored by the authors is *loss of vision sufficient to prevent one from being self-supporting in an occupation, making the individual dependent on other persons, agencies, or devices in order to live.*

"Industrial blindness" is said to be present when a worker can no longer pursue an occupation because of poor vision; "automobile blindness" when vision is so poor that the responsible licensing agency in that state will not issue a driver's license. The term color blindness is a misnomer since this genetically transmitted disorder is not blindness as that term is generally understood and is only a minor handicap to a few people. Loss of vision may affect only the central fields, only the peripheral fields, or only specific portions of the peripheral fields in one or both eyes. Total loss of vision in one eye is said to reduce visual capacity by only 10%, though it makes the other eye infinitely more valuable.

The World Health Organization defines visual impairment as shown in Table 26–1. WHO officials encourage investigators and reporting agencies in all countries to report blindness and near blindness according to the categories defined in this table.

All of the disorders that may cause blindness are discussed more fully in other parts of this book. This chapter is an attempt to summarize some pertinent information about the epidemiology of blindness as a worldwide health problem with emphasis on those categories of blindness that are preventable by the combined efforts of physicians and health agencies.

INCIDENCE OF BLINDNESS THROUGHOUT THE WORLD

Table 26–2 lists some countries where fairly reliable data are available about the incidence of blindness. Even where health statistics are most reliable, the methods of counting the blind are often crude and may be applied according to different criteria in different places and at different times within any extensive geographic area. Note that Table 26–2 has no data for China, India, Mexico, Canada, Argentina, or Australia. If Pakistan has 1000 blind people per 100,000 population, that is 1% of a population of 65,000,000. If the incidence of blindness in India (population 600,000,000) and China (800,000,000) is half what it is in Pakistan, the number of blind in the unlisted countries alone is already many millions. In the countries listed in Table 26–2, there are either somewhat more or somewhat less than 3 million blind people depending on whether the data are thought to be exaggerated or conservative. The kind of effort it

Table 26–1. Categories of visual impairment. (Adapted from the International Classification of Diseases, World Health Organization, 1977.)

Category of Visual Impairment	Visual Acuity (Best Corrected)
Low vision 1	6/18 3/10 (0.3) 20/70
Low vision 2	6/60 1/10 (0.1) 20/200
Blindness 3	3/60 (finger counting at 3 m) 1/20 (0.05) 20/400
Blindness 4	1/60 (finger counting at 1 m) 1/50 (0.02) 5/300
Blindness 5	No light perception

Visual Field

Patients with a visual field radius no greater than 10 degrees but greater than 5 degrees around central fixation should be placed in category 3 and patients with a field no greater than 5 degrees around central fixation in category 4—even if the central acuity is not impaired.

Table 26–2. Blind persons per 100,000 inhabitants.
(Estimates based on WHO surveys.)*

Saudi Arabia	3000
Uganda	1842
Pakistan	1000
Tunisia	450
Japan	248
Indonesia	239
England and Wales	200
Italy	200
USA	200
Sweden	196
Brazil	147
Switzerland	145
France	107
Russia	90
Poland	66
Germany	60
Belgium	51

*Data reproduced, with permission, from Bietti GB: *World Health Magazine* (Feb–March) 1976:4. Based on global figures obtained in 1970 (including some figures of earlier provenance). Some of the data were only rough estimates when obtained and may have changed markedly since then.

would take to make a substantial reduction in any of these figures is almost too vast to contemplate. The same was true years ago when the public health profession set out to eradicate smallpox as one of the scourges of humanity. Smallpox formerly caused much blindness, but it is most unlikely that anyone will ever again be blinded, disfigured, or killed by what was an almost universal public health concern only a few decades ago. Fortunately, it is not necessary in the health professions that success be unqualified and total to earn the label of "success." Eliminating one cause of blindness would be a magnificent victory even if the other causes were unaffected. It is precisely because the numbers are so great that partial success in the effort to treat and prevent blindness must be sought by all available means.

WHO estimates that 10 million people are totally blind today and that millions more have loss of sight sufficient to prevent them from living a normal life. These numbers are increasing rapidly.

CAUSES OF BLINDNESS

The leading causes of preventable blindness in the world are trachoma, leprosy, onchocerciasis, and xerophthalmia. About 2 million people are blind from trachoma, at least 1 million from leprosy, 1 million from onchocerciasis, and 100,000 from xerophthalmia. Glaucoma, cataract, retinal detachment, and diabetic retinopathy have not been separately identified in WHO's statistical compilations, but many ophthalmologists believe that each of these disorders would rank ahead of onchocerciasis and xerophthalmia as a cause of blindness. Since some form of treatment is

available for all 3 disorders, there is no reason why they should not be included among the preventable causes of blindness.

Trachoma

Trachoma is an infectious disease caused by *Chlamydia trachomatis*. It can be prevented by adequate diet, proper sanitary facilities, and education and can be cured by sulfonamides or tetracycline drugs. About 400 million people have trachoma, most of them in Africa, the Middle East, and Asia. Trachoma is a form of bilateral keratoconjunctivitis that causes corneal scarring. When the scarring is severe, blindness results.

Leprosy

Leprosy (Hansen's disease) affects 15–16 million people in the world and has a higher percentage of ocular involvement than any other systemic infection. The type and frequency of ocular involvement differ in different parts of the world, and surveys of leprosy hospitals reveal that 6–90% of patients have ocular involvement. Many investigators feel that all leprosy patients will have ocular manifestations if the disease persists long enough. Reports on the prevalence of blindness among such patients indicate that up to 10% of leprosy patients may be blind from the disease, which means that over 1 million people are blind from leprosy worldwide. Such figures would place leprosy as the second leading cause of blindness resulting from an infectious disease, and it may thus be a greater visual threat than onchocerciasis.

Onchocerciasis

Onchocerciasis (due to *Onchocerca volvulus*, a roundworm) is transmitted by bites of the blackfly *Simulium damnosum* in Africa and other species of *Simulium* in Central and South America. The larvae are deposited in clear running streams (hence the name river blindness), and the adult female discharges large numbers of microfilariae that may enter the eyes and destroy them, causing total blindness. Onchocerciasis is endemic in the greater part of tropical Africa and Central and South America. The most heavily infested zone is the Volta River basin, which extends over parts

Table 26–3. Areas of eye afflicted by major blinding diseases.

Anterior segment diseases
Trachoma
Leprosy
Onchocerciasis
Xerophthalmia
Cataract
Herpes simplex keratitis
Posterior segment diseases
Glaucoma
Retinal degeneration
Retinal detachment

Note: In general, the anterior segment diseases are more preventable than the posterior segment diseases.

of Dahomey, Ghana, Ivory Coast, Mali, Niger, Togo, and Upper Volta. Drug treatment (diethylcarbamazine) is not very effective, and the best hope for control of the disease is insect eradication and personal protection by screening.

Xerophthalmia

Xerophthalmia is due to avitaminosis A and is exacerbated by protein-calorie malnutrition. It is a common cause of blindness in infants in India, Bangladesh, Java, and other countries where malnourishment (especially avitaminosis A) is a severe problem. Inadequate dietary vitamin A causes the cornea to become soft and necrotic. Perforation of the cornea with or without bacterial infection may occur secondarily. Affected babies usually do not reach adulthood and die from malnutrition or pneumonia. Xerophthalmia can be prevented by providing vitamin A supplementation wherever dietary restriction occurs as a result of poor economic conditions. If the problems of distribution and administration were solved, the cost of a quantity of the vitamin sufficient to prevent blindness in 1000 infants would be only about $20.

Other Causes

Glaucoma, cataract, retinal detachment, and diabetic retinopathy are discussed in greater detail elsewhere in this text. The incidence of blindness due to glaucoma has decreased in recent years as a result of earlier detection, improved medical and surgical treatment, and a greater awareness and understanding of the disorder by the lay population.

It is not known why the incidence of cataract is so high in India and Pakistan, and there is a great need for more cataract surgeons in these areas. In these countries, cataract can be listed as a common cause of blindness. In most of the western countries, on the other hand, the relative incidence of cataract is low, there is an oversupply of cataract surgeons, and any person with a cataract, regardless of economic circumstances, has easy access to surgery, which has a 90–95% success rate. For this reason many ophthalmologists, especially in the USA, take the view that cataract is not a cause of blindness in their experience.

Diabetic retinopathy is an increasingly more common cause of blindness everywhere in the world. Recent advances in surgical treatment (vitrectomy, laser therapy) are of some help, but many patients still suffer from progressive retinal hemorrhages, proliferative retinopathy, and eventual bilateral blindness. A vast research effort directed at all aspects of diabetes is in progress, and there is justification for hoping that the next generation of diabetics will benefit greatly from what is being done now.

Hereditary conditions are important causes of blindness but should gradually decrease in incidence in response to the efforts of genetic counselors to increase public awareness of the preventable nature of these disorders.

As is true also in other countries where medical care and social services are widely available, blindness in the USA is to a great extent related to the aging process, and about half of the legally blind people in this country are over age 65. The leading causes of blindness in this age group are glaucoma, diabetes, vascular diseases, and degenerative retinal disorders.

Amblyopia ("lazy eye") is decreased visual acuity in one eye in the absence of any organic eye disease responsible for the visual impairment. The function of vision develops from birth to age 7. If vision has not developed (because of disuse of the eye) by age 7, there is no chance that it will develop later.

PREVENTION OF BLINDNESS

It should be obvious from the foregoing discussion of the incidence and causes of blindness that the solution to the problem of blindness lies in prevention rather than treatment. Little has been done where much could be done, particularly in the developing countries, and there, most especially, in children. If a choice must be made, it would be a simple one between (a) spending millions on organ transplant research to keep a few people alive a few years longer and (b) using that money to solve some of the truly desperate problems of the earth's people. In some cases simple remedies are available and are not being used.

Some examples of what can be achieved for modest outlays of scarce funds are as follows:

(1) To cure one person of trachoma in Saudi Arabia: $1.00.

(2) To restore vision to one person in Pakistan blinded by cataracts: $20.

(3) To prevent blindness due to xerophthalmia in one infant in Java: 24 cents.

Recently, on the advice of WHO experts, the World Council for the Welfare of the Blind and several international professional ophthalmic societies and agencies agreed to take the initiative, which led to the establishment in 1974 of the International Agency for Prevention of Blindness (Vision International), with Sir John Wilson, a blind barrister, as president. The aim of this agency is to work with groups formed for the purpose of preventing blindness. Its theme, Foresight Prevents Blindness, was brought into prominent display when WHO celebrated the first World Health Day on April 7, 1976. Its goal is as follows: "In every donor country during 1976, every family should be asked—in thanksgiving for sight—to give $10 to save the sight of its fellow countrymen or of the millions in the third world. If we can raise this campaign to that degree of universal appeal, the result could be spectacular."

REHABILITATION OF THE BLIND

Technologic developments in recent years have created new opportunities for richer and more productive lives for blind people. In assessing these advances it is necessary to be aware of the blind population one is dealing with. Different categories of the blind have different needs, and some blind people simply cannot benefit from some of the more glamorous technical achievements. It has been said that over half of the blind people in the USA are over age 65. The elderly widowed housewife may need or want no more than mobility training in home care and a steady supply of Talking Books. A young person facing blindness in later life due to retinitis pigmentosa requires the full range of social services, including educational assessment, job rehabilitation, and psychologic counseling. The physician's role is to know what referral sources are available and how to use them skillfully. This means personally investigating the quality of services offered. Medical social workers, public health nurses, and counseling services and agencies serving the blind and visually handicapped are common sources of reliable information.

Low Vision Aid Clinics

Persons characterized as visually handicapped or partially sighted probably exceed in numbers those defined as legally blind by at least 3:1. Because these people have the potential for improved vision, low vision clinics have been established in many large medical centers and in special centers for the blind and visually handicapped. These clinics offer better refraction techniques and a wider range of optical aids, particularly for improved near vision, than would be available in the office of the practicing ophthalmologist.

A number of eye problems require nothing more than simple magnification. This is especially true of central field losses and macular lesions and disorders characterized by dimness of vision. Magnification is less useful for extensive peripheral field losses and large central or sector scotomas. In visual loss due to vascular disease the value of magnification is unpredictable, but this means of improving vision should be tried.

Patients rarely accept telescopic eyewear for long periods. Spectacle magnifiers for near vision up to +10 diopter sphere for both eyes and +40 diopter sphere for one eye are fairly well accepted.

The importance of adequate illumination should not be underestimated, since older patients even with vision normal for age need at least twice as much light for reading as younger persons. A hand magnifier for use when needed may be the best and most practical optical aid for many people.

Braille

This remarkably effective system of reading for the blind was introduced in 1825 by Louis Braille, a 16-year-old blind French youth living near Paris, who adapted it from a more complicated system of "point writing" devised by Charles Barbier. The Braille characters consist of raised dots arranged in 2 columns of three. The system is so simple that a blind child can quickly learn to read Braille, and proficient readers can

learn to read Braille as fast as they can talk. The system has been adapted to musical notation and technical and scientific uses also.

A Braille printing press was established in London in 1868, and soon thereafter the advantages of Braille reading became available in every important language in the world. Attempts to modify the alphabet culminated in an impressive display of international cooperation led by a talented group of Braillists working with UNESCO. In 1951 they produced an international Braille code that continues to be used.

Blinded adults learn Braille less easily than children, but with adequate motivation anyone can learn the system. The alphabet is shown in Fig 26–1.

Braille is used less commonly now than formerly, since many blind people prefer auditory aids both for informational and recreational purposes. For the partially sighted, large print editions may be easier to use and are more readily available. Braille continues to be essential on tags attached to items in common personal use even for people who do not wish to use it for reading.

All of the paper money in the Netherlands is Braille-printed to show the denomination in the lower left-hand corner. Switzerland is converting to the same system as old bills are taken out of circulation and replaced with new ones.

Mobility Training

Many state commissions for the blind offer a wide variety of mobility training courses, either directly or in cooperation with private agencies. The courses are offered on an outpatient and residential basis and have varied objectives according to the special needs of the people who apply for help. The curriculum commonly includes self-care, home functions, and mobility within the community.

Guide Dogs

The popular concept of the guide dog is somewhat unrealistic and no doubt colored by the natural affection most people have for these handsome animals. The guide dog is not trained to think and thus help its master function better in a strange and hostile world; its major function is to obey commands, and its usefulness is therefore directly related to the competence of its master. It may be said that a cane is not much of a companion, but neither does it have to be fed or housed or taken to the veterinarian when it gets sick. Older patients have trouble with the dogs because considerable physical strength is required to hold them in check. Guide dogs are most useful for students and professional men and women in good health who lead fairly well organized lives. At this time less than 2% of blind people in the USA use guide dogs. Sonar sensor canes may ultimately be a better answer to the mobility problem even for those who are now using a dog successfully.

Electronic Devices

Optacon is an electronic device that converts vis-

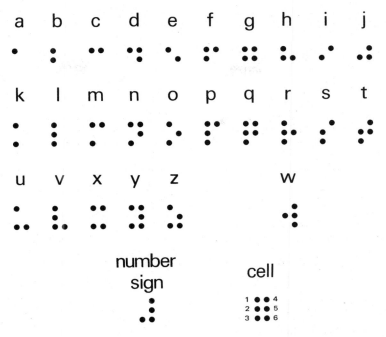

Figure 26–1. The Braille alphabet. The "cell" at bottom shows the numbering of the 6 raised dots used to make up the 26 letters of the Latin alphabet. Note that the first 10 letters use neither dot 3 nor dot 6. The second row of 10 letters is the same as the first row except dot 3 has been added (lower left-hand corner). The third row of 5 letters is the same as those above it except that dot 6 has been added (lower right-hand corner). The letter *w* is out of place because it is not part of the basic French alphabet, although it is used in loan-words from other languages (eg, wagon). Note that it is the mirror image of *r*. The number sign indicates that a numeral will follow; the end of a number is signified by a space. Punctuation marks are represented by combinations of dots other than those used to represent letters. What is shown here is grade 1 Braille, in which all words are spelled out in their entirety. Other more complicated grades of Braille utilize contractions and shortened forms of frequently used words. (Data based on information provided by Lighthouse for the Blind, San Francisco, California, and by the Sixth District, California State PTA Braille Transcription Project, San Jose, California.)

ual images of letters into tactile forms. It is easily portable and can be used with almost any kind of reading matter. A Talking Calculator is now available that offers the usual calculator functions and converts input signals into audible responses. There are a variety of optical enlargers, some of them based upon closed television circuitry. The Apollo electronic visual aid includes a camera with zoom lens, scanning table, and illuminator. Many of these systems are gradually becoming cheaper, but at current prices (about $1500) they are beyond the means of all but a few of the people who could use them.

FINANCIAL ASSISTANCE PROGRAMS

It is unfortunate that over half of the blind people in the USA are essentially dependent upon Social Security and whatever local supplemental aid may be available to them. For the younger blind population, rehabilitation programs are commonly administered at the state level by a division of the department of educa-

tion specifically set up to serve blind people in the state. Some of these programs are better than others, and all physicians should support efforts to increase the effectiveness of such programs in their geographic area of influence. The programs are of wide scope and offer preliminary counseling followed by academic or vocational training as the circumstances warrant. Once a realistic vocational objective has been established, full financial support is commonly available. This single resource is probably the most crucial referral available to the ophthalmologist, particularly in the case of young patients. Counseling services are available as early as the junior high school years to assure compliance with a curriculum consistent with measured aptitudes and interests. In many states, such rehabilitation programs as mobility training are administered under state auspices but contracted to private agencies for operational purposes.

In many countries of the world, the blind receive no financial or other support from their governments and are either cared for by their families or left to manage by themselves in any way they can.

References

General

Baghdassarian SA, Tabbara KF: Childhood blindness in Lebanon. *Am J Ophthalmol* 1975;**79**:827.

Belfort R Jr, Moraes MAP: Oncocercose ocular no Brasil. *Rev Assoc Med Brasil* 1979;**25**:123.

Brand M: The care of the eye. In: *The Star*. National Hansen's Disease Center, 1980.

Choyce DP: Blindness in leprosy. *Trop Doct* (Jan) 1973:16.

Faye E: Chapter 6 in: *The Low Vision Patient: Clinical Experience With Adults and Children*. Grune & Stratton, 1970.

Ffytche TJ: Blindness in leprosy. *Br J Ophthalmol* 1982; **65**:221.

Hobbs HE, Choyce DP: The blinding lesions of leprosy. *Lepr Rev* 1971;**42**:131.

Jones BR: Bowman lecture, 1975: The prevention of blindness from trachoma. *Trans Ophthalmol Soc UK* 1975;**95**:16.

Jones BR: General obstacles to the prevention of blindness. *Trans Ophthalmol Soc UK* 1978;**98**:316.

Law FW: World health day: 7 April 1976. *Br J Ophthalmol* 1976;**60**:231.

Lim ASM, Jones BR (editors): World's major blinding conditions. *Vision* 1982;**1**:1. [Entire issue.]

MacKay DM: The psychology of seeing. *Trans Ophthalmol Soc UK* 1973;**93**:391.

Nizetic B: Prevention of blindness: Potentialities of a systems analysis approach. *Sight Sav Rev* 1974; **44**:89.

Onchocerciasis. (Editorial.) *Br J Ophthalmol* 1976;**60**:1.

The Prevention of Blindness: Report of a WHO Study Group. World Health Organization Technical Report Series 518, 1973. [Entire issue.]

Roper-Hall MJ: Prevention of blindness from trauma. *Trans Ophthalmol Soc UK* 1978;**98(Part 2)**:313.

Roy FH: World blindness: Definition, incidence and major treatable causes. *Ann Ophthalmol* 1974; **6**:1049.

Sommer A et al: Xerophthalmia and anterior segment blindness among preschool-age children in El Salvador. *Am J Ophthalmol* 1976;**80**:1066.

Stetten D Jr: Coping with blindness. *N Engl J Med* 1981;**305**:458.

Additional References & Sources (See also p 387.)

Division for the Blind and Physically Handicapped, Library of Congress.

National Society for the Prevention of Blindness: *Estimated Statistics on Blindness and Vision Problems – 1970*.

Recording for the Blind, New York.

World Health Magazine (Feb–March) 1976.

Appendices

First Appendix: Ophthalmoscopic Examination

Hermann von Helmholtz, a German physicist and physiologist, invented the ophthalmoscope in 1851. In so doing, he provided the medical practitioner—ophthalmologist, internist, or neurologist—with an instrument that has become indispensable to the study of eye diseases and systemic diseases with ocular manifestations. Nowhere else in the body is it possible to examine living vascular and nerve tissue under magnification, and the information gained in this way can be of great diagnostic importance. It can also be of value in the management of a recognized disease process, providing a ready means of estimating changes in established lesions.

The principal contribution of the ophthalmoscope is of course the remarkable view of the inner eye it provides. Ophthalmoscopy, or examination of the fundus—optic disk, retina, retinal vessels, macula, and choroid—is therefore of prime ophthalmoscopic importance. However, examination of other ocular tissues—cornea, iris, lens, and vitreous—with the ophthalmoscope also yields valuable information. Although the slit lamp is a better instrument for this purpose, it is often not available, since it is used principally by the ophthalmologist. Inspection of the anterior ocular structures with the ophthalmoscope may alert the examiner to a wide variety of changes that are indicative of ocular or systemic diseases. It is possible in this way to recognize vascular changes and opacities in the cornea; hemorrhages and exudates in the anterior chamber; the location and nature of opacities in the lens; irregularities of the pupil; and opacities, detachments, and degenerative changes in the vitreous.

For all of these reasons, ophthalmoscopy should be an integral part of every general physical examination; and since both the ocular media and the fundus can be examined quickly and easily with the modern ophthalmoscope once its principles are understood, everyone doing general physical examinations—medical students, interns, general practitioners, internists, pediatricians, and others—should feel obliged to master the use of this extraordinary but essentially quite simple instrument.

The Use of Mydriatics

For the purposes of routine physical examination, it is almost always possible to visualize the ocular media and fundus adequately without dilating the pupil if the lighting in the examining room is sufficiently subdued and the light in the ophthalmoscope is strong (fresh batteries). If mydriasis is indicated, however (eg, to investigate impaired vision of unknown cause), the mydriatic should be short-acting and should not affect accommodation.

Phenylephrine hydrochloride (2.5–10%) is an excellent mydriatic for this purpose.* Topical use produces no systemic side-effects; the drug acts rapidly; and dilatation of the pupil can be accomplished by one or 2 instillations. A heavily pigmented iris is less responsive than a lightly pigmented one to phenylephrine alone, and such a patient may require the use of a cycloplegic, such as homatropine or cyclopentolate, along with phenylephrine.

Since any mydriatic agent can precipitate acute angle-closure glaucoma in an eye with a shallow anterior chamber, mydriatics must always be used with caution. In young patients the danger is negligible, but in adults the depth of the anterior chamber should be estimated by oblique illumination with a flashlight (Fig 14–7).

TYPES OF OPHTHALMOSCOPY

There are 2 types of ophthalmoscopy: indirect and direct (see accompanying diagrams). Each has special uses as well as special advantages and disadvantages (see table on p 345). Both require a darkened room and an ophthalmoscope supplied with an electrical source strong enough to produce a bright light. As a rule, the patient is sitting down and the examiner is standing—at the right side of the patient and holding the ophthalmoscope in the right hand when the right eye is examined; at the left side and using the left hand when the left eye is examined (see photos on p 346).

*Others are mentioned briefly on p 372.

1. INDIRECT OPHTHALMOSCOPY

Indirect ophthalmoscopy has been performed for many years by holding a convex lens (objective) between the ophthalmoscope and the patient's eye. The ophthalmoscope, with a +3 or +4 diopter lens in the aperture to neutralize the observer's accommodation, is held several centimeters from the patient's eye.

The disk is brought into view by having the patient look over the examiner's right shoulder at ear level when examining the right eye, and over the left shoulder at the same level when examining the left eye. Areas of interest near the disk can then be examined by having the patient move the eyes slightly in various directions.

Indirect ophthalmoscopy has 2 distinct advantages over direct ophthalmoscopy: It provides a large field of vision that gives the examiner a good view of the fundus even through an undilated pupil and in spite of opacities in the media, and it is not affected by major refractive errors in the patient's eyes. The disadvantages are the lower magnification and the inverted image. In making and recording observations, the observer must never forget that the image is inverted.

Binocular Indirect Ophthalmoscopy

The binocular indirect ophthalmoscope began to come into wide use among ophthalmologists in the 1950s. Its use is now being taught to all students of ophthalmology, and in the specialist's hands, it is being used almost to the exclusion of the standard monocular ophthalmoscope. Its advantages are a more powerful light source that can cut through cloudy media (eg, incipient cataract); its binocularity; and the fact that the entire peripheral retina can be viewed with it. It is unlikely, however, that this instrument will meet the needs of medical students and other physicians doing general physical examinations since it is relatively cumbersome and expensive, the technique of using it is difficult to master, and the pupil must be widely dilated because of its very strong light.

This instrument is further discussed and illustrated in Chapter 3.

2. DIRECT OPHTHALMOSCOPY

The use of the direct ophthalmoscope is the principal subject matter of this Appendix. Unless otherwise specified, all further references are understood to be to direct ophthalmoscopy.

The instrument has been greatly improved since Helmholtz published the first description of the ophthalmoscope, but the principle is the same. The basic unit is a strong light that can be directed into the patient's eye by reflection from a small mirror. The light is then reflected from the fundus of the patient's eye back through a small aperture in the ophthalmoscope to the examiner's eye. Various models of electric and battery-powered ophthalmoscopes are available.

In direct ophthalmoscopy, the aperture of the instrument is held as close as possible to the observer's eye and the subject's eye. The details of the inner eye will then be in focus if both eyes (examiner's and patient's) are emmetropic. If either eye is ametropic, a graduated series of convex (plus) or concave (minus) lenses can be moved into the aperture (by rotating the lens wheel with one finger) to bring the details into focus.

As the examiner directs the beam of the ophthalmoscope into the patient's eye and moves the plus lenses successively into the aperture (from +20 diopters down to about +4 diopters), the magnified details of the anterior segment of the eye (cornea, iris, and

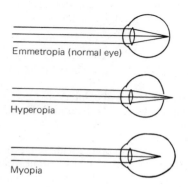
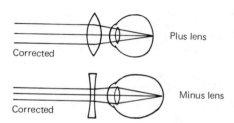

Common defects of the optical system of the eye. In hyperopia the eyeball is too short, and light rays come to a focus behind the retina. A biconvex lens corrects this by adding to the refractive power of the lens of the eye. In myopia the eyeball is too long, and light rays focus in front of the retina. Placing a biconcave lens in front of the eye causes the light rays to diverge slightly before striking the eye, so that they are brought to a focus on the retina. (Modified and reproduced, with permission, from Ganong WF: *Review of Medical Physiology,* 10th ed. Lange, 1981.)

lens) will first be visualized. As the examiner gradually reduces the strength of the plus lenses, the focus of observation gradually extends posteriorly through the vitreous until the retinal and other fundus details come into view.

The fundi of aphakic eyes (eyes without lenses) are examined with a lens in the range of +8 to +12 in the aperture or with the patient's own corrective lenses in place.

Red Fundus Reflection

The first step in ophthalmoscopy is to look for the red fundus reflection, which can be seen without magnification from a comfortable distance of 25–40 cm. The experienced examiner, when seeing the fundus reflection, can immediately rule out gross corneal lesions, dense opacities of the media, and complete detachment of the retina.

If opacities are present, they will appear as black forms against the red background.

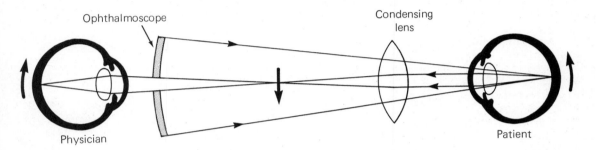

Indirect ophthalmoscopy. Arrow at focal point represents inverted image of patient's ocular fundus.

Comparison of Indirect and Direct Ophthalmoscopy

	Indirect	Direct
Area of field examined	Eight disk diameters	Two diameters
Area accessible to view	Up to ora serrata	Up to equator
Stereopsis	Yes	No
Image	Inverted, virtual	Erect, true
Magnification	2–4 ×	15–15 ×

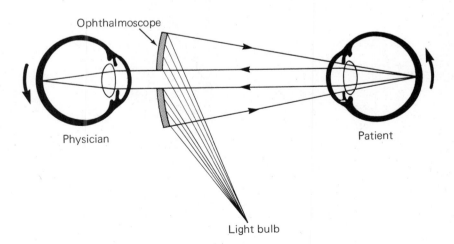

Direct ophthalmoscopy. Arrows show spatial orientation of images in examiner's and patient's eyes. (Modified and reproduced, with permission, from Nover A: *The Ocular Fundus,* 2nd ed. Lea & Febiger, 1971.)

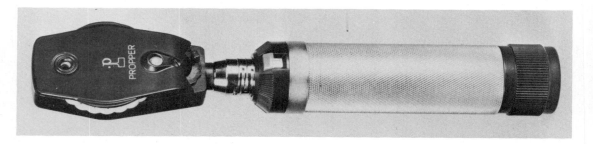

Ophthalmoscope. (Courtesy of Propper Manufacturing Co., Inc.)

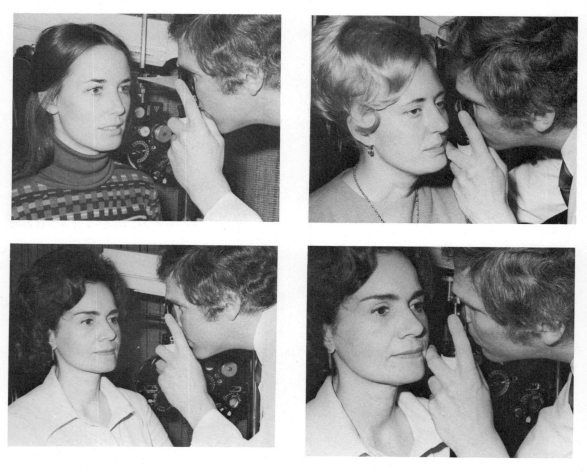

Position of patient and examiner for direct ophthalmoscopy

Cornea, Aqueous, Iris, & Lens

A. Cornea: In order to examine the cornea at close range, a strong plus lens is introduced into the aperture of the ophthalmoscope. For example, a dendritic lesion of the cornea is easy to see with a +20 diopter lens from a distance of approximately 2 cm, and with the same lens one can see corneal scars, ulcers, foreign bodies, pterygiums, and vascularization.

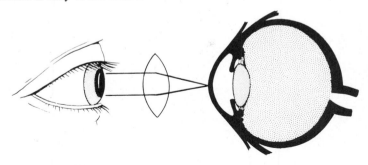

Examination of the cornea with a strong convex lens at close range

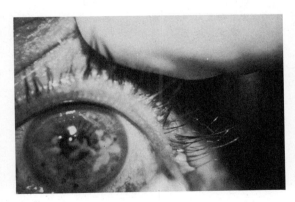

Dendritic figures seen in herpes simplex keratitis

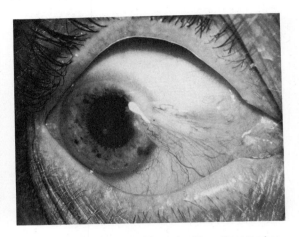

Pterygium, right eye. (Photo by Diane Beeston.)

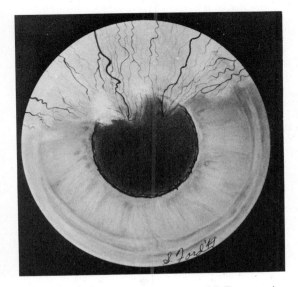

Trachomatous pannus. (Courtesy of P Thygeson.)

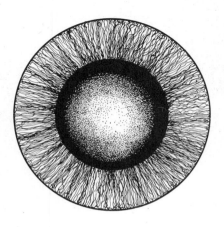

Disciform herpes simplex keratitis

B. Aqueous: The examiner can get a magnified view of abnormalities in the aqueous with the ophthalmoscope, eg, blood (hyphema) resulting from trauma or pus (hypopyon) in association with bacterial corneal ulcer.

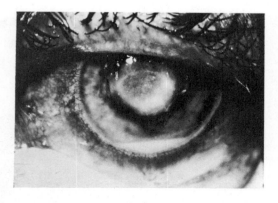

Hypopyon. (Courtesy of K Tabbara.)

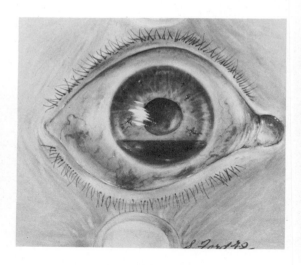

Blood in the anterior chamber (hyphema). (Courtesy of M Hogan.)

C. Iris: Since the iris is behind the cornea, a weaker lens is required in the ophthalmoscope to make it clearly visible. With a +15 diopter lens, for example, such disorders of the iris as tumors, nodules, pigmentary abnormalities, and synechiae can be seen in adequate detail.

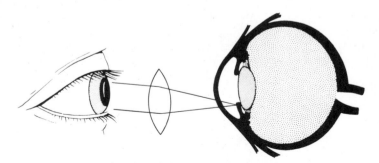

Examination of the iris with a strong convex lens

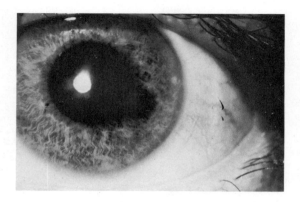

Tumor of iris. (Courtesy of K Tabbara.)

D. Lens: The lens is still farther posterior and can be seen quite well with a lens in the range of +8 to +12 diopters. If there are lens opacities, their location, shapes, sizes, and degrees of density can all be clearly viewed.

Examination of the lens with a weaker convex lens

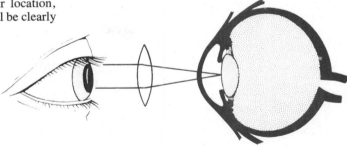

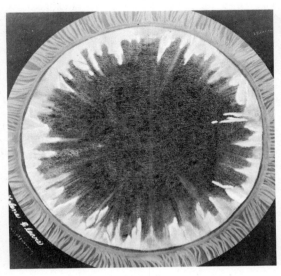

Senile cataract, "cuneiform" type. (Reproduced, with permission, from Cordes FC: *Cataract Types,* 3rd ed. American Academy of Ophthalmology and Otolaryngology, 1965.)

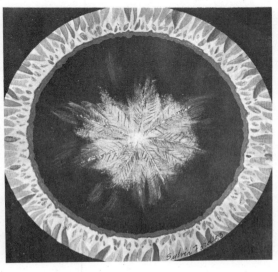

Traumatic "star-shaped" cataract in the posterior lens. (From Cordes FC: Ibid.)

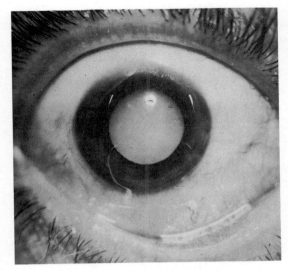

Mature senile cataract. (Courtesy of A Rosenberg.)

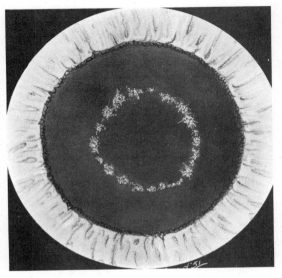

"Vossius' ring." (From Cordes FC: Ibid.)

Vitreous

As the examiner gradually rotates the lens wheel to bring lenses of from +8 to +4 diopters into the aperture, the focus extends posteriorly into the vitreous. Cloudiness of the vitreous may occur as a result of various inflammatory diseases of the optic disk, retina, and uvea. Vitreous hemorrhages give a very dark picture. Even a small amount of blood in the vitreous may appear almost black and can completely obstruct the view of the fundus. Fibrovascular proliferation in the vitreous can be seen in patients with advanced diabetic retinopathy. Degenerative changes—asteroid hyalosis and synchysis scintillans—can easily be seen with the ophthalmoscope.

Fundus

Examination of the fundus includes inspection of the optic disk, macula, retina, retinal vessels, choroid, and sclera. These structures can be brought into clear focus with a wide range of lenses depending on the refractive error of the patient and the examiner. If the patient has high myopia, the size of the image is greatly increased; with high hyperopia, it is greatly decreased. The retina can be examined by direct ophthalmoscopy as far anteriorly as the equator of the eyeball in patients with widely dilated pupils; but the area from the equator to the ora serrata can be examined adequately

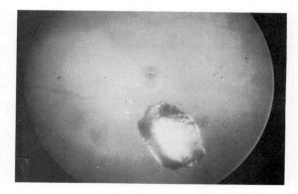

Metallic foreign body in vitreous as seen with ophthalmoscope

only with the binocular indirect ophthalmoscope.

Examination of the fundus must proceed systematically if lesions of diagnostic importance are not to be overlooked. A sketch of the disk, macula, and major blood vessels will help to localize the lesions, and all fundus lesions should be described and sketched for the case record. If the lesion is one that should be observed periodically, fundus photographs are highly desirable.

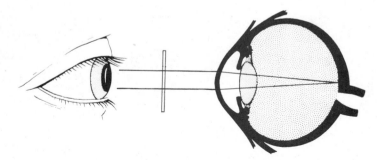

Examination of retina with a zero lens (assuming that the physician is emmetropic)

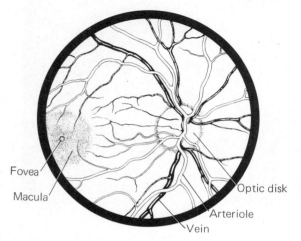

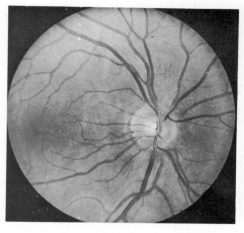

Fovea

Macula

Optic disk

Arteriole

Vein

The normal fundus. Diagram at left shows landmarks of the photograph at right. (Photo by Diane Beeston.)

A. Optic Disk: Under the strong light of an oph-thalmoscope and with adequate magnification, observation of the optic disk can yield clinical information that is not available about any other nerve in the body. As a first step in the examination, the disk's size, color, and vascularity and the degree of cupping should be assessed.

Although the diameter of the normal optic disk in adults averages only about 1.5 mm, with the ophthalmoscope it appears quite large. All of the details are clearly visible, including the central artery and vein and the numerous capillaries on the disk's surface that produce the pink color.

The disk is round or oval, and the nasal edge is less distinct than the temporal edge. A white crescent may appear around the temporal edge, especially in myopic patients. This is bare sclera exposed by a normal break in the choroid.

The optic disk usually has a white central depression (cup) whose diameter averages approximately one-third of the disk diameter. This is referred to as the cup/disk ratio and should be noted on the patient's record (eg, 0.3 cup). In normal individuals the cup/disk ratio ranges from 0.0 (flat disk) to 0.9 (huge cup). In some patients, the disk is elevated, and if the eleva-tion is significant the condition is referred to as pseu-dopapilledema. In patients with glaucoma, recording the cup/disk ratio is especially important, since the breadth and depth of the cup increase in uncontrolled glaucoma with the death of the nerve fibers. In this situation, the cup/disk ratio becomes a measure of the progress of the disease.

In optic neuritis the disk becomes abnormally vascular and slightly elevated. Small hemorrhages are sometimes seen.

In papilledema, the essential feature is bulging forward (elevation) of the disk due to pressure (usually intracranial) from behind. The vessels on the disk's surface are engorged, and hemorrhages may occur.

In optic atrophy, there is reduction in the vascularity of the optic nerve head. With reduction in vascularity, the normal pink color of the healthy disk turns white.

In central retinal artery occlusion, the disk immediately becomes pale. Weeks to months later, the nerve whitens.

Occlusion of the central retinal vein produces a dramatic clinical picture. Extensive hemorrhages in the region of the optic disk make the area look as if it had been "slapped with a red paintbrush."

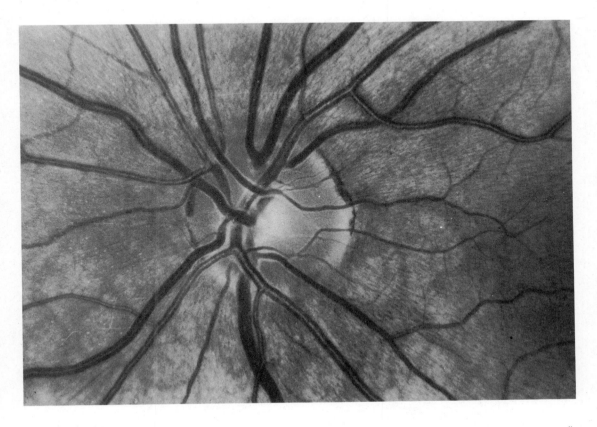

Normal optic disk and peripapillary retina. Note rich vascular network supplying the retinal nerve fiber layer surrounding the disk. (Courtesy of WF Hoyt.)

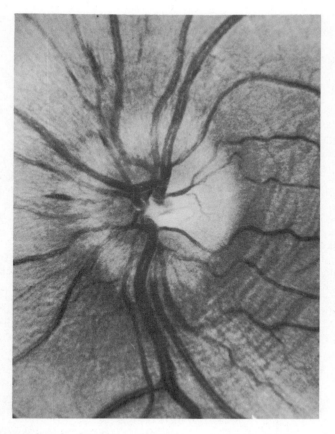

Early papilledema showing blurring of disk margins and peripapillary nerve fiber layer. Vessels are buried (blurred by surrounding edema), resulting in absence of highlights and fine detail in retina. (Courtesy of WF Hoyt.)

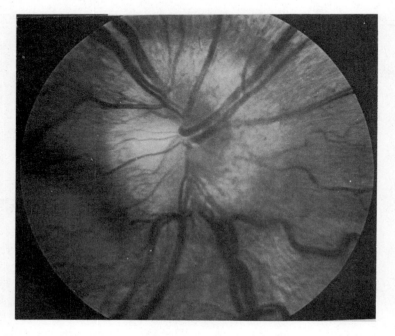

Papilledema causing moderate disk elevation without hemorrhages. (Courtesy of WF Hoyt.)

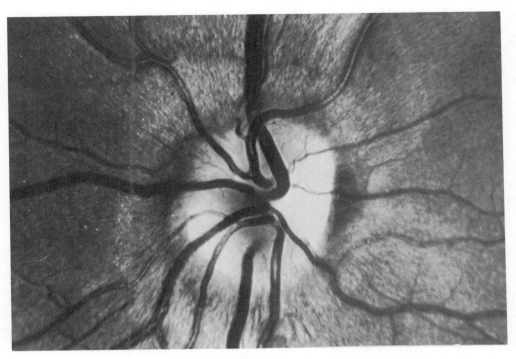

Pseudopapilledema. Note vessels on top (not buried). (Courtesy of WF Hoyt.)

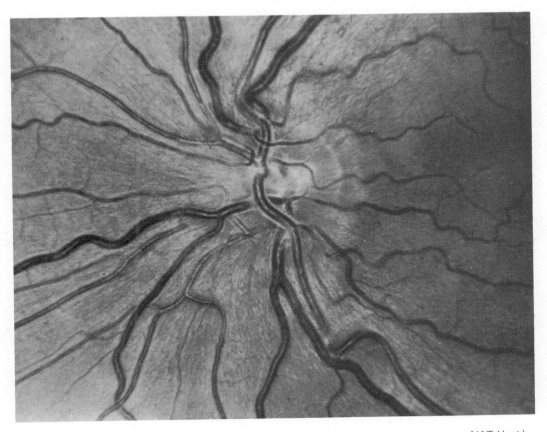

Congenitally "full" optic disk. There is no edema, and the disk is not choked. (Courtesy of WF Hoyt.)

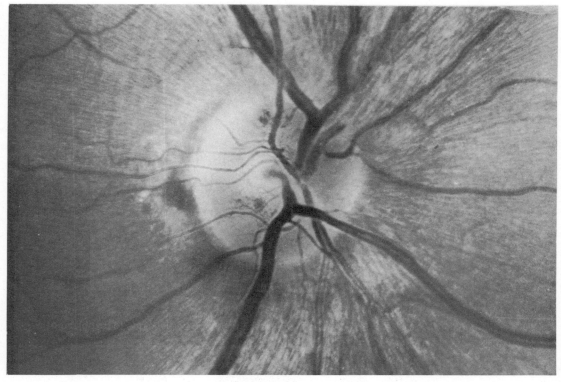

Optic neuritis (papillitis) with disk changes, including capillary hemorrhages and minimal edema. (Courtesy of WF Hoyt.)

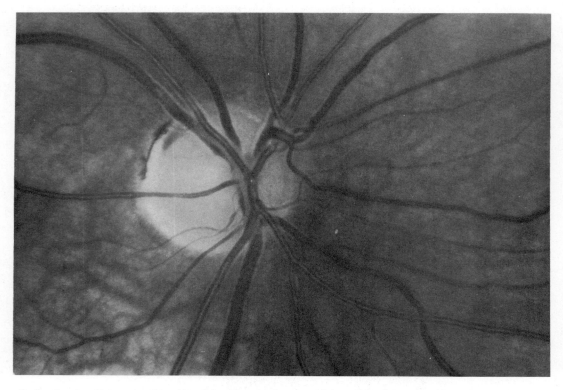

Optic atrophy. Note avascular white disk and avascular network in surrounding retina. (Courtesy of WF Hoyt.)

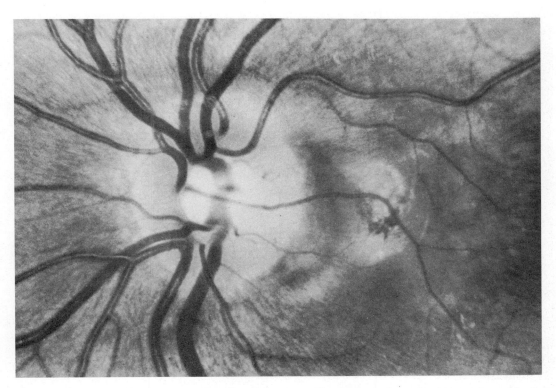

Chorioretinal peripapillary scar with atrophy of overlying nerve fiber layer, perhaps due to toxoplasmosis. Central vision was defective. (Courtesy of WF Hoyt.)

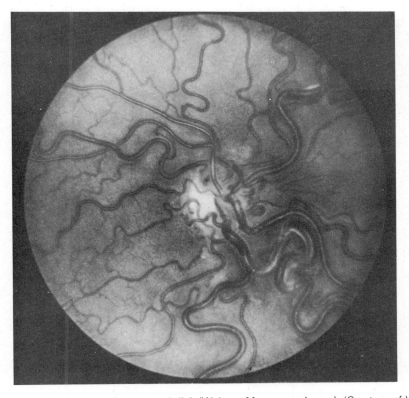

Arteriovenous malformation of retina and disk (Wyburn-Mason syndrome). (Courtesy of WF Hoyt.)

B. Macula: The macula is an oval area situated about 2 disk diameters temporally to and slightly below the optic disk. It is devoid of blood vessels and appears to be darker than the surrounding retina. There is a central light reflection from the centrally located, slightly depressed fovea.

The commonest affliction of the macula is disciform macular degeneration. In its end stage this appears as a round, fairly well circumscribed, elevated white mass. Other types of macular degeneration (hereditary, cystic, circinate, etc) are described in Chapter 13.

In central retinal artery occlusion, the macula is edematous and ischemic. With the choroidal blood supply showing through, the fovea, in contrast to the ischemic retina, appears as a "cherry-red spot."

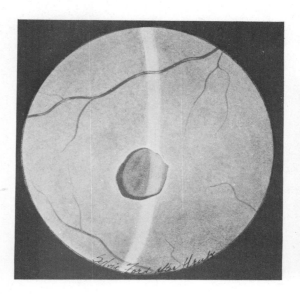

Hole in retina, macular area, posttraumatic

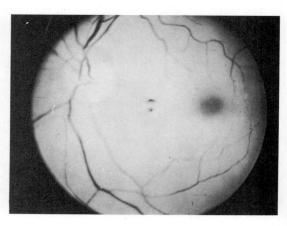

Twenty-four hours after closure of central retinal artery, left eye. The macular area shows a "cherry-red spot."

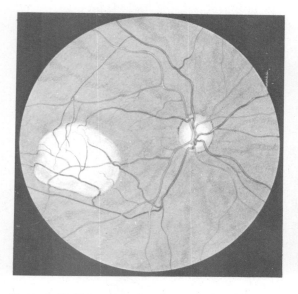

Healed disciform macular degeneration (drawing). (Courtesy of F Cordes.)

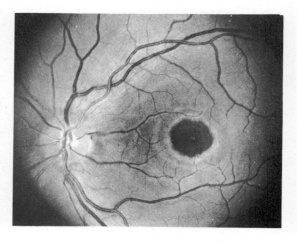

Juvenile macular degeneration (hereditary). (Courtesy of WF Hoyt.)*

*This photograph and those on pp 351–355 are by Ron Eckelhoff.

C. Retina: Retinal detachment appears ophthalmoscopically as a gray, elevated cloud affecting part or all of the retina. Detachments are associated with one or more orange-red retinal tears.

A variety of retinal disturbances (eg, those associated with retinitis pigmentosa) can be seen with the ophthalmoscope.

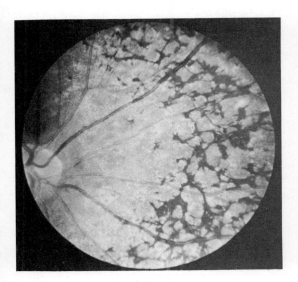 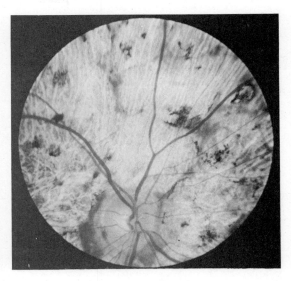

Retinitis pigmentosa. *Left:* Typical "bone spicule" arrangement of pigmentary changes. *Right:* Clumped, scattered pigment, attentuated arteries, and choroidal sclerosis. (Photos by L Arlinghaus.)

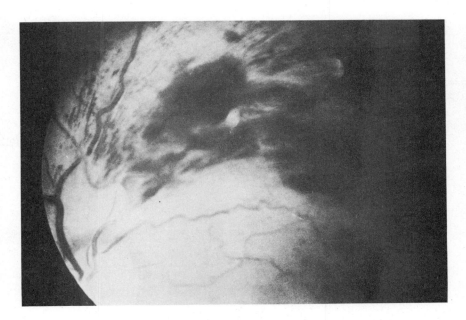

Thrombosis of superior temporal retinal vein. (Courtesy of K Tabbara.)

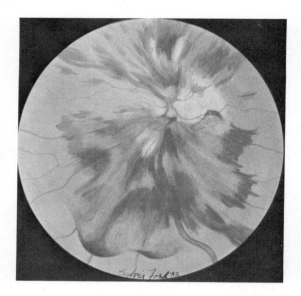

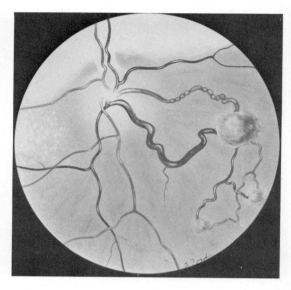

Subhyaloid hemorrhage around optic disk associated with subarachnoid hemorrhage (drawing).

Hemangiomas of the retina (drawing). (Courtesy of F Cordes.)

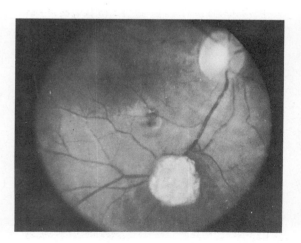

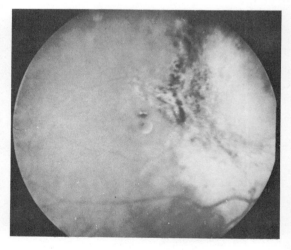

Tuberous sclerosis

Retinoblastomas after x-ray radiation

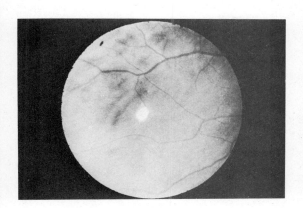

Retinal fat embolism. (Courtesy of K Tabbara.)

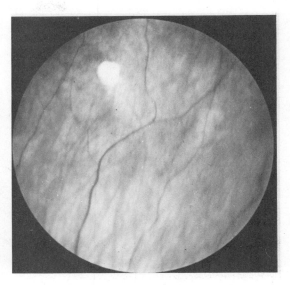

"Histo spot"—a depigmented area in peripheral retina. (Courtesy of K Tabbara.)

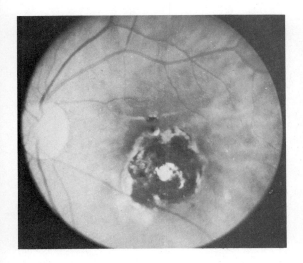

Healed toxoplasmic chorioretinitis. Note scarring in left macular area.

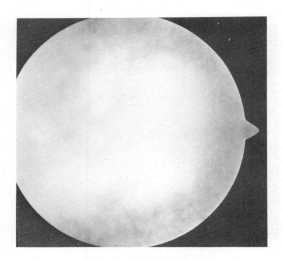

Acute toxoplasmic chorioretinitis. (Courtesy of K Tabbara.)

D. Retinal Vessels: The retinal arteries and veins can be seen clearly with the ophthalmoscope. After the first bifurcation of the central retinal artery, the vessels are called arterioles. They should be examined for caliber, occlusion, color of the blood column, course and contour, light reflection from the blood column, pulsation, compression, and aneurysms.

In arteriosclerosis, the walls of the retinal arterioles are infiltrated with lipids and cholesterol. Sclerosis supervenes, and the sclerotic changes are easy to see ophthalmoscopically.

In hypertension, the changes in the retinal arterioles include vasospasm, narrowing, sclerosis, and eventually occlusion. If severe enough, hypertensive retinopathy can lead to retinal edema, cotton wool patches, hemorrhages, and eventually papilledema.

Retinal changes associated with diabetes mellitus are similar to the changes associated with hypertension but more devastating. They include microaneurysms, dilated veins, hemorrhages and exudates, and neovascularization. When major hemorrhages are absorbed, fibrous tissue forms along with the neovascularization. This gives the picture of proliferative diabetic retinopathy, which is usually destructive enough to cause blindness. Retinal hemorrhages and exudates can also be caused by other systemic disorders, including lupus erythematosus and blood dyscrasias.

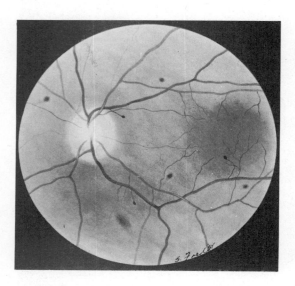

Diabetic retinopathy stage I (drawing)

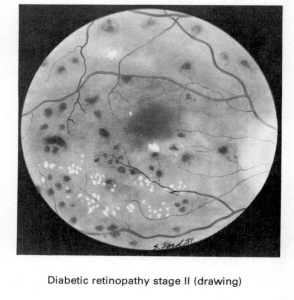

Diabetic retinopathy stage II (drawing)

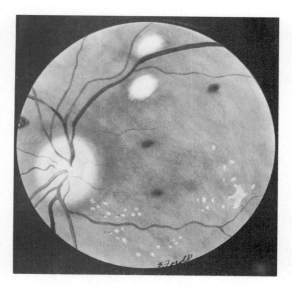

Diabetic retinopathy stage III (drawing)

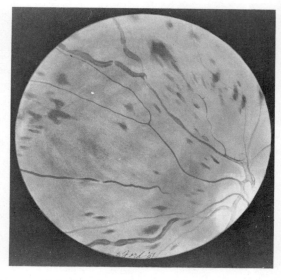

Diabetic retinopathy stage IV (drawing)

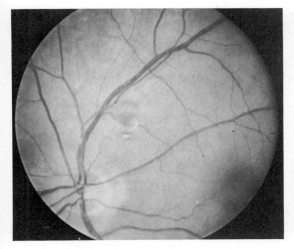

Keith-Wagener retinopathy stage I

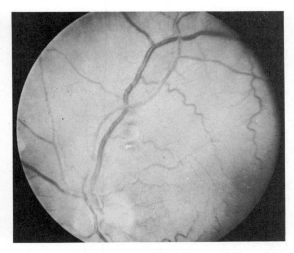

Keith-Wagener retinopathy stage II

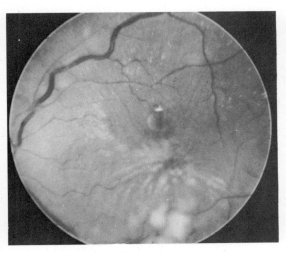

Keith-Wagener retinopathy stage III

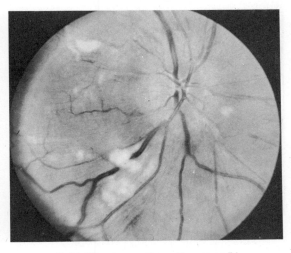

Keith-Wagener retinopathy stage IV

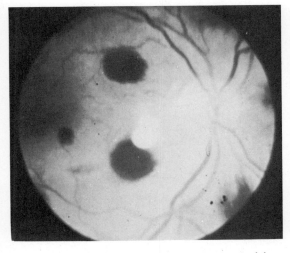

Retinal hemorrhages associated with severe pernicious anemia

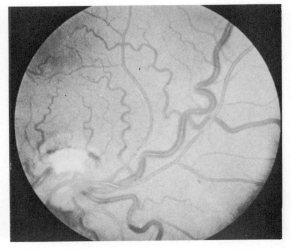

Engorged and markedly tortuous veins of polycythemia vera. (Photo by L Arlinghaus.)

E. Choroid and Sclera: If the pigment epithelium, which normally precludes visualization of the choroidal vessels and sclera, is congenitally absent or has degenerated, the vessels can be easily seen. In some myopic individuals, the sclera is visible near the temporal edge of the optic disk. In individuals who have punched-out lesions of the retina and choroid, which follow focal necrotizing retinochoroiditis (eg, toxoplasmosis, histoplasmosis), the sclera can be seen in the vicinity of the lesions surrounded by pigmentary proliferation.

Sclerosis of the choroidal vessels is seen in association with thinning and degeneration of the retina. A choroidal tear is quite likely to occur after a severe contusion of the globe.

Malignant melanoma appears ophthalmoscopically as a pigmented, elevated mass located most commonly in the posterior choroid on the temporal side.

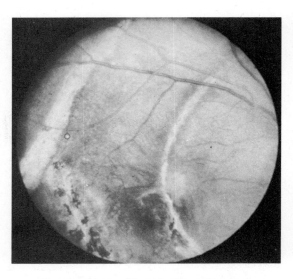

Choroidal tears. (Photo by Diane Beeston.)

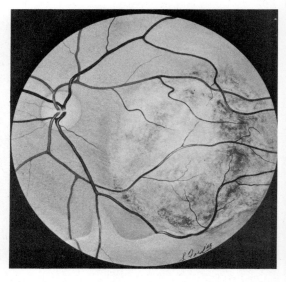

Malignant melanoma of choroid, macular area, left eye (drawing). (Courtesy of F Cordes.)

•   •   •

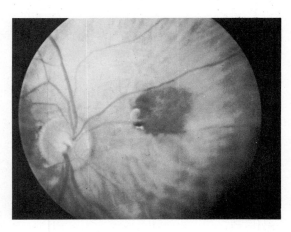

Nevus of choroid. (Photo by Diane Beeston.)

Ballantyne AJ, Michaelson IC: *Textbook of the Fundus of the Eye,* 2nd ed. Livingstone, 1970.

Cogan DG: *Ophthalmic Manifestations of Systemic Vascular Disease.* Saunders, 1974.

Jensen PE, Kalina RE: Congenital anomalies of the optic disk. *Am J Ophthalmol* 1976;**82:**27.

Keeney AH: *Ocular Examination: Basis and Techniques,* 2nd ed. Mosby, 1976.

More light through the ophthalmoscope. *Lancet* 1974;**1:**489.

Nover A: *The Ocular Fundus,* 2nd ed. Lea & Febiger, 1971. [Translated from German by F Blodi.]

Rucker CW: *History of the Ophthalmoscope.* Whiting Printers & Stationers, 1971.

Stetten D Jr: Coping with blindness. *N Eng J Med* 1981; **305:**458.

Vilas CH: *The Ophthalmoscope: Its Theory and Practical Uses.* Duncan Brothers, 1882.

Second Appendix:
The CT Scan
in Ophthalmologic Diagnosis

The development of a safe, rapid, and noninvasive technique for examination of the orbit and brain has led to revolutionary improvements in ophthalmologic diagnosis. Computer-assisted tomography (CT) in the transverse axial plane was developed in 1967 by G.N. Hounsfield at the Central Research Laboratories of EMI Ltd. The ease of diagnosis of intracranial lesions without dependence on cerebral angiography and air encephalography has been of outstanding benefit to neurologists and ophthalmologists.

The orbit has proved to be a particularly appropriate subject for CT evaluation because of the great differences in density between the main orbital structures and the surrounding orbital fat. Eye muscles, the optic nerve, and the major orbital vessels can be demonstrated, as well as the adjacent compartments of the head such as the paranasal sinuses and the intracranial space. This proved to be most helpful in the evaluation of visual loss, proptosis, oculomotor disorders, and visual field defects. More recently, the introduction of thin section computed tomography with higher spatial and contrast resolution has greatly facilitated detailed examination of intracranial and orbital structures. Thin section CT has also provided the technologic basis for high-quality computer reconstructions—ie, the capacity to reconstruct images in any desired plane based on information contained in one stack of axial sections. The number of reconstructions is unlimited, and additional radiation is not required. The use of computer-derived reconstructions allows comparison of structures such as the optic nerve, eye muscles, or optic canal independently of plane of section or head position. Simultaneous demonstration of intracranial and intraorbital soft tissue structures together with the demonstration of bony fissures and canals reduces the number of radiologic procedures necessary for accurate diagnosis of orbital disease. Computed tomography has thus become the primary procedure for x-ray diagnosis of orbital disorders.

PRINCIPLES & TECHNIQUE

A conventional x-ray is obtained by passing an x-ray beam through a structure and measuring the emergent rays by their ability to expose photographic film. Tissues of high density have higher absorption values, so that a 2-dimensional record is obtained of a 3-dimensional structure. Only when component tissues differ markedly in density can they be satisfactorily examined. These limitations have led to the use of contrast media administered into the arterial or venous systems or by direct infusion into specific anatomic areas. The complications of these invasive techniques are well known.

Computer-assisted tomography (CT scan) replaces photographic film with a sodium iodide crystal that functions as an x-ray detector. The crystal gives off visible light when exposed to x-rays, and a photomultiplier system generates an electrical signal. A large number of individual readings are taken of a collimated x-ray beam scanning transverse axial slices of the head. The readings are then processed by a computer, and the anatomy of the slice is mathematically reconstructed. The resolution attained demonstrates soft tissues, and the series of transverse axial slices allows 3-dimensional reconstruction.

CT SCAN IN ORBITAL DIAGNOSIS

Optic Nerve

The course and size of the optic nerve can be well demonstrated by CT, particularly with the aid of computer reconstructions. However, the appearance of the optic nerve depends to a great extent on the plane of the section and eye position, and these variables must always be considered before quantitative conclusions are reached. Moderate symmetric enlargement of both optic nerves between the optic canal and the globe is seen in cases of increased intracranial pressure due to distention of the optic nerve sheath. Diffuse enlargement can also be demonstrated in inflammatory lesions, eg, sarcoidosis. Localized areas of enlargement are noted with optic nerve sheath meningiomas and optic gliomas.

Extraocular Muscles

The appearance of the extraocular muscles is important in the differential diagnosis of orbital lesions. Muscle enlargement is seen in Graves's disease, orbital pseudotumor, congestion of the orbital veins, and neoplastic infiltration. Reduction of muscle size may indicate atrophy due to congenital or acquired nerve

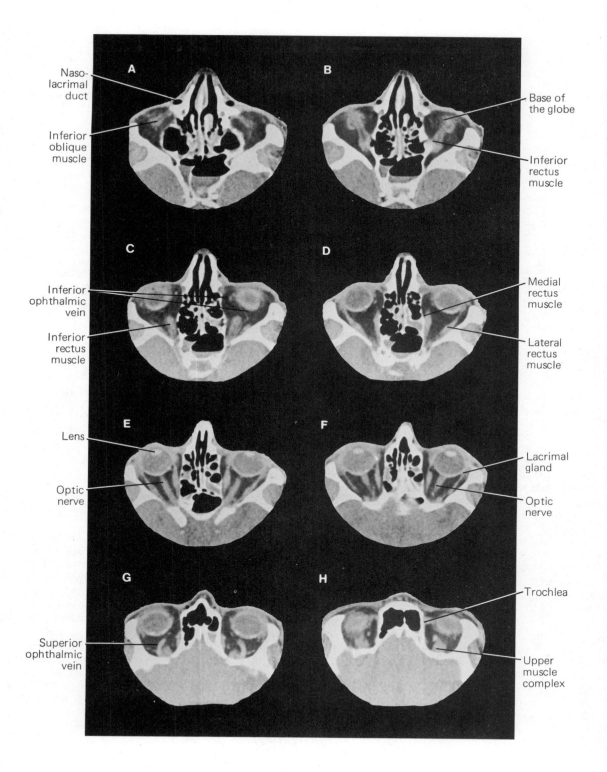

Figure 1. Normal CT scan showing the anatomy of the orbit. Axial CT sections, thickness 1.5 mm. *A,* lowest section; *H,* highest section. Note clear delineation of individual muscles, optic nerve, and major veins within the orbital fat.

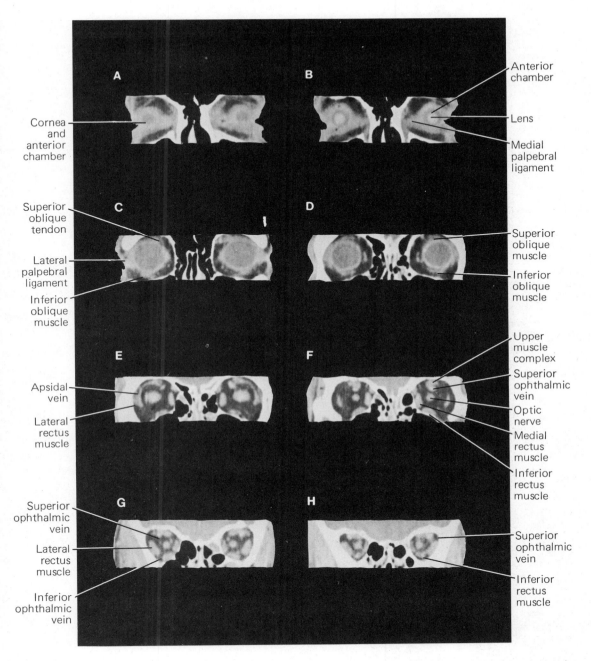

Figure 2. Coronal computer reconstructions from axial CT sections. **A,** most anterior section; **H,** most posterior section. Note detailed demonstration of ocular and orbital structures.

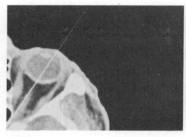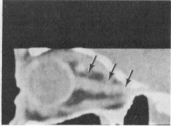

Figure 3. Para-axial computer reconstruction through the optic nerve. *Right,* plane of reconstruction on axial section; *left,* reconstructed image.

palsy or secondary fibrotic changes within the muscle itself.

Mass Lesions

CT scan demonstrates the location and extent of orbital masses, their anatomic relationships to other soft tissue structures, and changes in the adjacent bony orbit. Simultaneous display of other cranial spaces such as the paranasal sinuses and the anterior and middle cranial fossae often helps to identify the origin of the lesion—eg, in the case of a mucocele or nasopharyngeal carcinoma. The location, shape, and degree of delineation of orbital mass lesions provide further differential diagnostic information. Cavernous hemangiomas, for example—the most common benign orbital tumors in adults—are typically well-delineated round or oval tumors within the upper outer muscle cone. Orbital masses in the upper outer extraconal space can often be shown to arise from the lacrimal gland. If the diagnosis cannot be made on the

basis of CT criteria, the procedure at least demonstrates the optimal approach for tissue biopsy.

Diffuse Infiltrative Lesions

Diffuse cellular infiltrations of the orbital contents occur in both specific and nonspecific inflammatory disorders, including orbital cellulitis and orbital pseudotumor as well as lymphomas and other neoplasms. If the history and clinical findings do not clearly indicate the inflammatory origin, tissue biopsy is mandatory.

Ocular Lesions

The use of CT scan in the diagnosis of ocular lesions is still being evaluated. Thin section reconstruction techniques have proved useful in the management of patients with intraocular hemorrhages or foreign bodies, large intraocular tumors, retinal detachments, and panophthalmitis. Further applications of CT scan in the diagnosis of lesions involving the eyeball will undoubtedly be developed within the next few years.

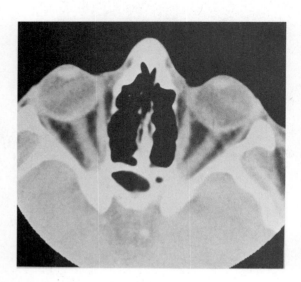

Figure 4. Bilateral optic nerve sheath distention due to increased intracranial pressure in a patient with pseudotumor cerebri.

CT SCAN IN THE DIAGNOSIS OF INTRACRANIAL LESIONS WITH OPHTHALMOLOGIC MANIFESTATIONS

Evaluation of Visual Loss

Various causes of unilateral or bilateral visual loss due to retro-orbital lesions such as intracanalicular or sphenoid ridge meningiomas, carotid aneurysms, and pituitary tumors can be demonstrated on the same CT scan that shows or excludes possible orbital causes (eg, optic nerve tumors or compression by orbital mass lesions).

Evaluation of Visual Field Defects

CT scan will identify the causes of optic nerve and chiasmal compression and lesions of the posterior optic pathway. A diagnosis achieved in this way has the added advantage of sparing the patient the morbidity associated with hazardous invasive procedures.

Evaluation of Oculomotor Disturbances

Treatable causes of cranial nerve palsies such as

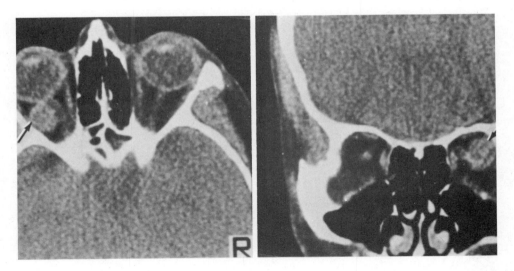

Figure 5. Cavernous hemangioma of the left orbit. Axial and coronal section at a midorbital level. The well-delineated, almost round tumor is demonstrated in the typical location within the upper outer quadrant of the muscle cone and displaces the optic nerve medially.

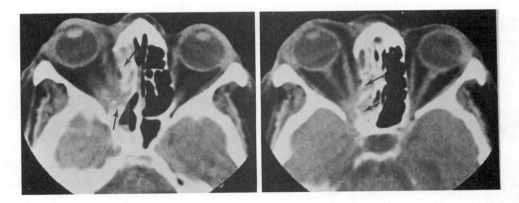

Figure 6. Granuloma due to fungal infection extending from the left paranasal sinuses into the orbit and middle cranial fossa. The medial bony wall of the orbit is partially destroyed. Clinical examination revealed minimal proptosis, slight inflammatory edema in the area of the left orbit, blindness, and dysaesthetic pain.

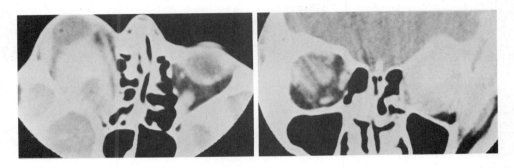

Figure 7. Biopsy-proved orbital schwannoma causing extreme proptosis, enlargement of the bony orbit, blindness, and pain. *A,* axial section; *B,* coronal section at a midorbital level.

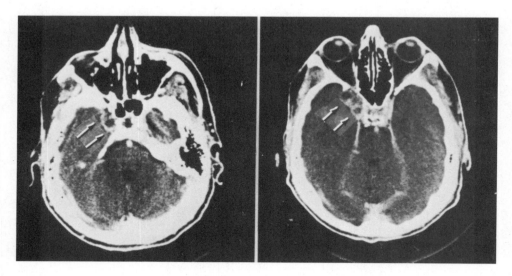

Figure 8. Right parasellar schwannoma extending into the orbital apex and cavernous sinus, causing progressive visual loss and cranial nerve signs. *A,* lower section; *B,* higher section.

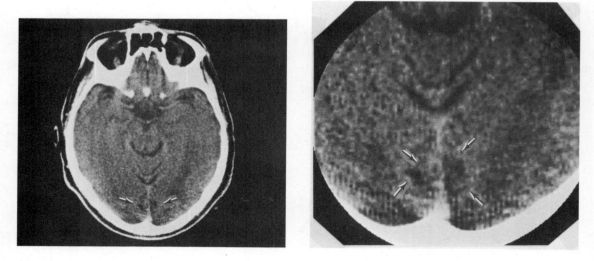

Figure 9. Bilateral small infarctions of the visual cortex causing a ringlike scotoma in the middle field of vision. *A,* axial section; *B,* magnified view of the occipital cortex. The infarcted areas appear as zones of low density between the splenium and the occipital pole.

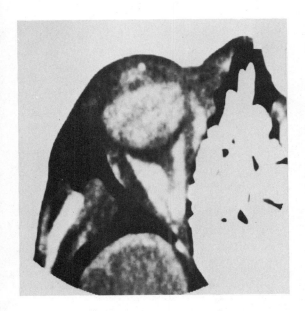

aneurysms of the circle of Willis and basal or parasellar tumors can usually be demonstrated by CT scan. Exclusion of these lesions can only increase the clinician's confidence in a conservative treatment regimen in cases where cranial nerve palsies are due to inflammatory diseases or local ischemic disorders. The demonstration of tumors, hemorrhages, infarctions, or atrophy by CT scan may also identify the causes of gaze palsies, nystagmus, Parinaud's syndrome, and other oculomotor abnormalities in the area of the brain stem, midbrain, cerebral aqueduct, and cerebellum.

Figure 10. Panophthalmitis. The vitreous space is filled with heterogeneous zones of increased density. The lid and adjacent muscle tissue appear swollen. There is increased density in Tenon's space. The retrobulbar fat appears almost normal.

•   •   •

References

Alper MG: Endocrine orbital disease. In: *Orbit Roentgenology*, Arger PH (editor). Wiley, 1977.

Aubin ML, Vignaud J: Computerized tomography of the eye: A study of 62 pathologic cases. *Neuroradiology* 1978;**16**:456.

Bernardino ME et al: Computed tomography in ocular neoplastic disease. *Am J Roentgenol* 1978;**131**:111.

Bernardino ME et al: Scleral thickening: A CT sign of orbital pseudotumor. *Am J Roentgenol* 1977;**129**:703.

Brismar JKR et al: Unilateral endocrine exophthalmos. Diagnostic problems in association with computed tomography. *Neuroradiology* 1976;**12**:12.

Byrd SE et al: Computed tomography of intraorbital optic nerve gliomas in children. *Radiology* 1978;**129**:73.

Cabanis EA et al: Computed tomography of the optic nerve. 2. Size and shape modifications in papilledema. *J Comput Assist Tomogr* 1978;**2**:150.

Cohen MM: Brain computer-assisted tomography. Chap 26, pp 350–372, in: *Neuro-ophthalmology*. Vol 2. Lessell S, Van Dalen JTW (editors). Excerpta Medica, 1982.

Danziger A, Price HI: CT findings in retinoblastoma. *Am J Roentgenol* 1979;**133**:695.

Enzmann D et al: Computed tomography in Graves's ophthalmology. *Radiology* 1976;**118**:615.

Enzmann D et al: Computed tomography in orbital pseudotumor: Idiopathic orbital inflammation. *Radiology* 1976;**12**:597.

Frisén L, Schöldström G, Svendsen P: Drusen in the optic nerve head: Verification by computed tomography. *Arch Ophthalmol* 1978;**96**:1611.

Gaster RN, Duda EE: Localization of intraocular foreign bodies by computed tomography. *Ophthalmic Surg* 1980;**11**:25.

Goldberg L, Danziger A: Computed tomographic scanning in the management of retinoblastoma. *Am J Ophthalmol* 1977; **84**:380.

Hammerschlag SB et al: Blow-out fractures of the orbit: A comparison of computed tomography and conventional radiography with anatomical correlation. *Radiology* 1982;**143**:487.

Hedges TR et al: Computed tomographic demonstration of ocular calcification: Correlations with clinical and pathologic findings. *Neuroradiology* 1982;**23**:15.

Hounsfield GN: Computerized axial scanning (tomography). 1. Description of system. *Br J Radiol* 1973;**46**:1016.

Lloyd GAS: Vascular anomalies in the orbit: CT and angiographic diagnosis. *Orbit* 1982;**1**:45.

McAuley DL, Ross Russell RW: Correlation of CAT scan and visual field defects in vascular lesions of the posterior visual pathways. *J Neurol Neurosurg Psychiatry* 1979;**42**:298.

Ostertag CB, Unsöld R: Correlation of infarctions of the visual cortex with homonymous visual field defects. *Arch Psychiatr Nervenkr* 1981;**230**:265.

Tadmor R et al: Computed tomography of the orbit with special emphasis on coronal sections. *Neuroradiology* 1978;**16**:591.

Trokel SL, Hilal S: Orbital computer-assisted tomography. Chap 24, pp 340–351, in: *Neuro-ophthalmology*. Vol 1. Lessell S, Van Dalen JTW (editors). Excerpta Medica, 1980.

Trokel SL, Hilal SK: Recognition and differential diagnosis of enlarged extraocular muscles in computed tomography. *Am J Ophthalmol* 1979;**87**:503.

Trokel SK, Hilal SK: Submillimeter resolution CT scanning of orbital diseases. *Ophthalmology* 1980;**87**:412.

Trokel SL, Sudec KH: Computerized tomography of orbit and optic nerve lesions. Chap 14, pp 111–118, in: *Neuroophthalmology Update*. Smith JL (editor). Masson, 1977.

Unsöld R: On the CT-diagnosis of optic nerve lesions: Differential diagnostic criteria. *Albrecht Von Graefes Arch Klin Exp Ophthalmol* 1982;**218**:124.

Unsöld R, DeGroot J, Newton H: Images of the optic nerve: Anatomic-CT-correlation. *Am J Roentgenol* 1980;**135**:767.

Unsöld R, Newton TH, Hoyt WF: CT examination technique of the optic nerve. *J Comput Assist Tomogr* 1980;**4**:560.

Unsöld R, Norman D, Berninger W: Multiplanar evaluation of the optic canal from axial transverse CT sections. *J Comput Assist Tomogr* 1980;**4**:418.

Unsöld R, Stanley JA, DeGroot J: The CT-topography of retrobulbar anesthesia: Anatomic-clinical correlation of complications and suggestion of a modified technique. *Albrecht Von Graefes Arch Klin Ophthalmol* 1981;**217**:125.

Unsöld R et al: *Computer Reformations of the Brain and Skull Base: Anatomy and Clinical Application*. Springer-Verlag, 1982.

Vignaud J, Aubin ML: Les coupes coronales (frontales) d'orbite en tomodensitometrie. *J Neuroradiol* 1978;**5**:161.

Third Appendix:
Commonly Used Eye Medications

The following is intended to serve as a brief formulary of commonly used ophthalmic drugs. Standard pharmacology and physiology texts should be consulted for more detailed information.

TOPICAL ANESTHETICS

Topical anesthetics are useful for several diagnostic and therapeutic procedures, including tonometry, removal of foreign bodies or sutures, gonioscopy, conjunctival scraping, and minor surgical operations on the cornea and conjunctiva. One or 2 instillations are usually sufficient, but the dosage may be repeated during the procedure.

Tetracaine, proparacaine, and benoxinate are the most commonly used topical anesthetics. For practical purposes, they can be said to have equivalent anesthetic potency.

Other available topical anesthetic solutions include piperocaine (Metycaine), 2%, and cocaine, 1–4%.

Tetracaine Hydrochloride (Pontocaine)
Preparations: Solution, 0.5–1%.
Dosage: 1 or 2 drops and repeat as necessary.
Onset and duration of action: Anesthesia occurs within 1 minute and lasts for about 15–20 minutes.
Comment: Stings considerably on instillation.

Proparacaine Hydrochloride (Ophthaine, Ophthetic)
Preparation: Solution, 0.5%.
Dosage: 1 or 2 drops and repeat as necessary.
Onset and duration of action: Anesthesia begins within 20 seconds and lasts 10–15 minutes.
Comment: Least irritating of the topical anesthetics.

Benoxinate Hydrochloride (Dorsacaine)
Preparation: Solution, 0.4%.
Dosage: 1 or 2 drops and repeat as necessary.
Onset and duration of action: Anesthesia begins within 1 or 2 minutes and lasts for 10–15 minutes.

Comment: Activity and duration of action are approximately equivalent to those of proparacaine. Benoxinate is the only anesthetic compatible with fluorescein. These 2 agents are available in a combined solution (Fluress) for use prior to applanation tonometry.

LOCAL ANESTHETICS FOR INJECTION

Lidocaine (Xylocaine), procaine, and mepivacaine (Carbocaine) are the most commonly used local anesthetics for eye surgery. Longer-acting agents such as bupivacaine (Marcaine) and etidocaine (Duranest) may be mixed with other local anesthetics to prolong the duration of effect. Local anesthetics are extremely safe when used with discretion, but the physician must be aware of the potential systemic toxic action when rapid absorption occurs from the site of the injection, with excessive dosage, or following inadvertent intravascular injection.

The addition of hyaluronidase encourages spreading of the anesthetic and shortens the onset to as little as 1 minute. For these reasons, hyaluronidase is commonly used in retrobulbar injections prior to cataract extraction. Up to 4 mL may be injected behind the globe with relative safety. Injectable anesthetics are used by ophthalmologists most commonly in older patients, who may be susceptible to cardiac arrhythmias; therefore, epinephrine is ordinarily omitted.

Lidocaine Hydrochloride (Xylocaine)
Owing to its rapid onset and longer action (1–2 hours), lidocaine has become the most commonly used local anesthetic. It is slightly more potent than procaine. Forty mL of 1% solution may be used safely. In cataract surgery, 20 mL are more than adequate. The maximum safe dose is 4.5 mg/kg without epinephrine and 7 mg/kg with epinephrine.

Procaine Hydrochloride
Preparations: Solution, 1 and 2%.

Dosage: Approximately 50 mL of a 1% solution can be safely injected without systemic effects. The maximum safe dose is 10 mg/kg.

Duration of action: 45–60 minutes.

Mepivacaine Hydrochloride (Carbocaine)

Preparations: Solution, 1 and 2%.

Dosage: Infiltration and nerve block, up to 20 mL of 1 or 2% solution.

Duration of action: Approximately 2 hours.

Comment: Carbocaine is thought to be slightly less potent than procaine and lidocaine. It is usually used in patients who are allergic to those agents. The maximum safe dose is 7 mg/kg.

MYDRIATICS & CYCLOPLEGICS

Mydriatics and cycloplegics both dilate the pupil. In addition, cycloplegics cause paralysis of accommodation (patient unable to see near objects, eg, printed words). They are commonly used drugs in ophthalmology, singly and in combination. Their prime uses are (1) for dilating the pupils to facilitate ophthalmoscopy; (2) for paralyzing the muscles of accommodation, particularly in young patients, as an aid in refraction; and (3) for dilating the pupil and paralyzing the muscles of accommodation in uveitis to prevent synechia formation and relieve pain and photophobia. Since mydriatics and cycloplegics both dilate the pupil, they should not be used in eyes with narrow anterior chamber angles since either a mydriatic or a cycloplegic can cause angle-closure glaucoma in such eyes.

1. MYDRIATICS

Phenylephrine is a mydriatic with little or no cycloplegic effect.

Phenylephrine Hydrochloride (Neo-Synephrine)

Preparations: Solution, 2.5–10%.

Dosage: 1 or 2 drops in each eye and repeat in 5–10 minutes.

Onset and duration of action: The effect usually occurs within 30 minutes after instillation and lasts 2–3 hours.

Comment: Phenylephrine is used both singly and with cycloplegics to facilitate ophthalmoscopy, in treatment of uveitis, and to dilate the pupil prior to cataract surgery. It is used almost to the exclusion of all other mydriatics. If a patient is allergic to phenylephrine, hydroxyamphetamine hydrobromide (Paredrine) or eucatropine hydrochloride (Euphthalmine) may be substituted. The 10% solution should not be used in newborn infants, in cardiac patients, or in patients receiving reserpine, guanethidine, or tricyclic antidepressants, because of increased susceptibility to the vasopressor effects.

2. CYCLOPLEGICS
(Parasympatholytics)

Atropine Sulfate

Preparations: Solution, 0.25–2%; ointment, 0.5 and 1%.

Dosage: For refraction in children, instill 1 or 2 drops of 0.25–0.5% solution in each eye twice a day for 1 or 2 days before the examination and then 1 or 2 drops 1 hour before the examination.

Onset and duration of action: The onset of action is within 30–40 minutes. A maximum effect is reached in about 2 hours. The effect lasts for up to 2 weeks in a normal eye, but in the presence of acute inflammation the drug must be instilled several times daily to maintain its effect.

Toxicity: Atropine drops must be used with caution to avoid toxic reactions resulting from systemic absorption. Restlessness and excited behavior with dryness and flushing of the skin of the face, dry mouth, fever, inhibition of sweating, and tachycardia are prominent toxic symptoms, particularly in young children.

Comment: Atropine is an effective and long-acting cycloplegic. In addition to its use for cycloplegia in children, atropine is applied topically several times daily in the treatment of iritis. Atropine is used by many eye surgeons to dilate the pupil for a few weeks after cataract surgery.

Scopolamine Hydrobromide

Preparation: Solution, 0.25%.

Dosage: 1 or 2 drops in each eye 2 or 3 times daily.

Onset and duration of action: Cycloplegia occurs in about 40 minutes and lasts 48–72 hours when scopolamine is used as an aid to refraction in normal eyes. The duration of action is much shorter in inflamed eyes.

Toxicity: Scopolamine occasionally causes dizziness and disorientation, mainly in older people.

Comment: Scopolamine is an effective cycloplegic. It is used in the treatment of uveitis, in refraction of children, and in postoperative cataract patients.

Homatropine Hydrobromide

Preparations: Solution, 1, 2, and 5%.

Dosage: 1 or 2 drops in each eye and repeat 2 or 3 times at intervals of 10–15 minutes.

Onset and duration of action: Maximal cycloplegic effect lasts for about 3 hours, but complete recovery time is about 36 hours. In certain cases, the shorter action is an advantage over scopolamine and atropine.

Toxicity: Sensitivity and side-effects associated with the topical instillation of homatropine are rare.

Cyclopentolate Hydrochloride (Cyclogyl)

Preparations: Solution, 0.5 and 1%.

Dosage: 1 or 2 drops in each eye and repeat after 10 minutes.

Onset and duration of action: The onset of dilatation and cycloplegia is within 30–60 minutes. The duration of action is less than 24 hours.

Comment: Cyclopentolate is more popular than homatropine and scopolamine in refraction because of its shorter duration of action. Occasionally, neurotoxicity may occur, manifested by incoherence, visual hallucinations, slurred speech, and ataxia.

Tropicamide (Mydriacyl)

Preparations: Solution, 0.5 and 1%.

Dosage: 1 or 2 drops of 1% solution in each eye 2 or 3 times at 5-minute intervals.

Onset and duration of action: The time required to reach the maximum effect is usually 20–25 minutes, and the duration of this effect is only 15–20 minutes; therefore, the timing of the examination after instilling tropicamide is important. Complete recovery requires 5–6 hours.

Comment: Tropicamide is an effective mydriatic with weak cycloplegic action and is therefore most useful for ophthalmoscopy.

DRUGS USED IN THE TREATMENT OF GLAUCOMA

The concentration used and the frequency of instillation should be individualized on the basis of tonometric measurements. Use the smallest dosage that effectively controls the intraocular pressure and prevents optic nerve damage.

1. DIRECT-ACTING CHOLINERGIC (PARASYMPATHOMIMETIC) DRUGS

Pilocarpine Hydrochloride

Preparations: Solution, 0.5–6%.

Dosage: 1 or 2 drops in each eye up to 6 times a day.

Comment: Pilocarpine was introduced in 1876 and is still the most commonly used antiglaucoma drug.

Carbachol (Doryl)

Preparations: Solution, 0.75–3%.

Dosage: 1 or 2 drops in each eye 3–4 times a day.

Comment: Carbachol is poorly absorbed through the cornea and so is used only if pilocarpine is ineffective. Its duration of action is 4–6 hours. If benzalkonium chloride is used as the vehicle, the penetration of carbachol is significantly increased.

2. INDIRECT-ACTING REVERSIBLE ANTICHOLINESTERASE DRUGS

Physostigmine Salicylate (Eserine)

Preparations: Solution, 0.25–0.5%.

Dosage: 1 or 2 drops in each eye 3 or 4 times a day.

Comment: A high incidence of allergic reactions has limited the use of this old but effective antiglaucoma drug. It can be combined in the same solution with pilocarpine.

Neostigmine Bromide

Preparations: Solution, 2.5–5%.

Dosage: 1 or 2 drops in each eye 2–6 times a day.

3. INDIRECT-ACTING IRREVERSIBLE ANTICHOLINESTERASE DRUGS

These drugs are strong and long-lasting and are used when pilocarpine, carbachol, and epinephrine fail to control the intraocular pressure. The miosis produced is extreme. Local irritation is common, and phospholine iodide is believed to be cataractogenic in some patients. Pupillary block may occur. (See p 164.)

Isoflurophate (DFP, Floropryl)

Preparations: 0.1% in peanut oil; 0.025% ophthalmic ointment.

Dosage: 1 or 2 drops in each eye twice daily.

Echothiophate Iodide (Phospholine Iodide)

Preparations: Solution, 0.03–0.25%.

Dosage: 1 or 2 drops in each eye once or twice daily or less often, depending upon the response.

Comment: Echothiophate iodide is a long-acting drug similar to isoflurophate that has the advantages of being water-soluble and causing less local irritation. Systemic toxicity may occur in the form of cholinergic stimulation, including salivation, nausea, vomiting, and diarrhea.

Demecarium Bromide (Humorsol)

Preparations: Solution, 0.12 and 0.25%.

Dosage: 1 or 2 drops in each eye once or twice a day.

Comment: Systemic toxicity similar to that associated with echothiophate iodide may occur.

4. ADRENERGIC (SYMPATHOMIMETIC) DRUGS

In the treatment of glaucoma, epinephrine has the advantages of long duration of action (12–72 hours) and no miosis, which is especially important in patients with incipient cataracts (effect on vision not accentuated). At least 25% of patients develop local allergies; others complain of headache and heart palpitation (less common with dipivefrin).

Epinephrine acts by both decreasing aqueous production and increasing outflow.

Some of the preparations available for use in open-angle glaucoma are listed below. The dosage is the same for all, ie, 1 or 2 drops in each eye once or twice daily:

Epinephrine bitartrate (Epitrate), 2%.
Epinephrine hydrochloride (Glaucon), 0.5, 1, and 2%.
Epinephryl borate (Epinal), 0.5 and 1%.
Epinephryl borate (Eppy), 0.5 and 1%.
Dipivefrin (Propine), 0.1%.

5. BETA-ADRENERGIC BLOCKING DRUGS

Timolol maleate is a beta-adrenergic blocking agent applied topically for treatment of open-angle glaucoma, aphakic glaucoma, and some types of secondary glaucoma. A single application can lower the intraocular pressure for 12–24 hours. Timolol has been found to be effective in some patients with severe glaucoma inadequately controlled by maximum tolerated antiglaucoma therapy with other drugs. The drug does not affect pupillary size or visual acuity. Although timolol is well tolerated and relatively free from systemic side-effects, it should be prescribed cautiously for patients with known contraindications to systemic use of beta-adrenergic blocking drugs (eg, asthma, heart failure).

Timolol Maleate (Timoptic)
  Preparations: Solution, 0.25 and 0.5%.
  Dosage: 1 drop of 0.25% solution in each eye twice daily. Increase to 1 drop of 0.5% solution in each eye twice daily if needed.

6. CARBONIC ANHYDRASE INHIBITORS

Inhibition of carbonic anhydrase in the ciliary body reduces the secretion of aqueous. The oral administration of carbonic anhydrase is especially useful in reducing the intraocular pressure in selected cases of open-angle glaucoma and can be used with some effect in angle-closure glaucoma.

The carbonic anhydrase inhibitors in use are sulfonamide derivatives. Oral administration produces the maximum effect in approximately 2 hours; intravenous administration, in 20 minutes. The duration of action is 4–6 hours following oral administration.

The carbonic anhydrase inhibitors are used in patients whose intraocular pressure cannot be controlled with eye drops. They are valuable for this purpose but have many undesirable side-effects, including potassium depletion, gastric distress, diarrhea, exfoliative dermatitis, renal stone formation, shortness of breath, fatigue, acidosis, and tingling of the extremities.

Acetazolamide (Diamox)
  Preparations and dosages:
    Oral: Tablets, 125 and 250 mg; give 1 or 2 tablets 4 times a day (dosage not to exceed 1 g in 24 hours). Sustained-release capsules, 500 mg; give 1 capsule twice a day, usually morning and evening.
    Parenteral: May be given intramuscularly or intravenously for short periods in patients who cannot tolerate the drug orally.

Dichlorphenamide (Daranide)
  Preparation: Tablets, 50 mg.
  Dosage: Give a priming dose of 100–200 mg followed by 100 mg every 12 hours until the desired response is obtained. The usual maintenance dosage for glaucoma is 25–50 mg 3–4 times daily. The total daily dosage should not exceed 300 mg daily.

Ethoxzolamide (Cardrase, Ethamide)
  Preparation: Tablets, 125 mg.
  Dosage: 125 mg 2–4 times daily.

Methazolamide (Neptazane)
  Preparation: Tablets, 50 mg.
  Dosage: 50–100 mg 2 or 3 times daily (total not to exceed 600 mg/d).

7. OSMOTIC AGENTS

Hyperosmotic agents such as urea, mannitol, and glycerin are used to reduce intraocular pressure by making the plasma hypertonic to aqueous humor. These agents are generally used in the management of acute (angle-closure) glaucoma and occasionally in pre- or postoperative surgery when reduction of intraocular pressure is indicated. The dosage for all is approximately 1.5 g/kg.

Urea (Ureaphil, Urevert)
  Preparation: 30% solution of lyophilized urea in invert sugar.
  Onset and duration of action: Maximum hypotensive effect occurs in about 1 hour and lasts 5–6 hours.
  Toxicity: Accidental extravasation at the injection site may cause local reactions ranging from mild irritation to tissue necrosis.

Mannitol (Osmitrol)

Preparation: 20% solution in water.

Onset and duration of action: Maximum hypotensive effect occurs in about 1 hour and lasts 5–6 hours.

Glycerin (Glyrol, Osmoglyn)

Preparations and dosage: Glycerin is usually given orally as 50% solution with water, orange juice, or flavored normal saline solution over ice (1 mL of glycerin weighs 1.25 g).

Onset and duration of action: Maximum hypotensive effect occurs in 1–2 hours and lasts 5–6 hours.

Toxicity: Nausea, vomiting, and headache occasionally occur.

Comment: Oral administration and the absence of diuretic effect are significant advantages of glycerin over the other hyperosmotic agents.

TOPICAL CORTICOSTEROIDS

Indications

Topical corticosteroid therapy is indicated for inflammatory conditions of the anterior segment of the globe. Some examples are allergic conjunctivitis, uveitis, episcleritis, scleritis, phlyctenulosis, superficial punctate keratitis, interstitial keratitis, and vernal conjunctivitis.

Administration & Dosage

The corticosteroids and certain derivatives vary in their anti-inflammatory activity. The relative potency of prednisolone to hydrocortisone is 4 times; of dexamethasone and betamethasone, 25 times. The side-effects are not decreased with the higher-potency drugs even though the therapeutic dosage is lower.

The duration of treatment will vary with the type of lesion and may extend from a few days to several months.

Initial therapy for a severely inflamed eye consists of instilling drops every 1 or 2 hours during waking hours. When a favorable response is observed, gradually reduce the dosage and discontinue as soon as possible.

Caution: The steroids enhance the activity of the herpes simplex virus, as shown by the fact that perforation of the cornea occasionally occurs when they are used in the eye for treatment of herpes simplex keratitis. Corneal perforation was an extremely rare complication of herpes simplex keratitis before the steroids came into general use. Other side-effects of local steroid therapy are fungal overgrowth, cataract formation (unusual), and open-angle glaucoma (common). These effects are produced to a lesser degree with systemic steroid therapy. Any patient receiving local ocular corticosteroid therapy or long-term systemic corticosteroid therapy should be under the care of an ophthalmologist.

A partial list of the available topical corticosteroids for ophthalmologic use is as follows:

Hydrocortisone acetate suspension, 0.5, 1, and 2.5%.

Prednisolone suspension, 0.2%.

Prednisolone sodium phosphate solution, 0.125 and 1%.

Dexamethasone suspension, 0.1%.

Medrysone suspension, 1%.

Fluorometholone suspension, 0.1%.

ANTI-INFECTIVE OPHTHALMIC DRUGS

1. TOPICAL ANTIBIOTIC SOLUTIONS & OINTMENTS

Antibiotics are commonly used in the treatment of external ocular infection, including bacterial conjunctivitis, sties, marginal blepharitis, and bacterial corneal ulcers. The frequency of use is related to the severity of the condition. Antibiotic treatment of intraocular infection is discussed on p 377.

Bacitracin, neomycin, polymyxin, erythromycin, tetracycline, and gentamicin are the most commonly used topical antibiotics. They are used separately and in combination as solutions and as ointments.

Bacitracin

Preparation: Ointment, 1000 units/g.

Comment: Most gram-positive organisms are sensitive to bacitracin. It is not used systemically because of nephrotoxicity.

Erythromycin

Erythromycin, 1% ointment, is an effective agent, particularly in staphylococcal conjunctivitis.

Neomycin

Preparations: Solution, 2.5 mg/mL; ointment, 5 mg/g.

Dosage: Apply ointment or drops 3 or 4 times daily. Solutions containing 50–100 mg/mL have been used for corneal ulcers.

Comment: Effective against gram-negative and gram-positive organisms. Neomycin is usually combined with some other drug to widen its spectrum of activity. It is best known in ophthalmologic practice as Neosporin, both in ointment and solution form, in which it is combined with polymyxin and bacitracin. Contact skin sensitivity develops in 5% of patients if the drug is continued for longer than a week.

2. TOPICAL PREPARATIONS OF SYSTEMIC ANTIBIOTICS

Topical use of the antibiotics commonly used systemically should be avoided if possible, because sensitization of the patient may interfere with future systemic use. However, in certain instances clinical judgment overrides this principle if the drug is particularly effective locally and the disorder is serious. A prime example of this is tetracycline in the treatment of trachoma, the commonest eye infection in the world.

Tetracyclines

Preparations: Solution, 5 mg/mL; ointment, 5–10 mg/g.

Comment: Tetracycline, oxytetracycline, and chlortetracycline have limited uses in ophthalmology because their effectiveness is so often impaired by the development of resistant strains. Solutions of these compounds are unstable with the exception of Achromycin in sesame oil, which is widely used in the treatment of trachoma.

Gentamicin (Garamycin)

Preparations: Solution, 3 mg/mL; ointment, 3 mg/g.

Comment: Gentamicin is rapidly gaining wide acceptance for use in serious ocular infections, especially corneal ulcers and intraocular infections caused by gram-negative organisms.

Penicillin

Preparation: Ointment, 1000 units/g.

Comment: May be used instead of silver nitrate in prophylaxis of gonorrheal ophthalmia neonatorum.

Chloramphenicol

Preparations: Solution, 5–10 mg/mL; ointment, 10 mg/g.

Comment: Chloramphenicol is effective against a wide variety of gram-positive and gram-negative organisms. It rarely causes local sensitization, but cases of aplastic anemia have occurred with long-term therapy.

3. SULFONAMIDES

The sulfonamides are the most commonly used drugs in the treatment of bacterial conjunctivitis. Their advantages include (1) activity against both gram-positive and gram-negative organisms, (2) relatively low cost, (3) low allergenicity, and (4) the fact that their use is not complicated by secondary fungal infections, as sometimes occurs following prolonged use of antibiotics.

The commonest sulfonamides employed are sulfisoxazole and sulfacetamide sodium.

Sulfacetamide Sodium (Sulamyd)

Preparations: Ophthalmic solution, 10 and 30%; ointment, 10%.

Dosage: Instill 1 or 2 drops frequently, depending upon the severity of the conjunctivitis.

Sulfisoxazole (Gantrisin)

Preparations: Ophthalmic solution, 4%; ointment, 4%.

Dosage: As for sulfacetamide sodium (above).

4. TOPICAL ANTIFUNGAL AGENTS

Natamycin (Natacyn)

Preparation: 5% suspension.

Dosage: Instill 1 or 2 drops in each eye every 1–2 hours.

Comment: Effective against filamentary and yeast forms. Initial drug of choice for most mycotic corneal ulcers.

Nystatin (Mycostatin)

Not available in ophthalmic ointment form, but the dermatologic preparation (100,000 units/g) is not irritating to ocular tissues and can be used with good results in the treatment of fungal infection of the eye.

Amphotericin B (Fungizone)

More effective than nystatin but not available in ophthalmic ointment form. The dermatologic preparation is highly irritating. A solution (1.5–5 mg/mL of distilled water in 5% dextrose) must be made up in the pharmacy from the powdered drug. Many patients have extreme ocular discomfort following application of this drug.

5. ANTIVIRAL AGENTS

Idoxuridine (Dendrid, Herplex, Stoxil)

Preparations: Ophthalmic solution, 0.1%; ointment, 0.5%.

Dosage: 1 or 2 drops every hour during the day and every 2 hours at night. With improvement (as determined by fluorescein staining), the frequency of instillation is gradually reduced. The ointment may be used 4–6 times daily, or the solution may be used during the day and the ointment at bedtime.

Comment: Used in the treatment of herpes simplex keratitis. Epithelial infection usually improves within a few days. Therapy should be continued for 3 or 4 days after apparent healing. Many ophthalmologists still prefer to denude the affected corneal epithelium and not use idoxuridine.

A Method of Treating Postoperative Bacterial Endophthalmitis

(1) Aspiration of aqueous and vitreous:
  (a) Giemsa's stain
  (b) Gram's stain
  (c) Cultures (blood agar, thioglycolate, Sabouraud's) and antibiotic sensitivity tests.
(2) Treatment prior to identification of causative organisms by smear and culture:
  (a) Systemic*–
    Nafcillin, 1 g intravenously every 4 hours, **plus**
    Gentamicin, 3–5 mg/kg intravenously in 3 divided doses

  (b) Subconjunctival*–
    Nafcillin, 100 mg daily as single injection
    Gentamicin, 20 mg daily as single injection
  (c) Topical–
    Gentamicin, 3 mg/mL, 2 drops every hour around the clock
    Atropine, 1%, 2 drops 4 times daily
(3) Specific antibiotic treatment in maximal doses should be started as soon as causative organisms are identified and sensitivity studies completed.
(4) Intravitreal injection of very low doses of antibiotics and vitrectomy may be indicated in severe cases.

*Nafcillin and gentamicin are to be administered in separate syringes.

Vidarabine (Adenine Arabinoside; Ara-A; Vira-A)

Preparation: Ophthalmic ointment, 3%.

Dosage: In herpetic epithelial keratitis, apply 4 times daily for 7–10 days.

Comment: Ara-A is effective against herpes simplex virus but not other RNA or DNA viruses. It is effective in some patients unresponsive to idoxuridine. Ara-A interferes with viral DNA synthesis. The principal metabolite is arabinosylhypoxanthine (Ara-Hx). The drug is effective against herpetic corneal epithelial disease and has limited efficacy in stromal keratitis or uveitis. It may cause cellular toxicity and delay corneal regeneration. The cellular toxicity is less than that of idoxuridine.

Trifluridine (Viroptic)

Preparation: 1% solution.

Dosage: One drop every 2 hours (maximum total, 9 drops daily).

Comment: Acts by interfering with viral DNA synthesis. More soluble than either idoxuridine or vidarabine and probably more effective in stromal disease.

Acyclovir (Investigational)

Acyclovir (acycloguanosine) is a new antiviral agent, still investigational for ophthalmologic use, which shows great promise in the treatment of herpes simplex infection. It is phosphorylated by virus-specified thymidine kinase and is converted to acyclovir triphosphate, which inhibits viral DNA polymerase. The drug is not phosphorylated by cellular kinase and does not affect host cells. It has low toxicity. No commercial ophthalmic preparation is currently available; a topical product available for treatment of genital herpes cannot be used in the eye.

DIAGNOSTIC DYE SOLUTIONS

Sodium Fluorescein

Preparations: Solution, 2%, in single-use disposable units; as sterile paper strips; as 10% sterile solution for intravenous use in fluorescein angiography.

Dosage: 1 or 2 drops.

Comment: Used as a diagnostic agent for detection of corneal injury, in applanation tonometry, and in fitting contact lenses.

Rose Bengal

Preparation: Solution, 1%.

Dosage: 1 or 2 drops.

Comment: Used in diagnosis of keratoconjunctivitis sicca; the mucous shreds and corneal epithelial changes stain more brilliantly than with fluorescein.

TEAR REPLACEMENT & LUBRICATING AGENTS

Methylcellulose and related chemicals, polyvinyl alcohol and related chemicals, and gelatin are used in the formulation of artificial tears, ophthalmic lubricants, contact lens solutions, and gonioscopic lens solutions. These agents are particularly useful in the treatment of keratoconjunctivitis sicca. (See Chapter 6.)

To increase viscosity and prolong corneal contact time, methylcellulose is sometimes added to eye solutions (eg, pilocarpine).

Fourth Appendix

VISUAL STANDARDS

INDUSTRIAL VISUAL EVALUATION*

The following mathematical calculation of loss of visual efficiency is used for legal and industrial cases, particularly in determination of compensation for injury.†

Calculation of total visual efficiency is based on 3 factors of equal importance: percentage loss of visual acuity, percentage loss of visual field, and percentage loss of coordinated ocular movements. Percentage loss of visual acuity in one eye does not represent the individual's total disability; even a total loss of one eye would not represent a 50% disability if the remaining eye were normal. Many people lead normal lives with one eye.

For evaluation of industrial visual efficiency, therefore, 3 visual functions are measured and mathematically coordinated: (1) visual acuity, (2) visual field, and (3) ocular motility (diplopia field, binocular field).

Visual Acuity

Distance and near vision are weighted evenly.

For purposes of calculating total visual acuity loss, near visual acuity is equally as important as distance acuity.

Example: If the distance acuity is 6/24 (20/80) and the subject can read Jaeger 6—

$$\frac{40 + 50}{2} = \begin{array}{l} \text{45\% visual acuity loss, or 55\%} \\ \text{visual acuity efficiency} \end{array}$$

Visual Field

A white test object is used in 8 meridians as

*Modified and reproduced, with permission, from *Arch Ind Health* 1955;**12**:439. For further explanation of the reasons behind the statistics and a legal discussion, see Spaeth EB: *Trans Am Acad Ophthalmol Otolaryngol* 1957;**61**:592.

†The method described here may differ from government standards for defining reduced vision in assessing eligibility for compensation, which vary from state to state. The State Department of Industrial Relations (or its equivalent) can be contacted for data.

AMA Method of Estimation of Percentage Visual Loss
(Using Best Correcting Spectacle Lens)

Distance	
Distance Visual Acuity	% Loss
20/20 (6/6)	0
20/25 (6/7.5)	5
20/40 (6/12)	15
20/50 (6/15)	25
20/80 (6/24)	40
20/100 (6/30)	50
20/160 (6/48)	70
20/200 (6/60)	80
20/400 (6/120)	90

Near	
Jaeger Test Type	% Loss
1	0
2	0
3	10
6	50
7	60
11	85
14	95

diagrammed on p 380. This can be done with a 3-mm object at 0.33 m, using a perimeter. A full field represents 100% function. (Illumination should be at least 7 footcandles.)

Ocular Motility

The extent of diplopia in the various directions of gaze is best determined using a tangent screen at 1 meter. A small test light is used and diplopia plotted along the 3 meridians above the horizontal 10, 20, and 30 degrees from fixation. Diplopia fields are also plotted on the horizontal meridians and the 3 meridians below, 10, 20, 30, and 40 degrees from the straight-ahead position. Diplopia within the central 20 degrees represents 100% loss of motility efficiency of one eye, since this condition usually requires patching one eye. If diplopia is not present in the central 20 degrees, loss of ocular motility is calculated from a field diagram showing percentage loss. This value is then subtracted

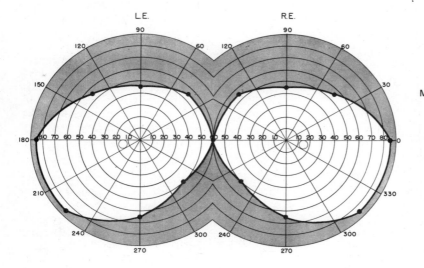

Minimum Legal Visual Field

Minimal Normal Field:

Temporally	85°
Down and temporally	85°
Down	65°
Down and nasally	50°
Nasally	60°
Up and nasally	55°
Up	45°
Up and temporally	55°
Full field	= 500°

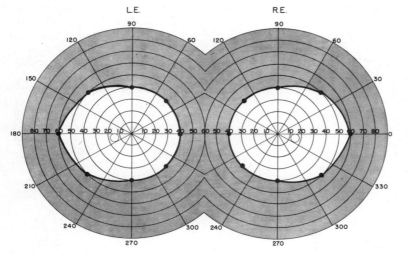

Twenty-eight Percent Loss

Moderate Loss of Field:

Temporally	60°
Down and temporally	50°
Down	40°
Down and nasally	40°
Nasally	40°
Up and nasally	40°
Up	40°
Up and temporally	50°
	360°

$$\frac{360 \times 100}{500} = \begin{array}{l} \text{72\% field remaining, or} \\ \text{28\% field loss} \end{array}$$

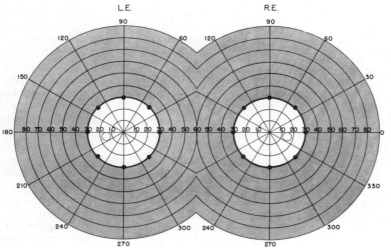

Fifty-two Percent Loss

Severe Loss of Field:

Temporally	30°
Down and temporally	30°
Down	30°
Down and nasally	30°
Nasally	30°
Up and nasally	30°
Up	30°
Up and temporally	30°
	240°

$$\frac{240 \times 100}{500} = \begin{array}{l} \text{48\% field remaining, or} \\ \text{52\% field loss} \end{array}$$

from 100 and expressed as "80% motility efficiency," etc.

The inferior fields are weighted heavily, since this is the position of the eyes in reading. Diplopia away from fixations in other quadrants is considered much less important.

Visual Efficiency (VE) of One Eye

The percentages of efficiency for the 3 measurements are multiplied to give the total visual efficiency.

>Example: Visual acuity = 73%
>   Visual field = 57%
>   Motility   = 90%
>
>0.73 × 0.57 × 0.90 = 37% VE or 63% loss

Visual Efficiency (VE) of 2 Eyes

The 2 eyes are calculated separately and the better eye is weighted 3 times and the poorer eye once. Thus, one blind eye and one normal eye gives 75% visual efficiency.

$$\frac{3 \times (\% \ VE \ better \ eye) + \% \ VE \ in \ worse \ eye}{4} = binocular \ VE \ (\%)$$

Example: RE = 90%; LE = 30%.

$$\frac{3 \times 90 + 30}{4} = 75\% \ binocular \ VE$$

VISUAL STANDARDS FOR THE ARMED FORCES*

The visual acuity requirements outlined below apply for all branches of the services. For aircraft pilots, service academy candidates, and some other officer assignments, the requirements are much more rigid.

Standards for Disqualification

Any strabismus of 40 prism diopters or more uncorrectable by lenses to less than 40 diopters is disqualifying, as is the presence of diplopia. Any active or progressive disease of the eyes is disqualifying even though the minimal visual standards can be met.

Minimal Standards

Distance visual acuity must correct to one of the following: (1) 6/12 (20/40) in one eye and 6/20 (20/70) in the other; (2) 6/9 (20/30) in one eye and 6/30 (20/100) in the other; (3) 6/6 (20/20) in one eye and 6/120 (20/400) in the other.

Near visual acuity must correct to at least J-6 in the better eye.

*Subject to change. Medical Officers for Recruitment at military hospitals or induction centers are supplied with the latest data.

VISUAL STANDARDS FOR DRIVERS' LICENSES IN THE USA

States have varying visual standards for persons applying for drivers' licenses. Failure to meet certain minimum standards may result in suspension of driving privileges or denial of license unless a certificate is obtained from an ophthalmologist or optometrist. In recent years there has been a trend toward higher standards and more periodic visual testing, especially in persons over age 70.

EDUCATIONAL VISUAL STANDARDS IN THE USA

Twelve percent of the pupils in elementary schools have significant eye difficulty, but no more than one in 1000 requires special educational facilities because of severe visual deficiencies. Although a medical examination is mandatory for school children in all states because of assessments required by Public Law 94-142, ophthalmologic examinations are seldom included. It has therefore been found necessary to devise procedures by which it will be possible, without a highly specialized staff, to give preliminary screening tests.

The Snellen test is the single most important test. Visual acuity tests may be given by nurses, parents, or trained volunteer teachers. Visual acuity testing of preschool children is far more important than visual acuity testing of school-age children. Testing should be performed as early as possible, preferably no later than 3½–4 years of age.

Even if a child has a significant visual handicap, it is best to try regular school. If the student cannot keep up with regular school work, special "sight-saving" classes are necessary.

Education of Visually Handicapped Children

Education must be provided for partially seeing pupils at all school levels. (For educational purposes, a partially seeing child is one who has a corrected visual acuity of 6/20 [20/70] or less in the better eye.) Experience indicates that it is best to establish the first class on an elementary school level, since the earlier help is given the better will be the prospect of success. In communities in which the school population is too small to warrant the establishment of more than one class, it may be advisable to give the advantages of the special class to children above the second grade, since much less close eye work is required in the first and second grades and a great deal of material in large, clear print is available for younger children. In general, well-motivated partially sighted children have good learning potential.

Education of Blind Children

Children with poor visual acuity who are unable to take advantage of ordinary visual educational methods are entered either in special schools for the blind, where emphasis is placed upon learning by touch (Braille), or (preferably) in integrated schools where facilities are available for special training but where the child is not deprived of all contact with normal persons in the same age group.

Allen MJ: *Vision and Highway Safety*. Chilton, 1970.

Blum HL et al: *Vision Screening for Elementary Schools*. Univ of California Press, 1968.

Cameron JH, Cameron M: Visual screening of pre-school children. *Br Med J* 1978;**1:**1693.

Committee on Rating of Mental and Physical Impairment: The visual system. Chap 7 in: *Guides to the Evaluation of Permanent Impairment*. American Medical Association, 1971.

Harrington DO: *The Visual Fields: A Textbook and Atlas of Clinical Perimetry*, 4th ed. Mosby, 1976.

Potts AM: *The Assessment of Visual Function*. Mosby, 1972.

PRACTICAL FACTORS IN ILLUMINATION

The physical aspects of illumination discussed below are of practical interest to the physician who may be called upon to evaluate the adequacy of light sources in factories, shops, schoolrooms, and homes. Of principal interest is light **intensity,** conventionally measured in footcandles (modernly, in lux). One footcandle is the intensity of light falling upon 1 square foot of a surface located 1 foot from a point source of one international candle. One footcandle equals 16.76 lux. Footcandles can be measured directly with special light meters.

Proper illumination minimizes eyestrain and increases the speed and efficiency of reading. Poor lighting does not cause eye disease but increases eye fatigue. The most common error students make in adjusting their lighting arrangement is to place a desk lamp opposite to them on the desk. From this position the light is reflected into the reader's eyes, causing glare. For reading, the best light source is an incandescent or fluorescent lamp coming from above that produces a diffuse light with a minimum of glare and shadows. For writing, the light source should be so adjusted that the shadow of the arm and hand on the page is eliminated.

The most common sources of light are daylight, incandescent light, and fluorescent light. Daylight is an excellent light source but quite variable, and it is difficult to control its intensity. Incandescent lamps simulate daylight and provide a steady, diffuse flow of light. Ordinary fluorescent tubes operate on an alternating current that causes flickering, but it is possible to link 2 fluorescent tubes in a couple so adjusted that when one is on the up-phase the other is on the down-phase, thus eliminating the flicker.

Illumination Factors Affecting Visibility

A. Intensity: The amount of illumination is directly related to reading efficiency. A reader employ-ing 5 footcandles reads much slower and less efficiently than if a 30-footcandle source were utilized. The following minimum intensities are recommended (assuming that all undue reflections resulting in glare have been eliminated): reading black print on white paper, 30–40 footcandles; schoolrooms, 30–40 footcandles at the desk and 40–50 footcandles at the blackboard; passageways, halls, and closets, 5 footcandles; eye charts, 80–100 footcandles; operating room illumination at the point of surgery, 300 footcandles.

There is a close relationship between a person's age and the magnification and illumination required. Because they have great powers of accommodation, children can read small print in semidarkness by holding the page close to their eyes. (This does not hurt the child's eyes although it may bother the parents.) On the other hand, a 48-year-old, slightly farsighted presbyope cannot read under ordinary illumination without magnifying glasses because the power of accommodation has been lost. Using a stronger light bulb or taking the printed material into sunlight makes reading possible in such cases. The presbyope also can improve visual performance by holding printed matter farther away. ("I need longer arms.")

The basic requirement in illumination is to have enough light to see by. Once this is accomplished, the intensity of illumination and the magnification (eyeglasses) can be adjusted to increase the efficiency of visual performance.

The intensity of light on an object is inversely proportionate to the square of the distance from the light source. Therefore, if a reading lamp 0.6 m (2 feet) from the page is moved to a distance of 1.2 m (4 feet), there will be 4 times less light on the page.

B. Contrast: It is much easier to read black letters on a white page than black letters on a blue page. Eye fatigue is minimized when the surroundings are about 30–40% darker than the object being observed. Thus, in watching a television screen it is best not to have a completely darkened room.

C. Diffuseness: Shadows and spotlight phenomena should be avoided. However, diffuseness is overdone by manufacturers of indirect lighting fixtures. Indirect "reading lamps" are usually inadequate because of the vastly decreased amount of illumination on the printed page. This can be demonstrated by observing the unwarranted amount of light cast on the ceiling by the average indirect reading lamp.

D. Age of Subject: Illumination requirements and age are closely related, as evidenced by the increased illumination required by the 45-year-old presbyope compared with a teenage daughter. Although it is not recommended, children in the 7–16 age group can read adequately in semidarkness, whereas the same person 30 years later may be able to read the telephone book only by "taking it to the window." Conversely, many people in the 50- to 65-year range who require full correction for their presbyopia can still read fine print without glasses in sunlight.

In general, illumination should be sufficient to perform the task at hand efficiently and comfortably.

REHABILITATION OF THE VISUALLY HANDICAPPED & SPECIAL SERVICES AVAILABLE TO THE BLIND

Although no completely reliable statistics are available, the most widely used estimates place the legally blind population of the USA at 2.24 per thousand (ie, approximately 500,000). Approximately 50,000 become legally blind annually, and many others have enough visual loss to constitute a serious employment problem.

Blindness does not necessarily imply helplessness. Individual adjustment to marked visual impairment or total blindness varies with age at onset, temperament, education, economic resources, and many other factors. The older patient, for example, may accept blindness quite stoically, whereas for the younger patient the vocational or social impact of blindness is often catastrophic. Blindness is accepted more easily by persons who are born blind and by persons of any age who lose their vision gradually rather than suddenly.

The responsibility of the physician clearly does not end with the diagnosis, prevention, and treatment of ocular disorders that might result in blindness. The physician caring for the patient who is suddenly faced with actual or imminent blindness is in a position to be of great assistance. When blindness is a possibility but is not inevitable (eg, during acute ocular inflammation), optimism and reassurance are warranted. However, it is unwise to offer false hopes or to delay "breaking the news" when blindness is inevitable. If it is certain that blindness will occur, it is important to extend to the distraught patient as well as to the patient's family the warmth, understanding, encouragement, and assistance so desperately needed. The physician should be alert to the severe depressive reactions that may occur.

It is especially important to assist the patient in making the adjustment to blindness while some vision is still present. Early referral to rehabilitation agencies is essential for recently blinded adults and those with irreversible progressive visual loss. Training programs or reeducation for the many changes involved in daily living and employment are greatly simplified if the patient has the partial support provided by even limited vision.

It may be valuable to have the patient talk with a blind person who has made a satisfactory adjustment to blindness.

Many special services are available for blind persons. The aim of the rehabilitation program is to enable the patient to lead as nearly normal a life as possible. Approximately 5000 blind persons in the USA are rehabilitated and obtain paid employment each year. An additional larger number of blind homemakers are able to perform their household duties without assistance or are able to live independently of others.

The physician should work actively with both the patient and the family and with other professional people concerned with rendering services to the blind.

Rehabilitation must be individualized. Guide dogs, for example, may be extremely valuable for certain persons but totally unsatisfactory for others. The methods of sightless reading and writing must be adapted to the capabilities, needs, and preferences of each patient. Mobility training is most important; several universities* have undergraduate and postgraduate programs in mobility training for the blind.

State Services

The physician should be familiar with the many special services available to the blind. Services vary from state to state but may be illustrated by the diversified programs for the blind conducted by the State of California.†

A. Educational Services for the Blind:

1. California School for the Blind–A residential school for general education from kindergarten through the secondary grades; also provides field service, guidance, and assistance to preschool children and students in advanced courses.

2. California State Library–A repository for magazines and books in raised type (Moon and Braille), talking books and machines for use with the books, casettes and tapes, games adapted for use by the blind, and writing appliances. These materials may be secured directly from the library or by mail (postage-free).

3. Office of Special Education–Coordinates the establishment and operation of special public school programs for visually handicapped children throughout the state. This program enables blind and partially seeing students to live at home and attend school with normal children.

4. Clearinghouse Depository for Handicapped Students–Instructional aids for visually handicapped students in public or nonprofit private schools that comply with the Civil Rights Act. Also serves as a referral service on educational materials for visually handicapped students.

B. Reader Services for Blind Students: Provides reader services for blind students in high schools, junior colleges, vocational training schools, colleges, and universities.

C. Rehabilitation Services for the Blind:

1. Field rehabilitation services–Counselor-teachers provide services to the blind within their

---

*Undergraduate level programs are at Cleveland State University in Ohio, Florida State University in Florida, and Stephen F. Austin University in Texas. Graduate programs are at Boston University, California State University (Los Angeles), Northern Colorado University, San Francisco State University, University of Arkansas, University of Wisconsin, and Western Michigan State University.

†The services referred to are those provided by public-sponsored agencies for the blind and do not include the many religious organizations, private or voluntary health and welfare agencies, sheltered workshops, and community and recreational facilities.

homes or in hospitals and other institutions so that individuals may learn the skills necessary to meet the demands of daily living. Counseling in adjustment to blindness is given to the visually disabled person and the family.

2. Orientation Center for the Blind (State of California Department of Rehabilitation)—Provides intensive orientation and prevocational training, including training in techniques of daily living and travel, physical conditioning, sensory training, instruction in Braille, typing, and business methods, and training in hand and machine work, homemaking, and other vocationally useful skills. Limited residence facilities are available.

3. Vocational Rehabilitation Service—Provides, for the adult blind, vocational counseling to help work out suitable employment objectives, supervised vocational training, and job placement. The following services may also be provided if needed for employment and if the applicant is unable to pay for them: medical and surgical treatment, including hospitalization; prosthetic appliances and glasses; maintenance and transportation while undergoing treatment or training; and tools or equipment needed in training, job placement, or self-employment.

4. Business enterprise program—Assists blind persons to establish and operate vending stands, snack bars, and cafeteria or other businesses they may be qualified to operate.

D. Social Welfare Programs for the Blind:

1. Supplemental Security Income (SSI)—Financial assistance paid by state and federal governments to blind persons who, because of loss or impairment of sight, are unable to provide themselves with the necessities of life.

2. Aid to Potentially Self-Supporting Blind—Financial assistance by the county and state to the adult blind who, because of loss or impairment of sight, are unable fully to provide themselves with the necessities of life but who are working on a plan for self-support.

3. Prevention of Blindness—A program designed to prevent blindness or restore vision by providing necessary medical or surgical treatment through MediCal (Medicaid in other states) and other federal, state, and local funds.

4. Counseling and support programs—County Social Service Departments provide help to visually handicapped persons through locating needed services and, when necessary, paying for in-home chore workers.

E. Provisions for Prevention of Blindness, Preventive Medicine Services Branch (California State Department of Health):

1. Prevention of blindness in newborn infants—Enforces legal requirement of (1) silver nitrate or penicillin prophylaxis for the eyes as a preventive measure against ophthalmia neonatorum; (2) prenatal serologic test of parents for syphilis; and (3) control of excessive use of oxygen in the care of premature infants as a preventive measure against retrolental fibroplasia.

2. Control of communicable diseases apt to cause loss of vision—Requires reporting, isolation, treatment, and control of ophthalmia neonatorum, trachoma, and syphilis.

3. Aid to Physically Handicapped Children (California Children's Service)—Provides for the necessary medical care of children suffering from eye conditions leading to loss of vision if the parents or legal guardians are unable to meet these costs in whole or in part.

F. Guide Dogs for the Blind: The State Board of Guide Dogs for the Blind (California State Department of Consumer Affairs) was established for the purpose of ensuring that guide dogs are trained and that their owners also are trained to use the dogs as guides. Minimum requirements, licensing, and supervision of Guide Dog Schools are functions of the Board.

National Services

The following organizations will provide information and send literature and catalogs upon request:

(1) American Foundation for the Blind, 15 West 16th Street, New York 10011. Provides information on almost all phases of problems of the blind; sells special watches, home appliances, etc, for the blind.

(2) American Printing House for the Blind, 1839 Frankfort Avenue, Louisville, Kentucky 40206. Prints and sells Braille publications.

(3) Guide Dogs for the Blind, Inc., PO Box 1200, San Rafael, California 94902. Training of guide dogs and training of blind persons to use dogs as guides.

(4) The Hadley School for the Blind, Inc., 700 Elm Street, Winnetka, Illinois 60093. Provides free home-study courses from elementary level into college, vocational and avocational training, Braille and other useful skills. Accredited by National Home Study Council, National Accreditation Council, and North Central Association of Colleges and Schools. Affiliate member of National University Extension Association.

(5) Howe Press of Perkins School for the Blind, Watertown, Massachusetts 02172. Manufactures and distributes internationally the Perkins Brailler (portable Braille typewriter) and Braille paper. Also children's stories in a special Braille edition, games, mathematical aids, Braille maps, music, and Braille writing appliances.

(6) Library of Congress. Extensive collection of books and magazines in Braille, on disk, and on cassette available free to visually impaired US citizens. Materials and playback equipment are distributed through a system of network libraries in each state. (Consult local library for specific addresses.) Music materials only are circulated directly from the Library (Division for the Blind and Physically Handicapped, 1291 Taylor Street, NW, Washington, DC 20542).

(7) Rehabilitation Services Administration, Bureau for the Blind and Visually Handicapped, US Department of Health, Education, and Welfare, Washington, DC 20201. Conducts a nationwide program for the vocational rehabilitation of the blind;

provides pamphlets and other information regarding rehabilitation services available to the blind.

(8) *Readers Digest*. Publishes *Readers Digest* in Braille and on records for the Talking Book; may be secured from the American Printing House for the Blind.

(9) Recording for the Blind, Inc., 215 East 58th Street, New York 10022. Records textbooks and educational materials free of charge for blind persons for educational, vocational, or professional use.

(10) The Seeing Eye, Inc., PO Box 375, Morristown, New Jersey 07960. First organization in USA to provide guide dogs for qualified blind persons (1929).

(11) Central Rehabilitation Section for Visually Impaired and Blinded Veterans (117A), Veterans Administration Hospital, Hines, Illinois 60141. Provides rehabilitation program lasting up to 18 weeks for veterans. Low vision and blind centers also located at Veterans Administration Hospitals in West Haven, Connecticut, and Palo Alto, California. Round trip transportation of veteran generally paid by Veterans Administration.

(12) Xavier Society for the Blind, 154 East 23rd Street, New York 10010, provides free periodical and library service in Braille, large print, and cassette or open reel tape recordings to any interested blind or partially sighted reader. Catalogs available on request.

(13) Louis Braille Foundation for Blind Musicians, Inc., 215 Park Avenue South, New York 10003. A national, nonprofit clearinghouse for professional blind musicians and composers. It transcribes and copyrights musical works; provides publicity and promotion; sponsors concerts; provides musical instruments, Braille music, and special equipment for needy musicians; sponsors the LBF Artists' Bureau; and provides scholarship aid.

American Foundation for the Blind. 1976–77 Catalog of Publications.

Carroll TJ: *Blindness*. Little, Brown, 1961.

Cholden L: *Psychiatric Aspects of Informing the Patient of Blindness*. American Academy of Ophthalmology and Otolaryngology, Instruction Section, Course No. 221, 1953.

Cholden L: *Some Psychiatric Problems in the Rehabilitation of the Blind*. Bulletin of the Menninger Clinic, Vol. 18, No. 3, May 1954.

If Blindness Occurs. The Seeing Eye, Inc.

Mallinson GG (editor): *Blindness 1977–78*. American Association of Workers for the Blind, Inc., 1978.

Stetten D Jr: Coping with blindness. *N Engl J Med* 1981; **305**:458.

US Department of Health, Education and Welfare: *Support for Vision Research: Interim Report of the National Advisory Eye Council, 1976*. National Institutes of Health, DHEW Publication No. (NIH) 76-1098.

VOCABULARY OF TERMS RELATING TO THE EYE*

Accommodation: The adjustment of the eye for seeing at different distances, accomplished by changing the shape of the lens through action of the ciliary muscle, thus focusing a clear image on the retina.

Agnosia: Inability to recognize common objects despite an intact visual apparatus.

Albinism: A hereditary deficiency of pigment in the retinal pigment epithelium, iris, and choroid.

Amaurosis fugax: Transient recurrent unilateral loss of vision.

Amblyopia: Uncorrectable blurred vision due to disuse of the eye with no organic defect.

Aniridia: Congenital absence of the iris.

Aniseikonia: A condition in which the image seen by one eye differs in size or shape from that seen by the other.

Anisometropia: Difference in refractive error of the eyes, eg, one eye hyperopic and the other myopic.

Anophthalmos: Absence of a true eyeball.

Anterior chamber: Space filled with aqueous bounded anteriorly by the cornea and posteriorly by the iris.

Aphakia: Absence of the lens.

Aqueous: Clear, watery fluid that fills the anterior and posterior chambers.

Asthenopia: Eye fatigue caused by tiring.

Astigmatism: Refractive error that prevents the light rays from coming to a single focus on the retina because of different degrees of refraction in the various meridians of the cornea.

Binocular vision: Ability of the eyes to focus on one object and to fuse the 2 images into one.

Blepharitis: Inflammation of the eyelids.

Blepharospasm: Involuntary spasm of the lids.

Blindness: In the USA, the usual definition of blindness is corrected visual acuity of 6/60 (20/200) or less in the better eye, or a visual field of no more than 20 degrees in the better eye.

Blind spot: "Blank" area in the visual field, corresponding to the light rays that come to a focus on the optic nerve.

Buphthalmos: Large eyeball in infantile glaucoma.

Canaliculus: Small tear drainage tube in inner aspect of upper and lower lids leading from the puncta to the common canaliculus and then to the tear sac.

Canal of Schlemm: A circular modified venous structure in the anterior chamber angle.

Canthus: The angle at either end of the eyelid aperture; specified as outer and inner.

Cataract: A lens opacity.

Chalazion: Granulomatous inflammation of a meibomian gland.

*Modified and reproduced, with permission, from Publication 172 of the National Society for the Prevention of Blindness, Inc.

Chemosis: Conjunctival swelling from any cause.

Choroid: The vascular middle coat between the retina and sclera.

Ciliary body: Portion of the uveal tract between the iris and the choroid. It consists of ciliary processes and the ciliary muscle.

Coloboma: Congenital cleft due to the failure of some portion of the eye or ocular adnexa to complete growth.

Color blindness: Diminished ability to perceive differences in color.

Concave lens: Lens having the power to diverge rays of light; also known as diverging, reducing, negative, myopic, or minus lens, denoted by the sign (−).

Cones and rods: Two kinds of retinal receptor cells. Cones are concerned with visual acuity and color discrimination; rods, with peripheral vision under decreased illumination.

Conjunctiva: Mucous membrane that lines the posterior aspect of the eyelids and the anterior sclera.

Convergence: The process of directing the visual axes of the eyes to a near point.

Convex lens: Lens having power to converge rays of light and to bring them to a focus; also known as converging, magnifying, hyperopic, or plus lens, denoted by the sign (+).

Cornea: Transparent portion of the outer coat of the eyeball forming the anterior wall of the aqueous chamber.

Corneal contact lenses: Thin lenses that fit directly on the cornea under the eyelids.

Corneal graft (keratoplasty): Operation to restore vision by replacing a section of opaque cornea with transparent cornea.

Cover test: A method of determining the presence and degree of phoria or tropia by covering one eye with an opaque object, thus eliminating fusion.

Crystalline lens: A semi-transparent biconvex structure suspended in the eyeball between the aqueous and the vitreous. Its function is to bring rays of light to a focus on the retina. (Now usually called simply the lens.)

Cycloplegic: A drug that temporarily puts the ciliary muscle at rest, paralyzes accommodation, and dilates the pupil.

Cylindric lens: A segment of a cylinder the refractive power of which varies in different meridians.

Dacryocystitis: Infection of the lacrimal sac.

Dark adaptation: The ability of the retina and pupil to adjust to decreased illumination.

Diopter: Unit of measurement of strength of refractive power of lenses or of prisms.

Diplopia: Seeing one object as two.

Ectropion: Turning out of the eyelid.

Emmetropia: Absence of refractive error.

Endophthalmitis: Extensive intraocular infection.

Enophthalmos: Abnormal retrodisplacement of the eyeball.

Entropion: A turning inward of the eyelid.

Enucleation: Complete surgical removal of the eyeball.

Epiphora: Tearing.

Esophoria: A tendency of the eyes to turn inward.

Esotropia: A manifest inward deviation of the eyes.

"E" test: A system of testing visual acuity in illiterates, particularly preschool children.

Exenteration: Removal of the entire contents of the orbit, including the eyeball and lids.

Exophoria: A tendency of the eyes to turn outward.

Exophthalmos: Abnormal protrusion of the eyeball.

Exotropia: A manifest outward deviation of one or both eyes.

Farsightedness; See Hyperopia.

Field of vision: The entire area that can be seen without shifting the gaze.

Floaters: Small dark particles in the vitreous.

Focus: The point to which rays are converged after passing through a lens; focal distance is the distance between the lens and the focal point.

Fornix: The junction of the palpebral and bulbar conjunctiva.

Fovea: Depression in the macula adapted for most acute vision.

Fundus: The posterior portion of the eye visible through an ophthalmoscope.

Fusion: Coordinating the images received by the 2 eyes into one image.

Glaucoma: Abnormally increased intraocular pressure.

Gonioscopy: A technique of examining the anterior chamber angle, utilizing a corneal contact lens, magnifying device, and light source.

Hemianopia: Blindness of one-half the field of vision of one or both eyes.

Heterophoria (phoria): A tendency of the eyes to deviate.

Heterotropia: See Strabismus.

Hippus: Spontaneous rhythmic movements of the iris; iridokinesia.

Hordeolum, external (sty): Infection of the glands of Moll or Zeis.

Hordeolum, internal: Meibomian gland infection.

Hyperopia, hypermetropia (farsightedness): A refractive error in which the focal point of light rays from a distant object is behind the retina.

Hyperphoria: A tendency of the eyes to deviate upward.

Hypertropia: A manifest deviation of one eye in relation to the other.

Hyphema: Blood in the anterior chamber.

Hypopyon: Pus in the anterior chamber.

Hypotony: Abnormally soft eye from any cause.

Injection: Congestion of conjunctival blood vessels.

Iris: Colored, circular membrane, suspended behind the cornea and immediately in front of the lens.

Ishihara color plates: A test for color vision based on the ability to trace patterns in a series of multicolored charts.

Jaeger test: A test for near vision using lines of various sizes of type.

Keratoconus: Cone-shaped deformity of the cornea.

Keratomalacia: Corneal softening, usually associated with avitaminosis A.

Lacrimal sac: The dilated area at the junction of the nasolacrimal duct and the canaliculi.

Lens: A refractive medium having one or both surfaces curved. (See also Crystalline lens.)

Leukoma: Corneal scar from any cause.

Limbus: Junction of the cornea and sclera.

Macula lutea: The small avascular area of the retina surrounding the fovea.

Microphthalmos: Abnormal smallness of the eyeball.

Miotic: A drug causing pupillary constriction.

Mydriatic: A drug causing pupillary dilatation without affecting accommodation.

Myopia: A refractive error in which the focal point for light rays from a distant object is anterior to the retina.

Nearsightedness: See Myopia.

Nystagmus: An involuntary, rapid movement of the eyeball that may be horizontal, vertical, rotatory, or mixed.

Oculist or ophthalmologist: Terms used interchangeably; a physician who is a specialist in diseases of the eye.

Ophthalmia neonatorum: Conjunctivitis in the newborn.

Ophthalmoscope: An instrument with a special illumination system for viewing the inner eye, particularly the retina and associated structures.

Optic atrophy: Optic nerve degeneration.

Optic disk: Ophthalmoscopically visible portion of the optic nerve.

Optician: One who makes or deals in eyeglasses or other optical instruments and who fills prescriptions for glasses.

Optic nerve: The nerve that carries visual impulses from the retina to the brain.

Optometrist: A nonmedical person trained in the measurement of refraction of the eye.

Orthoptist: One who gives training to those with ocular muscle imbalances.

Oscillopsia: The subjective illusion of movement of objects that occurs with some types of nystagmus.

Palpebral: Pertaining to the eyelid.

Pannus: Infiltration of the cornea with blood vessels.

Papilledema: Swelling of the optic disk.

Partially seeing child: For educational purposes, a partially seeing child is one who has a corrected visual acuity of 6/20 (20/70) or less in the better eye.

Perimeter: An instrument for measuring the field of vision.

Peripheral vision: Ability to perceive the presence, motion, or color of objects outside of the direct line of vision.

Photocoagulation: A method of causing artificial inflammation of the retina and choroid for treatment of certain types of retinal disorders, particularly retinal detachment.

Photophobia: Abnormal sensitivity to light.

Posterior chamber: Space filled with aqueous anterior to the lens and posterior to the iris.

Presbyopia ("old sight"): Physiologically blurred near vision, commonly evident soon after age 40.

Pseudoisochromatic charts: Charts with colored dots of various hues and shades forming numbers, letters, or patterns, used for testing color discrimination.

Pterygium: A triangular growth of tissue that extends from the conjunctiva over the cornea.

Ptosis: Drooping of the eyelid.

Puncta: External orifices of the upper and lower canaliculi.

Pupil: The round hole in the center of the iris that corresponds to the lens aperture in a camera.

Refraction: (1) Deviation in the course of rays of light in passing from one transparent medium into another of different density. (2) Determination of refractive errors of the eye and correction by glasses.

Refractive error (ametropia): A defect that prevents light rays from being brought to a single focus on the retina.

Refractive media: The transparent parts of the eye having refractive power.

Retina: Innermost coat of the eye, formed of light-sensitive nerve elements.

Retinal detachment: A separation of the retina from the choroid.

Retinitis pigmentosa: A hereditary degeneration and atrophy of the retina.

Retinoscope: An instrument especially designed for the objective aspect of refraction.

Rods: See Cones and rods.

Sclera: The white part of the eye—a tough covering that, with the cornea, forms the external protective coat of the eye.

Scotoma: A blind or partially blind area in the visual field.

Slit lamp: A combination light and microscope for examination of the eye, principally the anterior segment.

Snellen chart: Used for testing central visual acuity. It consists of lines of letters or numbers, in graded sizes drawn to Snellen measurements.

Strabismus (tropia): A manifest deviation of the eyes.

Sty: External hordeolum.

Sympathetic ophthalmia: Inflammation in one eye following traumatic inflammation in the fellow eye.

Synechia: Adhesion of the iris to cornea (anterior synechia) or lens (posterior synechia).

Tonometer: An instrument for measuring intraocular pressure.

Trachoma: Serious infectious keratoconjunctivitis.

Uvea (uveal tract): The iris, ciliary body, and choroid.

Uveitis: Inflammation of one or all portions of the uveal tract.

Visual acuity: Detailed central vision, as in reading.

Vitreous: Transparent, colorless mass of soft, gelatinous material filling the eyeball behind the lens.

Zonule: The numerous fine tissue strands that stretch from the ciliary processes to the lens equator (360 degrees) and hold the lens in place.

Zonulolysis: Lysis of the zonule, as with chymotrypsin, to facilitate removal of the lens in cataract surgery.

SELECTED REFERENCE BOOKS

Apple DJ: *Clinicopathologic Correlation of Ocular Disease: A Text and Stereoscopic Atlas*, 2nd ed. Mosby, 1978.

Aronson SB, Elliott JH: *Ocular Inflammation*. Mosby, 1972.

Beard C: *Ptosis*, 2nd ed. Mosby, 1976.

Beard C, Quickert MH: *Anatomy of the Orbit: A Dissection Manual*. Aesculapius, 1969.

Blodi FC, Allen L, Frazier DO: *Stereoscopic Manual of the Ocular Fundus in Local and Systemic Disease*. 6 vols. Mosby, 1964–1979.

Brockhurst RJ et al (editors): *Controversy in Ophthalmology*. Saunders, 1977.

Cant JS (editor): *The Optic Nerve: Proceedings of the Second William Mackenzie Memorial Symposium Held in Glasgow, September 1971*. Mosby, 1973.

Cant JS (editor): *Vision and Circulation: Proceedings of the Third William Mackenzie Memorial Symposium Held in Glasgow, July 1st–4th, 1974*. Mosby, 1976.

Cogan DG: *Neurology of the Visual System*, Seventh Printing. Thomas, 1977.

Cogan DG: *Ophthalmic Manifestations of Systemic Vascular Disease*. Saunders, 1974.

Current Concepts in Ophthalmology. 5 vols. Mosby, 1967–1976. [Various editors.]

Davson H: *The Eye*, 2nd ed. Academic Press, 1969–1977.

Dawson C, Schacter J: *Human Chlamydial Infections*. PSG Publishing Co, 1978.

Deutman AF (editor): *New Developments in Ophthalmology: Symposium Held at Nijmegen, October 16–18, 1975*. W. Junk, 1976.

Duane T: *Clinical Ophthalmology*. 5 vols. Harper & Row, 1976. [Looseleaf reference service with annual revision pages.]

Duke-Elder S (editor): *System of Ophthalmology*. 15 vols. Mosby, 1958–1976.

Dunlap EA (editor): *Gordon's Medical Management of Ocular Disease*, 2nd ed. Harper & Row, 1976.

Ellis PP: *Ocular Therapeutics and Pharmacology*, 5th ed. Mosby, 1977.

Emery JM: *Phacoemulsification and Aspiration of Cataracts*. Mosby, 1979.

Fasanella RM: *Eye Surgery: Innovations and Trends, Pitfalls, Complications*. Thomas, 1977.

Fedukowicz HB: *External Infections of the Eye*, 2nd ed. Appleton-Century-Crofts, 1978.

Fine BS: *Ocular Histology*, 2nd ed. Harper & Row, 1979.

Fonda G: *Management of the Patient With Subnormal Vision*, 2nd ed. Mosby, 1970.

Fraunfelder FT: *Drug-Induced Ocular Side-Effects and Drug Interactions*. Lea & Febiger, 1976.

Friedlaender MH: *Ocular Immunology*. Proctor Foundation, 1979.

Ganong WF: *Review of Medical Physiology*, 10th ed. Lange, 1981.

Girard LJ: *Advanced Techniques in Ophthalmic Microsurgery*. Vol 1. Mosby, 1979.

Golden B: *Ocular Inflammatory Disease*. Thomas, 1974.

Harley RD: *Pediatric Ophthalmology*. Saunders, 1975.

Harrington DO: *The Visual Fields: A Textbook and Atlas of Clinical Perimetry*, 5th ed. Mosby, 1981.

Havener WH: *Ocular Pharmacology*, 4th ed. Mosby, 1978.

Havener WH: *Synopsis of Ophthalmology*, 5th ed. Mosby, 1979.

Helveston EM: *Atlas of Strabismus Surgery*, 2nd ed. Mosby, 1977.

Henderson JW: *Orbital Tumors*. Saunders, 1973.

Henkind P et al (editorial consultants): *Physicians' Desk Reference (PDR) for Ophthalmology*, 11th ed. Medical Economics, 1983.

Hogan MJ, Zimmerman LE: *Ophthalmic Pathology*, 2nd ed. Saunders, 1962.

Hogan MJ et al: *Histology of the Human Eye*. Saunders, 1972.

Hornblass A: *Tumors of the Ocular Adnexa and Orbit*. Mosby, 1979.

Huber A (translated by Blodi FC): *Eye Signs and Symptoms in Brain Tumors*, 3rd ed. Mosby, 1976.

Hughes WF (editor): *The 1982 Year Book of Ophthalmology*. Year Book, 1982.

Hurtt J, Rasicovici A, Windsor CE: *Comprehensive Review of Orthoptics and Ocular Motility*, 2nd ed. Mosby, 1977.

Jaffe NS: *Cataract Surgery and Its Complications*, 3rd ed. Mosby, 1981.

Jaffe NS et al: *Pseudophakos*. Mosby, 1978.

Jawetz E, Melnick JL, Adelberg EA: *Review of Medical Microbiology*, 15th ed. Lange, 1982.

Jones IS: *Diseases of the Orbit*. Harper & Row, 1979.

Keeney AH: *Ocular Examination: Basis and Technique*, 2nd ed. Mosby, 1976.

Kempe CH, Silver HK, O'Brien D (editors): *Current Pediatric Diagnosis & Treatment*, 7th ed. Lange, 1982.

King JH, Wadsworth JAC: *Atlas of Ophthalmic Surgery*, 2nd ed. Lippincott, 1970.

Kinney R: *Independent Living Without Sight and Hearing*. Hadley School for the Blind, 1972.

Kolker AE, Hetherington J Jr: *Becker-Shaffer's Diagnosis and Therapy of the Glaucomas*, 5th ed. Mosby, 1982.

Kwitko ML: *Surgery of the Infant Eye*. Appleton-Century-Crofts, 1979.

Leopold IH (editor): *Symposium on Ocular Therapy*. Vol 10. Mosby, 1977.

Locatcher-Khorazo D, Seegal BC: *Microbiology of the Eye*. Mosby, 1972.

Lowenfeld B: *The Changing Status of the Blind: From Separation to Integration*. Thomas, 1975.

McCord CW: *Oculoplastic Surgery*. Raven Press, 1981.

Machemer R: *Vitrectomy*, 2nd ed. Grune & Stratton, 1979.

Mann I: *Culture, Race, Climate, and Eye Disease: An Introduction to the Study of Geographical Ophthalmology*. Thomas, 1966.

Miller NR (editor): *Walsh & Hoyt's Clinical Neuro-ophthalmology*, 4th ed. Vol 1. Williams & Wilkins, 1982.

Miller SJH: *Parsons' Diseases of the Eye*, 16th ed. Churchill-Livingstone, 1978.

Moses RA: *Adler's Physiology of the Eye: Clinical Application*, 7th ed. Mosby, 1981.

Newell FW: *Ophthalmology: Principles and Concepts*, 5th ed. Mosby, 1982.

New Orleans Academy of Ophthalmology: *Symposium on Strabismus*. Mosby, 1978.

Parks MM: *Ocular Motility and Strabismus*. Harper & Row, 1975.

Paton D, Goldberg MF: *Management of Ocular Injuries*. Saunders, 1976.

Pau H: *Differential Diagnosis of Eye Diseases*. Saunders, 1978.

Pavan-Langston D: *Manual of Ocular Diagnosis and Therapy*. Little, Brown, 1980.

Perkins ES: *Scientific Foundations of Ophthalmology*. Heinemann, 1977.

Perkins ES, Dobree JH: *The Differential Diagnosis of Fundus Conditions*. Mosby, 1972.

Perkins ES, Hill DW (editors): *Scientific Foundations of Ophthalmology*. Year Book, 1979.

Reese AB: *Tumors of the Eye*, 3rd ed. Harper & Row, 1976.

Rose FC: *Medical Ophthalmology*. Chapman & Hall, 1976.

Salzmann M: *Anatomy and Histology of the Human Eyeball in the Normal State*. Chicago Medical, 1912.

Scheie HG, Albert DM: *Textbook of Ophthalmology*, 2nd ed. Saunders, 1977.

Schlaegel T: *Ocular Histoplasmosis*. Grune & Stratton, 1977.

Schlaegel T: *Ocular Toxoplasmosis and Pars Planitis*. Grune & Stratton, 1978.

Shaffer RN, Weiss DI: *Congenital and Pediatric Glaucomas*. Mosby, 1970.

Sorsby A: *Diseases of the Fundus Oculi*. Butterworth, 1975.

Sorsby A (editor): *Modern Ophthalmology*. 4 vols. Lippincott, 1972.

Trevor-Roper PD: *Lecture Notes on Ophthalmology*, 6th ed. Blackwell, 1980.

Unsöld R et al: *Computer Reformations of the Brain and Skull Base: Anatomy and Clinical Application*. Springer-Verlag, 1982.

Von Noorden GK, Maumenee AE: *Atlas of Strabismus*, 3rd ed. Mosby, 1977.

Walsh FB, Hoyt WF: *Clinical Neuro-ophthalmology*, 3rd ed. 3 vols. Williams & Wilkins, 1969.

Warwick R (editor): *Eugene Wolff's Anatomy of the Eye & Orbit*, 7th ed. Saunders, 1976.

Wilmer WH: *Atlas Fundus Oculi*. Macmillan, 1934.

Wilson LA: *External Diseases of the Eye*. Harper & Row, 1979.

Index